Introduction to Basics of Pharmacology and Toxicology

Avinash Arivazhahan • Neel Shah
Selvarajan Sandhiya • Gerard Marshall Raj
Editors

Introduction to Basics of Pharmacology and Toxicology

Volume 4: Pharmacology and Therapeutics

Springer

Editors
Avinash Arivazhahan
Medical Affairs & Medical Education
Novo Nordisk India Ltd.
Bengaluru, Karnataka, India

Neel Shah
Regulatory Affairs
Concept 2 Clinic Inc. (C2C)
Richmond Hill, ON, Canada

Selvarajan Sandhiya
Clinical Pharmacology
Jawaharlal Institute of Postgraduate Medical Education and Research (JIPMER)
Puducherry, Pondicherry, India

Gerard Marshall Raj
Pharmacology
All India Institute of Medical Sciences (AIIMS) Bibinagar
Hyderabad, Telangana, India

ISBN 978-981-95-1919-4 ISBN 978-981-95-1920-0 (eBook)
https://doi.org/10.1007/978-981-95-1920-0

This Springer imprint is published by the registered company Springer Nature Singapore Pte Ltd.
The registered company address is: 152 Beach Road, #21-01/04 Gateway East, Singapore 189721, Singapore

*Every single **mentor** in my life, personal and professional...*
*Every single **contributor** involved...*
*Every single **reader** because this has been written with **YOU** in mind...*
Forever with gratitude,

Avinash Arivazhahan
Chennai, Tamil Nādu, India
August 2024

I dedicate this book to my teachers, alma mater at JIPMER for making me capable, to my family who anchors me through storms that frequently visit the sea called life. Most of all, to Gerard Marshall Raj whose enthusiasm was infectious enough to compel me to finish writing what we once dreamt of and started many years ago.

Neel Shah
Mississauga, ON, Canada
August 2024

Dedicated to all my mentors including my parents and my sister Diana (for their love, care, and affection), my darling "chinnu" @ Dr. Rekha (for her unconditional love and exceptional support; especially on our 10th wedding anniversary), and finally to our little wonders "Gershin," "Riyaana," "Adelina," "Riya," and "Ivaan."

Gerard Marshall Raj
Hyderabad, Telangana, India
August 2024

Foreword

Dr. Gerard Marshall Raj was one of the best pharmacology postgraduates of JIPMER, Pondicherry, during my period. He embarked on writing textbooks of Pharmacology at the Postgraduate level. Earlier, he had edited and published three volumes of textbooks in Pharmacology, namely, (1) General and Molecular Pharmacology, (2) Systemic Pharmacology, and (3) Experimental Pharmacology. Now, he and his team have written the fourth volume of the book on Clinical Pharmacology. To the best of my knowledge, these four volumes put together is the first Indian Pharmacology Text Book, which covers comprehensively the entire pharmacology, catering to the needs of postgraduates and researchers in Pharmacology.

The fourth volume of the book is divided into four major sections, viz., Clinical Pharmacology, Drug Discovery and Development, Drug Regulations, and Novel Drug Therapies. All chapters are well-written, up to date, and easy to comprehend. The contributors are from academia and the pharma industry from India and abroad. I could see the blend of academia and industrial collaboration resulting in writing this excellent book. Editing a multiauthor book is challenging, which Dr. Gerard and his team have done commendably. What is missing is the nascent field of Artificial Intelligence and Machine Learning in drug discovery and development.

I am proud of the contributions of Dr. Gerard and other eminent authors whose publications meet the unmet needs of Indian postgraduate pharmacology students and researchers. The postgraduate students of clinical pharmacology, drug researchers, and developers will find this book extremely useful in India and abroad.

C. Adithan, MD, DNB (Clin. Pharmacol), PhD, FAMS, FIMSA, FIPS
(Retd) Dean Research, Sri Balaji Vidyapeeth President, Indian Pharmacological Society (2007) Chief Editor, Indian Journal of Pharmacology (1992–2000)
Puducherry, Puducherry, India

(Retd.) Faculty Research and HOD-Pharmacology
and Clinical Pharmacology, JIPMER
Puducherry, Puducherry, India

Preface

This four-volume textbook series kicked off with identifying the unmet need of not having a single resource that can help students access anything and everything that they would need for appearing in their examinations. This thought initiated by Dr. Gerard Marshall Raj was then fueled by the other editors and authors. When I received the first phone call from Dr. Gerard inviting me to collaborate on this project, I honestly felt that this would be a Himalayan task, and half-heartedly agreed to take this up, considering the workload that I had back then. Today, we stand at a point where all of us can proudly pat ourselves on the shoulder and present to you this final volume in a meticulously written and curated educative series (I still stand by my initial thought of this being a Himalayan task! It is just that the view we have from the top of the Himalayas today is something beyond comparison!). This has truly been a remarkable journey for me personally, with several learnings along the way.

Volume 4 is quite different from the rest of the volumes in that it holds immense clinical and therapeutic value, and hence can be relevant not just to students of Pharmacology but also to current and budding clinical pharmacologists, pharmaceutical physicians, and practicing clinicians. This volume spans across a wide spectrum of topics including clinical pharmacology, drug discovery, drug development, global and Indian regulatory landscapes, and novel drug therapies, among others. The chapters, as with the other three volumes, are written in a simple, clear language with excellent "easy recall" value, thanks to the crisp pointers.

All the chapters in this volume are written by authors who have experience and exposure in the respective fields, thus making this very pertinent, credible, and contemporary. Latest advancements in the field of Pharmacology are covered in the utmost detail, including perspectives on what the near future holds for us.

The key features of our review book include:

- Point-wise listing of facts
- Inclusion of around 187 figures, tables, and boxes

No preface is complete without thanking and acknowledging the names involved. Huge shout-out to the key contributors of this series: Dr. Gerard, Dr. Abialbon, Dr. Mageshwaran, Dr. Neel, and Dr. Nishanthi. My sincere kudos to all the chapter authors who have dedicated their time and efforts in penning down these beautifully written manuscripts, which have then been reviewed multiple times by legends and giants in Pharmacology. Hugs and kisses to my lovely better half, Dr. Jhananey, who was accommodative of the hours that this journey required me to sit in front of my laptop screen.

I sincerely hope and wish that this volume serves useful to the wide readership that we have generated over the past three volumes. In case you have not explored the other three volumes, I would strongly recommend you to check them out as well! Happy reading!

P.S.: Please do share your valuable feedback to the editors or chapter authors as appropriate. This would surely help us become better writers and teachers!

Forever with gratitude

Bengaluru, Karnataka, India Avinash Arivazhahan

Preface to Volume 1

General and Molecular Pharmacology: Principles of Drug Action (https://link.springer.com/book/10.1007/978-981-32-9779-1)

It was in the mid-2016s, when I had been in the phase of transformation from a post-graduate student to a teaching-faculty, this idea of writing a book especially for M.D. Pharmacology post-graduates came out from no-where. Though it was a light-bulb thought, I had been ruminating on that since then.

And it was in the late 2017s and early 2018s, I had actually started working on this herculean task. The first thing I did was to browse through the various syllabi of Indian Universities imparting M.D. Pharmacology course. I could retrieve (online search) around 20 syllabi of Universities in India from the States of Bihar, Delhi, Karnataka, Kerala, Madhya Pradesh, Maharashtra, Odisha, Puducherry (UT), Punjab, Tamil Nadu, Uttar Pradesh, and West Bengal. Then, I sifted through the course contents and also the recommended reference books & textbooks to finalize the topics to be covered.

The ultimate goal of this book is to cater to a prospective M.D. Pharmacology post-graduate appearing for his/her formative or summative (final) assessment examinations. Hence, I had divided the book into exam paper-wise volumes,

Volume 1: General and Molecular Pharmacology: Principles of Drug action
- *deals about General Pharmacology*

Volume 2: Essentials of Systemic Pharmacology: From Principles to Practice
- *deals about Systemic Pharmacology*

Volume 3: Experimental Pharmacology: Research methodology and Biostatistics
- *deals about Experimental Pharmacology*

Volume 4: Pharmacology and Therapeutics
- *deals about Clinical Pharmacology*

For this project, I had included five other contributors from the field of Pharmacology, namely, Dr. Mageshwaran, Dr. Abialbon, Dr. Avinash, Dr. Neel and Dr. Nishanthi. They are the major contributors of this four-volume book and also serve as the primary editors of the other three volumes. I know them both personally and professionally for the past 8 to 10 years. They are a bunch of young-yet-proficient and enthusiastic academicians whom I suppose could satisfy the demands of this project. They are currently working in different medical institutes and pharmaceutical industries around the globe.

The present book **(Volume 1: General and Molecular Pharmacology: Principles of Drug action)** is divided into the following five parts.

Part I on *Historical Aspects of Drug Discovery* comprises renowned contributions to the field of Pharmacology by personalities both from the Indian arena and from world over – including the Nobel Laureates.

Part II on *General Pharmacological Principles* discusses in detail about the various facets of general pharmacology ranging from sources of drugs; routes of drug administration; basic pharmacokinetics including drug transporters and pharmacodynamics including adverse effects; drug interactions to structure-activity relationships.

Special Topics in Pharmacology encompassing drug information; pharmacogenetics; chrono- and ethno-pharmacology; pharmaco-epidemiology and -economics; orphan drugs; fixed-dose combinations; translational and reverse pharmacology; gene and stem cell therapy and principles of prescription writing are compiled under **Part III**.

Part IV is about *Toxicology* including two chapters on environmental toxicology and basic principles of management of drug poisoning.

Part V deals about *Molecular Biology in Pharmacology* with chapters on PCR, blotting techniques, antisense oligonucleotides among others.

The M.D. Pharmacology post-graduates rely on multiple texts for their assessment examinations which could be highly time-consuming especially during the preparation period. Moreover, by referring to different texts of varied patterns can at times be extremely distracting to a potential exam-going student. Hence, a review book of this sought can be in a way lessen the arduous task of referring to numerous books or materials with mixed patterns.

The book could be also of use to young pharmacologists working in different job portfolios ranging from teaching-research faculty in academia, pursuing medical advisory roles in pharmaceutical industry to drug safety physicians in pharmacovigilance sectors.

The key features of our review book are

- Point-wise listing of facts.
- Inclusion of around 187 figures, tables and boxes.

These features make the book more concise and precise. Thereby, they make the reading all the more easier and reproducible.

Wishing you all a very happy reading!

Puducherry, Puducherry, India
April 2019

Gerard Marshall Raj

Preface to Volume 2

Essentials of Systemic Pharmacology: From Principles to Practice (https://link.springer.com/book/10.1007/978-981-33-6009-9)

This book aims to present the most important information and concepts relating to the clinical use of drugs in a concise yet comprehensive way. The use of chemical substances to modify altered pathophysiology towards normalcy has been one of the major modes of clinical management of human diseases. A good understanding of pharmacodynamic mechanisms of actions would not only be helpful to understand a drug's use in a particular disease but also to theorize possible adverse drug reactions and possible off-label uses. Pharmacokinetic aspects of a drug help select an appropriate drug in relevant conditions and thereby personalize the treatment based on the disease, patient, and drug factors.

In the words of the Late Dr. Steven A Dkhar, my professor, getting to know a drug is akin to getting to know a person. A drug has its positives and its negatives. While the positives are what we desire and shun the negatives, the fact that you really cannot separate both will eventually dawn on you. Understanding the negatives helps better utilize drugs or, rather, avoid the unnecessary use of drugs. Hence a balanced approach to understanding the drugs would benefit the budding pharmacologist.

The properties of clinically useful drugs (both pharmacokinetic and pharmacodynamic) have been presented in concise form rather than verbose text. Concepts related to drugs' use have been explained with diagrams whenever needed. Considerations that would help put the knowledge obtained to clinical practice are listed whenever possible. The drugs are dealt with based on organ systems whose pathology they are most likely to treat. Since most of them have actions on multiple organ systems, care has been taken to present the spectrum of action of a drug on multiple systems and how it contributes to the adverse drug profile of the drug.

This book is possible owing to the result of many brilliant minds working together as a team. This book along with three other volumes has been the result of the passion and hard work of Dr. Gerard Marshall Raj. He has been instrumental in bringing the project to fruition. The other main contributors are Dr. Magheshwaran, Dr. Nishanthi, Dr. Neel Shah, and Dr. Avinash. Various others have also contributed individual chapters. The accumulation of such knowledge and wisdom is not possible if not for the numerous great minds who have toiled to discover/study these pharmacological phenomena and record them diligently.

The key features of our review book are:

- Point-wise listing of facts.
- Inclusion of around 417 figures, tables, and boxes.

While this book is primarily targeted to postgraduates specializing in pharmacology, it can be a handy and useful reference to anyone who is involved in clinical medicine. We hope this book is of special use to postgraduates for their exam preparation.

Saint Kitts and Nevis, West Indies
January 2020

Abialbon Paul

Preface to Volume 3

Experimental Pharmacology: Research Methodology and Biostatistics (https://link.springer.com/book/10.1007/978-981-19-5343-9)

Experimental pharmacology is an ever-evolving branch of pharmacology. From traditional animal experimentation to modern high throughput screening techniques, the subject of experimental pharmacology has seen drastic progression in research medicine. In addition, various international ethical regulations and guidelines have been implemented over the past five decades to improve the quality of research. This book has up-to-date information regarding the recent developments in various fields of experimental pharmacology and standard guidelines for the same.

Besides experimental pharmacology, a budding pharmacologist should also acquire sufficient knowledge in analytical pharmacology, research methodology, and biostatistics to carry out research work in flawlessly scientifically valid methods. Thus, this book has been designed to integrate various research sector topics as a primary goal. All the topics have been discussed in-depth and written point-wise for easy recollection of postgraduates during exam preparation.

The chapters of various sectors in research in this book were written by experts in respective fields. Prof. Shewade, Dr. Gerard, and I have scrutinized all the chapters and made them into concise, apothegmatic, and absorbing texts.

The key features of our review book are:

- Point-wise listing of facts.
- Inclusion of around 270 figures, tables, and boxes.

I hope you enjoy the book and recollect the points efficiently.

Thanjavur, Tamil Nadu, India
November 2021

Mageshwaran Lakshmanan

Acknowledgments

I place my wholehearted gratitude to the publisher Springer for having given the due shape to this proposal. Foremost, I wish to express my special thanks to Dr. Gaurav Singh (the former Acquisition Editor) who provided valuable suggestions during the initial stages of this project. I would also wish to extend my sincere regards to Swati Sharma, the Associate Editor (Books), Aishwarya Thyagarajan, the Production Editor (Books), and their team for their patience and concerted efforts in preparing this book.

As the corresponding editor, I am greatly indebted to my friends and co-editors Dr. Avinash Arivazhahan and Dr. Neel Shah, who took the primary responsibility of editing this volume and to the editors of other volumes of this book, namely, Dr. Abi, Dr. Nishanthi, and Dr. Magesh—but for them, the whole proposal would not have seen the light of the day. I am equally indebted to all the 38 contributors of this book for extensively devoting their precious time and mind.

I also place my sincere regards to Additional Professor and Head (Dr.) Sandhiya Selvarajan from the Department of Clinical Pharmacology, Jawaharlal Institute of Postgraduate Medical Education and Research (JIPMER), Puducherry, India, for her guidance as a senior editor of this book.

I would also like to acknowledge Retd. Professor (Dr.) Adithan Chandrasekaran from the Department of Pharmacology, Mahatma Gandhi Medical College and Research Institute, Puducherry, India, for readily accepting to write a Foreword for this book. He also served as the Director, Central Inter-Disciplinary Research Facility (CIDRF), Sri Balaji Vidyapeeth (SBV), Puducherry, and also as Faculty (Research)-cum-Professor and Head, Department of Clinical Pharmacology, JIPMER, Puducherry.

I would like to extend my deep sense of gratitude to Prof. (Dr.) Vikas Bhatia, Executive Director, AIIMS Bibinagar, Hyderabad, for being a patron of par-excellence and constantly guiding us in all our endeavors including this book. I would also like to sincerely thank Prof. (Dr.) Rahul Narang, Dean (Academics), Prof. (Dr.) Sangeetha Sampath, Dean (Research), Prof. (Dr.) Nitin Ashok John, Dean (Examination), and Prof. (Dr.) Abhishek Arora, Medical Superintendent, AIIMS Bibinagar, Hyderabad, for their continuous motivation in all our academic pursuits. I would also like to acknowledge my colleagues Dr. Radhika, Dr. Madhavi, Dr. Debasis, and Dr. Rekha for supporting me in this venture.

Nothing is possible without the Divine Grace ("Glory be to the FATHER!"). Therefore, I thank the Almighty for showering good health and well-being to complete this book.

Hyderabad, Telangana, India
October 2024

Gerard Marshall Raj

Contents

Editors and Contributors

About the Editors

Avinash Arivazhahan completed his M.B.B.S. at Pondicherry University and M.D. in Pharmacology from Manipal University. He has been affiliated with the pharmaceutical industry as a Medical Affairs professional since then. Currently, he is a Senior Medical Manager at Novo Nordisk India Ltd., heading a team of vibrant and dynamic Senior Medical Advisors and Medical Advisors for the Diabetes & Insulins portfolio. Prior to this assignment, he has worked at Sanofi India Ltd. in the Medical Affairs department. He has authored over 65 articles in indexed national and international medical journals. He has also co-authored textbook chapters, including several in the current four-volume textbook series. In addition, he holds an MBA in Marketing Management and a dual certification in medical writing and clinical research. Manipal University has recognized him with the prestigious "PRAISE" award for excellence in research during his postgraduation tenure. Apart from contributing to scientific projects, he is also an invited speaker and a resource person for several industry and academia talks.

Neel Shah, MBBS and MD in Pharmacology from JIPMER, is working as the VP of a regulatory consulting firm in Canada with their in-house brand of mental health supplements. He finds regulatory solutions for unique and innovative healthcare products to enter the market and serve unmet needs. He does product applications summarizing safety and efficacy evidence for agencies such as Health Canada and manages life cycle for around 20 drug products, 30 Natural Health Products, 20 medical devices, and around 40 cosmetics at a given time. He also brings to compliance promotional material that enters the highly regulated Canadian market. He has also worked in clinical research and medico-marketing and is now leading this start-up into a growth phase. He received the prestigious M.N. Ghosh gold medal, 2015 batch, JIPMER, and won Excellence award at Regulatory Affairs course at Humber College, Ontario, Canada, in 2020.

Selvarajan Sandhiya, M.B.B.S., M.D. (Pharmacology), D.N.B., D.M. (Clinical Pharmacology), is currently the Head of Department of Clinical Pharmacology at JIPMER, Puducherry. She is involved in teaching D.M. Clinical Pharmacology residents and guiding Ph.D. scholars. She is currently the Member Secretary of the Institutional Ethics Committee (Interventional Studies) at JIPMER. She is also the coordinator of the Adverse Drug Reaction Monitoring Centre in JIPMER, functioning under the Pharmacovigilance program of India. To her credit, she has nearly 70 articles in indexed journals, both national and international.

Gerard Marshall Raj holds an M.B.B.S. and M.D. in Pharmacology. Currently, he is working as an Associate Professor in the Dept. of Pharmacology, AIIMS Bibinagar, Hyderabad, Telangana, India. He has contributed and co-edited the Springer Book Volumes, "Introduction to Basics of Pharmacology and Toxicology—Volume 1: General and Molecular Pharmacology: Principles of Drug action," "Volume 2: Essentials of Systemic Pharmacology: From Principles to Practice," and "Volume 3: Experimental Pharmacology: Research Methodology and Biostatistics." He has also contributed book chapters in other books. He has received multiple prizes for academic and research activities, including the Dr. Peter Sleight Memorial Award for outstanding individual performance and Dr. Salim Yusuf Team Award for best team performance during a course on "RCTs" organized by St. John's Medical College and Research Institute, recently. He has acted as a resource person in various workshops, training programs, CMEs, and delivered invited talks as a guest speaker. He was awarded the "Prof. M. N. Ghosh Gold Medal" for his outstanding performance during the M.D. Pharmacology course at JIPMER, Puducherry, and has published many research articles, reviews, commentaries, and other papers in peer-reviewed and indexed journals. He has received extramural research grants from ICMR and Anusandhan National Research Foundation (ANRF). He has acted as a reviewer for several elite journals and for the National Institute for Health Research (NIHR), UK—Global Health Research Unit scrutinizing funding research proposals.

Contributors

Nishanthi Anandabaskar Department of Pharmacology, Sri Manakula Vinayagar Medical College and Hospital, Puducherry, Puducherry, India

Vinothini Anandabaskar Department of Obstetrics and Gynaecology, Sri Ramachandra Institute of Higher Education and Research (SRIHER), Chennai, Tamil Nadu, India

Vimala Ananthy Department of Pharmacology, Mahatma Gandhi Medical College and Research Institute (MGMCRI), Sri Balaji Vidyapeeth, Pondicherry, India

J. Arifunhera Department of Pharmacology, Chettinad Hospital & Research Institute, Chennai, Tamil Nadu, India

Avinash Arivazhahan Medical Affairs & Medical Education, Novo Nordisk India Ltd., Bengaluru, Karnataka, India

Sarjana Atal Sanofi India Ltd., Bhopal, India

Shubham Atal Department of Pharmacology, All India Institute of Medical Sciences (AIIMS), Bhopal, Madhya Pradesh, India

Porkodi Ayyar Department of Pharmacology, SRM Medical College Hospital and Research Centre, SRM Institute of Science and Technology, Chennai, Tamil Nadu, India

K. Mythili Bai Government Siddhartha Medical College, Vijayawada, India

Santenna Chenchula All India Institute of Medical Sciences (AIIMS), Bhopal, India

Saibal Das Indian Council of Medical Research – National Institute for Research in Bacterial Infections, Kolkata, India

Department of Global Public Health, Karolinska Institutet, Stockholm, Sweden

Snehalata Gajbhiye Department of Pharmacology, All India Institute of Medical Sciences (AIIMS), Nagpur, Maharashtra, India

Vikneswaran Gunaseelan Department of Clinical Research, Narayana Health, Bengaluru, India

Jigar Katwala Medical University of Americas, Nevis, Saint Kitts and Nevis

Swaminarayan Institute of Medical Sciences & Research, Kalol, Gandhinagar, Gujarat, India

Vishnoukumaar Sivaji Teliatry Inc, Richardson, Texas, USA

Sushil Kiran Kunder Novo Nordisk India Ltd, Bengaluru, Karnataka, India

Mageshwaran Lakshmanan Department of Pharmacology, Thanjavur Medical College, Thanjavur, Tamilnadu, India

C. Madhavrao All India Institute of Medical Sciences (AIIMS), Mangalagiri, India

Kalpana Ramanna Mali Department of Pharmacology, All India Institute of Medical Sciences (AIIMS) Bibinagar, Hyderabad, India

Bikash Ranjan Meher Department of Pharmacology, All India Institute of Medical Sciences, Bhubaneswar, Odisha, India

Arup Kumar Misra Department of Pharmacology, All India Institute of Medical Sciences, Mangalagiri, Andhra Pradesh, India

Anusha Natarajan Department of Pharmacology, Jawaharlal Institute of Postgraduate Medical Education & Research (JIPMER), Puducherry, India

Priyadharsini Raman Palanisamy Department of Pharmacology, Jawaharlal Institute of Postgraduate Medical Education and Research (JIPMER), Karaikal, Puducherry, India

Ashwini Patil Sanofi India Ltd., Pune, India

Indumathi Prabath Department of Pharmacology, Chettinad Hospital and Research Institute, Chettinad Academy of Research and Education, Kelambakkam, Tamil Nadu, India

Rekha Priyadarshini Department of Pharmacology, All India Institute of Medical Sciences (AIIMS), Bibinagar, Hyderabad, India

Gerard Marshall Raj Department of Pharmacology, All India Institute of Medical Sciences (AIIMS) Bibinagar, Hyderabad, Telangana, India

Venkateswaran Ramanathan Department of Medicine, Jawaharlal Institute of Postgraduate Medical Education and Research (JIPMER), Puducherry, India

Mirunalini Ravichandran Department of Pharmacology, Jawaharlal Institute of Postgraduate Medical Education and Research (JIPMER), Puducherry, Puducherry, India

Neel Shah Regulatory Consultant, Concept2Clinic Inc., Richmond Hill, ON, Canada

M. Shanthi Department of Pharmacology, Sri Manakula Vinayagar Medical College and Hospital, Puducherry, India

Sushil Sharma Department of Pharmacology, All India Institute of Medical Sciences (AIIMS), Mangalagiri, Andhra Pradesh, India

Santhosh Shivabasappa Senior Clinical Research Scientist, Qure.ai, Bengaluru, Karnataka, India

Surya Singaravelu Department of Pharmacology, Indira Gandhi Medical College & Research Institute (IGMC & RI), Puducherry, India

Akila Srinivasan Department of Pharmacology, Mahatma Gandhi Medical College and Research Institute (MGMCRI), Sri Balaji Vidyapeeth, Pondicherry, India

Shravan Venkatraman Department of Clinical Pharmacology, Jawaharlal Institute of Postgraduate Medical Education and Research (JIPMER), Puducherry, India

Mourouguessine Vimal Department of Pathology, Sri Manakula Vinayagar Medical College and Hospital, Puducherry, India

Anuhya Vinayaka Novartis Healthcare Pvt. Ltd., Hyderabad, India

Part I

Clinical Pharmacology

Clinical Pharmacokinetics

1

Surya Singaravelu and Venkateswaran Ramanathan

Abstract

Pharmacokinetics involves the study of how a drug moves across the body with time, and various parameters are used to describe this process of drug disposition. An understanding of these pharmacokinetic parameters is essential in the optimization of drug therapy. Clinical pharmacokinetics particularly deals with the factors responsible for the inter-individual variations in the kinetics of drugs. At a fundamental level, it is important to appreciate the differences between zero-order and first-order elimination kinetics. Further, pharmacokinetic analytical methods are available that help us to appreciate the relation between various parameters and thereby enable us to understand, predict and optimize the drug kinetics. These analytical methods primarily include compartmental modelling, non-compartmental analysis and physiologically based pharmacokinetic modelling. They fundamentally differ in their assumptions and are preferentially used in different contexts based on their advantages. While the above-mentioned methods are described at an individual level, population pharmacokinetics studies summarize the kinetic parameters at a population level. In addition to the understanding of pharmacokinetic principles, the availability of therapeutic drug monitoring services plays a major role in optimizing the day-to-day clinical management of patients on drugs with narrow therapeutic index.

S. Singaravelu (✉)
Department of Pharmacology, Indira Gandhi Medical College & Research Institute (IGMC & RI), Puducherry, India
e-mail: drsurya05@gmail.com

V. Ramanathan
Department of Medicine, Jawaharlal Institute of Postgraduate Medical Education and Research (JIPMER), Puducherry, India

A. Arivazhahan et al. (eds.), *Introduction to Basics of Pharmacology and Toxicology*, https://doi.org/10.1007/978-981-95-1920-0_1

Keywords

Zero-order · First-order · Steady-state concentration · Clearance · Volume of distribution · Half-life · Elimination rate constant

The sequence of events occurring in the human body following administration of a drug can be divided into two broad categories, namely, pharmacokinetics and pharmacodynamics.

- In simple terms, ***pharmacokinetics*** can be explained as 'The effects of the body on the drug administered'; in other words, 'How the body handles the drug following its administration?'
- On the other hand, ***pharmacodynamics*** refers to 'The effects of the drug on the body' which can be both desirable (**therapeutic effects**) or undesirable (**adverse effects**). In other words, 'What the drug does to the body?'
- Variations in both pharmacokinetics and pharmacodynamics can contribute to variabilities in the action of a particular drug.

1.1 Pharmacokinetics

- It is the study of the ***time course*** of the amount of drug in the body and thus it deals with the processes that determine the events ranging right from the ingestion of the drug to its removal from the body.
- Therefore, it can also be defined as the study dealing with the processes of ***absorption, distribution, metabolism*** and ***elimination*** of a drug from the body. In other words, it is the study of time course of drug absorption, distribution, metabolism and excretion in the body. Thus, pharmacokinetics gives a ***relationship between the drug concentration and time*** in the body.

1.2 Clinical Pharmacokinetics

- The interindividual variations in the action of a drug can be due to various underlying conditions which differ from person to person.
- The branch of ***clinical pharmacology*** aims to describe the various underlying conditions that affect drug actions among individuals and also aims to determine the mechanisms behind the variations in the drug effects. Thus, it helps in improving the effectiveness of therapy with the available drugs as well as paves the way for identifying more effective molecular targets for development of newer drugs with improved efficacy.
- ***Clinical pharmacokinetics*** is the discipline that applies pharmacokinetic concepts and principles in humans in order to design individualized dosage regimens

which optimize the therapeutic response of a medication while minimizing the chance of an adverse drug reaction.

- Thus, it aims to determine a quantitative relationship between the dose administered and plasma concentrations of the drug.
- Applying the principles of clinical pharmacokinetics helps in choosing or modifying dosage regimens for patients in order to optimize efficacy and minimize the untoward effects.
- It is obvious that most of the drugs act via specific receptors, and the receptors are vastly distributed in the body. However, these receptor sites are often inaccessible, and it is not practical to directly measure the concentration of the drugs at these sites. For example, The receptor site for antiepileptic such as phenytoin is located within the brain making it quite difficult to measure the phenytoin levels at this site.
- Since it is difficult to directly measure the drug concentration at the neural tissue, we resort to the alternative method wherein it can be easily measured in body fluids such as blood, plasma, serum, urine or saliva. Thereby, by using the different body fluid concentrations of a particular drug as a proxy for its concentration at the site of action (receptor site), we can predict the pharmacodynamic effect (beneficial/unwanted).
- An individual description of the pharmacokinetic processes of absorption, distribution, metabolism and elimination, and the various factors affecting them are dealt in detail in volume 1 of this book.

1.3 Plasma Concentration vs Time Curve

- The graph of plasma concentration vs time is obtained by plotting the values of plasma concentration of a particular drug in the y-axis (ordinate) against the time since administration on the x-axis (abscissa). The curve thus obtained is usually an exponential decay curve and it can be made linear in a semilogarithmic graph wherein the plasma concentration values are plotted in a logarithmic scale along the y-axis.
- The plasma concentration vs time curve is used in the determination of various pharmacokinetic metrics such as the maximum concentration (Cmax), minimum concentration (Cmin), steady-state concentration (Css), average concentration at steady state (Css,avg), area under the curve (AUC), time corresponding to maximum concentration (Tmax) and time corresponding to minimum concentration (Tmin).
- The plasma concentration vs time curve varies according to the route, dose, duration and frequency of administration of a particular drug.
- The plasma concentration vs time profile of a drug administered by oral route is given in Fig. 1.1a. This curve can be obtained by continuously measuring the drug concentration at various time points following administration.

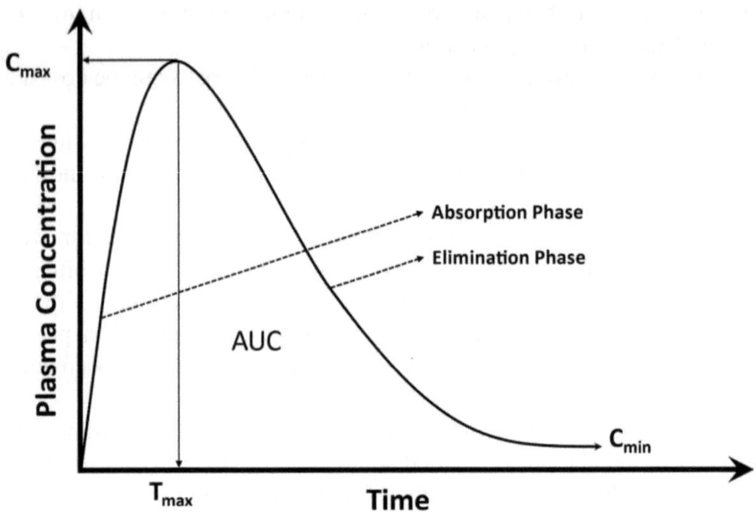

Fig. 1.1a Schematic diagram of 'plasma concentration vs time curve' of drug administered by oral route. *Cmax* Maximum concentration of drug in plasma, *Tmax* Time since the last dose corresponding to Cmax, *Cmin* the lowest concentration measured in plasma before the subsequent dose, and *AUC* Area under the curve of plasma concentration-time curve

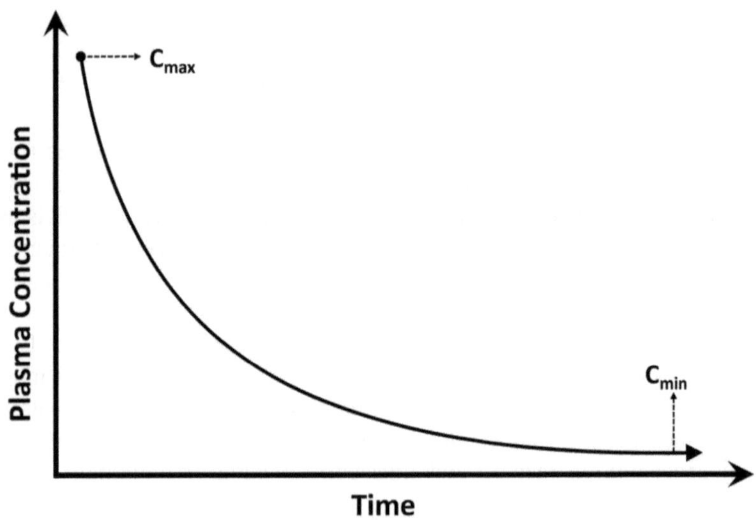

Fig. 1.1b Schematic diagram of 'plasma concentration vs time curve' of drug administered by intravenous route. *Cmax* Maximum concentration of drug in plasma, *Cmin* the lowest concentration measured in plasma before the subsequent dose

- The plasma concentration vs time curve for a drug given as intravenous bolus is shown in Fig. 1.1b. This curve can be obtained by continuously measuring the drug concentration at various time points following administration. The maximum plasma concentration in this plot will be seen immediately following the administration of the drug. However, in actual clinical settings, it is impractical to collect multiple samples from the patients to make these plots.

1.4 Cmax

- It is the highest concentration achieved in the plasma or at the compartment of reference in the period following drug administration and before the administration of the subsequent dose. This is usually expressed as mg/L (which is equivalent to µg/mL). When the drug concentration is much lower, ng/mL or pg/mL may be used. It can be directly obtained from the plasma concentration vs time profile curve of a drug.

1.4.1 Clinical and Pharmacological Implication

- Cmax can account for some of the short-term adverse effects of the drug.
- It is also useful in BA/BE (Bioavailability and Bioequivalence) studies to show pharmacological equivalence between two similar products such as generic vs novel drug product.
- In case of antibiotics that follow *concentration-dependent killing* (CDK), the ratio of Cmax to minimum inhibitory concentration (MIC) is considered as an indicator of antibacterial efficacy. The peak concentration should be at least 8 to 10 times greater than the MIC at the focus of infection in order to achieve an optimal antibacterial effect.
- The time point corresponding to Cmax is the **Tmax** for the drug and it is expressed in hours or minutes depending on the unit of measure of x-axis.

1.5 Cmin

- It is also known as the trough concentration. It is the concentration at which the drug is lowest within a particular dosing interval. Usually, it is the systemic concentration of the drug just before the administration of the subsequent dose. This is also expressed as mg/L (which is equivalent to µg/mL). When the drug concentration is much lower, ng/mL or pg/mL may be used. The time point corresponding to Cmin is considered as **Tmin** and it is expressed in hours or minutes depending on the unit of measure of x-axis.

1.5.1 Clinical and Pharmacological Implication

- It is useful in therapeutic drug monitoring (TDM) as an indicator of therapeutic efficacy or toxicity. This is mainly indicated in case of drugs with narrow therapeutic index where minor changes in the drug concentration can significantly affect the drug's efficacy or safety.
- It is also another important measure like Cmax in case of BA/BE studies.

1.6 Css

- It is defined as the concentration of a drug during the period when the concentration remains relatively constant following repeated drug administration at fixed dosing intervals. It is seen when the rate of drug absorption is in *dynamic equilibrium* with the rate of drug elimination.
- On repeated administration at regular intervals, the plasma concentration of a drug goes through a series of peaks and troughs and it reaches a point where the concentration achieves a steady state *(*Fig. 1.2*)*.
- The time to reach steady state is dependent on the half-life (t1/2) of a drug and in general, any drug takes approximately 4–5 half-lives to attain steady state. There are minimal fluctuations in the peak and trough levels of a drug at steady state; therefore, the therapeutic effects of the drug are predictable and consistent at steady state.
- **Css,max**, also known as the maximum steady-state concentration, is the maximum concentration that can be achieved in the steady state following repeated

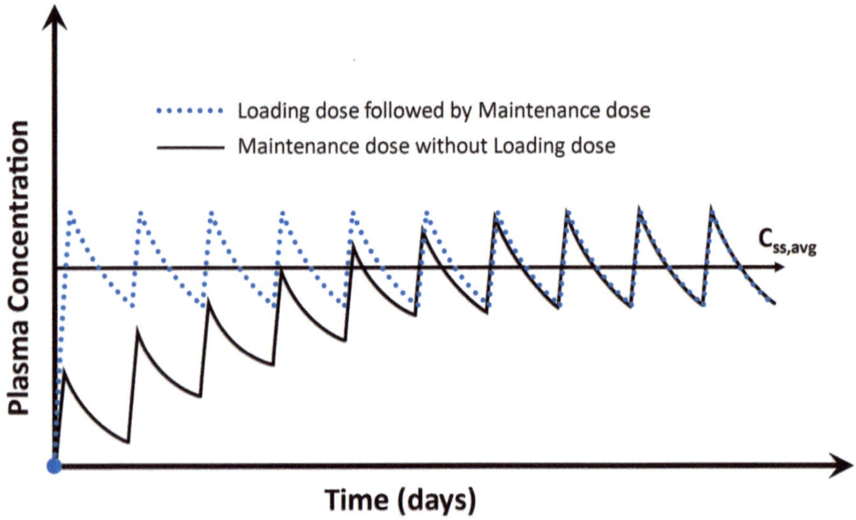

Fig. 1.2 Schematic representation of Css,avg. in the 'plasma concentration vs time curve' achieved during the maintenance dosing with and without loading dose

maintenance dose administration, whereas **Css,min** is the lowest concentration in the steady state, which is measured just before the next scheduled maintenance dose. The values of Css,min and Css,max are constant for a given dosing interval at steady state.

- **Css,avg** is the average concentration achieved by the drug at steady state. It approximates the arithmetic mean of the maximum (Css,max) and minimum (Css,min) concentrations during the steady state. The exact value may be calculated by using the formula, **Css,avg = AUC(0-t)/t.**
- Where AUC(0-t) refers to the area under the curve in a plasma concentration vs time profile between two consecutive doses. It is expressed as mg × h/L and 't', the dosing interval, refers to the time interval between two consecutive and it is expressed in hours (h). The unit for Css,avg is mg/L.

1.6.1 Clinical and Pharmacological Implication

- The knowledge of steady-state concentration helps in deciding the optimal dosing regimen of a drug which is required to maintain a reliable concentration within the therapeutic range, especially in case of drugs with narrow therapeutic index.
- The concept of steady-state concentration is applicable only in case of drugs showing first-order kinetics wherein there is a predictable relationship between the dose administered and the plasma concentration.

1.7 Order of Elimination Kinetics

- The kinetics of elimination of drugs can follow different orders such as zero-order, first-order and mixed-order kinetics based on the relationship between the rate of elimination and the plasma concentration of the drugs.

Rate of elimination α [plasma concentration]^{order}.

- The order of the kinetics refers to the exponent taken by the plasma concentration in the above formula. Rate of elimination is directly proportional to the plasma concentration in first-order kinetics. Whereas, in zero-order kinetics the rate of elimination is independent of plasma concentration wherein the exponent taken by the plasma concentration is zero, reducing it to one, and hence the rate of elimination remains a constant.
- The zero-order and first-order elimination kinetics are explained in this chapter by using the example of elimination of drug following a one-compartment model when given as an intravenous bolus dose.

1.7.1 First-Order Elimination Kinetics

- In this type of elimination kinetics, the rate of elimination of the drug is directly proportional to the plasma concentration of the drug at any given time. At higher plasma concentrations more amount of drug will be eliminated and the amount of drug eliminated will be lesser at lower plasma concentrations.
- In other words, a ***constant fraction*** of the drug is eliminated from the body per unit time. Unlike zero-order kinetics, in this type, the elimination processes do not get saturated and can get adapted to the body's needs to prevent the accumulation of the drug.
- Table 1.1 shows the example of a **drug X** which follows first-order elimination when given at a dose of 100 mg by IV bolus.
- Thus, in case of a drug following first-order kinetics, the fraction of drug eliminated will be constant over time, whereas the amount of drug eliminated varies at each time interval since administration. First-order elimination kinetics is seen in more than 95% of the drugs when given at normal therapeutic doses.
- Figure 1.3a shows the plasma concentration vs time curve of a drug following first-order elimination kinetics when the X and Y axes are plotted in a normal scale.
- Figure 1.3b shows the plasma concentration vs time curve for the same drug which is linearized when plotted on a semilogarithmic scale with the plasma concentration of the drug on the logarithmic y-axis.
- By applying mathematical principles, linearizing the plasma concentration vs time curve makes it easier for us to predict the plasma concentrations at different time points since the concentration at any time point will be on the straight line rather than a curve, i.e. the plasma concentration at any particular time point can be predicted by selecting a time point and then correspondingly matching plasma concentration for that particular time.

Table 1.1 Drug X following first-order elimination on IV bolus administration

Time since drug administration (hours)	Amount of drug in the body (mg)	Amount of drug eliminated during each time interval (mg)	Fraction of drug eliminated during each time interval
0	100	–	–
1	88	12	0.12 (=12/100)
2	77.4	10.6	0.12 (=10.6/88)
3	68.1	9.3	0.12 (=9.3/77.4)
4	59.9	8.2	0.12 (=8.2/68.1)

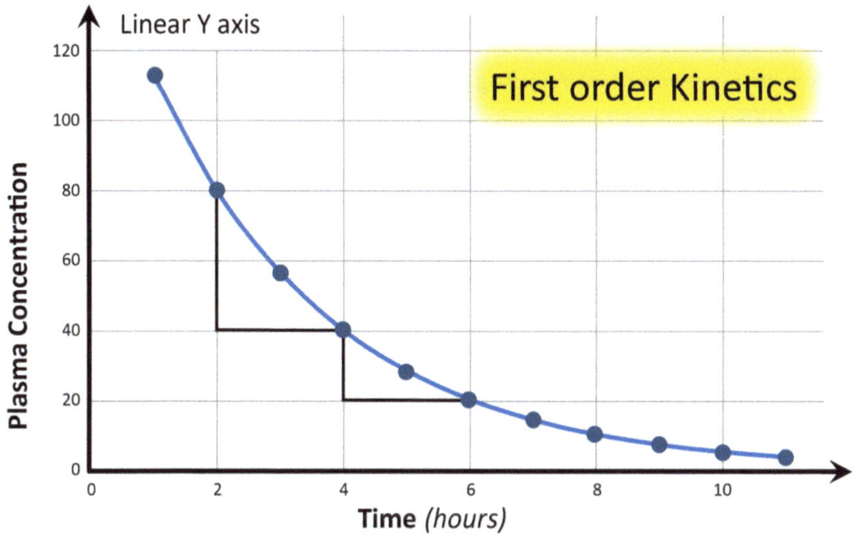

Fig. 1.3a Schematic representation of the 'plasma concentration vs time curve' for a drug following first-order kinetics when represented on a standard graph sheet

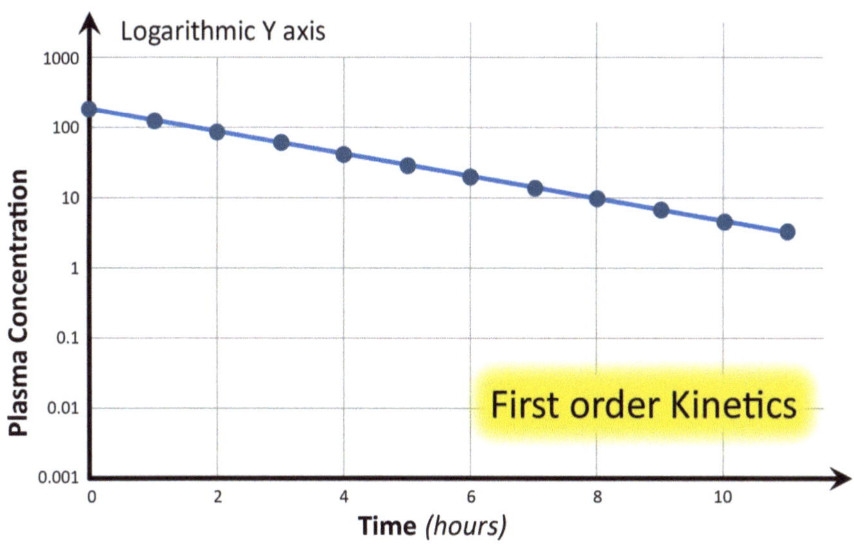

Fig. 1.3b Schematic representation of the 'plasma concentration vs time curve' for a drug following first-order kinetics when represented on a semilogarithmic graph sheet

1.7.2 Zero-Order Elimination Kinetics

- A ***constant amount*** of the drug is eliminated from a biological system per unit time.
- The rate of elimination is independent of the total plasma concentration of the drug in the body at any given time. Therefore, zero-order kinetics can also be called as *concentration-independent* in drug disposition.
- Table 1.2 shows the example of a drug Y which follows zero-order elimination when given at a dose of 100 mg by IV bolus.
- From Table 1.2, it can be appreciated that the *amount of drug* eliminated per unit time is constant in the case of a drug following zero-order kinetics.
- The elimination phase is linear in a graph of plasma concentration (y-axis) vs time (x-axis) when both the axes are linear as in Fig. 1.4, whereas logarithmic transformation of the concentration in the y-axis gives a non-linear graph and therefore zero-order kinetics is also known as non-linear kinetics.
- Zero-order kinetics is ***rare*** and it can occur in the following settings:
  - When the elimination system of a drug with respect to metabolic pathways or enzymes gets saturated or used up due to increased concentrations of the drug in the body. Therefore, zero-order kinetics is also called as ***saturation kinetics***.
  - For example, a classic example of zero-order kinetics is the metabolism of ethanol in the liver. Ethanol undergoes sequential oxidation steps in the liver by the enzymes, namely alcohol dehydrogenase (ADH) and aldehyde dehydrogenase (ALDH) to be converted to acetaldehyde and acetic acid, respectively. Each of the oxidation steps requires a molecule of NAD^+ in the liver. Therefore, beyond a particular blood ethanol concentration, the elimination kinetics of ethanol gets switched from first order to zero order due to the inability of the liver to supply adequate NAD^+ for the oxidation process.
  - The other drugs which often follow zero-order kinetics owing to saturation of their elimination process are: Phenytoin, aspirin, cisplatin and fluoxetine.
  - Zero-order kinetics can be seen with any drug in the setting of ***drug overdosage*** which leads to saturation of the elimination pathways (Table 1.3).

Table 1.2 Drug Y following zero-order elimination following IV bolus administration

Time since drug administration (hours)	Amount of drug eliminated (mg)	Amount of drug eliminated during each time interval (mg)	Fraction of drug eliminated during each time interval
0	100	–	
1	85	15	0.15 (=15/100)
2	70	15	0.18 (=15/85)
3	55	15	0.21 (=15/70)
4	40	15	0.27 (=15/55)

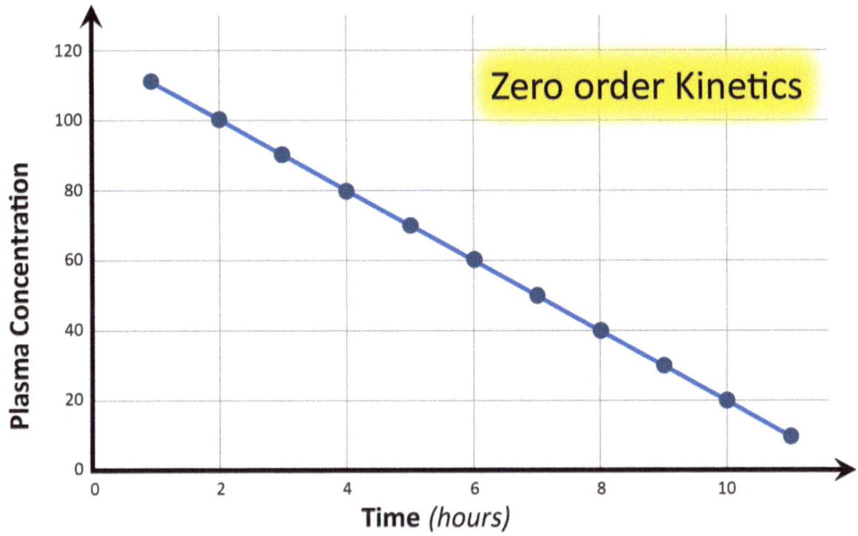

Fig. 1.4 Schematic representation of the 'plasma concentration vs time curve' for a drug following zero-order kinetics when represented on a normal graph sheet

Table 1.3 Differences between first-order and zero-order kinetics

First-order kinetics	Zero-order kinetics
Drug concentration shows an exponential decrease over time. It is called linear kinetics.	Drug concentration shows a non-exponential decrease over time.
Linear relation in semilogarithmic plasma concentration vs time graph	Linear relation in normal plasma concentration vs time graph
The fraction of drug eliminated per unit time is constant	The amount of drug eliminated per unit time is constant
Rate of elimination is directly proportional to the plasma concentration of the drug at a given time point	Rate of elimination is independent of plasma concentration of the drug
Half-life is constant	Half-life is not a constant, but increases with plasma concentration.
Clearance is constant	Clearance varies with plasma concentration. It increases with reducing plasma concentration.
Majority of drugs at therapeutic doses follow first-order kinetics	Followed by most of the drugs at higher concentrations due to saturation of metabolic/elimination pathways

1.8 Kinetic Homogeneity

- It is the term which describes a ***predictable relationship*** between the plasma drug concentration and the concentration of the drug at the site of receptors where the drug produces the desired therapeutic effects. Since the plasma drug concentration is directly proportional to the concentration of drug at receptor

site, it is assumed that any change in the plasma concentration can reflect the changes in the receptor sites as well as in the tissues.
- The assumptions in clinical pharmacokinetics are based on the property of kinetic homogeneity which is the basis on which the plasma concentrations of a drug for therapeutic efficacy and toxicity are established.

1.9 Pharmacokinetic Models

- These are *hypothetical mathematical models* used to describe the disposition of drug within the biological system. They are used to establish quantitative relationships by estimating the various pharmacokinetic (PK) parameters such as volume of distribution and clearance.
- PK models can act as tools that aid in model-based drug development by determining the absorption, distribution, metabolism and elimination characteristics of a new drug.
- ***Types of pharmacokinetic models:***

  (i). Compartmental models.
  (ii). Non-compartmental models.
  (iii). Physiologically based pharmacokinetic models (PBPK).

1.9.1 Compartmental Models

- This type of mathematical model describes the drug disposition by dividing the body into one or more individual compartments.
- The most commonly used method for the pharmacokinetic characterization of a drug is to portray the body as a system of compartments and to assume the rate of transfer of drug to happen between the compartments as well as the rate of drug elimination to occur from the compartments.
- The compartments are *pharmacokinetically homogenous, theoretical, imaginary* and are not tangible in nature and can range from a simple one-compartment model to more complex multi-compartment models which can even comprise of hundreds of compartments.
- In general, additional compartments can be added to the basic one or two-compartment models based on the nature of the drug and its applications. However, the commonly used pharmacokinetic models have $\leq$3 compartments.
- In multicompartment models, the individual compartments are connected in either series (*catenary model*) or parallel (*mamillary model*) wherein the central compartment is connected to all the peripheral compartments but there is no connection between the individual peripheral compartments. The drugs are distributed uniformly within each individual compartment and they can move in and out of these compartments in a reversible fashion.

1.9.1.1 One-Compartment Model

- In this type of pharmacokinetic model, the whole body is considered as a single central compartment in which the drug is well mixed and pharmacokinetically homogenous.
- The central compartment corresponds to the blood and the highly perfused organs such as liver and kidneys where the drug gets distributed immediately following administration.
- This type of pharmacokinetic model is cost-efficient, easy to construct and simple in estimating the required pharmacokinetic parameters.
- It is suitable for drugs that do not distribute extensively throughout the body. Since the distribution is considered to be uniform within the compartment, the elimination can be assumed to be linear.
- The major limitation is that the majority of the drugs do not distribute uniformly throughout the body, thus challenging the assumption of uniform distribution for one-compartment models.
- A one-compartment model (Fig. 1.5) is described to be ***open*** when the input and output with respect to the single compartment are unidirectional, i.e. a drug moving out of the compartment will get eliminated from the body. The recirculation of the drug does not occur within the body. The open model gives a visual representation of the plasma concentration of a drug following a one-time administration.

1.9.1.2 Two-Compartment Models

- This type of pharmacokinetic model also accounts for drug distribution with respect to the two compartments which are classified based on the rate of blood flow and the affinity towards the particular drug. The vascular compartment and other highly perfused organs and tissues such as liver and kidney are treated as a common pharmacokinetically homogenous unit referred to as the ***central compartment***.
- The other poorly perfused tissues such as muscle, lean tissue and fat are grouped into a hypothetical single peripheral compartment. The drug in the central compartment can move either to the peripheral compartment or outside the body. Whereas, the movement of drug between the central and peripheral compartments is generally bidirectional thus helping in recirculation.
- Unlike the one-compartment model in this type, the drug is not assumed to be uniformly distributed within the entire body. At the same time, the drug distribution within an individual central or peripheral compartment is assumed to be uniform and instantaneous.

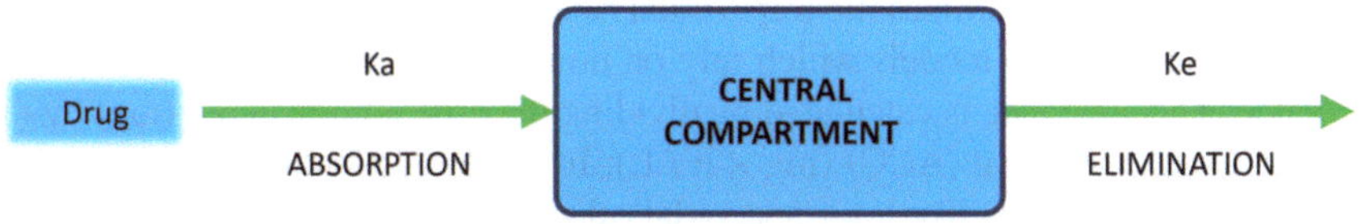

Fig. 1.5 Schematic representation of a one-compartment open model of drug disposition. Ka—Rate of absorption of the drug, and Ke—Rate of elimination

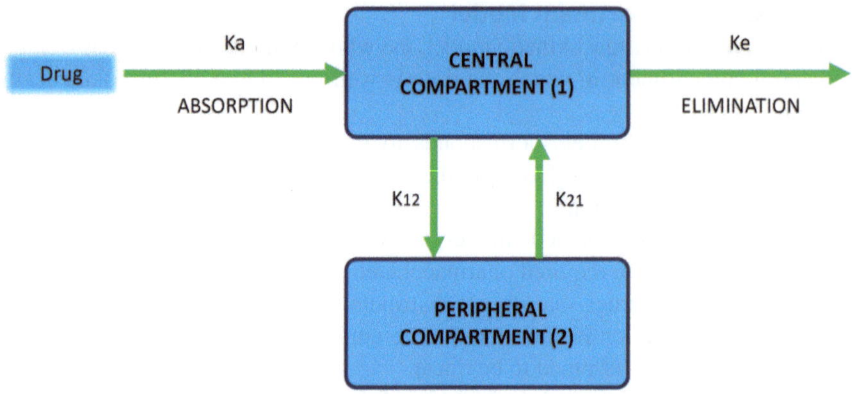

Fig. 1.6 Schematic representation of a two-compartment model of drug disposition. *Ke* rate of elimination, and K_{12} *and* K_{21} rates of drug transfer between the 2 compartments

- A two-compartment model cannot be sufficient for those drugs with more than two distinct elimination phases thus mandating the need for models with additional compartments (Fig. 1.6).

1.9.2 Non-compartmental Analysis

- Non-compartmental analysis (NCA) is a ***model-independent method*** and different from compartmental models due to the fact that it does not make assumptions regarding compartments within the body. In other words, NCA does not require the assumption of a specific compartmental model for either drug or metabolite and can be easily done for any drug which follows first-order elimination kinetics.
- This type of analysis is useful in evaluating drug exposure when the assumption of a particular compartment model is not valid due to the **complexity of the drug distribution**. Non-compartmental analysis is quicker, cost-efficient, less complex and employs simple algebraic equations to estimate the PK parameters. The important PK parameters obtained using this method are elimination rate constant (ke), clearance (Cl), mean residence time (MRT) and volume of distribution (Vd). These PK parameters are derived from AUC and area under the moment curve (AUMC).
- The time course of drug concentration in plasma is regarded as a statistical distribution curve and the statistical moments such as MRT and $AUC_{0\text{-}\infty}$ can be determined using this method.
- The NCA method utilizes the trapezoidal rule for the calculation of AUC unlike the compartmental models which rely on non-linear regression analysis for the same. The clearance is calculated by dividing the dose administered (mg) by the area under the curve (AUC) (mg × h / L). In NCA, AUC may be estimated by using other methods like log-trapezoidal rule, splines and Lagrangians.
- Thus, **Clearance (L/h) = Dose administered (mg) / AUC (mg × h / L).**

- The **area under the moment curve** or **AUMC** can be obtained by determining the area under the curve from a plot of time (from zero to infinity) along the x-axis versus product of plasma concentration of the drug at a particular time point and time (Cp*t) along the y-axis. The trapezoidal rule is again used in the determination of AUMC, and the unit of AUMC is (mg × h^2)/L.
- The mean residence time (MRT) is defined as the average time spent by a drug molecule in the body before getting eliminated. It can be calculated using the following equation:

$$MRT\,(h) = AUMC\left(mg \times h^2\right) per\ L\,/\,AUC\left(mg \times h\right) per\ L$$

- Non-compartmental analysis can give a better description of the plasma concentration vs time profile when the time points of sampling following a drug administration in pharmacokinetic studies are closer (intense sampling) compared to the sparse sampling with fewer sampling time points involved in model-based analysis or population pharmacokinetic studies.

1.9.3 Compartmental vs Non-compartmental Analysis

- In terms of utility, compartmental analysis can be used to determine the pharmacokinetics of a drug across multiple studies, whereas non-compartmental analysis is the preferred method for establishing the initial exposure characteristics of the drug in preclinical and toxicology studies, and is best used to characterize the PK within a single study.
- Non-compartmental analyses require 'intense sampling' across the entire concentration versus time profile and are therefore most commonly utilized in early phase of clinical trials or clinical pharmacology studies. Compartmental models can integrate both rich and sparse sampling and are often utilized to analyse phase 2 and 3 clinical trials with fewer samples per subject.
- Unlike NCA, compartmental analysis can be used for dose adjustment in subjects by accounting for variability in the PK estimates due to factors such as age, gender or derangement in the hepatic and renal functions.

1.9.4 Physiologically Based Pharmacokinetic (PBPK) Model

- These are physiologically based pharmacokinetic models in the sense that they describe the various processes involved in drug disposition such as absorption, distribution, metabolism and elimination by taking into account the *anatomical and physiological aspects* of the biological system along with the individual properties of the drug being studied.
- It was first proposed by a Swedish physicist and biochemist named Teorell in the year 1937.

- The PBPK model classifies the body into different individual compartments of different organs or tissues with inclusion of details regarding the size of the organ, its tissue composition (including lipid content) and the rate of blood flow to the organ.
- Thus, PBPK models are in general multicompartment models wherein the individual compartments, i.e. organs or tissues are interconnected by blood vessels or lymphatic vessels.
- The model comprises of *individual differential equations* for each organ/tissue compartment which takes into account the organ size, blood flow, other physiological parameters (e.g. pulmonary ventilation for lungs) and the concentration of enzymes or receptors related to the particular organ.
- The PBPK model also considers the various physical and chemical characteristics of the drug such as its molecular weight, size, lipid solubility and water solubility which can play a major role in its distribution and elimination from the body.
- The PBPK models can serve as a robust and cost-effective tool in characterizing the pharmacokinetic parameters with accounting for the physiological variations specific to a population.
- This method is especially useful in characterizing the pharmacokinetics of a drug in vulnerable and sensitive populations such as elderly, children, pregnancy and cancer patients.

1.10 Pharmacokinetic Parameters

The various pharmacokinetic parameters for a drug such as clearance (CL), volume of distribution (Vd), half-life (t1/2), elimination rate constant (Ke) and area under the curve (AUC) and their clinical and pharmacological implications are discussed below.

1.10.1 Half-Life

- Half-life is the time required to decrease the concentration of the drug in plasma by one-half of its initial concentration. For example, if the initial plasma concentration of a drug A given as an intravenous bolus is 100 mg/L, the time duration that is necessary for the concentration to fall to 50 mg/L is called the half-life.
- The knowledge about half-life is useful in understanding the duration of action and the optimal dosing regimen for a particular drug.
- The half-life is constant for a drug following a first-order kinetics of elimination whereas the half-life of the drug decreases as the plasma concentration decreases for a drug following zero-order kinetics.
- Half-life can be determined as follows:

$$T1/2 = \ln 2 / Ke \text{ (where (ln) is the natural logarithm \& } \ln 2 - 0.693\text{)}.$$

(or)

$$T1/2 = 0.693/Ke$$

(or)

$$T1/2 = 0.693 \times (Vd/CL)$$

- Thus, half-life is a ***secondary pharmacokinetic parameter*** which is dependent on other primary pharmacokinetic parameters such as CL (Clearance) and Vd (Volume of distribution).
- The half-life and elimination rate constant of a drug denote how early a drug is removed from the plasma and thus helps us in deciding the appropriate dose required for the drug.
- The half-life can vary between seconds, minutes, hours to days depending on the nature of the drug.

1.10.1.1 Clinical/Pharmacokinetic Implications of Half-Life

- It gives an idea about the duration of stay of the drug in the biological system.
- Half-life gives an idea about the time required (in general 4–5 half-lives) for a drug to attain steady-state concentrations in the body *or* to get eliminated completely if therapy is stopped *or* to attain a new steady state if dosing rate is changed.
- It is useful in the management of drug toxicity or overdose.
- To determine the frequency of dosing for a particular drug: The half-life gives a rough idea of the amount and frequency of maintenance dose since it is roughly half of the initial dose with the dosing interval corresponding to the half-life of the drug. For example, for a drug having a t1/2 of 12 hours if the initial/priming dose to achieve the desired plasma concentration is 100 mg then the maintenance dose will be approximately 50 mg every 12 hours. However, this approach would be impractical for drugs with very short t1/2 (< 3 hours) because of the requirement of frequent maintenance dosing, therefore these drugs need to be given as a continuous intravenous infusion instead.

1.10.2 Volume of Distribution, Vd

- It is the ***apparent volume*** in the body that is required to contain the amount of drug administered if distributed homogeneously at the concentration measured in plasma.
- It is called as *apparent Vd* because it accounts for the *hypothetical volume* within the biological system that is required for containing the entire dose administered if the drug concentration were to be the same in the entire body as that measured in the plasma. Thus, Vd is an indirect measure of the extent to which a drug is distributed in the body fluids and tissues.

- **Vd = Dose administered/Plasma concentration.** The unit of Vd is in litres; L. It can also be expressed as L/kg body weight of the individual.
- In case of drugs whose Vd is more or less equal to the total volume of plasma, it is implied that these drugs are mostly contained within the blood vessels and are therefore poorly distributed to the extravascular tissues. The Vd is relatively low in case of such drugs and these drugs can also be bound to plasma proteins which can further hamper their distribution to the surrounding tissues.
- A large Vd is seen in case of drugs which are widely distributed in tissues and body fluids other than blood/plasma.

1.10.2.1 Factors Determining the Vd of a Drug

- **Lipid solubility:** Hydrophobic/non-polar/unionized drugs are more likely to have a higher Vd since they can more readily cross the biological membranes and get distributed in the body beyond the vascular compartment.
- **Tissue binding:** Drugs with high tissue binding can have increased Vd.
- **Plasma protein binding:** Drugs with lower plasma protein binding are less likely to be confined to the vascular compartment and thus have higher Vd.
- **Molecular size:** Vd is inversely proportional to the molecular size of a drug because drugs with increased molecular size can less readily cross the biological membranes and vice versa.
- Disease conditions such as burns and sepsis which can lead to **third spacing of fluids** can lead to a false increase in Vd.
- Concentration of drug transporters in a particular tissue/organ can also affect the Vd.
- Physiological factors such as age, body weight and body composition can also affect the Vd of drugs.

1.10.2.2 Clinical/Pharmacokinetic Implications of Volume of Distribution

- Haemodialysis can be used in the management of drug overdose due to drugs with low Vd and low plasma protein binding which are primarily confined to the vascular compartment, e.g. Lithium, metformin and salicylates.
- In case of the removal of drugs of high molecular weight or high plasma protein binding, a technique of extracorporeal blood purification such as **hemadsorption** or **hemoperfusion** is used, e.g. Barbiturates, carbamazepine, valproate and theophylline.
- Volume of distribution can be used to calculate the amount of loading dose and this is generally used for drugs with higher Vd which are predominantly distributed in the tissues. Administration of loading dose in the case of these drugs helps in achieving an adequate plasma concentration for optimal therapeutic efficacy and desired concentration at the site of its action after distribution to the other tissues.

$$Loading\ dose = Vd \times Desired\ plasma\ concentration$$

- Drugs with high Vd also have higher half-life due to their extensive tissue distribution and drugs with lower Vd that are primarily confined to the vascular compartment are cleared quickly from the body via renal route and hence such drugs have lower half-life.

1.10.3 Clearance

- Clearance of the drug can be defined as the *amount of plasma that is cleared of a particular drug per unit time*. Thus, it should be interpreted as a rate and not simply as the amount of drug that is removed from the body.
- Drugs can be cleared from the body by either metabolism or by elimination. While clearance due to metabolism indicates the conversion of drug into metabolites, the clearance due to elimination refers to removal of the drug from the body by excretion via urine or stools due to renal or hepatic elimination, respectively.
- In case of drugs which do not undergo exclusive clearance via one particular route (renal/hepatic), the total clearance can be calculated using the following formula:

$$CL\,total = CL\,renal + CL\,nonrenal$$

(or)

$$CL\ total = CL\ renal + CL\ hepatic + CL\ other\ routes$$

- The nonrenal routes of clearance include predominantly hepatic with or without minor elimination through other routes such as the skin via sweat (e.g. phenobarbitone), lungs via breath (e.g. volatile anaesthetics & alcohol), saliva (phenytoin, theophylline) and breast milk (e.g. propylthiouracil, ethanol, morphine). However, the minor routes of elimination are not clinically significant except for very few drugs.
- Since the clearance is constant for drugs following first-order elimination kinetics, the clearance for such drugs can be expressed mathematically as follows:

$$CL_{total} = Ke \times Vd$$

- i.e. the clearance is the elimination rate constant (fractional rate of drug loss) times the volume of distribution of the drug.
- In case of single dose of drug with 100% bioavailability as in the case of drug administered via intravenous route with first-order kinetics of elimination, the clearance can be calculated using the following formula:

$$CL = Dose\,administered\,/\,AUC$$

- **Clearance of an organ** can be calculated using the formula given below

$$CL\,organ = Q\left[\left(Ca - Cv\right)/\,Cv\right] = Q \times E$$

- In the above equation, **Q** refers to the rate of blood flow through the organ expressed in mL/minute and **Ca** refers to the concentration of drug in the blood vessel entering the organ or the arterial blood and **Cv** refers to the concentration of drug in the blood vessel exiting the organ or the venous blood.
- **E** is the *extraction ratio* which is a measure of an organ's ability to remove the drug from the body. The value of extraction ratio can be any number ranging from 0 to 1. By definition, an organ with an extraction ratio of 1 for a particular drug is 100% efficient in clearing the drug.
- The above equation helps us to understand the concept of clearance and is generally not useful in clinical practice for drug monitoring. Clearance of a drug is generally calculated as model model-independent parameter by non-compartmental analysis and hence no assumptions regarding the compartments have to be made.

1.10.3.1 Factors Affecting Clearance of a Drug

- **Age:** Clearance of drugs generally declines with increase in age due to comorbidities and normal age-related decline in the hepatic and renal functions.
- **Hepatic impairment:** The liver plays an important role in clearance of drugs by increasing its metabolism via the microsomal and non-microsomal enzymes which converts them into metabolites suitable for elimination. Therefore, any compromise in liver function can drastically affect the clearance.
- **Renal impairment:** The drugs and their metabolites are mainly eliminated by the kidneys and therefore renal impairment can lead to reduction in rate of removal of drug from the body thus leading to accumulation of drugs and prolongation of their half-lives.
- **Plasma protein binding:** Acidic drugs bind mainly with albumin and basic drugs bind mainly to alpha-1-acid glycoprotein. Drugs with high plasma protein binding tend to stay in the body for longer durations since they are less readily excreted by the kidneys.
- **Rate/amount of blood flow to organ of elimination:** Certain disease states which affect the rate of blood flow to the organs such as liver and kidney can also affect the clearance of drugs.
- **Drug interactions:** When more than one drug is taken together it can interact with one another, thus leading to increased or decreased clearance.
- For example, a combined therapy of thiazide diuretics and lithium leads to lithium toxicity by increasing the reabsorption of sodium and lithium at proximal convoluted tubule. Lithium has a narrow therapeutic index. The concomitant use of these two drugs together thus results in lithium toxicity due to elevated plasma concentrations. Hence, combining lithium with thiazide diuretics should be avoided.
- **Microsomal enzyme induction/inhibition:** Drugs that can induce the microsomal enzymes such as CYP3A4 and CYP2D9 can increase the metabolism and clearance of other drugs which are metabolized by these enzymes. Similarly, drugs inhibiting microsomal enzymes can decrease the clearance of drugs metabolized by these enzymes.

1.10.3.2 Clinical/Pharmacokinetic Implications of Clearance

- The clearance of the drug is used to calculate the maintenance dose of the drug as a part of the ***2-dose strategy*** *of drug* (followed by the loading dose).

  $$\textit{Maintenance dose} = \textit{Clearance of the drug} \times \textit{Target plasma concentration}$$

  Thus, for drugs having more clearance, the amount of maintenance dose will also increase and vice versa.

- **Dosage modification/adjustment** will be done for patients with renal or hepatic impairment in case of the drugs excreted by renal or hepatic routes, respectively.

1.10.4 Area Under the Curve

- The area under the curve in pharmacokinetics is a *definite integral* of the concentration of a drug as measured in blood/plasma over a time period. The concentration of the drug can be measured using chromatographic techniques such as high-performance liquid chromatography (HPLC). It gives a measure of total exposure of the body to a drug following its administration (Fig. 1.7a).
- The AUC can be calculated from clearance by the following formula.

  $$AUC = \left(\textit{Dose administered} / \textit{Clearance}\right)$$

- When the clearance of a drug is very high, the duration of stay of the drug in the body is relatively lesser and hence the AUC also gets smaller.
- In case of a drug following first-order kinetics, if the clearance is constant then the AUC can be said to be directly proportional to the dose of administration of the drug and thus as the dose increases the AUC will also increase.

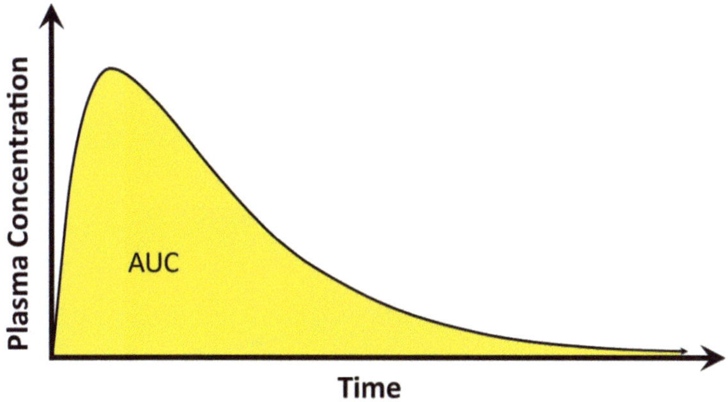

Fig. 1.7a Schematic representation of the area under the curve of a 'plasma concentration vs time plot' of a drug

- The AUC can also be calculated from the elimination rate constant as follows:

$$AUC = \left(Initial\ concentration\left(C0\right)/\ Ke\right)$$

The unit of C0 is mg/L and the unit of Ke is 1/h; therefore, the unit of AUC is (mg × h/L).

For a drug following first-order kinetics, the AUC can be calculated by dividing the entire area into small trapezoids Figs. 1.7b and 1.7c and then summating the areas of the individual trapezoids.

$$AUC = AUC_{0-2} + AUC_{2-4} + AUC_{4-6} + AUC_{6-8} + AUC_{8-10} + AUC_{10-12} + AUC_{last-\infty}$$

The area of individual trapezoid can be calculated using the formula

$$Area = \left[\left(C1 + C2\right)/2\right] \times \left(t2 - t1\right)$$

- By applying the above equation, the areas of the individual trapezoids can be summated to obtain the AUC as follows:

The entire area under the curve can be obtained by summating the individual areas of each trapezoid.

- However, this method is useful only for estimating the AUC till the last measured concentration but in order to calculate the clearance using AUC we have to find the $AUC_{0-\infty}$, this can be obtained by calculating the area beyond the last concentration using the equation

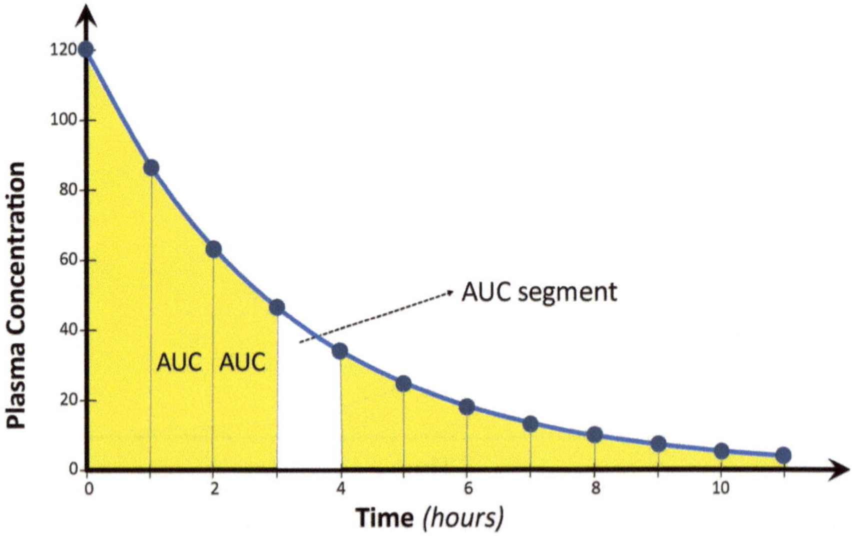

Fig. 1.7b Schematic representation of the trapezoidal rule of area under the curve of a 'plasma concentration vs time plot' of a drug

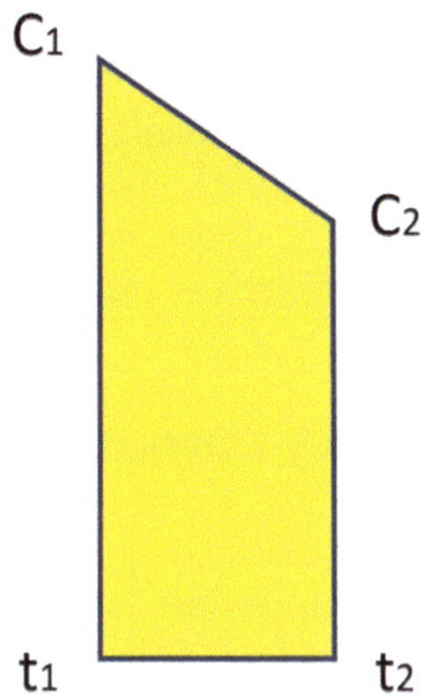

Fig. 1.7c Showing an individual trapezoid from the AUC

$$Terminal\ area = C_{last} / Ke$$

- Wherein C_{last} is the last concentration measured and Ke is the elimination rate constant. The area obtained using the above equation when added to the area obtained using trapezoidal method gives the $\mathbf{AUC_{0\text{-}\infty}}$.
- It is a good practice to calculate the AUC from time 0, i.e. the time corresponding to just before the administration of the drug to infinity after single drug administration, and within the dose interval after multiple dose treatment. In the first case the extrapolation from the last measurable concentration to infinity is computed assuming that the wash-out in the terminal phase follows a mono-exponential profile, and for this calculation the terminal half-life is also needed. In the second case, extrapolations are not necessary, provided the beginning and the end of the dosing intervals are also sampled.

1.10.4.1 Clinical/Pharmacokinetic Implications of Measuring AUC

- It can be used to calculate the ***fractional or relative bioavailability*** of a drug when given by a non-intravenous route and this can be obtained by dividing the AUC of the drug when given by a particular route such as intramuscular, subcutaneous or intradermal, by the AUC of the drug following an intravenous administration.

$$\begin{aligned}&Relative\ bioavailability\ of\ a\ drug\ given\ by\ intramuscular\ route\\&= AUC(intramuscular\ route) / AUC(intravenous\ route).\end{aligned}$$

Thus, AUC plays an important role in determining the bioequivalence of a drug in case of BA/BE studies.

- AUC can also be used to determine the drug exposure between two different formulations of the same drug viz. oral capsule vs oral tablet. The relative bioavailability can be calculated by dividing the AUC of the two different formula-

tions. If the percentage of relative bioavailability is within the accepted limits (80–125%) then the formulations are said to be bioequivalent.
- AUC determination is useful in toxicology to determine the amount of drug exposure to the body.
- AUC determination can also help in calculating other pharmacokinetic parameters such as clearance and bioavailability.

1.10.5 Elimination Rate Constant (Ke)

- In case of drugs following first-order elimination kinetics, the plasma concentration vs time curve can be linearized by plotting the data in a semilogarithmic graphical scale with y-axis containing the drug concentration in the logarithmic scale.
- The slope of the elimination phase of the plasma concentration vs time curve thus obtained is called the elimination rate constant. It is denoted as **Ke or Kel or λ**. The elimination rate constant describes the fraction of drug eliminated per unit time. In case of first-order kinetics, if 50% of a drug is eliminated every 1 h, then the Ke for the drug would be 0.5/h. It can be described as the rate at which plasma concentrations will decline during the elimination phase. It is a proportionality constant relating to the rate of change in plasma concentration of a given drug.
- In case of drugs following linear or first-order kinetics, the elimination rate constant is independent of the initial plasma concentration or the dose in which the drug was administered.
- Ke can be calculated from the half-life (t1/2) of a drug, wherein

$$Ke = 0.693 / t1/2 \tag{1.1}$$

- Since t1/2 can be calculated from (0.693*Vd)/ CL; substituting this Eq. 1.1 gives

$$Ke = CL / Vd \tag{1.2}$$

- Thus, the Ke value can be calculated directly from the slope of the elimination phase of a semilogarithmic plasma concentration vs time plot.
- It is important to distinguish between the elimination rate and the elimination rate constant. The rate of any reaction (tangent or slope, *d*Cp/*d*t) changes as the concentration changes; however, for a drug following first-order kinetics the rate constant (ke) does not change.

1.11 Pharmacokinetic Studies

These can be broadly classified into two main types: traditional/non-population pharmacokinetic methods and population pharmacokinetics.

1.11.1 Non-population Pharmacokinetics

- This is also known as the ***traditional method*** of pharmacokinetic study. It is usually used as a part of phase 1 of clinical trial for testing the safety and establishing the pharmacokinetics of a trial drug and for comparing the pharmaceutical equivalence of two drugs as in case of BA/BE studies.
- These studies involve a relatively small number of patients of around 8 to 16 and it follows a fixed design with respect to the time points for sampling following the administration of the drug of interest.
- The traditional pharmacokinetic studies follow a ***two-staged approach*** in the first stage of which the important pharmacokinetic parameters such as the elimination rate constant, clearance and volume of distribution are determined in each individual and the second stage comprises of descriptive statistics of the individual pharmacokinetic parameter summarized as arithmetic or geometric mean along with its standard deviation.
- The major drawback of these traditional pharmacokinetic studies is the wide interindividual variabilities which can lead to overestimation of the parameters studied. It is also difficult to determine the important covariates such as age, gender and body mass index (BMI) which can lead to pharmacokinetic variability and it cannot be achieved when the data is sparse involving very few sampling time points.
- If the traditional PK data is adequate, it can be further used for PK modelling by fitting into specific compartment models but there can always be some level of uncertain precision in estimating the parameters.

The advantages and disadvantages of traditional PK methods are given below:

Advantages
Less time-consuming and can be done in healthy subjects
Can be done with small number (8–16) of participants
Does not require complex mathematical models or equations
Lesser chances of sampling errors since sampling time points are fixed
Useful to understand basic PK as a part of phase 1 study

Disadvantages
Study participants are not representative of the actual patient population
Requires intensive sampling; minimum 10 samples per participant
Not convenient to be performed on paediatric age group
Has high interindividual variability among the PK parameters studied
Does not account for effect of covariates such as age, BMI and gender on the values obtained
Not suitable for simulations or predictions if the number of patients studied are very less

1.11.2 Population Pharmacokinetics

- As the name suggests, these methods involve PK modelling within a population, i.e. a greater number of participants (minimum 40–50) as compared to the traditional method. Therefore, it also accounts for the *inter-subject* and *inter-occasion variability* compared to the traditional methods.
- Population pharmacokinetics (Pop PK) methods study the population as a whole rather than the individuals in it. They depend on concentration vs time data from many individuals and can also utilize pooled data from multiple studies.
- In contrast to traditional PK methods, it also offers flexibility with recruiting patients with different doses and different time points of sampling and sparse sampling (4–5 samples per patient) with proper documentation of the variations.
- Pop PK methods are thus technically more complex as compared to the traditional PK since they depend on proper fitting into appropriate compartment models and complex mathematical equations to obtain the results. The interindividual variability within the study population can be addressed by incorporating appropriate covariate data such as age, body mass index (BMI) and kidney/liver function.
- In contrast to traditional PK methods, here the individual PK parameters are usually expressed as the mean and variability estimates at the end of parametric modelling.
- It should be clear that pop PK methods are not a fallback option when the concentration vs time data of the patient is sparse; rather they should be utilized to construct mathematical models with maximum covariates in order to enable the physician to decide the dosing of a drug for a particular patient who comes under similar population. Thus, pop PK methods can be used for predictions and simulations and are thus helpful in deciding dose at various stages of drug development.

The advantages and disadvantages of population PK methods are given below:

Advantages
Usually done on patients who are taking the drug of interest
Allows flexible timings and doses during sampling
Requires only few samples from each patient (4–5)
Can account for effect of covariates on the PK parameters obtained
Can explain both inter- as well as intraindividual variability

Disadvantages
More time-consuming
Increased chance of sampling errors due to differences in the timing of sampling
Requires a greater number of study participants
Involves complex mathematical model building and complex equations
Increased chance of missing data with respect to the covariates studied

1.12 Therapeutic Drug Monitoring

- It is a branch of clinical pharmacology that deals with measurement of drug levels in the blood or plasma. Therapeutic drug monitoring offers *personalized medicine* to an individual by helping to tailor the dose according to each person. Thus, it is useful in improving the clinical outcomes especially for drugs with narrow therapeutic index where even a minimal increase in plasma concentration can lead to toxicity.
- The dosage adjustment for such drugs can be made a priori based on the already available information from pharmacogenetic, demographic and clinical data.
- *A posteriori* dosage adjustment can be made by pharmacokinetic monitoring which involves measurement of plasma concentration of the drug of interest or by pharmacodynamic monitoring of surrogate biomarkers for drug response.
- The plasma concentration measured can be influenced by various factors such as the timing of administration, dosing regimen, route of administration, method of sample collection, storage of samples before assessment, the robustness and validity of the assay and the type of instrument used for TDM.
- The drug concentrations measured can also be affected by the patient factors such as presence of other comorbidities including hepatic or renal impairment and history of concomitant medications.
- In order to avoid errors in drug concentration measurement it is necessary to take precautions at all 3 stages: (1) **Pre-analytical** (sample collection, storage of samples), (2) **Analytical** (sample processing, running the assay and calculating the drug levels), and (3) **Post-analytical** (interpreting of the values for the particular patient and giving an opinion).
- Thus, therapeutic drug monitoring is a multidisciplinary process which involves contributions from the clinicians, nurses, clinical pharmacists, pharmacologists and laboratory technical staff.
- **The following criteria are to be met to perform therapeutic drug monitoring for a particular drug:**
  - The drug of interest should have a consistent pharmacodynamic relationship between the plasma concentration and the pharmacological effects in terms of safety and efficacy.
  - The drug should have a significant interpatient variability with respect to its pharmacokinetics.

- The drug should have a narrow therapeutic index.
- In general, for drugs which are given as a fixed dosage, the sampling for TDM should ideally be done after the elapse of 4–5 elimination half-lives. In case the samples are taken before this period, the values may not reflect steady-state concentration and the actual clearance of the patient thus making it difficult for the physician to make dosage adjustments.
- The drug should not have any easy and objectively measurable surrogate markers for assessing its therapeutic outcome.
- The drugs which are administered for chronic conditions where patient compliance needs to be verified in the background of lack of improvement, e.g. immunosuppression in organ transplant patients and valproate in patients with psychiatric disorders such as bipolar disease.
- The analytical instruments such as high-performance liquid chromatography (HPLC), liquid chromatography tandem mass spectrometry (LC-MS/MS) and chemiluminescence immunoassay are some of the commonly used methods to determine drug levels.
- Some of the drugs for which TDM is done routinely are: antiepileptics such as phenytoin, carbamazepine, valproic acid and phenobarbitone; immunosuppressants such as tacrolimus, cyclosporin and mycophenolate mofetil; antipsychotics such as clozapine; mood stabilizer lithium; digoxin and antimicrobials such as gentamicin, amikacin and vancomycin.

1.12.1 Application of TDM for Patient Care

- In case of drugs following linear or first-order kinetics, the new dose required for the patient in achieving the desired plasma concentration can be obtained from the equation:

$$Css(measured) / Css(desired) = Dose(previous) / Dose(new)$$

(or)

$$Dose(new) = Dose(previous) \times Css(desired) / Css(measured)$$

- In case of drug overdose or poisoning, serial monitoring of drug levels after initiation of treatment will help to decide the further course of management for the patient.
- Monitoring of trough concentration in case of drugs with serious toxicity such as ototoxicity or nephrotoxicity can help in modifying the dose to maintain the plasma concentration within the therapeutic range, e.g. antibiotics such as vancomycin, amikacin and colistin.

Bibliography

1. Rowland M, Tozer TN (2011) Clinical pharmacokinetics and pharmacodynamics: concepts and applications, 4th edn. Wolters Kluwer Health/Lippincott William & Wilkins, Philadelphia
2. Katzung BG (2017) Basic and clinical pharmacology, 14th edn. McGraw-Hill, New York
3. Gibaldi M, Perrier D (1975) Route of administration and drug disposition. Drug Metab Rev 3(1):185–199. https://doi.org/10.3109/03602537408993742
4. Brown MJ, Sharma P, Mir FA, Bennett PN (2018) Clinical pharmacology, 12th edn. Churchill Livingston Elsevier, London
5. DiPiro Joseph T and American Society of Health-System Pharmacists (2002) Concepts in clinical pharmacokinetics, 3rd edn. American Society of Health-System Pharmacists, Bethesda
6. Ritter J, Lewis L, Mant T, Ferro A (2008) A textbook of clinical pharmacology and therapeutics, 5th edn. CRC Press, Florida
7. Egbelowo O (2018) Nonlinear elimination of drugs in one-compartment pharmacokinetic models: nonstandard finite difference approach for various routes of administration. Math Comput Appl 23(2):27. https://doi.org/10.3390/mca23020027
8. Foster DM (2007) Noncompartmental versus compartmental approaches to pharmacokinetic analysis. In: Principles of clinical pharmacology. Academic Press, pp 89–105

Bibliography

1. Rowland M, Tozer TN (2011) Clinical pharmacokinetics and pharmacodynamics: concepts [illegible]

[illegible]

Essential Medicines and Rational Use of Drugs

2

Rekha Priyadarshini

Abstract

The essential medicines list (EML) is a fundamental pillar in promoting the rational use of medicines, grounded in the principle of the "right to health." Essential medicines are those that should be consistently available in sufficient quantities, in appropriate dosage forms, with guaranteed quality, and at a cost that is affordable to both individuals and communities across all levels of the healthcare system. The main aim of the WHO's efforts to promote rational medicine use is to ensure that both healthcare providers and patients use medicines in a clinically appropriate and cost-effective manner. Access to essential medicines remains uneven, especially in low- and middle-income countries (LMICs), where healthcare equity is still a significant challenge. Improving the rational use of medicines is crucial for reducing morbidity and mortality, while also helping to contain healthcare costs. Addressing these gaps requires a multidisciplinary and collaborative approach, involving stakeholders from across the healthcare spectrum. Efforts must focus on strengthening existing health infrastructure, enhancing workforce capacity, and implementing evidence-based policies that promote universal access to essential medicines and support the effective application of rational drug use at all levels of care.

Keywords

Essential medicines · Essential drugs · Essential medicines list · National List of Essential Medicines of India · Rational Use of Drugs · Rational Drug Use

R. Priyadarshini (✉)
Department of Pharmacology, All India Institute of Medical Sciences (AIIMS) Bibinagar, Hyderabad, India
e-mail: rekha.pharma@aiimsbibinagar.edu.in

A. Arivazhahan et al. (eds.), *Introduction to Basics of Pharmacology and Toxicology*,
https://doi.org/10.1007/978-981-95-1920-0_2

2.1 Essential Medicines

2.1.1 Introduction

Essential medicines have been established on the grounds of "the right to health" concept. The International Conference on Primary Health Care adopted the Alma-Ata Declaration way back in 1978, during which "health" was affirmed as a fundamental human right and underscored the global commitment to achieving the highest possible level of health—"Health for All"—through primary healthcare. It also recognized the provision of essential medicines as one of the eight core components of primary healthcare.

The principles behind the formulation of essential medicines are easy accessibility, availability, appropriateness, and guaranteed quality of goods and services. Essential medicines also promote cost-effective use of resources to enhance the quality and accessibility of healthcare. This is particularly important for resource-limited countries.

Essential medicines list (EML) is one of the key components of rational use of medicines. The WHO model list of essential medicines stands as a guide to formulate countries' own essential medicine lists as per the country-specific disease prevalence, priorities, and also treatment guidelines.

2.1.2 Definition of Essential Medicines

Definition for "essential medicines" was given by the World Health Organization's Expert Committee on the Selection and Use of Essential Medicines.

> Essential medicines (EMs) are those that satisfy the priority healthcare needs of the population and are chosen with regard to disease prevalence and public health relevance, evidence of clinical efficacy and safety, as well as comparative costs and cost-effectiveness

Essential medicines must be consistently available in adequate quantities, in suitable dosage forms, with assured quality, and at a price that is affordable to individuals and the community. Their accessibility across all levels of healthcare is crucial to enhancing public health outcomes.

2.1.3 Concept of EML Evolution

2.1.3.1 World Health Organization's Model List of Essential Drugs

- The concepts of "essential drugs" and "national drug policy" was introduced in 1975 by the World Health Assembly to address inequities in global health. These ideas swiftly became integral part of the global public health terminology. The World Health Assembly was founded to provide a solution to seal the huge gap which was created between benefiters and non-benefiters of pharmaceutical harvest of the mid-1900s.

- The World Health Assembly urged the WHO to assist member states in selecting essential medicines that align with their specific healthcare priorities, and to ensure their consistent availability, assured quality, and affordability.
- The World Health Organization (WHO) published the **first Model List of Essential Drugs in the month of October 1977, which contained 186 medicines**. Subsequently, "Provision of essential drugs" is recognized as one of the key elements of primary healthcare by the Declaration of Alma-Ata.
- The intention behind the WHO's EML was to serve as a template to member countries to prepare their own national essential medicines list because essential medicines are utmost important, basic, indispensable, and necessary for the health and needs of the population.

2.1.3.2 National List of Essential Medicines (NLEM)

- In India, essential medicines list was first developed by the Tamil Nadu state in early 1994. Later, Delhi developed a comprehensive Drug Policy in 1994 with an objective to improve the availability and accessibility of quality essential drugs for the needy.
- The First National List of Essential Medicines (NLEM) of India was prepared in 1996 with 279 medicines, almost after 20 years of inception of essential medicines list (1977) by the World Health Organization.
- Expert Committee is the one which evaluates the scientific evidence with respect to comparative effectiveness, safety, and cost-effectiveness, to make a decision on inclusion or exclusion of the medicines from the list, and also to review the therapeutic alternatives and update on AWaRe (Access–Watch–Reserve) classification of antibiotics.
- The revised versions of NLEM were brought out subsequently, in 2003 (with 354 medicines), 2011 (with 348 medicines), 2015 (with 376 medicines), and the latest 2022 (with 384 medicines).
- In 2022, essential medical devices were included in the National List of Essential Medicines (NLEM) for the first time. Some of the essential medical devices including diagnostic kits, glucometers, and blood pressure apparatus were incorporated in the present list.

2.1.4 Core Principles of Essential Medicines (Fig. 2.1)

2.1.5 Selection of Essential Medicines

The selection of limited number of medicines as essential is a critical process, which is governed by several principles set forth by the World Health Organization (WHO) and individual national healthcare authorities (Box 2.1).

Promote Equity in Healthcare access:

- Reduce health disparities by ensuring that vital treatments are accessible to all, particularly underserved populations by promoting the transparent sharing of health and medicines information by governments, national health systems, and the pharmaceutical industry.

Promote Evidence-Based Selection:

- Medicines included in the EML undergo rigorous evaluation for efficacy, safety, and cost-effectiveness. This ensures that only drugs with a favourable benefit-risk ratio are prioritized.

Promote Affordability and Accessibility:

- It is very fundamental to ensure essential medicines are available at reasonable costs. This goal can be achieved by strategies like bulk procurement, generic substitution, and price controls with effective pricing policies.

Promote Sustainable Healthcare Systems:

- Policies to optimize resource allocation and focusing on cost-effective interventions must be implemented by governments and national health systems, so as to reduce the amount of out-of pocket spending on medicines

Fig. 2.1 Principles of essential medicines

2.1.5.1 Criteria for Selection and Inclusion of Medicines in Essential Medicines List

1. Public health relevance based on the prevalence of diseases and conditions within a population.
2. As per the Standard Treatment Guidelines (STGs).
3. Evidence-based efficacy and safety of medicines.
4. Cost-effectiveness.
5. Availability in suitable Dosage Forms and Strengths for the local healthcare context.
6. Stability under typical storage conditions and easy to transport.

Box 2.1 Different Lists of Essential Medicines

WHO model list of essential medicines (EML)	National Lists	Periodic Review and Updates
Serves as a global guide	Individual countries customize the WHO list of essential medicines as per their needs	Revise periodically to reflect new evidence, emerging health threats, and the availability of new medicines
WHO updates the model list every two years	Essential medicine committees decide the number of medicines that need to be included in the list after assessing local epidemiological data, availability, and affordability	

Table 2.1 The WHO AWaRe classification

	Access group	Watch group	Reserve group
Antibiotics include	Recommended first/second-line treatments for common microbial infections	High risk of antimicrobial resistance and should be used cautiously	Last-resort antibiotics
Clinical significance	Increased availability and use of these antibiotics is very much encouraged within the framework of functioning health systems to reduce the use of more potent drugs for common microbial infections and combat resistance	To avoid resistance limit the use of these medicines to certain serious infections	Use of these medicines is highly restricted to severe, multi-drug-resistant infections to prevent resistance
Examples	Amoxicillin	Ciprofloxacin	Colistin

2.1.6 Access–Watch–Reserve (AWaRe) Classification

The Access–Watch–Reserve (AWaRe) classification of antibiotics, introduced by the WHO in 2017, is a great initiative aimed at promoting the responsible use of antibiotics and combating antimicrobial resistance. Widely accepted by stakeholders, AWaRe supports the development of country-specific antibiotic stewardship programs, facilitates the rational selection of antibiotics for essential medicine lists, and helps shape effective public health policies by ensuring balanced access while preventing overuse.

This classification categorizes the antibiotics into three groups: Access group, Watch group, and Reserve group (Table 2.1).

2.1.7 Components of Essential Medicines List

2.1.7.1 Components of the WHO's Essential Medicines List

It contains core list and Complementary list:

Core and Complementary Medicines

- **Core List**: These are essential medicines that satisfy the health needs of the majority of the population. They should be **available at all times** in appropriate amounts and dosage formulations.
- **Complementary List**: Includes medicines that require **specialized diagnostics or facilities**, or are used for rare conditions.

Symbols

The list contains certain **symbols or annotations** to convey specific meanings about medicines included on the list (Table 2.2).

2.1.7.2 Components of NLEM

All the essential medicines that are listed in the NLEM are categorized into Primary Care facility, Secondary care facility, and Tertiary care facility and presented as (P), (S), and (T) respectively besides each individual medicine to satisfy the healthcare needs of population.

Symbols in NLEM (Table 2.3)

2.1.8 Purposes that can be served by the National List of Essential Medicines

- Promotion of rational use of medicines.
- Ensure safe and effective treatment of priority disease conditions of a population and optimize the available healthcare resources of the country.
- It can also serve as a guiding document for:
  - State governments to formulate their own essential medicines lists

Table 2.2 Symbols in the WHO EML

Symbol	Significance
[c]	• This symbol in core list signifies that there is a specific indication for restricting its use to children
[c]	• This symbol in the complementary list of medicines indicates that these drugs require specialist diagnostic or monitoring facilities, specialist medical care, or specialized training for their use in children
□ (square box)	• This symbol in the core list signifies therapeutic equivalents to the listed medicine, for consideration in national essential medicines lists • Therapeutic equivalents can include single medications, or multiple medicines medications within a specific pharmacological class or chemical subgroup. These are categorized at the fourth level of the anatomical therapeutic chemical (ATC) classification system, and they demonstrate comparable clinical effectiveness and safety profiles
[a]	• This symbol indicates that there is an age or weight restriction on use of the medicine
*	• It signifies a clinical concern related to the medicine, with further details provided in the footnote

Table 2.3 Symbols in NLEM

Symbol	Significance
(P)	• Primary care facility
(S)	• Secondary care facility
(T)	• Tertiary care facility

- Development of standard treatment guidelines
- Help in preparing hospital formularies
- Effective procurement and supply of medicines in both public and private sectors
- Health insurance providers in determining reimbursement policies
- Defining the "MUST KNOW" competencies for the education and training of healthcare professionals, including those in medicine, dentistry, pharmacy, and nursing

The major impediments in implementing the Essential Medicines concept are listed in Fig. 2.2.

2.1.9 Conclusion

The main purpose of selection of essential medicines is to make sure that the populations at large have access to all life-saving vital drugs. By means of making affordable and high-quality medicines available in all healthcare settings, the process of selection of essential medicines also wards of health inequities, improves public health outcomes, and also increases overall health coverage.

2.2 Rational Use of Drugs

2.2.1 Definition and Importance

- The Definition of ***Rational Use of Medicines*** (RUM) as per WHO is.

> Patients receive medications appropriate to their clinical needs, in doses that meet their own individual requirements, for an adequate period of time, and at the lowest cost to them and their community.

- The WHO's goal in promoting rational medicine use is to ensure that health professionals and consumers utilize medicines in a therapeutically effective and cost-efficient manner.
- The rational use of drugs is critical to the effective functioning of healthcare systems.

Economic Barriers

- Although many essential medicines are relatively low-cost, financial constraints continue to pose a major challenge in low- and middle-income countries (LMICs). Out-of-pocket expenses often restrict access, especially for those requiring long-term treatment for chronic diseases.

Supply Chain Issues

- Inefficient supply chains lead to frequent stockouts, delays, and medicine wastage. These issues are further aggravated by weak logistics systems, inadequate forecasting, and corruption.

Patent and Intellectual Property (IP) Rights

- Patents on newer essential medicines can limit affordability. Although the Trade-Related Aspects of Intellectual Property Rights (TRIPS) agreement offers flexibilities for public health emergencies, many countries face challenges in effectively implementing them.

Lack of Political Will

- Strong political commitment is crucial for enforcing policies that enhance access to essential medicines. However, weak governance and competing priorities often push health initiatives to the sidelines

Inadequate Healthcare Infrastructure

- In many LMICs, a lack of trained healthcare workers and poorly equipped facilities impede the delivery of essential medicines.

Fig. 2.2 Key challenges in implementing the essential medicines concept

- Enhancing the rational use of medicines among healthcare professionals and the public is crucial for controlling drug costs and reducing morbidity and mortality associated with both communicable and non-communicable diseases.
- Irrational use of medicines is a significant global concern. WHO estimates indicate that more than half of all medications are improperly prescribed, dispensed, or sold, and nearly 50% of patients fail to use them as recommended.
- Inappropriate medicine use can occur at any stage of the four main phases in the medicines use cycle (Fig. 2.3).
- Any kind of misuse, overuse, or underuse will lead to wastage of resources, expose to widespread health hazards (toxicity/adverse drug reactions), and even antimicrobial resistance.
- An effective rational drug use program in any country is built upon three core elements, as illustrated in Fig. 2.4.

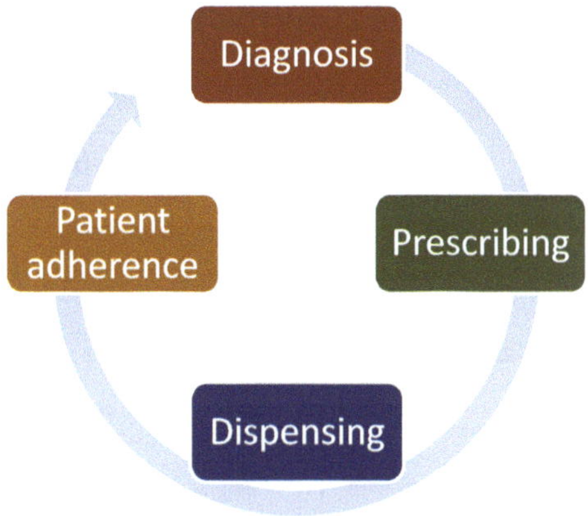

Fig. 2.3 Medicines use cycle

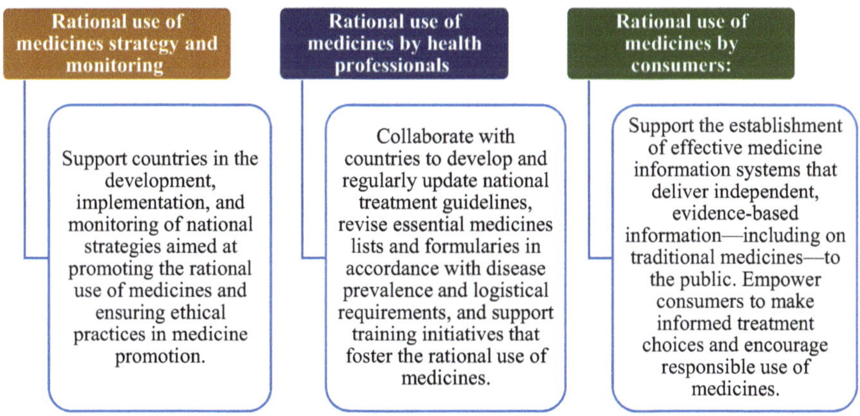

Fig. 2.4 Elements of rational drug use

- The above elements were structured to reflect the core responsibilities of a national essential medicines programme and were developed in close collaboration with regional and country offices.

2.2.2 Irrational Use of Medicines

Examples of irrational use of medicines

- Inappropriate polypharmacy
- Inappropriate use of drugs (incorrect dose, route, and duration)
- Use of antimicrobials for non-microbial infections & excessive use of the parenteral route over available appropriate oral formulations
- Failure to comply with Standard Treatment Guidelines while prescribing.
- Inappropriate self-medication
- Non-adherence to dosing regimes

2.2.2.1 Factors Contributing to Irrational Use of Medicines

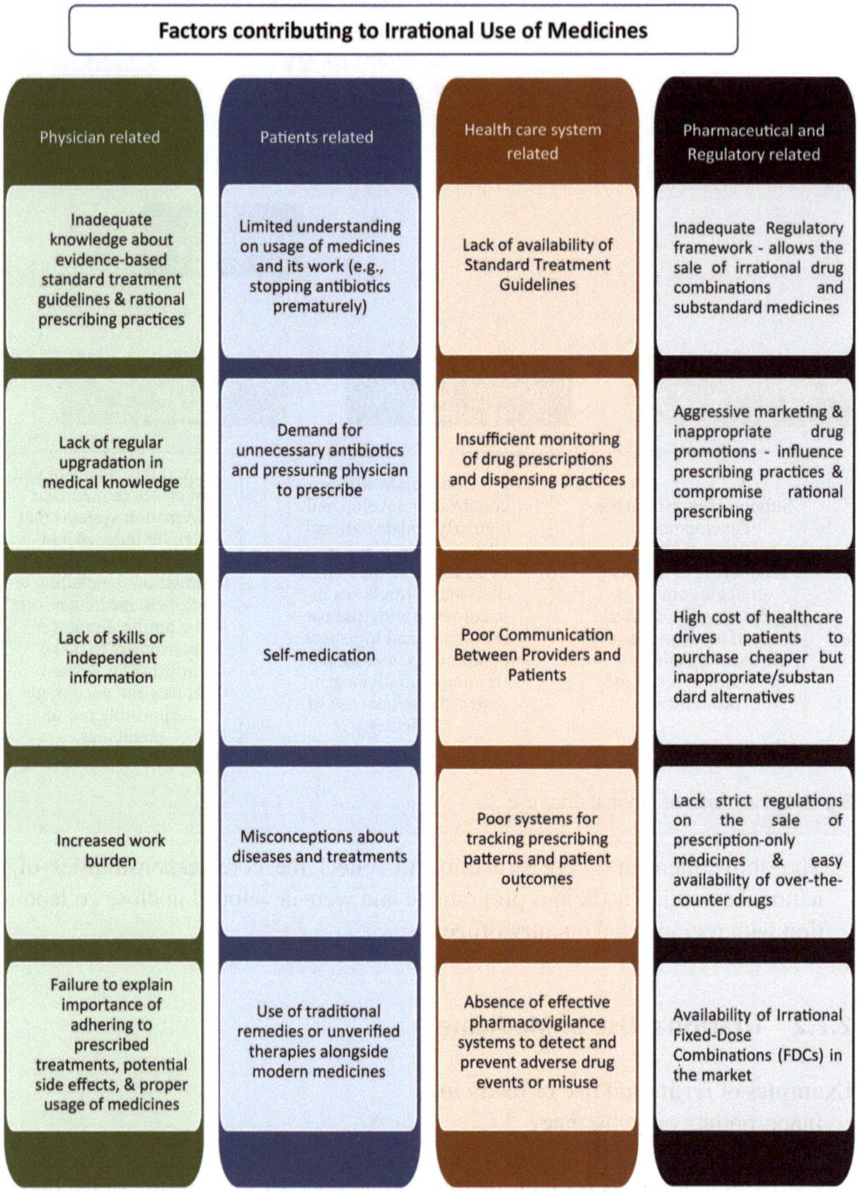

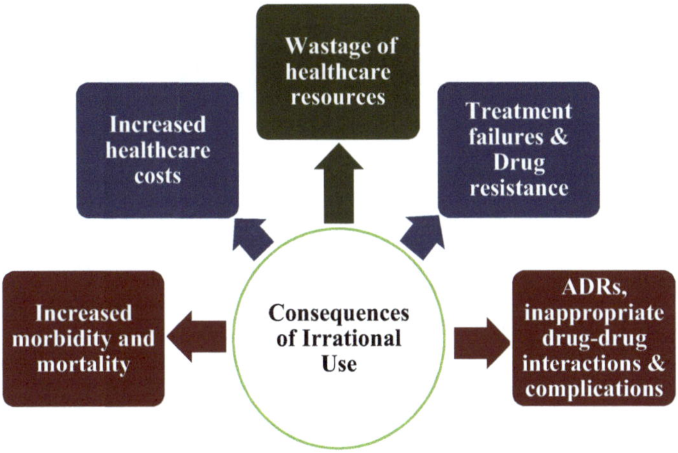

Fig. 2.5 Consequences of irrational drug use

2.2.2.2 Consequences of Irrational Use (Fig. 2.5)

2.2.3 Methods to Measure Irrational Use of Medicines

There are various established methods to measure irrational use of medicines. Selection of method will be based on the specific problem (e.g., overuse of antibiotics, polypharmacy, or inappropriate prescribing) and the target population (e.g., hospitals, pharmacies, or community settings).

The various methods are listed in Fig. 2.6.

2.2.4 Important Indicators of Rational Drug Use

2.2.4.1 WHO Drug Use Indicators

International Network for the Rational Use of Drugs

The mainstay indicators to assess drug usage are Core drug indicators (Prescribing indicators, Patient care indicators, Health facility indicators and Complementary indicators.

(a) **Core drug indicators**

- **Prescribing Indicators:**
  - Average number of drugs per prescription
  - Percentage of generic drugs prescribed
  - Percentage of antibiotics prescribed per prescription
  - Percentage of injectables prescribed per prescription

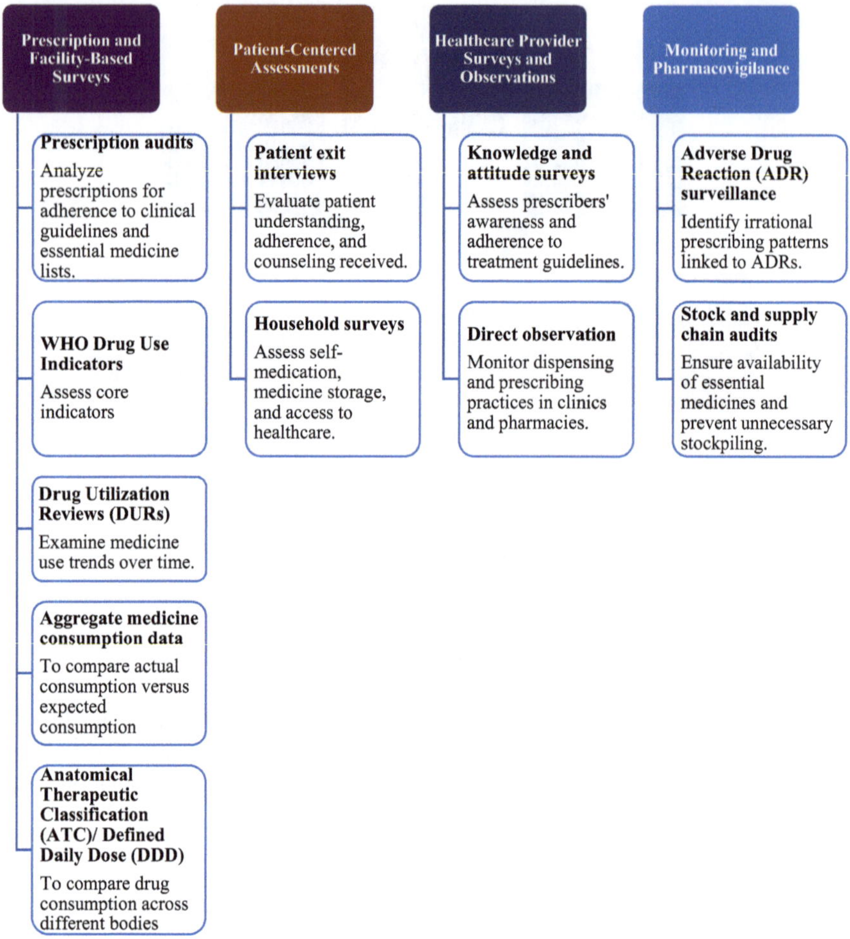

Fig. 2.6 Methods to measure irrational drug use

  - Percentage of drugs prescribed from essential medicines list of the hospital/ institution
- **Patient care Indicators:**
  - Average consultation of time
  - Average dispensing time
  - Percentage of drugs actually dispensed
  - Percentage of drugs adequately labelled
  - Patient's knowledge of correct dosage
- **Health Facility Indicators:**
  - Availability of essential medicines list or formulary
  - Availability of key drugs for some general health problems

(b) **Complementary indicators**

- Average medicine cost per encounter
- Percentage prescriptions in accordance with clinical guidelines

2.2.4.2 Anatomical Therapeutic Classification (ATC) and Defined Daily Dose (DDD)

Anatomical Therapeutic Classification (ATC)

- It is an internationally recognized framework for classifying medicines according to their therapeutic use, pharmacological action, and chemical structure.
- It is maintained by the World Health Organization (WHO) and classifies drugs into five hierarchical levels:

  (a) Anatomical Main Group—Indicates the organ or system the drug affects.
  (b) Therapeutic Subgroup—Defines the drug's main therapeutic purpose.
  (c) Pharmacological Subgroup—Specifies the mechanism of action.
  (d) Chemical Subgroup—Groups drugs based on their chemical structure.
  (e) Chemical Substance—Identifies the specific active ingredient.

- The ATC system is widely used for drug regulation, research, and monitoring medicine use, ensuring consistency in pharmaceutical classification worldwide.

Defined Daily Dose (DDD)

- It is the assumed average maintenance dose per day of a drug for its main indication in adults.
- World Health Organization (WHO) developed it as a standardized unit of measurement to facilitate the comparison of drug consumption across various settings, populations, and time periods.
- It is a technical unit and does not necessarily reflect the actual prescribed dose.
- Helps in monitoring and analysing drug utilization trends globally.
- Facilitates comparison of medicine use between hospitals, regions, and countries.
- The DDD system is widely used in pharmacovigilance, healthcare policy-making, and assessing rational drug use.

  Addressing the irrational use of medicines demands a comprehensive strategy that includes enhanced education, stricter regulations, strengthened healthcare systems, and patient empowerment. Hence, promoting rational drug use requires a collaborative effort involving healthcare professionals, policymakers, patients, and the pharmaceutical industry.
  WHO promotes rational use of medicines by supporting key interventions.

2.2.5 Interventions Supported by WHO

There are 12 key interventions supported by WHO

1. **Establishment of a multidisciplinary national body to coordinate policies on medicine use:**

- A multidisciplinary national body which coordinates with various important stakeholders, both public and private, is essential to promote rational use. Best results will pop up when the interventions are implemented in a coordinated way.

2. **Use of clinical guidelines:**
   - Every country should have evidence-based standard treatment guidelines developed based on their disease prevalence and the skills of available prescribers. And also development and adherence to evidence-based standard treatment guidelines are critical and vital in promoting rational use of medicines.
3. **Development and use of the national essential medicines list:**
   - Every country should establish its own National Essential Medicines List (EML), as it is a fundamental component of promoting the rational use of medicines. The EML supports equity in healthcare access, facilitates evidence-based medicine selection, enhances affordability and availability, and contributes to a sustainable healthcare system.
4. **Establishment of drug and therapeutics committees in districts and hospitals:**
   - Drugs and therapeutic committees promote rational use of medicines by ensuring the safe and effective use of medicines in the appropriate medical setups.
5. **Inclusion of problem-based pharmacotherapy training in undergraduate curricula:**
   - Problem-based pharmacotherapy training, centred on common clinical conditions and aligned with clinical guidelines and essential medicines lists, is an effective approach to instilling rational prescribing habits. This method has proven highly successful in training undergraduate medical and paramedical students.
6. **Continuing in-service medical education as a licensure requirement:**
   - CMEs are most effective when conducted face-to-face in a problem-based, targeted format, extending beyond medical and paramedical professionals to include medicine retailers. Making CME participation a mandatory requirement for license renewal would further enhance its impact. Government support is essential to ensure the organization of unbiased, independent CMEs, free from the influence of pharmaceutical companies, whose involvement often introduces bias.
7. **Supervision, audit and feedback:**
   - Supervision through prescription audits and feedback (drug use evaluation), peer reviews, and group processes (such as identifying medicine use issues and developing, implementing, and evaluating corrective strategies) are essential for ensuring high-quality care.

8. **Use of independent information on medicines:**
   - Drug Information Centres (DICs) and drug bulletins play a vital role in providing healthcare practitioners with unbiased, evidence-based information about medicines, helping to counter the influence of pharmaceutical companies.
9. **Public education about medicines:**
   - Governments have a critical responsibility to ensure the quality of medicines and the accuracy of information provided to consumers. Clear and comprehensive labelling, with accurate, legible, and easily understandable product information, is essential for effective public understanding. In addition, strict regulation and monitoring of pharmaceutical advertising are necessary to prevent misleading influences on both prescribers and the public. Public education campaigns should be implemented to dispel common myths surrounding modern medicine and to curb irrational treatment demands across all age groups, including children, adults, and the elderly.
10. **Avoidance of perverse financial incentives:**
    - One of the potential causes of irrational use of medicines is financial incentives and any kind of such incentives should be seriously avoided. Examples include prescribing expensive medications for financial gain when more affordable alternatives are available or adding unnecessary drugs to a prescription. To promote the rational use of medicines, insurance policies should be designed to reimburse only essential medicines, excluding non-essential ones.
11. **Use of appropriate and enforced regulation:**
    - Adequately funded and judicially supported regulatory authorities will enforce the regulations effectively. This will have a great positive impact on promotion of rational use of medicine.
12. **Sufficient government expenditure to ensure availability of medicines and staff:**
    - Essential medicines and public health facilities with trained medical professionals and staff are the minimum mandatory requirements to promote rational use of medicines. The government should at least increase public expenditure on the health sector to 3% of the GDP and on drugs to at least 1% of the GDP along with the implementation of a rational drug policy would be mandatory to achieve the goals of universal access to essential drugs.

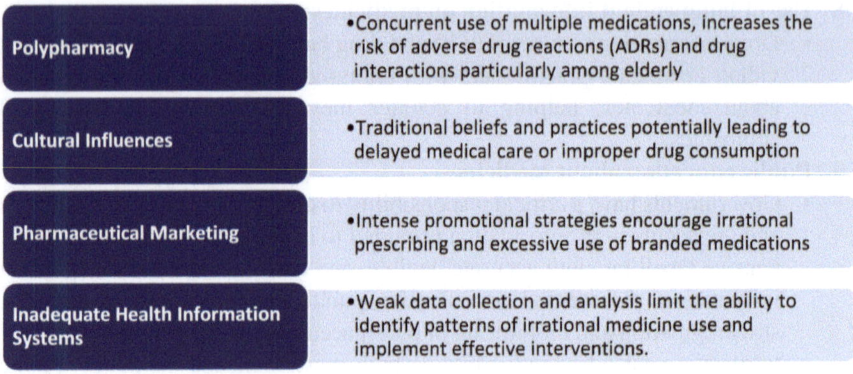

Fig. 2.7 Challenges in rational drug use

2.2.6 Challenges in Rational Drug Use (Fig. 2.7)

2.2.7 Role of Stakeholders

(a) **Healthcare Professionals:** Physicians, pharmacists, and nurses play a central role in rational prescribing, dispensing, and patient education. Training in clinical pharmacology and adherence to treatment guidelines is essential.
(b) **Government and Policymakers:** Governments must prioritize essential medicines in healthcare budgets and implement robust regulatory frameworks to promote rational drug use.
(c) **Pharmaceutical Industry:** Manufacturers should focus on producing high-quality, affordable generics and refrain from unethical marketing practices.
(d) **Patients:** Educated and empowered patients can act as a check against irrational prescribing and demand accountability from healthcare providers.

2.2.8 Conclusion

Availability of essential medicines along with rational use of drugs forms the basis for delivery of effective and equitable healthcare to the masses. However, the affordability and availability of essential medicines are not uniform particularly in the low- and middle-income countries (LMIC) where equitable healthcare is still a question mark. And the provision of optimal healthcare is disparate and discrete in these regions.

All these call for a multidisciplinary and collaborative approach involving representations from a variety of healthcare stakeholders—with a special focus on upliftment of existing infrastructure, increasing manpower effectively, and also to implement evidence-based policies. The ultimate vision should be for universal access of essential medicines and also for effective implementation of rational use of drugs at all levels of healthcare.

Bibliography

Akhmad AD, Satibi, Endarti D, Kristina SA. Factors Related to the Evaluation of Essential Medicines Use in Health Facilities in Indonesia. Pharmacy Practice 2024 Jan–Mar;22(1):2907

Chambers P. Rational use of medicines. Vet Rec. 2011 Aug 27;169(9):226–7

Dugani S, Wasan KM, Kissoon N. World Health Organization and Essential Medicines. J Pharm Sci. 2018 May;107(5):1261–1262

Kar SS, Pradhan HS, Mohanta GP. Concept of essential medicines and rational use in public health. Indian J Community Med. 2010 Jan;35(1):10–3

Kshirsagar NA. Rational use of medicines: Cost consideration & way forward. Indian J Med Res. 2016 Oct;144(4):502–505

Laing R, Hogerzeil H, Ross-Degnan D. Ten recommendations to improve use of medicines in developing countries. Health Policy Plan. 2001 Mar;16(1):13–20

Levy M, Reidenberg MM. What has been the impact of the concept of essential drugs? Clin Pharmacol Ther. 2003 Apr;73(4):275–8

Magrini N, Robertson J, Forte G, Cappello B, Moja LP, de Joncheere K, Kieny MP. Tough decisions on essential medicines in 2015. Bull World Health Organ. 2015 Apr 1;93(4):283–4

Mhlanga BS, Suleman F. Price, availability and affordability of medicines. Afr J Prm Health Care Fam Med. 2014;6(1), Art. #604, 6 pages

Mohanta GP, Manna PK. Rational use of medicines - Indian perspective! Int J Risk Saf Med. 2015;27 Suppl 1:S47–8

Myhr K. Access to and price of medicines globally. Tidsskr Nor Laegeforen. 2011 Oct 18;131(20):2019–21

National List of Essential Medicines 2022 [Internet]. 2022 [cited 2025 April 29] Available from: https://cdsco.gov.in/opencms/resources/UploadCDSCOWeb/2018/UploadConsumer/nlem2022.pdf

Nguyen HTT, Dinh DX, Nguyen TD, Nguyen VM. Availability, prices and affordability of essential medicines: A cross-sectional survey in Hanam province, Vietnam. PLoS One. 2021 Nov 18;16(11):e0260142

Ofori-Asenso R, Agyeman AA. Irrational Use of Medicines-A Summary of Key Concepts. Pharmacy (Basel). 2016 Oct 28;4(4):35

Peacocke EF, Myhre SL, Foss HS, Gopinathan U. National adaptation and implementation of WHO Model List of Essential Medicines: A qualitative evidence synthesis. PLoS Med. 2022 Mar 11;19(3):e1003944

Perehudoff SK, Laing RO, Hogerzeil HV. Access to essential medicines in national constitutions. Bull World Health Organ. 2010 Nov 1;88(11):800

Promoting rational use of medicines saves lives and money, WHO experts say. Saudi Med J. 2004 Sep;25(9):1309–10

Quick JD, Hogerzeil HV, Velasquez G, Rago L. Twenty-five years of essential medicines. Bull World Health Organ. 2002;80(11):913–4

Quick JD. Essential medicines twenty-five years on: closing the access gap. Health Policy Plan. 2003 Mar;18(1):1–3

Rational use of medicines. Lancet. 2010 Jun 12;375(9731):2052

Sofat R, Cremers S, Ferner RE. Drug and therapeutics committees as guardians of safe and rational medicines use. Br J Clin Pharmacol. 2020 Jan;86(1):10–12

T Anjali, S Suvedha, S Karunavardhan, M Apoorva, S Saran Kumar and D Hepcy Kalarani. Rational use of medicines. Int. J. Pharmacognosy Pharm. Sci. 2021;3(2):39–43

THSTI | Promoting the Rational Use of Medicines [Internet]. 2015 [cited 2025 April 29] Available from: https://lms.thsti.in/wp-content/uploads/2024/04/Awareness-in-public-about-medicines-concerning.pdf

World Health Organization. How to Investigate Drug Use in Health Facilities. Selected Drug Use Indicators. Geneva: WHO; 1993

World Health Organization| Promoting rational use of medicines [Internet]. 2025 [cited 2025 April 29] Available from: https://www.who.int/activities/promoting-rational-use-of-medicines

World Health Organization| WHO Model List of Essential Medicines – 23rd list, 2023 [Internet]. 2023 [cited 2025 April 29] Available from: https://www.who.int/publications/i/item/WHO-MHP-HPS-EML-2023.02

Drug Information Centre

3

Santhosh Shivabasappa and Akila Srinivasan

Abstract

Drug information centre (DIC) is a facility that provides independent and unbiased information on drugs to healthcare professionals for the benefit of patients. DICs critically assess the relevant literature and provide timely response to drug-related queries. A well-functioning DIC has access to information database and tools. Being medically qualified, clinical pharmacologists are well-suited to provide recommendations to treating physicians in the management of adverse drug reactions (ADRs), detection of drug-drug interactions, and medication reconciliation in patients on polypharmacy. DICs contribute to rational drug use by providing accurate and independent information. DICs can also help in minimizing risk of ADRs and reducing healthcare costs incurred due to management of ADRs. Antimicrobial resistance is a global threat and DICs can play their part by guiding antibiotic selection and judicious use of designated antimicrobials.

Keywords

Drug information centre · DIC · rational drug use · clinical pharmacologist

S. Shivabasappa (✉)
Senior Clinical Research Scientist, Qure.ai, Bengaluru, Karnataka, India
e-mail: santhosh.srs@gmail.com

A. Srinivasan
Department of Pharmacology, Mahatma Gandhi Medical College and Research Institute (MGMCRI), Sri Balaji Vidyapeeth, Pondicherry, India

A. Arivazhahan et al. (eds.), *Introduction to Basics of Pharmacology and Toxicology*,
https://doi.org/10.1007/978-981-95-1920-0_3

3.1 Introduction

- Drug information centres (DICs) are defined as "institutions dedicated to provide objective, independent and current information on drugs and their use, and communicate to the different categories of users for better understanding and benefit of patients".
- The availability of accurate, unbiased information contributes to safe and effective pharmacotherapy while minimizing adverse drug events. The World Health Organization (WHO) has also emphasized the key role of DIC in promoting rational drug use.
- The lack of independent, unbiased drug information is a key contributing factor to irrational drug use in the community and health facilities. With growing research on drugs and their effects, the information continues to expand at a rapid pace. Though technological advancements (internet and smartphones) have enhanced the accessibility of drug information, accuracy is a concern. This necessitates independent and critical assessment of drug information to guide pharmacotherapy.

3.2 Brief History

- The first DIC was established at the University of Kentucky in the United States in 1962. Several DICs became operational in the Unted States and Europe from the 1960s to 1980s.
- Today, DICs are functioning throughout the world including in India and several developing countries. WHO has encouraged establishment of DICs across the world through technical support and funding.
- Independent medicine information services are recognized as a key component of the National Health Plan by the WHO for promoting rational drug use.

3.3 Staff Composition and Workflow of DIC

- A DIC usually provides services to healthcare providers (HCPs) including clinicians, nurses, and pharmacists. Some DICs could also provide information on drugs use to the general public.
- A DIC should have databases and trained professionals to provide the requisite information relevant to the queries raised.
- The staff composition varies widely across the countries. While in many of the European countries, DICs are led by a clinical pharmacologist and run jointly by physicians and pharmacists, in the United States, DICs are led by clinical pharmacists. Many DICs in India are run by a team consisting of senior pharmacologists, resident trainees, and nurses.
- A point to note is that the clinical pharmacist and the clinical pharmacologist bring complementary skill sets in running successful DICs. While clinical

pharmacists are more adept in handling drug-specific queries, clinical pharmacologists can address patient-specific and diagnostic problems.
- While the nature of queries could vary widely, they can be grouped into the following categories:
  - Therapeutic choice (in cases of drug allergy, resistance, multimorbidity, etc.)
  - Therapeutic approach in case of drugs with low safety margin or therapeutic window, and high interaction potential.
  - Dosage and duration of therapy.
  - Adverse drug reaction (ADR) evaluation.
  - ADR management.
  - Request for drug levels or interpretation based on drug levels.
- The timeframe of drug-related queries could also vary.
  - Some are of emergent nature, which need to be answered quickly over a telephone or advise provided within minutes.
  - Few are urgent, which need to be responded within an hour or two.
  - For a routine query, the opinion can be arrived at much later (e.g., hours).
- A typical workflow in a DIC is depicted in Fig. 3.1. The workflow would vary depending on the urgency of the drug-related query, as mentioned above.
- The relevant patient and disease factors should always be taken into consideration while addressing the drug-related query. Wherever possible, a printed response should be provided to the clinician with links to online resources and additional references as needed. Ideally, DIC should function as a two-way communication between the HCP and the DIC team. Any additional issues or concerns should be discussed in the wards during therapeutic rounds. The response has to be specific and any explicit action, if required, should be suggested.
- While DIC can provide suggestions, the ultimate responsibility to accept or modify the treatment regimens rests with the primary clinician in charge of the patient. When an advice is not implemented, feedback has to be obtained for identifying possible reasons for not accepting the advice. Additional clinical information on patient outcomes is crucial for strengthening future drug information services.
- The literature sources of a DIC could be categorized into.
  - **Primary:** These form the original basis on which all drug-related information is constructed (original publications on drugs such as clinical trials, case series, case reports, and related pharmacological research).
  - **Secondary:** In this type, there is synthesis of drug information based on primary sources (review Articles, meta-analyses, drug monographs, national formulary, standard treatment guidelines, therapeutic guidelines from professional societies, drug indices, etc.).
  - **Tertiary**: These are extracted summaries of information from other sources (textbooks, general reference books, drug bulletins, etc.).

In addition to the above, each DIC should have an internal database of queries and responses provided, which serves as a useful reference for future queries.

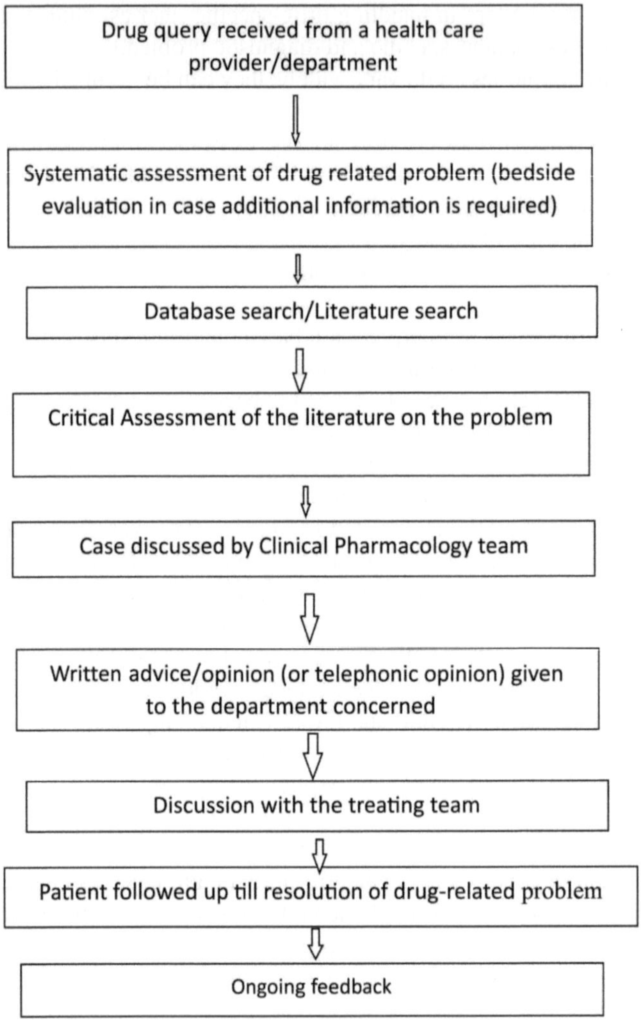

Fig. 3.1 A typical workflow of drug information centre (DIC) in a hospital

3.4 Dissemination to the General Public

- Some DICs provide drug information to the general public. The information has to be tailored to the needs of the population and should be easily understood by a non-scientific layperson.
- The information is usually generic and provided only as a guidance and not as a substitute for professional advice. Several DICs in India have been providing information on drug overdose and toxins to the general public. This could raise awareness amongst the general public on the rational use of medicines and the importance of reporting ADRs.

3.5 Role of Clinical Pharmacologists in DICs

- Clinical pharmacologists are medically qualified with training and experience in patient care, which makes them ideally suited to suggest patient-specific recommendations to the treating physician.
- Their therapeutic knowledge and skill can contribute in identifying ADRs, drug-drug interactions, and intervening in case of therapeutic failure.
- Their extensive knowledge on pharmacokinetics, pharmacodynamics, and pharmacogenetics could aid in dosage optimization and selection of alternative agents.
- Clinical pharmacologists are also actively involved in research.
- Their expertise in literature search and critical assessment of literature is of immense value in providing accurate drug information services.
- Clinical pharmacologists possess knowledge of standard treatment guidelines for various diseases and hence can make informed decisions for initiating, titrating or intensifying therapy.
- They can work together with the treating physician in the pharmacotherapy of patients with renal or hepatic dysfunction, pregnant women, lactating mothers, pediatric and geriatric populations.
- They can also evaluate patients on polypharmacy ($\geq$ 5 medications) and provide their expert advice to reduce treatment burden and costs.
- Clinical pharmacologists' advice is frequently sought in the management of adverse events and ADRs. They can proactively support in dosage optimization or therapy modification in addition to treatment of an adverse drug reaction.
- Clinical pharmacologists are actively involved in ADR monitoring activities. They can support reporting of ADR-related queries. They can also collect follow-up information on the individual patient to evaluate the response following therapy optimization.
- Clinical pharmacologists running therapeutic drug monitoring (TDM) services can integrate TDM interpretation into drug information services. A timely identification and management of toxic level of drug can prevent serious adverse events.

While many online tools exist for checking interactions, medically qualified pharmacologists will be better placed to distinguish between important and less important interactions. The tools prompt a high number of interactions and the clinical pharmacologist can interpret the interaction checklist in light of the particular patient.

3.6 Potential Impact of DIC

- DICs play a key role in promotion of rational drug use. The unbiased, accurate, and independent information empowers healthcare professionals and enhances quality of care. DICs can decrease the impact of marketing influence of the pharmaceutical industry by providing independent and unbiased information.

- Therapeutics forms a core component of patient care and very often, HCPs need to spend a great amount of time and effort to find the relevant information. DICs can assist clinicians in finding reliable information.
- DICs can reduce ADRs in the hospital and community at large. A well-functioning DIC can also reduce medication errors using regular feedback and working closely with prescription monitoring systems. These advantages translate to reduced healthcare costs incurred on the management of ADRs. DICs can also report and complement ADR monitoring activities in the institution.
- DICs can work closely with the Drugs and Therapeutics Committee (DTC) of the hospital or institution and provide key inputs at the time of formulary development and medication management.
- DICs have tremendous potential to conduct training activities aimed at specific drug-related problems. They can bring out newsletters aimed at junior doctors, interns, and postgraduate trainees to promote rational therapy.
- Some DICs have extended their role and participate in bedside therapeutic rounds and contribute to exchange of knowledge between DIC team and treating clinician. DICs have also developed additional expertise in optimizing drugs with low safety margin like phenytoin, cyclosporine, and tacrolimus.

3.7 Role of DICs in Fighting Antimicrobial Resistance

Antimicrobial resistance (AMR) is a global threat and is of great public health importance. One of the key components of fighting AMR is rational use of antimicrobial.

- While advising on antimicrobial choice and optimization, DIC takes into account possible causes, organisms involved, antibiotic susceptibility patterns, severity of the infection, need for source control, and therapy monitoring. These measures can reduce irrational use of antibiotics and reduce the emergence of resistant organisms. DICs can help formulate policies for use of designated drugs and treatment of multi-drug resistant organisms (MDRs).
- Several centres in India have highlighted how clinical pharmacologist-led DICs with adequate training in knowledge of essential medicines, therapeutic drug monitoring, and rational use of medicines can contribute to Antimicrobial Stewardship Programme.
- DICs can actively work with key stakeholders like clinical microbiologist, clinician, pharmacist, and nursing staff.

3.8 Illustrative Examples Are Depicted in Box 3.1

Box 3.1 Some Examples on Drug-Related Query and the Response Given with Comments

Drug-related query	Response	Comment
Drug allergy 22-year-old male with headache, joint pain presents with itching and rashes all over the body after taking naproxen. Advice with regard to the choice of analgesic?	In cases of hypersensitivity to NSAIDs, cross-reactivity rate to other NSAIDs may occur in up to 36% cases. Option of COX-2 inhibitors under close medical supervision Paracetamol for pain management in future Tramadol or opioids can be used as alternatives in exceptional circumstances	Drug allergy is not uncommon. Prior history of allergy to same or similar group of drugs needs to be evaluated DICs need to develop expertise to evaluate drug allergy and suggest alternate therapy options
Drug-drug interactions A 32-year-old male patient of TB meningitis on isoniazid, rifampicin, pyrazinamide, ethambutol (HRZE) with seizures develops worsening of motor symptoms (ataxia, diplopia) after being started on phenytoin for seizures	Phenytoin drug levels to be tested by therapeutic drug monitoring (level was noted to be 32 mcg/mL; normal range 10–20 mcg/mL) Phenytoin TDM must be done when the patient is on multiple medications including phenytoin Monitor serum albumin levels as hypoalbuminemia can affect phenytoin binding and increase free phenytoin levels Phenytoin to be replaced by alternate antiepileptics to avoid drug-drug interactions	Isoniazid inhibits phenytoin metabolism leading to phenytoin toxicity. In case there is also hypoalbuminemia, Sheiner-Tozer equation must be used to derive adjusted phenytoin concentration for hypoalbuminemia correction
Antimicrobial optimization 37-year-old male with polytrauma and multiple fractures has a prolonged ICU stay due to an infected implant. Wound discharge culture shows growth of *Klebsiella Pneumoniae* resistant to multiple antibiotics. What is the appropriate choice of antibiotic?	Patient condition should be assessed at bedside. General condition, immune status, comorbidities like diabetes mellitus, presence of fever, CRP and pro-calcitonin level, wound condition are to be noted Carbapenem and piperacillin-tazobactam can be used even in MDR settings if the minimal inhibitory concentration is found to be close to breakpoint levels and the patient is not immunocompromised, diabetic or toxic	Empirical antibiotic usage in patients with prolonged hospital stay can increase the risk of hospital-acquired infection Careful consideration to be given to the patient's immune condition and local susceptibility pattern

(continued)

Box 3.1 (continued)

Drug-related query	Response	Comment
Genomics-guided prescribing A 38-year-old female patient with cardiac valve replacement on anticoagulation with 5 mg warfarin per day (INR target 2–3) reported constantly increasing INR values (from 2.8 on day 2 to 4.2 on day 5 to 5.6 on day 8). Even after withholding warfarin for 3 days, INR remained high (4.5). Opinion on anticoagulant dose titration and suggestion of alternative anticoagulants was sought from DIC	Genotyping for VKORC1 and CYP2C9 polymorphisms could help in assessing if the patient was carrying CYP2C9*1*1 (wild genotype) or variant genotypes (*1*2 or *1*3). Those with variant genotypes often require lesser warfarin dose to attain target INR. Once-daily INR determination needs to be performed until INR becomes stable in therapeutic range. Once INR reaches therapeutic range, warfarin could be restarted at 1 mg/day if the patient carries variant genotypes in CYP2C9 or VKORC1	Warfarin sensitivity could be seen in some Asians where even routinely prescribed doses (5 mg/day) can cause disproportionate increase in INR

3.9 Research Potential of DIC

- The database maintained by DICs can provide tremendous opportunities to conduct research and training activities. DICs can collaborate with referring departments and identify focus areas that need further research.
- Postgraduate students, interns, junior staff, and nurses posted in DIC can learn key skills of critical appraisal of literature.
- The analysis of DIC queries can help devise educational content and interventions to different departments for promoting rational drug use.
- The DIC database can identify drivers of the use of antimicrobials, and a prospective audit and feedback can be instituted based on the needs of different specialities.
- Measurement of performance of DIC in terms of queries addressed, time taken to respond and any challenges faced can provide feedback for improving DIC services. DICs can also conduct studies on impact of their services on patient outcomes.
- There could be instances where a response provided by DIC is not implemented. Documenting possible reasons and patient course in such instances provides a useful learning resource.

3.10 Future Trends and Upcoming Research

- The need for reliable and unbiased information on drugs will increase as the drug research landscape evolves. With the ageing population, polypharmacy and complex pharmacotherapy, DICs have to adapt to manage the growing complexity of queries.
- Currently, there exist several online tools for checking drug-drug interactions, and many more are being developed. DICs have to constantly update themselves of new databases, tools, technologies, and critically evaluate them for their usefulness.
- The use of EMRs and electronic prescriptions is gaining momentum in countries like India. There is a push towards digitalization in care delivery. Going forward, digital reviews and advice will become more mainstream. DIC services could be integrated with EMR platforms for smooth referral process. This could throw some challenges for smaller centres with limited resources.
- Artificial intelligence and machine learning have been greatly discussed lately. The ability of AI models to provide reliable information on drugs will be an intense area of research. While large language models (LLMs) have shown some promise in answering general health-related queries from a patient, their capability to answer patient-related drug query is still unproven as several concerns exist with regard to their application in clinical practice.
- The data which have been used to train these models is mainly from a different population, and responses provided by the current models are frequently vague and non-specific. We also have to keep in mind the limitations of AI responses, and the need for verification by a professional prior to making decisions.
- The services provided by DICs have to be more patient-centric. With the advent of precision medicine, consideration of individual patient's comorbidity, biomarkers, pharmacogenomics and prediction models could become more mainstream.
- AMR is a global threat. All possible measures are to be explored to tackle this challenge. Going forward, DICs are perfectly placed to curb the irrational use of antibiotics and promote the rational use of agents.
- As demonstrated by a few studies from tertiary care centres in India, DIC could take up an active role in guiding antibiotic selection, avoiding redundant antibiotic cover and judicious use of designated antimicrobials.
- We live in the era of information overload and the information on drugs is expanding every day. COVID-19 demonstrated the critical role that DICs can play in these times. While the information was easily accessible, much of it was in the form of unverified information and from unreliable sources. DICs can step up in those circumstances to perform rigorous review and deliver accurate, unbiased information.
- DICs can support development of prescription monitoring systems and clinical decision support tools by providing constant feedback.
- The future will see collaboration between members with diverse skill sets like clinical pharmacologists, pharmacists, clinicians and nurses working in a

multidisciplinary DIC team. As more allied professionals gain prescribing rights, the queries to DIC can also see an uptrend from professionals with diverse backgrounds.

- Existing DICs can form a network to exchange best practices, share knowledge and learn from each other. The database from DICs can help in local practice guidelines.
- Integration of ADR services, pharmacokinetics, TDM, and DIC services could strengthen the quality of services offered. This would optimize the utilization of services while also enhancing quality of care provided.
- DICs educating the public will use more of social media tools. This could raise ethical and social concerns surrounding information dissemination. The regulation is still evolving about the optimal use of social media for drug-specific information.

3.11 Challenges and Limitations

- The efficient functioning of DIC requires institutional commitment through sufficient funding, allocation of human resources and critical infrastructure. DICs in many developing countries frequently face lack of support and manpower to provide optimal service. A round-the-clock service by DIC would need dedicated staff and resources to function.
- Access to recent updates, online databases, and information sources is a challenge in many resource-constrained settings. With the advent of open-access publishing, certain barriers have been lifted with regard to access. However, efforts are needed at the institutional and policy level to support and nurture independent DICs.
- Low awareness prevails among clinicians and other healthcare providers on the services provided by DICs. DICs should actively engage with all stakeholders to raise awareness.
- The clinical pharmacologist needs to understand the patient-level information, apply sound clinical skills and interpret the data. A hospital DIC at the core is a patient-level service. The ability to develop these skills might be limited in some centres in India.
- Many queries might be beyond the scope of clinical pharmacologists and pharmacists. For example, in case of suspected toxic effects of drug, a clinical toxicologist's expertise might be required.
- In the Indian context, many patients use alternative and complementary therapies, where the literature on efficacy and safety of these agents may be sparse.
- At present, many DICs provide responses and suggestions that are purely recommendations. The treating physician has the final say in accepting or rejecting the advice. A two-way communication needs to be established to understand the barriers to adopting these suggestions. Measurement of performance of hospital DIC requires feedback from the treating team. This is very important for successful implementation of any DIC today and in the future.

- Advice is contextualized and specific to health system and geographical region. A "one size fits all" approach does not help. DIC services have to be tailored to the local context.

3.12 Conclusion

- DIC is a facility established for providing authentic, unbiased, and organized information on specialized queries relating to the rational use of medications to other healthcare professionals or general public.
- DICs help in objective and timely dissemination of technical and scientific information on drugs.
- While pharmacists are well suited to deliver the descriptive query on a drug, clinical pharmacologists can provide patient-oriented response to a query.
- Future medical pharmacologists have to move away from the traditional concept of drug information services and contribute in ways that would add value to patient care and referring teams.

Bibliography

Ahmad R, Rehman S (2018) Antimicrobial stewardship: need of the hour. Int J Basic Clin Pharamacol 7:1444–1449

Ali AA, Yusoff SM, Joffry SM, Wahab MSA (2013) Drug information service awareness program and its impact on characteristics of inquiries at DIS unit in Malaysian public hospital. Arch Pharm Pract 4:9

Behera SK, Xavier AS, Gunaseelan V, Ravindra BK, Selvarajan S, Chandrase-karan A, Dkhar SA (2017) Drug information center as referral service in a south Indian tertiary care hospital. Int J Pharm Investig 7:182–187

Chauhan N, Moin S, Pandey A, Mittal A, Bajaj U (2013) Indian aspects of drug in-formation resources and impact of drug information Centre on community. J Adv Pharm Technol Res 4:84–93

Dager WE, Inciardi JF, Howe TL (1995) Estimating phenytoin concentrations by the Sheiner-Tozer method in adults with pronounced hypoalbuminemia. Ann Pharmacother 29(7–8):667–670

Geneva: World Health Organization 2004. "WHO medicines strategy: Countries at the core", 2004–2007

Heck J, Stichtenoth DO, Sabau R, Schröder C, Engeli S, Pape T et al (2022) Clinical-pharmacological drug information center of Hannover Medical School: experiences and analysis from a tertiary care university hospital. Sci Rep 12:19409

Kakkar AK, Shafiq N, Singh G, Ray P, Gautam V, Agarwal R et al (2020) Antimicrobial stewardship programs in resource constrained environments: understanding and addressing the need of the systems. Front Public Health 8:140

Krishna Kumar D, Shewade DG, Loriot MA, Beaune P, Balachander J, Sai Chandran BV, Adithan C (2014) Effect of CYP2C9, VKORC1, CYP4F2 and GGCX genetic variants on warfarin maintenance dose and explicating a new pharmacogenetic algorithm in south Indian population. Eur J Clin Pharmacol 70:47–56

Nova Manosalva MA, López Gutiérrez JJ, Cañas M (2016) Drug information centers: an overview to the concept. Rev Colomb Cienc Quím-Farma 45:243–255

Ontario H (2021) DPYD genotyping in patients who have planned cancer treatment with fluoropyrimidines: a health technology assessment. Ont Health Technol Assess Ser 21:1–86

Panditrao A, Shafiq N, Kumar-M P, Sekhon AK, Biswal M, Singh G et al (2021) Impact of an antimicrobial stewardship and monitoring of infection control bundle in a surgical intensive care unit of a tertiary-care hospital in India. J Glob Antimicrob Resist 24:260–265

Silas JH, Lennard MS, Tucker GT, Smith AJ, Malcolm SL, Marten TR (1978) The role of the clinical pharmacologist in district general hospitals. Br J Clin Pharmacol 5(1):3–5

Tett SE (2008) Clinical pharmacology: opportunities for educating new practitioners—an Australian perspective. Clin Pharmacol Ther 83:921–924

Varghese D, Ishida C, Patel P, Koya HH. Polypharmacy. StatPearls [Internet]. Accessed 24 Oct 2024. Last updated 2024 Feb 12

Evidence-Based Medicine

4

Gerard Marshall Raj

Abstract

Evidence-based medicine (EBM) is a science in itself which paves way for effective utilization of healthcare literature in medical practice. EBM is not only about overcoming subjective judgment, tradition, and authority in medical practice, but to impart other values such as patient preferences and choices along with best-available evidence. Hence, EBM can be considered as a "patient-centred" approach to clinical decision-making. Currently, EBM lies at the core of clinical practice. EBM tends to integrate "clinical epidemiology" and "biomedical research" – by imbibing and applying their concepts, "statistical analysis" and "scientific methodology", respectively. The real purpose of EBM was to harness the incremental increase in biomedical data and ever-expanding medical knowledge – with far few "real" breakthroughs – and make the "busy" clinicians to adopt and implement the "best" available evidence efficiently in day-to-day clinical practice. Initially, EBM was essentially focused on three major domains, namely, critical appraisal of available literature, development of systematic reviews, and clinical practice guidelines. All along these years, it is observed that EBM had contributed heavily to clinical medicine in the following ways, as quoted by Guyatt *(the scientist who had introduced the term "Evidence-Based Medicine", 35 years ago)* himself, shifting the practice of medicine on the base of scientific judgement, delineating the complex evidence hierarchies, prioritizing the patient values and preferences in clinical decision-making, and in the development of more robust methodologies for producing trustworthy guidelines and recommendations. In this chapter, the definitions, evolution, current status, progress, and future of EBM are deliberated extensively.

G. M. Raj (✉)
Department of Pharmacology, All India Institute of Medical Sciences (AIIMS) Bibinagar, Hyderabad, Telangana, India
e-mail: gerard.pharma@aiimsbibinagar.edu.in

A. Arivazhahan et al. (eds.), *Introduction to Basics of Pharmacology and Toxicology*,
https://doi.org/10.1007/978-981-95-1920-0_4

Keywords

Evidence-Based Medicine (EBM) · Evidence-Based Practice (EBP) · Critical appraisal · Evidence pyramid · GRADE (Grading of Recommendations, Assessment, Development, and Evaluation system) approach · Evidence-Based Clinical Practice (EBCP) · PICO · Shared-Decision-Making (SDM) · Cochrane collaboration

> The first two years of medical school have got to be changed. Students are spending more and more time understanding the difficult aspects of molecular biology, but we are kidding ourselves to think they use their knowledge of DNA – in my day it was the Krebs cycle – in making clinical decisions at the bedside. They do not. They make clinical decisions based on how the last patient did, how their friends are treating patients and what the latest article by an authority says they should do. And we have got repeated evidence now that authorities are way behind with regard to the data in clinical trials – Dr. Tom Chalmers (1993)

> Half of what you'll learn in medical school will be shown to be either dead wrong or out of date within five years of your graduation; the trouble is that nobody can tell you which half—so the most important thing to learn is how to learn on your own – Dr. David Sackett (2003)

> Evidence-Based Medicine was ranked 7th among the top 15 most important medical advances (innovations) in healthcare since the journal's inception in 1840 – BMJ (2007)

> Research that leads to neither new insights nor new applications is wasted. Research that is poorly done is wasted. Research that nobody reads is wasted. Research that has been done before is wasted – Sir Iain Chalmers (2009)

4.1 Introduction

Evidence-Based Medicine (EBM) is rightfully placed alongside the discovery of antibiotics and vaccines as one of the most significant medical advances in the past 150 years. It can be considered as a strategic alliance between medical science and clinical experience for a more modern and ideal application of clinical practice. The basis behind EBM is to guide clinical practice by systematic biomedical research. In literal parlance, EBM can be considered as "medicine practiced on the basis of evidence".

The term EBM is sometimes referred to as "evidence-based practice (EBP)", "evidence-based clinical practice (EBCP)", or "evidence-based healthcare (EBHC)".

4.1.1 Evidence-Based Medicine—*The Definitions*

Evidence-Based Medicine can be defined as "the conscientious, explicit, and judicious use of current best evidence from healthcare research in making decisions about the care of individual patients and populations". Here, "evidence" (scientific) is "the evidence that serves to either support or counter a scientific theorem or hypothesis" *[Encyclopedia of Public Health]*.

The above definition of EBM was put forth by Sackett et al in 1996. In this paper, Sackett et al state that practising EBM entails the integration of "individual clinical expertise" with the "best available external clinical evidence (from systematic research)"—what they refer to as the "bottom-up" approach. And both these tenets are not mutually exclusive—i.e., a good doctor needs to use both. Hence, Sackett wanted integration of systematic research with expert judgement.

As per the above definition, the practicing physician must keep himself abreast with the current relevant research and should continuously seek for the optimal course of care for the patients under his treatment. Hence, EBM can be considered to possess the following characteristics: "explicit search for the best evidence", "fair judgment for the benefit of the patient", "complementary participation of patient in the decision-making process", and "gradual practice-based fine-tuning of clinical experience"). By this way, EBM keeps the stakes of all participants of healthcare delivery at ideal levels—for the physicians, EBM reduces the chances of committing errors; for the patients, EBM provides opportunity to self-contribute in the process that deals with their own life; and for the payers, EBM instills a sense of certainty and surety. Hence, the practice of EBM demands the integration of individual clinical expertise with the best available external clinical evidence generated from systematic research along with the patients' values and preferences (Fig. 4.1).

And the BMJ Best Practice defines EBM as, "the application of the best available research to clinical care, which requires the integration of evidence with clinical expertise and patient values". The best available research refers to clinically relevant (i.e., patient oriented) research that: illuminates the accuracy and precision of diagnostic tests; highlights the importance of prognostic markers; establishes the efficacy and safety of therapeutic, rehabilitative, or preventive healthcare strategies; or seeks to understand the patient experience. Hence, it is the physician-patients' values, preferences, concerns, expectations, circumstances, and settings that dictate the administration of the best available care—hence, EBM is not so-rigid as it is construed and always looks for the "best-tailored fit" in therapy for the individual patient.

And sometimes, EBM is considered as a combination of three components, namely, "clinical state and circumstances", "patients' preferences and actions", and "research evidence"—in that order; and the integration of the "physician's clinical expertise" with all of the above three components—as the fourth element.

The basic elements of EBM include (i) framing (defining) a clinical question—the four components of which are the "PICO: patient (or population), intervention (or exposure), comparison (or control), outcomes"; (ii) finding (searching) the best available evidence—MEDLINE (accessed through PubMed), Embase, and CINAHL are some of the notable medical research databases comprising millions of references to journal articles; (iii) assessing the certainty (quality) of the evidence—which includes ascertaining both internal validity (bias or "systematic" error and chance or "random" error) and external validity (generalizability); and (iv)

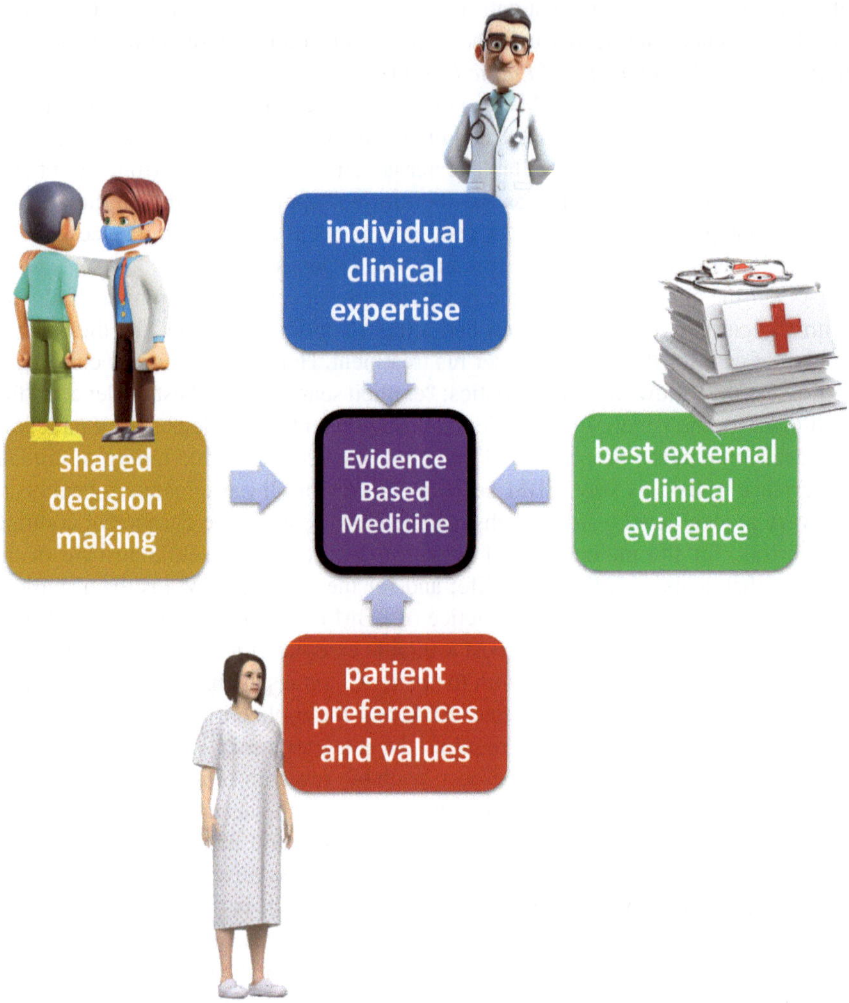

Fig. 4.1 Components of evidence-based medicine (EBM)

applying the evidence in practice, along with complementary clinical expertise and patient preferences—acting on the evidence to make a clinical decision. By following this framework in a sequential order, the EBM cycle comprises the following steps, namely, (i) "Asking" the question, (ii) "Acquiring" the evidence, (iii) "Appraising" the evidence, (iv) Incorporating "patient values and preferences", and (v) "Applying" to the patient. And this practice framework was put forth by Sackett himself in 1997. He also added that "the practice of EBM is a "process of life-long, self-directed learning" in which caring for our own patients creates the need for clinically important information about diagnosis, prognosis, therapy, and other clinical and healthcare issues". The above discussed "Sackett process" involves the following steps, namely, (1) structure a researchable question, (2) select the most likely resource, (3) design an effective search strategy, (4) summarize and critique the evidence, (5) apply the evidence to the patient of interest, and (6) evaluate the process and outcome.

UpToDate® (Wolters Kluwer), DynaMed® (EBSCO), ClinicalKey® (Elsevier), and Essential Evidence Plus (Wiley) are some of the notable point-of-care EBM tools which support in clinical decision-making for healthcare professionals.

The application of EBM in actual clinical practice requires a series of focused efforts and the "scientific study of methods to promote the systematic uptake of research findings and other evidence-based practices into routine practice, and, hence, to improve the quality and effectiveness of health services and care" is referred to as the "implementation research". Sometimes, also denoted as "implementation science"—which "aims to accelerate the adoption and integration of evidence-based practices, interventions, and policies into routine healthcare and public health practice to improve the impact on population health". Hence, through implementation science the gap between research and practice can be abridged.

Ultimately, by application of EBM, the healthcare delivery becomes better, safer, and cost-effective. And EBM can also be considered as "an evolutionary progression of knowledge based on the basic and clinical sciences and facilitated by the age of information technology".

4.2 Evidence-Based Medicine—*The History and Evolution*

The term Evidence-Based Medicine first appeared in an editorial (1991) by Dr. Gordon Guyatt. In that single-author paper, he describes that EBM requires skills of "literature retrieval", "critical appraisal", and "information synthesis". Hence, additional strategies like quickly tracking down publications of studies that are directly relevant to the clinical problem, critically appraising these studies, and applying the results of the best studies to the clinical problem at hand are the crucial steps in EBM. He also goes on to add that EBM requires judgement of the applicability of evidence to the patient on focus and follow systematic approaches to make decisions when direct evidence is not available.

And in "The Rational Clinical Examination" series in *JAMA* (1992), the Evidence-Based Medicine Working Group discoursed that the EBM as a new approach in teaching the practice of medicine. A paradigm shift from "purely" expertise-based, content (knowledge)-oriented, or clinical experience-based medical practice to more systematic assumptions (observations)-based, critical review of current medical literature, and application of rules of evidence before embarking on diagnostic/therapeutic options on a case-to-case basis was proclaimed. It is also stated that critical appraisal of literature is not merely an academic exercise rather it forms the crux for practical implementation of EBM. And further, critical appraisal would be the new way of doing medical practice by moving it to bedside.

Twenty years later, in an interview for *JAMA Network*, Dr. Guyatt fondly recollects the initial name coined for "evidence-based medicine" as "scientific medicine"—which then (early 1990s) created a huge uproar among the basic medical scientists and was not received well.

And Dave Sackett recollects how the term "critical appraisal" was requiring the much-needed rechristening to "evidence-based medicine"—as it involves science and literature integrated with best clinical skills to get the diagnosis right. So, EBM is a more broader term than critical appraisal—and it also involves evidence in the context of patient values and preferences.

And often, alignment with patient priorities with regard to clinical decision-making in care delivery has done wonders in improving healthcare outcomes. This process of "Shared-Decision-Making (SDM)" is now considered as a distinct entity in medical practice evolving from the roots of EBM. In SDM, the patient becomes the centre of clinical activity and this recent transformative collaboration of patients with doctors is referred to as the "patient revolution" in medical practice. The Mayo Clinic has even released freely accessible tools in the public domain for ready implementation of SDM; as actual implementation of SDM is generally considered as tough and challenging.

4.2.1 The Cochrane Collaboration and Archie Cochrane

Ian Chalmers was the forerunner for the establishment of the Cochrane Centre in Oxford (UK) in 1992 which was later transformed into The Cochrane Collaboration. Cochrane is an international independent network of researchers and healthcare professionals that perform systematic reviews of the evidence. These systematic reviews are high-quality literature reviews (unlike the narrative reviews) performed using systematic methods and are referred to as the "Cochrane Reviews". The Cochrane Reviews and the protocols for Cochrane Reviews ("Cochrane Protocols") can be retrieved through the *Cochrane Database of Systematic Reviews (CDSR)* which is a key component of the Cochrane Library. As on date, the CDSR includes more than 9000 Cochrane Reviews and stands as the leading database for systematic reviews in healthcare.

Cochrane recluses itself from commercial funding and is a not-for-profit organization with over 50 thousand collaborators (including patients, carers, and anyone interested in improving health outcomes) originating from more than 190 countries. And currently, the cochrane.org can be accessed in 20 different languages. The flourishing of The Cochrane Collaboration is a testimony for the perceived need to utilize EBM by healthcare professionals.

The stalwart epidemiologist Archie Cochrane was a fervent patron for conduct of randomized controlled trials (RCTs) despite the then accusations that were raised by medical ethicists against RCTs. He went on to reaffirm that good controlled clinical trials should replace other pseudoscientific studies undertaken by drug industry. Thanks to the positive influence from his mentor Sir Austin Bradford Hill (the great biostatistician) at the London School of Hygiene and Tropical Medicine—who had performed one of the first RCTs in medical history. He was also fully onto maintaining 100% response rate in epidemiological studies and even coined the self-eponymous term, namely, the "Cochrane units"—one Cochrane unit refers to a response rate of 91%, two Cochrane units refers to a response rate of 95%, and so on.

Cochrane's 50-year-old treatise titled *"Effectiveness and Efficiency: Random Reflections on Health Services* (1972)" discourses about "effectiveness" ("confirmed benefits of healthcare interventions – preferably by RCTs"), "efficiency" ("optimal delivery and utilization of available health resources for achieving positive outcomes"), and also about "equity/equality" ("assessment of the variation in healthcare delivery") in healthcare services. The book had a resounding reception and was later translated to eight languages. He also emphasized the need for systematic and scientific collation of all available RCTs ("critical summary"). He had assumptions on the concepts of cost-effectiveness and cost-benefit too (extension of the "effectiveness" component). And the setting up of The Cochrane Collaboration by Iain Chalmers and his colleagues in 1993 was a fitting tribute to the scientific envisions of Cochrane. And the Cochrane Collaboration was perceived on par to the Human Genome Project in its potential implications for modern medicine.

Medicine continues to be an undiscernible mixture of "science" and "art". EBM, in a way, helped in transcending the branch of Medicine away from its "uncertainty" and "probability" qualms—as Sir Willian Osler quoted medicine as a science of uncertainty and an art of probability.

However, there are some arguments speculating against the evolution of EBM like—EBM is not only about the RCTs as deciphered through the Cochrane's book and the confines of EBM should not be as narrow and restrictive as it is construed. Moreover, the reliance on the RCTs and the database of systematic reviews (including that of the Cochrane Collaboration) should not override the facets of clinical intuition and care dimension of clinical work including to bank on more humanistic doctor-patient relationship ["no RCTs, no real scientific evidence"—is false]. And RCTs should not only be considered as the universal gold standard of medical evidence but rather as means of detecting ineffective treatments; and consequently, redirecting the cost-saved to improve the healthcare system as a whole. It is emphasized that the "quality of care (living)" is equally important as that of the "quality of treatment" if not more. And also, the "recuperative power of the human body" should never be underestimated compared to the existing "therapies". This reverting back to "traditional" aspects of healthcare was even referred to as the "renaissance" movement of clinical practice—by the critics of EBM. The critics also go on to add that EBM is trying to "purify" medicine by letting out the "care" aspect of medicine and rather focusing more on the "scientific cure" part of medicine ("curative medicine").

In line with the motto of "critical appraisal" or rather forthright "criticisms" of scientific evidence and also doubled up with direct onslaught on some of the lacunae of the Cochrane Collaboration, the Collaboration itself came up with an innovative award, namely, the "Bill Silverman Prize". The award is given annually to the individual with the best critique "either through evaluating any aspect of the preparation, maintenance or dissemination of Cochrane Reviews or about the work of Cochrane more generally". Bill Silverman was a paediatrician who always asserted that, "criticism (including self-criticism) is a form of troublemaking that can help to drive progress"—hence, it is implied that, "all criticisms are helpful, and there are no such thing called 'negative' criticisms".

Like some philosophers who state that "evidence" in EBM (medical practice) should be viewed differently to that of the "evidence" in medical sciences—as the former is an exercise of identifying "something meaningful for someone" (e.g., in clinical decision-making) and the latter is an exercise of identifying "a sign of something" (e.g., in a scientific inquiry).

And even after two decades of its inception, there is wide variation in the implementation of EBM. Even now, it is sometimes emphasized that evidence that led to EBM should be considered only in the context of the patients—and not as a sole approach. This context is derived from the experience of practitioners—both individually and collectively. Hence, it is stated that EBM needs to complement experience-based medicine (ExBM) and can be more appropriately called as "Evidence-Informed Care".

Nevertheless, EBM is built on the base of conventional medical training and skills which includes a strong background of understanding of pathophysiological principles, meticulous history taking and physical examination, and also the need for compassionate attitude of the physician towards his/her patients.

4.3 Progress and Current Status of Evidence-Based Medicine

The proponents of EBM faced the brutal backlash from *The Lancet* anonymous editorial (1995) which scathingly stated, "…we deplore attempts to foist evidence-based medicine on the profession as a discipline in itself…". The editorial also rebuked the statement proclaimed by the EBM-group during the launch of the new *Evidence-Based Medicine* journal – "publish the gold that intellectually intense processes will mine from the ore of about 100 of the world's top journals". Of the many responses to this editorial, the notable ones are, how "one-way" consultant rounds would be transformed with "two-way" learning-cum-teaching at the bedside; compensate for the lack of time by busy clinicians in critically searching and appraising medical literature ("a general physician would need to examine 19 articles a day, 365 days a year, just to keep abreast of that specialty"); medical knowledge (evidence) should be based on scientific discourse and not on expertise—the former is "democratic and open to debate" and the latter would be "oligarchic and closed"; deficient scientific reasoning by the exponents of EBM—it is not about "choosing adjectives" or "prophesizing"; the advocates of EBM tend to be arrogant and denigrate the alternate views of others; "systematic observation" is not new to medical training, the same was existent since the times of Osler, Virchow, and Koch; in line with Godel's incompleteness theorem, EBM is "built on some shaky logical foundations: it will always be incomplete". Truth will not be contained in a recipe book; and unlike Archie Cochrane himself, "the Cochrane collaborators sit comfortably at their desk reviewing endless studies". All these views revealed the then prevailing ambiguity around EBM.

EBM was initially considered as a threat to "physician's autonomy" and was even adjudged as a new way of "dogmatic authoritarianism" originating from the Cochranian Oxford (like in parlance from the erstwhile Galenic Rome). But later, rather it disentangled the then plaguing "clinical freedom and democracy" for "evidence-based clinical practice"—as yearned by Cochrane himself.

And some scientists consider "evidence" as a weaker definition of actual "truth"—and as such evidence is only a reason or support for an opinion and not based on actual knowledge-derived "proof".

Further, EBM was assumed to concentrate only on the rationing of healthcare and equitable distribution of available facilities thereby aiding in cost-cuttings—so EBM had the negative monicker of "rationed medicine" rather than "rational medicine". One more argument is EBM is shifting focus "from the bedside to the medical libraries or computer terminals". And as it always said that "statistical significance" does not equate to "clinical significance"—similarly, EBM's initial "big" gains of the low hanging fruits have now been relegated to only "marginal" benefits in clinical practice.

Then, it was also a general impression that most of available literature (evidence) were for individuals with single isolated conditions and not for the complex comorbidities which are more prevalent. And the developed evidence-based guidelines are often mapped poorly to complex multimorbid states. Additionally, as much of the evidence is not disseminated through formal peer-reviewed publications, hence, we are forced to rely on biased irrelevant evidence for complex disease states.

Even in the introductory paras of the *JAMA* (1992) EBM paper, it was emphasized that neither mere intuition, unsystematic clinical experience, nor sole pathophysiological reasoning should be considered for clinical decision-making; rather, EBM entails the evaluation of evidence from existing clinical research. The same principle holds true even today and skillsets proclaimed then—like efficient literature searching and application of predefined rules in evidence assessment—are indispensable for any practicing clinician of today's era.

Initially, the EBM Working Group had asserted that only two set of populations (among healthcare providers) could take on application of EBM in clinical practice; one would be those who are overtly convinced about the positive outcomes of EBM on patient care and the other would be those who are quite sceptical about the intended benefits of EBM but even then, they still believe that EBM would not largely deteriorate patient health. The Working Group also concluded that the implementation of EBM would also aid in countering the exploding barrage of medical information, harnessing new technologies, controlling healthcare costings, and ultimately improving quality of medical care.

The "quality seal" embossed on the evidence-based medicine is sometimes misappropriated through vested interests—what is sometimes referred to as the "hijacking of EBM". Some arguments against the development of evidence-based practice are that most of the evidence is generated through trials funded by for-profit pharmaceutical companies. And the industry's selective publication of positive results over and above the negative results had been reported on multiple occasions ["publication bias" or "selective (non-) reporting bias"]. All these point towards a more of a "finance-based medicine" compromising the sanctity of EBM. Hence, the authenticity of such studies is always questioned and the necessity for more academia-funded studies are encouraged. In their pursuit to restrain the participation of the money-minting pharma and maintaining utmost ethical rigor for conduct of clinical trials, Sackett and Oxman satirically proposed (in the *BMJ*) for a company named the "HARLOT plc"—what they confess that would achieve positive results without lying in the fields of biomedical research—by merging the oldest and the second-oldest professions in the world. They wittingly state that through this company "we can protect your worthless product ("drug") as we shepherd it through the mine-fields sewn by objective scientists, fussy ethics committees, conscientious journal editors, writers of evidence-based guidelines, and licensing bodies".

The practice of EBM in the surgical fields is even more difficult compared to that in medical specialities. And the surgeons, in general, were all the more sceptical in the practical feasibility of application of EBM in surgical practice. Previously, lack of well-controlled trials in evaluating various surgical interventions and disinterest from funding bodies (particularly from the for-profit agencies) were considered as hurdles in generating hard evidence in the surgical specialties and hence, compromising on the "quality" of the evidence generated. In the start of the twenty-first century, only about 7% of the surgical interventions were found to be assessed in a randomized study design. The "IDEAL recommendations" was one such approach proposed to improve surgical evidence—which stand for Stage 1: **i**nnovation, Stage 2a: **d**evelopment, Stage 2b: **e**xploration, Stage 3: **a**ssessment, and Stage 4: **l**ong-term study. However, in the past two decades (i.e., 1999–2009 and 2009–19), the number of surgical interventions being evaluated through RCTs has greatly increased. Despite the increase in the quantity and quality, the ethical and logistic issues surrounding the conduct of these (surgical) RCTs still exist. And the inherent practice variability among the surgeons is another concern. Hence, the process and application of "evidence-based surgery" are far more intricate than the practice of EBM.

From the 1988 Commentary in JAMA (the year of passing of Cochrane) which envisaged the advent of "new Cochranes" in the field of medical practice (in the Americas)—echoing the need for well-tested and validated health services interventions, EBM as a whole has metamorphosed to such an extent that clinical practice without evidence is futile.

In the pre-EBM period, it is a usual assertion that the physicians practice only 10% of what they know. This sentence underlines the difficulty of putting EBM into actual practice. In the initial period of EBM establishment, there was an outcry that the contents in the drug label—particularly the so-called "contraindications" were given more weightage despite the inherent lack of strong evidence based on which they are brought out. Further, the practicing physicians were in a way coerced to strictly adhere to these label "contraindications" rather than on best-available evidence and/or patient preferences. All the more there is lack of publications of studies with the so-called "negative" results/conclusions—therefore the available evidence becomes biased. Hence, from the above discussion, it is pertinent that systematic reviewers are at the mercy of researchers of primary studies (RCTs and others). Therefore, it is the sole responsibility of the primary researchers to undertake trials with utmost care and make systematic reviews and meta-analyses more credible; otherwise, we may land up in the infamous "garbage-in, garbage-out (GIGO)" phenomenon.

"Drugs don't work in patients who don't take them", as opined by Everett Koop in the 1980s, was troubling the implementation of EBM. Nearly 30 to 50% of the patients do not take their prescribed medications and as such even with availability of hard evidence the delivery of appropriate healthcare is at abeyance. And what is even more disheartening is that clinical trials (including RCTs) are marred with compromised medication adherence—i.e., nearly 50% of trial participants do not comply with the dosing regimens specified in the study protocol. Consequently, the evidence generated is also at stake.

The process of making scientific peer review (of biomedical publications) more robust and credible and more so the registering of clinical trials prior to their commencement would make the evidence garnered more accountable. Peer reviewing system is the backbone of medical advances and registries would aid in reducing publication bias ("non-reporting of negative studies"). The "International Peer Review Congress"—which is held every 4 years and the "International Clinical Trials Registry Platform (ICTRP)"—which is maintained by the WHO, are testament for this affirmation.

Not all evidence that is being generated are equal and there are different levels of evidence. Fig. 4.2 illustrates the evidence hierarchy pyramid—wherein controlled biomedical research is placed at a higher level of evidence and compared to information generated from other sources. And some critics say that, in contrast to EBM, for achieving the goals of "precision medicine" the hierarchy of evidence pyramid must yield to a "more horizontal conception of medical knowledge". In precision medicine, the "individual treatment effect" *(patient-centred)* is considered to be more important compared to EBM which relies on the "average treatment effect" *(population-level)*. Whereas some state that "precision medicine" itself is a spinoff of EBM—and the final healthcare model should be rather a unified pluralistic approach with "evidence-based precision medicine". And a novel "medicine-based evidence (MBE)" approach was also proposed—wherein an archive of different patient profiles would be built up and a treating physician could match his current patient with those in the archive and contemplate managing on similar ways based on the accumulated evidence base.

Further, a "6S Hierarchy of Evidence-Based Resources" is suggested for searching and retrieving evidence for guiding clinical decision-making. The model recommends six layers of evidence sources, namely, ***Systems*** (Computerized Decision Support Systems), ***Summaries*** (Evidence-based clinical practice guidelines or textbooks), ***Synopses of Syntheses*** (Evidence-based abstraction journals, Database of Abstracts of Reviews of Effects [DARE]), ***Syntheses*** (Systematic reviews), ***Synopses of Studies*** (Evidence-based abstraction journals), and ***Studies*** (Original journal articles)—and hence, to proceed from the top to the bottom. The 6S approach can be considered under three broad categories, i.e., the "Systems" and the "Summaries" can be considered under "Summaries and Guidelines", the "Synopses of Syntheses",

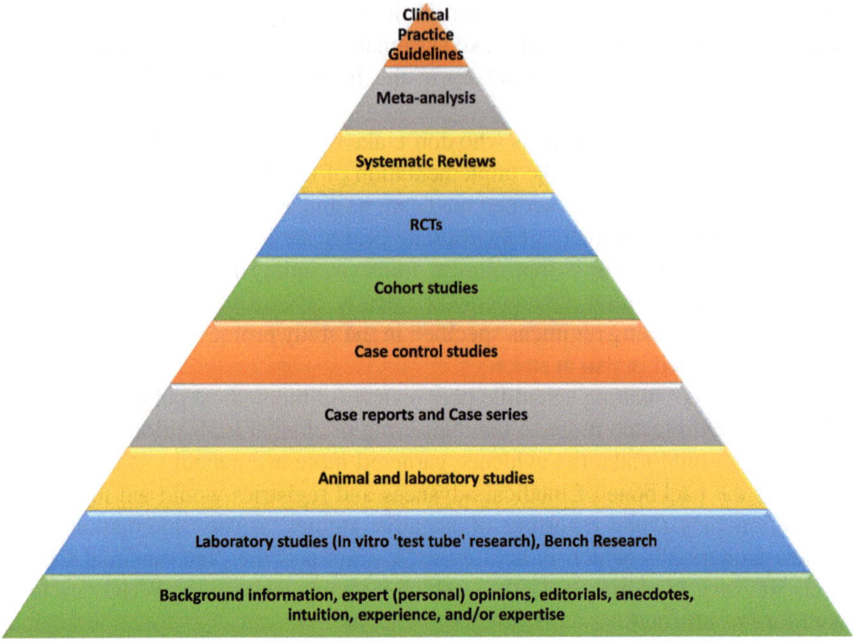

Fig. 4.2 The evidence hierarchy pyramid

"Syntheses", and "Synopses of Studies" can be considered under "Pre-Appraised Resources", and the "Studies" can be considered under "Non-Appraised Primary Studies". The TRIP (Turning Research into Practice) (www.tripdatabase.com), Epistemonikos (https://www.epistemonikos.org/en/), and ACCESSSS—Access to Evidence-based Summaries, Synopses, Syntheses, and Studies (https://www.accessss.org/) are some of the metasearch engines available for retrieving evidence from multiple levels of resources.

4.4 Future of Evidence-Based Medicine

The concept of EBM is easily one of greatest revolution in clinical practice of modern medicine and the *New York Times Magazine* hailed EBM as one of the most influential ideas of the year (2001). And for like any sudden shift in medical practice, EBM was initially fraught with scepticism among physicians, medical students, patients, and others. The acrimonious sobriquet "cookbook medicine" was tagged to EBM—where EBM was considered alike the recipe books and to be followed verbatim in spirit and letter ("slavish"). And even some referred to it as "ego-based medicine".

Previously, time constraints and ready access to latest medical literature were considered as some of the barriers to implementation of EBM in actual practice. However, with the advent of cutting-edge information technology systems these impediments have been cut short. And real-world studies have categorically proven that evidence-based practice improves patient outcomes and physician performance compared to the conventional standard practice.

In the Americas, the incorporation of evidence-guided medical decisions (EBM) was considered as the "fourth revolution" of healthcare following "introduction and expansion of health insurance", the "backlash of payers to reduce costs", and "outcomes-based research".

Like when Guyatt in his seminal editorial paper on EBM mentioned that clinicians need to look beyond the expertise of an expert lecturer or a local senior physician, or a textbook (compiled sometime back) to resolve patient management issues—hence, like the transition from "authoritative expertise-based medicine" to "evidence-based medicine", the onus lies with the clinicians to keep all the senses wide-open to imbibe further rational transformations of this discipline.

The spread of EBM and its applications to multiple disciplines of medical sciences showcases the broader impact of EBM. EBM, like discussed above, is a decisive tool to bring in social justice and health policy making.

The overconcentration of EBM on drugs and devices has left the other areas of healthcare in an "evidence vacuum"—and hence, more and equal evidence needs to be generated in the areas of health policy, health management, and health reforms.

EBM has progressed by leaps and bounds although it be with some expected hiccups; similar to how Cochrane had to struggle in executing his first "randomized" and "controlled" trial (1941) *[what he states as his first, worst, and most successful clinical trial]*, the successful accomplishment of the RCT on aspirin in secondary prevention of mortality in post-MI patients, and ultimately, culminating in the inception of the Cochrane Collaboration (1993).

As of now, though RCTs are considered as the "gold standard" of all clinical study designs in assessing therapeutic effectiveness, we could expect a change of views with inclusion of better type of trial methods—hopefully! And recently, it has been noted that, "on average, the effect estimates of RCTs and observational studies differ only very slightly". Hence, it is not only about the study design, i.e., RCTs vs other observational study designs (including retrospective and prospective cohort, case-control and cross-sectional studies).

As Gordon Guyatt envisages the need for highest level of easily accessed, easily understood, and preprocessed evidence is more than a basic requirement currently considering the burgeoning medical literature. More than 23 million articles published in over 5600 medical journals in the past 40 years; and around 25,000 to 30,000 randomized trials are being published every year in the last decade—what is referred to as the "bibliometric explosion". And a study in 2010, reported that 75 RCTs and 11 systematic reviews are being published every day. However, the good news is that a clinician needs to be aware of only 20 new articles per year to keep himself up to date in his area of expertise.

And Guyatt goes on to add that how succinct evident summaries (along with underlying patient preferences and values) of Standard Treatment Guidelines (STG) would come in handy for a busy primary care practitioner. The generated evidence is translated to applicable recommendations. The introduction of the "Grading of

Recommendations, Assessment, Development, and Evaluation (GRADE) system" is one such approach (a science for guidelines-making) for developing and presenting summaries of evidence ["quality or certainty of evidence"] and providing a systematic approach for making clinical practice recommendations ["strength of recommendations"]. This GRADE approach has been adopted by over 100 organizations—including the WHO and the NICE (National Institute for Health and Care Excellence, UK). And the Appraisal of Guidelines, Research and Evaluation (AGREE) Instrument is another such tool to assess the process of guideline development and reporting. Hence, a "trustworthy" clinical practice guideline should not only show the direction ("for" or "against") but also needs to quantify the strength ("strong" or "weak") of the provided recommendations.

Further, it should be noted that the generated evidence-based guidelines are not mere hard-fast directives and are not supposed to be overtly prescriptive—rather they should be considered as "guidance" document to a practicing physician. All guidelines and recommendations should only be considered in light of the relevant local factors that were involved by the guideline panel. So, while we need to "globalize the evidence", we need to "localize the recommendations". And the focus on EBM is getting rightfully shifted from more of a sphere of academic excellence yearning for the "ideal evidence" to implementation research, knowledge translation, and shared decision-making.

There are different critical appraisal tools for quality assessment of studies, such as the JADAD scale or the Revised Cochrane risk-of-bias (RoB 2) tool for "randomized trials" and the Newcastle-Ottawa Scale (NOS), Risk Of Bias In Non-randomized Studies - of Interventions (ROBINS-I), or the Methodological Index for Non-Randomized Studies (MINORS) for "non-randomized studies". And the AMSTAR 2 (A MeaSurement Tool to Assess systematic Reviews—2) critical appraisal tool can be used for "systematic reviews" that include randomized or non-randomized studies of healthcare interventions, or both. Additionally, critical appraisal checklists are being provided by the Critical Assessment Skills Programme (CASP) which was started (1980s) with prime objective of getting research into actual practice.

Currently, the "narrative reviews" are less relied upon and for obvious reasons the "systematic reviews" (and in some cases, "scoping reviews") have become more credible for evidence generation—what is sometimes referred to as the transformation from "eminence-based medicine" to "EBM". As the "narrative descriptive reviews" are generally written by the so-called subject experts and hence, are largely influenced by the expert's perception, experience, and also bias. In the beginning, to perform a systematic review it took nearly 2 years and now the same has been fast-tracked and the execution time is cut-short to almost by 75% (6 months) and sometimes, even to 2 weeks (by using automation tools); and the pioneers of EBM are quite confident that systematic reviews would be completed in a matter of 2 minutes in the near future. The Systematic Review Accelerator (SRA) is one such tool developed for the same purpose by Paul Glasziou and his team from the Bond University.

As expected, EBM is becoming more complex with the proposals such as the "next-generation 'deep' evidence-based medicine" which incorporates the various facets of advanced digital technologies (including machine learning and deep learning components), biomarkers, real-world data, and also out-of-the-box clinical trial designs. Study designs such as basket (or bucket) trial, umbrella trial, platform trial (e.g., the Recovery Platform Study), and master observational trial (MOT) [a combination of the master interventional trial and prospective observational trial] are being explored which could drastically cut short the time, efforts, and cost involved in development of novel drugs. And recently, the large language models (LLMs) such as ChatGPT have been found to accurately and consistently predict the RoB assessment of RCTs.

Table 4.1 enlists the contributions made towards EBM by some of the stalwarts of EBM.

4.5 Conclusion

Let us say no to "GOBSAT"— "Good Old Boys Sat Around the Table"—a process by which many guidelines were in fact developed previously—wherein a set of self-proclaimed subject experts discuss their often-subjective biased opinions and pontificating the same which may boil down as "consensus statements" or "expert opinions".

Ever since EBM was taking foothold, the transition of centre stage from treating physicians to care-receiving patients was highly perceptible. It is not only about how "clinicians" access, evaluate, and interpret the existent medical literature but also how this rigorous systematic exercise transforms "patient" lives. And it is a known fact that not all medical queries are always answered leading to implied uncertainty in clinical practice. In this context, EBM helps to maintain the much needed equipoise in patient care by providing extra cushion in acknowledging the dearth in current existing knowledge and how to tackle the same diligently. So, EBM not only considers high-quality evidence but also gives equal weightage for lack of robust evidence (low-quality evidence).

As it was discussed earlier, the healthcare of the twentieth century was more from the "doctors" (physician-centric) whereas from the start of the twenty-first century the attention has shifted towards the "patients" (patient-centric; *"no decision about me without me"*) and presently, the focus is on how to mutually consider each other's inputs so as to attain optimal therapeutic outcomes—"participatory medicine".

Like how Cochrane admonished against "God complex" as a terrible affliction of the then physicians—which is an absolutely overwhelming belief that their solutions to complex medical conditions are infallibly right, we need to move from this complex to a more "Human complex" (as the term indicates, humans are prone to errors and less autonomous) but rather with a "divine touch" (the thirst for an "ideal" state). Thanks to EBM—which rightfully embraces uncertainty with available evidence on par with good quality evidence—and hence, pushes for accruing more evidence!

Table 4.1 Pioneers of evidence-based medicine (EBM)

Name	Notable Affiliation(s)	Contributions and Accolades
Sir Austin Bradford Hill (1897, London, England –1991, Cumbria, London)	Reader, Epidemiology and Vital Statistics, London School of Hygiene and Tropical Medicine (LSHTM) Dean, LSHTM Chair and Director, Statistical Research Unit, Medical Research Council (MRC) Secretary and President, Royal Statistical Society	Hill's criteria for causation Hill AB. The environment and disease: association or causation? Proc R Soc Med 1965;58:295–300. https://doi.org/10.1177/003591576505800503 First scientist to prove a correlation between cigarette smoking and lung cancer (along with Richard Doll) Doll R, Hill AB. Smoking and carcinoma of the lung; preliminary report. Br Med J 1950;2:739–748. https://doi.org/10.1136/bmj.2.4682.739 Introduced randomization; pioneered the first modern RCT (use of streptomycin in treating tuberculosis) Hill AB. Principles of Medical Statistics. London: Lancet, 1937 Book: *Bradford Hill's Principles of Medical Statistics* *Honours:* Guy Medal in Gold (1953) Harben Gold Medal of the Institute of Public Health and Hygiene Commander of the Order of the British Empire (CBE)
Archibald (Archie) Cochrane (1909, Galashiels, Scotland—1988, Dorset, UK)	David Davies Professor of Tuberculosis and Chest Diseases, Welsh National School of Medicine (University of Wales College of medicine), Cardiff, Wales Director, Epidemiology Research Unit, UK Medical Research Council (MRC), Cardiff, Wales	Wrote a monograph titled, *"Effectiveness and Efficiency: Random Reflections on Health Services"* (1972) Father of Evidence-Based Medicine (EBM) Father of modern clinical epidemiology First President of the Faculty of Community Medicine (Pubic Health) of the Royal College of Physicians in the UK (1972–1975) Promulgated randomised clinical trials (RCTs) Broadly proposed the following themes, namely, epidemiological research, critical thinking and controlled clinical trials, health services assessment/ research, systematic reviews, and humanist care

Thomas C. Chalmers (1917, New York City, US—1995, New Hampshire, US)	Associate Director for Clinical Care and Director of the Clinical Center at the National Institutes of Health (NIH) in Bethesda, Maryland President, Mount Sinai Medical Center, New York Dean, Mount Sinai medical school, New York Harvard School of Public Health, Boston, MA MetaWorks	A pioneer of RCTs and systematic reviews (champion of RCTs) "The acknowledged leader in the design, conduct and evaluation of clinical trials" [as quoted by New York Academy of Medicine] *Notable publications:* Chalmers TC. Randomize the first patient! N Engl J Med 1977;296:107. https://doi.org/10.1056/NEJM197701132960214 Chalmers TC, Matta RJ, Smith H Jr., Kunzler AM. Evidence favoring the use of anticoagulants in the hospital phase of acute myocardial infarction. N Engl J Med 1977;297:1091–1096. https://doi.org/10.1056/NEJM197711172972004 [one of the first meta-analyses in clinical sciences textbooks are often seriously inconsistent with existing evidence, according to cumulative meta-analyses] Lau J, Antman EM, Jimenez-Silva J, Kupelnick B, Mosteller F, Chalmers TC. Cumulative meta-analysis of therapeutic trials for myocardial infarction. N Engl J Med 1992;327:248–254. https://doi.org/10.1056/NEJM199207233270406 Antman EM, Lau J, Kupelnick B, Mosteller F, Chalmers TC. A comparison of results of meta-analyses of randomized control trials and recommendations of clinical experts. Treatments for myocardial infarction. JAMA 1992;268:240–248 [a landmark paper that showed authoritative medical evidence for management of MI] Started the "Department of Geriatrics" in Mount Sinai Medical School in New York City [which was one of the first of its kind at an American medical school] Forerunner who sought for clinical trial registries ("better method of centrally recording the sporadic individual trials now going on") Proposer of the checklist for assessment of trial quality (even before the now established CONSORT checklist) [A proposal for structured reporting of randomized controlled trials. The Standards of Reporting Trials Group. JAMA 1994;272:1926–1931] "Thomas C. Chalmers prize student scholarship program" established by the Society for Clinical Trials (SCT) "Thomas C. Chalmers prize" awarded each year by the Cochrane collaboration for addressing methodological issues related to systematic reviews given to lead early career investigators (authors)

(continued)

Table 4.1 (continued)

Name	Notable Affiliation(s)	Contributions and Accolades
Alvan R. Feinstein (1925, Philadelphia, Pennsylvania, US—2001, Toronto, Ontario, Canada)	Medical Director at Irvington House Professor of Medicine and Epidemiology at Yale University School of Medicine Founding Director and Director (emeritus), Robert Wood Johnson Clinical Scholars Program at Yale	Father of modern clinical epidemiology Founder of clinical epidemiology Founder and editor of the *Journal of Clinical Epidemiology* Coined the words, 'comorbidity' [1970], 'trohoc' (cohort spelled backwards) [1973], and many others Bestowed with the following awards *Francis Gilman Blake award* as outstanding teacher to Yale medical students (1969) *Richard and Hinda Rosenthal Foundation Award* from the American College of Physicians (1982) *Robert J. Glaser Annual Award* from the Society for General Internal Medicine (1987) *J. Allyn Taylor International Prize* in Medicine (1987) *Gairdner Foundation (Canada) International Award* (1993) *"Sterling Professor of Medicine and Epidemiology"*, Yale University (1991) *"Distinguished teacher award"* by the American College of Physicians in 1998 *Oscar B. Hunter Award* from the American Society for Clinical Pharmacology and Therapeutics (1999) *Notable books:* "Clinical Judgment" (©1967): *Described the goals and methods of clinical reasoning* "Clinical Biostatistics" (©1977): *Presented the structure and contents of clinical research with groups* "Clinical Epidemiology: The architecture of clinical research" (©1985): *Described the strategies used to form clinical indexes and rating scales for important clinical phenomena such as pain, distress and disability* "Clinimetrics" (ISBN 978–0300038064) (©1987) "Multivariable analysis" (ISBN 978–0300062991) (©1996) "Principles of Medical Statistics" (ISBN 9781032477947) (©2002) Alvan R. Feinstein memorial award *(the award is to be given to an American physician who has made a major contribution to the science of patient care in activities that Dr. Feinstein has broadly defined as clinical epidemiology or clinimetrics, involving the direct study of patients' clinical conditions. This award is given every other year.)*

Name	Notable Affiliation(s)	Contributions and Accolades
David L. Sackett (1934, Chicago—2015, Canada)	Director, Trout Research and Education Centre at Irish Lake, Markdale, Ontario, Canada Founding Chair, Clinical Epidemiology and Biostatistics, McMaster University Chief Teaching Fellow, Harvard School of Public Health Physician-in-Chief, Medicine, Chedoke-McMaster Hospitals	Champion of EBM Father of EBM Organized a series of Health Care Evaluation Seminars at most of the Canadian Health Science Centres (1970s) Developed cost-utility analysis (1972) [along with Torrance GW, and Thomas WH] Initiated the journal titled, *"Evidence-Based Medicine"* (1995) [along with Davidoff F, Haynes B, and Smith R] [currently known as the *"BMJ evidence-based medicine (BMJ EBM)"*] Founding Director (1994) of the Centre for Evidence-Based Medicine (CEBM), Nuffield Department of Primary Care Health Sciences, University of Oxford First chair of the Cochrane Collaboration (foundation chair of the Cochrane Collaboration Steering Group) Inducted into the Canadian Medical Hall of Fame (2000) Appointed Officer of the Order of Canada (2001) Awarded Canada Gairdner Foundation Wightman Award (2009) *Notable publications:* Sackett DL. Bias in analytic research. J Chronic Dis 1979;32:51–63. https://doi.org/10.1016/0021-9681(79)90012-2 Sackett D. How to read clinical journals: I. Why to read them and how to start reading them critically. Can Med Assoc J 1981;124:555–558 Sackett DL. Rules of evidence and clinical recommendations on the use of antithrombotic agents. Chest 1986;89:2S–3S Laupacis A, Sackett DL, Roberts RS. An assessment of clinically useful measures of the consequences of treatment. N Engl J Med 1988;318:1728–1733. https://doi.org/10.1056/NEJM198806303182605 *[the concept "number needed to treat" was introduced]* Sackett DL, Rosenberg WM, Gray JA, Haynes RB, Richardson WS. Evidence based medicine: what it is and what it isn't. BMJ 1996;312:71–72. https://doi.org/10.1136/bmj.312.7023.71 Wrote a book titled, *"Clinical Epidemiology: A Basic Science for Clinical Medicine"* (1985) [along with Haynes RB and Tugwell P.] Book: *Evidence Based Medicine: How to Practice and Teach EBM* (1997) {"the bible of evidence-based medicine"}

(continued)

Table 4.1 (continued)

Name	Notable Affiliation(s)	Contributions and Accolades
Walter Spitzer (1937, Asuncion, Paraguay –2006)	Emeritus Professor of Epidemiology at McGill University Assistant and then as Associate Professor of Clinical Epidemiology and Biostatistics at McMaster University	Founding Co-Editor (along with Feinstein) and Editor Emeritus of the *Journal of Clinical Epidemiology* Founder of the Kellogg Centre for Advanced Studies in Primary Care, McGill University Introduced one of the first instruments for measuring the 'quality of life'. Established an Institute of Pharmacoepidemiology and Technology Assessment. Leader of the Canadian Task Force on the Periodic Health Examination which introduced grading of evidence to back up each recommendation and "Grade A" was only assigned if the recommendation was based on evidence from randomized trials. *Notable publications:* Spitzer WO, Sackett DL, Sibley JC, et al. The Burlington randomized trial of the nurse practitioner. N Engl J Med 1974;290:251–256. Spitzer WO, Feinstein AR, Sackett DL. What is a health care trial? JAMA 1975;233:161–163. Ibrahim MA, Spitzer WO. The case control study: the problem and the prospect. J Chronic Dis 1979;32:139–144. Spitzer WO, Kergin DJ, Yoshida MA, Russell WA, Hackett BC, Goldsmith CH. Nurse practitioners in primary care. 3. The southern Ontario randomized trial. Can Med Assoc J 1973;108:1005–1016
Sir Iain Chalmers (b. 1943, Liverpool, Lancashire, England)	Worked for United Nations in a Palestinian refugee camp (UN Relief and Works Agency) in the Gaza Strip (1969–1970) Coordinating editor, the James Lind library (https://www.jameslindlibrary.org/) and testing treatments interactive (https://en.testingtreatments.org/), Oxford, UK Articles editor, Centre for Evidence-Based Medicine, University of Oxford, UK British health services researcher	Performed the first systematic review (meta-analysis) of RCTs (1976) Created the National Perinatal Epidemiology Unit at Oxford University (1978) [funded by the World Health Organization and the UK Department of Health] Wrote the two-volume book titled, *"Effective Care in Pregnancy and Childbirth"* (1989) *(widely recognized as being the first evidence-based text book in any medical specialty)* Founding Director of the National Perinatal Epidemiology Unit (NPEU), Oxford (1978) First Director of the UK Cochrane Centre (1992) Co-founder of the Cochrane collaboration Sobriquets: "Maverick master of medical evidence", "systematic review man" Lifetime Achievement Award 2014 (BMJ) Knighted for services to healthcare [Knight Bachelor] (2000) C.-E. A. Winslow Award by Yale School of Public Health (2010) *Notable publications:* Chalmers I, Dickersin K, Chalmers TC. Getting to grips with Archie Cochrane's agenda. BMJ 1992;305:786–788. https://doi.org/10.1136/bmj.305.6857.786 Chalmers I. The Cochrane collaboration: preparing, maintaining, and disseminating systematic reviews of the effects of health care. Ann N Y Acad Sci 1993;703:156–165. https://doi.org/10.1111/j.1749-6632.1993.tb26345.x Schulz KF, Chalmers I, Hayes RJ, Altman DG. Empirical Evidence of Bias: Dimensions of Methodological Quality Associated With Estimates of Treatment Effects in Controlled Trials. *JAMA* 1995;273:408–412. https://doi.org/10.1001/jama.1995.03520290060030 Chalmers I, Bracken MB, Djulbegovic B, et al. How to increase value and reduce waste when research priorities are set.

Peter Tugwell (b. 1944, Egypt)	Senior Scientist, Methodological & Implementation Research, Ottawa Hospital Research Institute Director, Centre for Global Health, University of Ottawa Co-Director, WHO Collaborating Centre for Knowledge Translation and Health Technology Assessment in Health Equity, Bruyere Research Institute Professor, Medicine and Epidemiology & Community Medicine, University of Ottawa Chair, Management Group member, OMERACT® - Outcome Measures in Rheumatology	One of the founders of EBM and founding member of Cochrane Founding Director of the International Clinical Epidemiology Network (INCLEN) Training Centre at McMaster University Co-Editor-in-Chief, *Journal of Clinical Epidemiology* (2001–2022) Supported in the development of the Newcastle-Ottawa Scale (NOS) for assessing the quality of nonrandomised studies in meta-analyses Fellow of the Canadian Academy of Health Sciences Officer of the Order of Canada (2013) Canadian Institutes of Health Research (CIHR) Barer-Flood Prize (2020) *Notable publications*: Tugwell P, Boers M, Simon L, Strand V, Wells G, Shea B, Brooks P. Evidence-based rheumatology. London: BMJ books, 2005 Sackett,D. L. and Haynes,R. B. and Tugwell,P., 19,862,027,657, English, Book, USA, 9780316765954, Boston, Clinical epidemiology: a basic science for clinical medicine., (xiii +370 pp.), Little, Brown and Company, Clinical epidemiology: a basic science for clinical medicine., (1985)

(continued)

Table 4.1 (continued)

Name	Notable Affiliation(s)	Contributions and Accolades
Sir Muir Gray (b. 1944?)	Executive Director, Oxford Value and Stewardship Programme Director, the Optimal Ageing Programme Director, Research and Development for Anglia and Oxford Regional Health Authority Director, UK National Screening Committee Director, Clinical Knowledge, Process, and Safety for the National Health Service (NHS) Director, National Knowledge Service Chief Knowledge Officer, NHS Visiting Professor, Nuffield Department of Surgical Sciences, University of Oxford Chair, NHS Social Care Digital Service Contractor, Public Health England	Establishment of the Cochrane Collaboration Founding Director, Critical Appraisal Skills Programme (CASP) Founder, National Library for health Founder, Centre for Sustainable Healthcare Co-director, Department of Health's Quality Innovation Productivity and Prevention (QIPP) Right Care Programme, NHS Founder Director, Better Value Healthcare Founder, Oxford Centre for Triple Value Healthcare Knighted in 2005 for the development of the foetal, maternal and child screening programme and the creation of the National Library for health CBE (2000) *Notable publications:* Gray M, Jani A. Money isn't the most critical resource-we need to consider time and carbon. BMJ. 2022;379:o3002. https://doi.org/10.1136/bmj.o3002 Gray M, Jani A, Collins A. Reduce waste in the NHS to deliver population health. BMJ. 2024;385:q949. https://doi.org/10.1136/bmj.q949 Gray M, Meakins JL. Evidence-based surgical practice and patient-centered care: Inevitable. Surg Clin North Am. 2006;86:217–220. https://doi.org/10.1016/j.suc.2005.11.005 Book: Sod seventy!: The guide to living well, © 2017 Book: Sod sitting, get moving!: Getting active in your 60s, 70s and beyond Book: Sod sixty!: The guide to living well Book: Sod it! Eat well: Healthy eating in your 60s, 70s and beyond

Drummond Rennie (b. 1945?)	Former Contributing Deputy Editor, JAMA Adjunct Professor of Medicine, P.R. Lee Institute for Health Policy Studies, University of California, San Francisco Editor, NEJM	Founder and Director Emeritus, Peer Review Congress (directed seven congresses on peer review in biomedical publication) Editor, JAMAevidence Co-Director, San Francisco Cochrane Center Member, Commission on Research Integrity to the Public Health Service President, World Association of Medical Editors Award for Scientific Freedom and Responsibility [by the American Association for the Advancement of Science (AAAS) in 2008] *Notable publications:* Book titled, *"The Rational Clinical Examination: Evidence-Based Clinical Diagnosis"* published by the American Medical Association (2009) Rennie D. Guarding the guardians: a conference on editorial peer review. JAMA 1986;256:2391–2392. Rennie D, Yank V, Emanuel L. When authorship fails: a proposal to make contributors accountable. JAMA 1997;278: 579–85. Rennie D. The present state of medical journals. Lancet 1998;352 Suppl 2:SII18-SII22. https://doi.org/10.1016/s0140-6736(98)90295-1 Rennie D. CONSORT revised—improving the reporting of randomized trials. JAMA 2001;285: 2006–7. Rennie D. Integrity in scientific publishing. Health Serv Res 2010;45:885–896. https://doi.org/10.1111/j.1475-6773.2010.01088.x Rennie D. Let's make peer review scientific. Nature. 2016;535(7610):31–33. https://doi.org/10.1038/535031a

(continued)

Table 4.1 (continued)

Name	Notable Affiliation(s)	Contributions and Accolades
Brian Haynes (b. 1945?)	Professor of Clinical Epidemiology and Biostatistics and Professor of Medicine, Faculty of Health Sciences, McMaster University Chief of the Health Information Research Unit (HiRU), McMaster University Professor Emeritus, Department of Health Research Methods, Evidence, and Impact, Faculty of Health Sciences, McMaster University	Founding Editor of ACP Journal Club Former Director, CEBM Director of the Canadian Cochrane Centre One of the founders of EBM Officer of Order of Canada (OC) Rosenthal Award of the American College of Physicians *Notable publications:* Haynes RB. Where's the meat in clinical journals? ACP Journal Club 1993;119: A22-A23 Haynes RB, Cotoi C, Holland J, et al. Second-order peer review of the medical literature for clinical practitioners. JAMA 2006;295:1801–1808. https://doi.org/10.1001/jama.295.15.1801 Book: Clinical epidemiology: A basic science for clinical medicine Book: Evidence-based medicine: How to practice and teach—Fifth edition (2018)

Peter C. Gøtzsche (b. 1949, Næstved, Denmark)	Head, Nordic Cochrane Centre Professor, Clinical Research Review and Design, University of Copenhagen Visiting Professor, Institute of Health and Society, Newcastle University	Founder, Institute for Scientific Freedom (2019) Co-founder of the Cochrane collaboration *Notable publications:* Gøtzsche PC, Olsen O. Is screening for breast cancer with mammography justifiable?. Lancet 2000;355:129–134. https://doi.org/10.1016/S0140-6736(99)06065-1 Gotzsche PC. Why we need a broad perspective on meta-analysis. It may be crucially important for patients. BMJ 2000;321(7261):585–586. https://doi.org/10.1136/bmj.321.7261.585 Hróbjartsson A, Gøtzsche PC. Is the placebo powerless? Update of a systematic review with 52 new randomized trials comparing placebo with no treatment. J Intern Med 2004;256:91–100. https://doi.org/10.1111/j.1365-2796.2004.01355.x Hróbjartsson A, Gøtzsche PC. Placebo interventions for all clinical conditions. Cochrane database Syst rev. 2010;2010:CD003974. https://doi.org/10.1002/14651858.CD003974.pub3 Gøtzsche PC, Kassirer JP, Woolley KL, et al. What should be done to tackle ghostwriting in the medical literature?. PLoS Med 2009;6:e23. https://doi.org/10.1371/journal.pmed.1000023 Book: Deadly medicines and organised crime: How big pharma has corrupted healthcare, CRC Press, © 2013 *[Winner, British Medical Association Annual Book Award, Basics of Medicine, 2014]* Book: Vaccines: Truth, lies, and controversy (2020) Book: Mammography Screening: Truth, Lies, and Controversy (2012) *[Winner, Prescrire Prize 2012]* Book: Survival in an overmedicated world: Look up the evidence yourself (2019) Book: Death of a whistleblower and Cochrane's moral collapse (2019) Book: Deadly psychiatry and organized denial (2015) Book: Rational Diagnosis and Treatment: Evidence-Based Clinical Decision-Making (2007)

(continued)

Table 4.1 (continued)

Name	Notable Affiliation(s)	Contributions and Accolades
Kay Dickersin (b. 1951, Philadelphia, Pennsylvania, US)	Professor Emeritus, Epidemiology, Johns Hopkins Bloomberg School of Public Health Director, Center for Clinical Trials and Evidence Synthesis, Johns Hopkins Bloomberg School of Public Health Center for Drug Safety and Effectiveness Director, Cochrane eyes and vision review group, US satellite (CEVG@US)	Founder, National Breast Cancer Coalition (NBCC) (1991) Founder, International Clinical Trials Registry Platform (ICTRP) [WHO] Director, US Cochrane Center (USCC) Development of Cochrane's Central Register of Controlled Trials (CENTRAL) Founder, Consumers United for evidence-based healthcare (CUE) Awards and Honours Women's Hall of Fame, Baltimore City Commission for Women (1996) "Maryland's Top 100 Women," Daily Record (2006) MAMM magazine's "50 who made a difference." (1998) "Exceptional advocate," National Breast Cancer Coalition. (2000) "Contributions and enduring commitment to the eradication of cancer," American Association for Cancer Research. (2007) Ingram Olkin award, from the Society for Research Synthesis Methods for lifetime contributions to the field (2014) *Notable publications:* Dickersin K, Chan S, Chalmers TC, Sacks HS, Smith H Jr. Publication bias and clinical trials. Control Clin Trials 1987;8:343–353. https://doi.org/10.1016/0197-2456(87)90155-3 Dickersin K. The existence of publication bias and risk factors for its occurrence. JAMA. 1990;263(10):1385–1389. https://doi.org/10.1001/jama.1990.03440100097014 Dickersin K, Berlin JA. Meta-analysis: State-of-the-science. Epidemiol rev. 1992;14:154–176. https://doi.org/10.1093/oxfordjournals.epirev.a036084 Dickersin K, Rennie D. Registering Clinical Trials. JAMA 2003;290:516–523. https://doi.org/10.1001/jama.290.4.516 Little RJ, D'Agostino R, Cohen ML, et al. The prevention and treatment of missing data in clinical trials. N Engl J Med 2012;367:1355–1360. https://doi.org/10.1056/NEJMsr1203730 Vedula SS, Bero L, Scherer RW, Dickersin K. Outcome reporting in industry-sponsored trials of gabapentin for off-label use. N Engl J Med 2009;361:1963–71. Dickersin K. To reform U.S. health care, start with systematic reviews. Science 2010;329:516–7. Dickersin K, Straus SE, Bero LA. Evidence based medicine: increasing, not dictating, choice. BMJ 2007;334:s10. https://doi.org/10.1136/bmj.39062.639444.94

Gordon Guyatt (b. 1953, Hamilton, Ontario, Canada)	Distinguished Professor in the Departments of Medicine and Clinical Epidemiology and Biostatistics, McMaster University Professor, Health Research Methods, Evidence, and Impact, Faculty of Health Sciences, McMaster University Director of the Internal Medicine Residence Program Medical Reform Group, the Canadian health care system Member, Michael G. DeGroote Cochrane Canada Centre at McMaster, Faculty of Health Sciences Member, Centre for Medicinal Cannabis Research (CMCR), Faculty of Health Sciences	Coined the term "Evidence-based medicine" (1991) One of the most-cited living scientists in the world (Google scholar: 607058 citations, h-index = 304) Spearheaded the formation of the Evidence Based Medicine Working Group Played a key role in the development of the Grading of Recommendations Assessment, Development and Evaluation (GRADE) approach, now adopted by more than 90 organizations worldwide Awards and Honours 2024: Henry G. Friesen International Prize in Health Research 2022: Einstein Foundation Award for promoting quality in research 2022: Honorary Doctorate at the Faculty of Medicine of the University of Helsinki, Helsinki, Finland 2016: Inducted into the Canadian Medical Hall of Fame 2013: CIHR researcher of the year 2012: Fellow of the Royal Society of Canada 2012: The Queen Elizabeth II Diamond Jubilee Medal 2011: Officer of the Order of Canada 2011: Fellow of the Canadian Academy of Health Sciences 2009: Jack Hirsh Award for outstanding academic achievement 1996: McMaster University President's award for excellence in teaching *Notable publications:* Evidence-Based Medicine Working Group. Evidence-based medicine. A new approach to teaching the practice of medicine. JAMA 1992;268:2420–2425. https://doi.org/10.1001/jama.1992.03490170092032 Guyatt GH, Rennie D. Users' Guides to the Medical Literature. JAMA 1993;270:2096–2097. https://doi.org/10.1001/jama.1993.03510170086037 Guyatt GH, Sackett DL, Sinclair JC, Hayward R, Cook DJ, Cook RJ. Users' guides to the medical literature. IX. A method for grading health care recommendations. Evidence-Based Medicine Working Group. JAMA 1995;274:1800–1804. https://doi.org/10.1001/jama.274.22.1800 Grading quality of evidence and strength of recommendations. BMJ 2004; 328: 1490. https://doi.org/10.1136/bmj.328.7454.1490 Guyatt G H, Oxman A D, Vist G E, Kunz R, Falck-Ytter Y, Alonso-Coello P et al. GRADE: an emerging consensus on rating quality of evidence and strength of recommendations. BMJ 2008; 336: 924. https://doi.org/10.1136/bmj.39489.470347.AD Moher D, Liberati A, Tetzlaff J, Altman D G. Preferred reporting items for systematic reviews and meta-analyses: the PRISMA statement BMJ 2009; 339: b2535. https://doi.org/10.1136/bmj.b2535 Schulz KF, Altman DG, Moher D; CONSORT Group. CONSORT 2010 statement: updated guidelines for reporting parallel group randomised trials. BMJ 2010;340:c332. https://doi.org/10.1136/bmj.c332 Users' guides to the medical literature: A manual for evidence-based clinical practice, third ed., 2014, Gordon Guyatt, Drummond Rennie, Maureen O. Meade, Deborah J. Cook

(continued)

Table 4.1 (continued)

Name	Notable Affiliation(s)	Contributions and Accolades
Paul Glasziou (b. 1954)	Director, Centre for Evidence-Based Medicine, Oxford (2003–2010) Director and Professor, Evidence-Based Practice, Bond University Director, Institute for Evidence Based Healthcare, Bond University Director, Faculty of Health Sciences & Medicine, Bond University	Chair, Handbook of Non-Drug Interventions (HANDI) [RACGP - the Royal Australian College of General Practitioners] (online formulary of non-drug interventions in healthcare) Founder, Systematic Review Accelerator (SRA) project, Bond University Co-founder, International Collaboration for the Automation of Systematic Reviews (ICASR) Fellow of the Australian Academy of Health and Medical Sciences (2015) Officer of the Order of Australia (2021) *Notable publications:* Book: Systematic reviews in health care: A practical guide Book: Decision making in health care and medicine: Integrating evidence and values Book: An evidence-based medicine workbook Book: Clinical thinking: Evidence, communication and decision-making Book: Evidence-based medicine: How to practice and teach EBM Book: Evidence-based medical monitoring: Principles and practice Chalmers I, Glasziou P. Avoidable waste in the production and reporting of research evidence. Lancet 2009;374:86–89. https://doi.org/10.1016/S0140-6736(09)60329-9 Bastian H, Glasziou P, Chalmers I. Seventy-five trials and eleven systematic reviews a day: how will we ever keep up?. PLoS Med 2010;7:e1000326. https://doi.org/10.1371/journal.pmed.1000326 Lane R. Paul Glasziou: surfing the wave of evidence-based medicine. Lancet 2014;383:209. https://doi.org/10.1016/S0140-6736(13)62386-7 Hoffmann TC, Glasziou PP, Boutron I, et al. Better reporting of interventions: template for intervention description and replication (TIDieR) checklist and guide. BMJ 2014;348:g1687. https://doi.org/10.1136/bmj.g1687 Glasziou P, Chalmers I. Research waste is still a scandal—an essay by Paul Glasziou and Iain Chalmers BMJ 2018; 363:k4645

John P.A. Ioannidis (b. 1965, New York City)	Co-director, Meta-Research Innovation Center at Stanford (METRICS) Professor of medicine, Stanford prevention research center Professor, epidemiology and population health Director/ C.F. Rehnborg chair at Stanford prevention research center Chair, Department of Hygiene and Epidemiology, University of Ioannina Medical School (1999–2010) Adjunct professor positions at Harvard, tufts, and Imperial college	One of the most cited scientists in history. *The Atlantic* magazine (2010): "One of the most influential scientists alive." Referred to as "the conscience of science" A meta-research enthusiast (meta-research: "Research on research" or "the science of science") Highly cited researcher (Clarivate) in clinical medicine, social sciences and psychiatry/psychology. h-index = 268 (Google scholar), current citation rate: 6000 new citations per month (among the 6 scientists worldwide who are currently the most commonly cited). *["when contrasted against my vast ignorance, these values offer excellent proof that citation metrics can be horribly unreliable."—As stated by Ioannidis himself]* President, Association of American Physicians (2023–24) President, Society for Research Synthesis Methodology Editorial board, Journal of the American Medical Association (JAMA), Journal of the National Cancer Institute (JNCI), PLoS, and the Lancet. Editor-in-Chief, European Journal of Clinical Investigation (2010–2019) *Awards and honors:* European Award for Excellence in Clinical Science (2007) Chanchlani Global Health Award (2017) Epiphany Science Courage Award (2018) Einstein fellow (2018) Gordon award (2019) Albert Stuyvenberg Medal (2021) Harwood Prize (2022) Founders' medal for lifetime contributions to meta-science (2024). *Notable publications:* Ioannidis JP, Lau J. On meta-analyses of meta-analyses. Lancet 1996;348:756. https://doi.org/10.1016/S0140-6736(05)65647-4 Ioannidis JP. Why most published research findings are false. PLoS Med 2005;2:e124. https://doi.org/10.1371/journal.pmed.0020124 *[most-accessed article in the history of public library of science (>three million hits)]* Ioannidis JP. Contradicted and initially stronger effects in highly cited clinical research. JAMA 2005;294:218–228. https://doi.org/10.1001/jama.294.2.218 Ioannidis JP. Evidence-based medicine has been hijacked: a report to David Sackett. J Clin Epidemiol 2016;73:82–86. https://doi.org/10.1016/j.jclinepi.2016.02.012

(continued)

Table 4.1 (continued)

Name	Notable Affiliation(s)	Contributions and Accolades
		Goodman SN, Fanelli D, Ioannidis JP. What does research reproducibility mean? Sci Transl Med 2016;8:341 ps12. https://doi.org/10.1126/scitranslmed.aaf5027 Ioannidis JPA. Meta-research: Why research on research matters. PLoS Biol 2018;16:e2005468. https://doi.org/10.1371/journal.pbio.2005468 Literary Books (in Greek): "Toccata for the Girl with the Burnt Face" (Kedros 2012) and "Variations on the Art of the Fugue and a Desperate Ricercar" (Kedros 2014) Ioannidis JPA, Baas J, Klavans R, Boyack KW. A standardized citation metrics author database annotated for scientific field. PLoS Biol 2019;17:e3000384. https://doi.org/10.1371/journal.pbio.3000384 *[World's top 2% scientists]* Ioannidis JPA. The end of the COVID-19 pandemic. Eur J Clin Invest 2022;52:e13782. https://doi.org/10.1111/eci.13782 Ioannidis JPA, Pezzullo AM, Boccia S. The Rapid Growth of Mega-Journals: Threats and Opportunities. JAMA 2023;329:1253–1254. https://doi.org/10.1001/jama.2023.3212 Ioannidis JP. Transparency, bias, and reproducibility across science: a meta-research view. J Clin Invest 2024;134:e181923. https://doi.org/10.1172/JCI181923

Richard Smith (b. 1968, UK)	Former Editor-in-Chief, BMJ (1991–2004) Director, UnitedHealth Chronic Disease Initiative Board of Directors, Public Library of Science Honorary Professor, Imperial College London and the University of Warwick Chair, UK Health Alliance on Climate Change	Chief Executive, BMJ Publishing Group Chair, Cochrane Library Oversight Committee Member, UK Panel on Research Integrity Founding Fellow, Academy of Medical Sciences Chairman, the Point of Care Foundation Chair, Lancet Commission on the Value of Death Chairman of the Board of Directors, Patients Know Best *(a company that gives patients access to and control over all their health and social care data, including all records and test results)* Chair, icddr,b (International Centre for Diarrhoeal Disease, Bangladesh) *Notable publications*: Richard Smith: Dying of cancer is the best death (31 December 2014) BMJ Blog Richard Smith: Medical research—still a scandal (31 January 2014) BMJ Blog Richard Smith: How medicine is destroying itself (19 February 2018) BMJ Blog Richard Smith: Is cancer still the best way to die? (4 December 2020) BMJ Blog Davidoff F, Haynes B, Sackett D, Smith R. Evidence based medicine. BMJ 1995;310:1085–1086. https://doi.org/10.1136/bmj.310.6987.1085 Smith R. What clinical information do doctors need? BMJ 1996;313:1062–1068. https://doi.org/10.1136/bmj.313.7064.1062 Smith R. Medical journals are an extension of the marketing arm of pharmaceutical companies. PLoS Med 2005;2:e138. https://doi.org/10.1371/journal.pmed.0020138 Smith R. Peer review: a flawed process at the heart of science and journals. J R Soc Med 2006;99:178–182. https://doi.org/10.1177/014107680609900414 Smith R. The trouble with medical journals. J R Soc Med 2006;99:115–119. https://doi.org/10.1177/014107680609900311 Sallnow L, Smith R, Ahmedzai SH, et al. Report of the Lancet Commission on the Value of Death: bringing death back into life. Lancet 2022;399:837–884. https://doi.org/10.1016/S0140-6736(21)02314-X

(continued)

Table 4.1 (continued)

Name	Notable Affiliation(s)	Contributions and Accolades
Carl Heneghan (b. 1968, UK)	Professor of Evidence-Based Medicine and Director, Centre for Evidence-Based Medicine (CEBM), Oxford Co-Director, Global Centre for Healthcare and Urbanisation (GCHU), Kellogg college	Among the top 1% most cited scientists in his field Over 450 peer-reviewed publications (current h-index 99) and published over 110 systematic reviews Former Editor-in-Chief of BMJ Evidence-Based Medicine Founder of the "AllTrials campaign" (https://senseaboutscience.org/alltrials/) Writes regularly at Trust the Evidence (https://trusttheevidence.substack.com/)

Bibliography

Askheim C, Sandset T, Engebretsen E (2017) Who cares? The lost legacy of Archie Cochrane. Med Humanit 43(1):41–46. https://doi.org/10.1136/medhum-2016-011037

Atallah AN (1998) Why Archibald Cochrane used to call for effectiveness and efficiency? Sao Paulo Med J 116(1):1601. https://doi.org/10.1590/s1516-31801998000100001

Bagli D, Herbst KW, Harper L, Beckers G, Kaefer M, Kalfa N, Fossum M (2020) ESPU research committee. Further medical experience will be required to validate these results: how experience -based medicine shapes the validity of medical evidence. J Pediatr Urol 16(1):112–113. https://doi.org/10.1016/j.jpurol.2019.10.022. Epub 2019 Nov 14

Baum M (1999) Reflections on randomised controlled trials in surgery. Lancet 353(Suppl 1):SI6–SI8. https://doi.org/10.1016/s0140-6736(99)90220-9

Blackstone EH (2019) Precision medicine versus evidence-based medicine: individual treatment effect versus average treatment effect. Circulation 140(15):1236–1238. https://doi.org/10.1161/CIRCULATIONAHA.119.043014. Epub 2019 Oct 7

Bonfill X (2023) Revisiting the value of Archie Cochrane's contributions. BMJ Evid Based Med 28(2):73–74. https://doi.org/10.1136/bmjebm-2022-112142

Borah R, Brown AW, Capers PL, Kaiser KA (2017) Analysis of the time and workers needed to conduct systematic reviews of medical interventions using data from the PROSPERO registry. BMJ Open 7(2):e012545. Published 2017 Feb 27. https://doi.org/10.1136/bmjopen-2016-012545

Brignardello-Petersen R, Carrasco-Labra A, Guyatt GH (2022) How to interpret and use a clinical practice guideline or recommendation: users' guides to the medical literature. JAMA 2021;326(15):1516–1523. https://doi.org/10.1001/jama.2021.15319

Brower V (2003) The ethics of innovation. Should innovative surgery be exempt from clinical trials and regulations? EMBO Rep 4(4):338–340. https://doi.org/10.1038/sj.embor.embor815. PMID: 12671674; PMCID: PMC1319170

Bulger RJ (1988) Archie Cochrane revisited. JAMA 260(9):1284

Chalmers I (2008) Archie Cochrane (1909-1988). J R Soc Med 101(1):41–44. https://doi.org/10.1258/jrsm.2007.071004. PMCID: PMC2235918

Chalmers TC (1996) Dr. Tom Chalmers, 1917–1995: the trials of a randomizer. Interview by Malcolm Maclure. CMAJ 155(6):757–760

Chung KC, Ram AN (2009) Evidence-based medicine: the fourth revolution in American medicine? Plast Reconstr Surg 123(1):389–398. https://doi.org/10.1097/PRS.0b013e3181934742

Clark J, Glasziou P, Del Mar C, Bannach-Brown A, Stehlik P, Scott AM (2020) A full systematic review was completed in 2 weeks using automation tools: a case study. J Clin Epidemiol 121:81–90. https://doi.org/10.1016/j.jclinepi.2020.01.008

Cochrane | About us [Internet] (2024) [cited 2024 May 23]. Available from: https://www.cochrane.org/about-us

Cochrane AL, Blythe M (1989) One man's medicine: an autobiography of Professor Archie Cochrane. British Med Journal, London. ISBN: 0727902776, 9780727902771

Davidoff F, Haynes B, Sackett D, Smith R (1995) Evidence based medicine. BMJ 310(6987):1085–1086. https://doi.org/10.1136/bmj.310.6987.1085. PMID: 7742666; PMCID: PMC2549494

Dicenso A, Bayley L, Haynes RB (2009) Accessing pre-appraised evidence: fine-tuning the 5S model into a 6S model. Evid Based Nurs 12(4):99–101. https://doi.org/10.1136/ebn.12.4.99-b

Dickersin K, Rennie D (2012) The evolution of trial registries and their use to assess the clinical trial enterprise. JAMA 307(17):1861–1864. https://doi.org/10.1001/jama.2012.4230

Djulbegovic B, Guyatt GH (2017) Progress in evidence-based medicine: a quarter century on. Lancet 390(10092):415–423. https://doi.org/10.1016/S0140-6736(16)31592-6

Elwood P (2001) The first, worst, and most successful clinical trial of Archie Cochrane. J Epidemiol Community Health 55(6):369. https://doi.org/10.1136/jech.55.6.369a. PMCID: PMC1731910

Elwood PC, Cochrane AL, Burr ML et al (1974) A randomized controlled trial of acetyl salicylic acid in the secondary prevention of mortality from myocardial infarction. Br Med J 1(5905):436–440. https://doi.org/10.1136/bmj.1.5905.436

Emparanza JI, Cabello JB, Burls AJ (2015) Does evidence-based practice improve patient outcomes? An analysis of a natural experiment in a Spanish hospital. J Eval Clin Pract 21(6):1059–1065. https://doi.org/10.1111/jep.12460. Epub 2015 Oct 29

Evidence-Based Medicine Working Group (1992) Evidence-based medicine. A new approach to teaching the practice of medicine. JAMA 268(17):2420–2425. https://doi.org/10.1001/jama.1992.03490170092032

Evidence-based medicine, in its place (1995) Lancet 346(8978):785

Feinstein AR, Horwitz RI (1997) Problems in the "evidence" of "evidence-based medicine". Am J Med 103(6):529–535. https://doi.org/10.1016/s0002-9343(97)00244-1

Fossum M, Herbst K, Harper L, Castagnetti M, Beckers G, Bagli D, Kalfa N (2019) Kaefer M; ESPU research committee. Evidence-based medicine 1: background. J Pediatr Urol 15(1):78–79. https://doi.org/10.1016/j.jpurol.2018.11.007. Epub 2018 Nov 22

Gerris J (2011) The legacy of Archibald Cochrane: from authority based towards evidence based medicine. Facts Views Vis Obgyn 3(4):233–237. PMID: 24753871; PMCID: PMC3987463

Greenhalgh T, Howick J, Maskrey N, Evidence Based Medicine Renaissance Group (2014) Evidence based medicine: a movement in crisis? BMJ 348:g3725. Published 2014 Jun 13. https://doi.org/10.1136/bmj.g3725

Guyatt G, Oxman AD, Akl EA et al (2011) GRADE guidelines: 1. Introduction-GRADE evidence profiles and summary of findings tables. J Clin Epidemiol 64(4):383–394. https://doi.org/10.1016/j.jclinepi.2010.04.026

Guyatt GH, Oxman AD, Kunz R, et al (2008) Going from evidence to recommendations. BMJ 2008;336(7652):1049–1051. https://doi.org/10.1136/bmj.39493.646875.AE

Guyatt GH (1991) Evidence-based medicine [editorial]. American College of Physicians (ACP) J Club A-16. Annals Internal Med 114(suppl. 2) Available from: https://doi.org/10.7326/ACPJC-1991-114-2-A16

Haynes RB, Devereaux PJ, Guyatt GH (2002) Clinical expertise in the era of evidence-based medicine and patient choice. ACP J Club 136(2):A11–A14

Haynes RB (2002) What kind of evidence is it that evidence-based medicine advocates want health care providers and consumers to pay attention to? BMC Health Serv Res 2:3. https://doi.org/10.1186/1472-6963-2-3

Horwitz RI, Singer BH (2017) Why evidence-based medicine failed in patient care and medicine-based evidence will succeed. J Clin Epidemiol 84:14–17. https://doi.org/10.1016/j.jclinepi.2017.02.003

Ioannidis JP (2016) Evidence-based medicine has been hijacked: a report to David Sackett. J Clin Epidemiol 73:82–86. https://doi.org/10.1016/j.jclinepi.2016.02.012

Ioannidis JPA, Berkwits M, Flanagin A, Bloom T (2023) Peer review and scientific publication at a crossroads: call for research for the 10th international congress on peer review and scientific publication. JAMA 330(13):1232–1235. https://doi.org/10.1001/jama.2023.17607

JAMA Network | Evidence-based medicine: an oral history. Available from: https://ebm.jamanetwork.com/index.html

Lai H, Ge L, Sun M, Pan B, Huang J, Hou L, Yang Q, Liu J, Liu J, Ye Z, Xia D, Zhao W, Wang X, Liu M, Talukdar JR, Tian J, Yang K, Estill J (2024) Assessing the risk of bias in randomized clinical trials with large language models. JAMA Netw Open 7(5):e2412687. https://doi.org/10.1001/jamanetworkopen.2024.12687. PMID: 38776081; PMCID: PMC11112444

Lima JP, Tangamornsuksan W, Guyatt GH (2023) Trustworthy evidence-based versus untrustworthy guidelines: detecting the difference. Fam Med Commun Health 11(4):e002437. https://doi.org/10.1136/fmch-2023-002437

Martini C (2021) What "Evidence" in Evidence-Based Medicine? Topoi 40:299–305. https://doi.org/10.1007/s11245-020-09703-4

McCulloch P, Altman DG, Campbell WB et al (2009) No surgical innovation without evaluation: the IDEAL recommendations. Lancet 374(9695):1105–1112. https://doi.org/10.1016/S0140-6736(09)61116-8

Montori VM, Kunneman M, Brito JP (2017) Shared decision making and improving health care: the answer is not in. JAMA 318(7):617–618. https://doi.org/10.1001/jama.2017.10168

Montori VM, Leung TW, Devereaux PJ et al (2006) Can contraindications compromise evidence-based, patient-centered clinical practice? Can J Clin Pharmacol 13(1):e92–e101

Montori VM, Ruissen MM, Hargraves IG, Brito JP, Kunneman M (2023) Shared decision-making as a method of care. BMJ Evid Based Med. 28(4):213–217. https://doi.org/10.1136/bmjebm-2022-112068

Pronk AJM, Roelofs A, Flum DR, Bonjer HJ, Abu Hilal M, Dijkgraaf MGW, Besselink MG, Ahmed AU (2023) Two decades of surgical randomized controlled trials: worldwide trends in volume and methodological quality. Br J Surg 110(10):1300–1308. https://doi.org/10.1093/bjs/znad160. PMID: 37379487; PMCID: PMC10480038

Puljak L (2022) The difference between evidence-based medicine, evidence-based (clinical) practice, and evidence-based health care. J Clin Epidemiol 142:311–312. https://doi.org/10.1016/j.jclinepi.2021.11.015. Epub 2021 Nov 13

Rennie D, Chalmers I (2009) Assessing authority. JAMA 301(17):1819–1821. https://doi.org/10.1001/jama.2009.559

Sackett DL, Oxman AD, HARLOT plc (2003) HARLOT plc: an amalgamation of the world's two oldest professions. BMJ 327(7429):1442–1445. https://doi.org/10.1136/bmj.327.7429.1442. PMID: 14684640; PMCID: PMC300797

Sackett DL, Rosenberg WM, Gray JA, Haynes RB, Richardson WS (1996) Evidence based medicine: what it is and what it isn't. BMJ 312(7023):71–72. https://doi.org/10.1136/bmj.312.7023.71. PMID: 8555924; PMCID: PMC2349778

Sackett DL (1997) Evidence-based medicine. Semin Perinatol 21(1):3–5. https://doi.org/10.1016/s0146-0005(97)80013-4

Shah HM, Chung KC (2009) Archie Cochrane and his vision for evidence-based medicine. Plast Reconstr Surg 124(3):982–988. https://doi.org/10.1097/PRS.0b013e3181b03928. PMID: 19730323; PMCID: PMC2746659

Stavrou A, Challoumas D, Dimitrakakis G (2014) Archibald Cochrane (1909–1988): the father of evidence-based medicine. Interact Cardiovasc Thorac Surg 18(1):121–124. https://doi.org/10.1093/icvts/ivt451. Epub 2013 Oct 18. PMID: 24140816; PMCID: PMC3867052

Subbiah V (2023) The next generation of evidence-based medicine. Nat Med 29(1):49–58. https://doi.org/10.1038/s41591-022-02160-z. Epub 2023 Jan 16

Sur RL, Dahm P (2011) History of evidence-based medicine. Indian J Urol 27(4):487–489. https://doi.org/10.4103/0970-1591.91438

Toews I, Anglemyer A, Nyirenda JLZ, Alsaid D, Balduzzi S, Grummich K, Schwingshackl L, Bero L (2024) Healthcare outcomes assessedwith observational study designs compared with those assessed in randomized trials: a meta-epidemiological study. Cochrane Database Sys Rev 1:MR000034. https://doi.org/10.1002/14651858.MR000034.pub3

Vidaeff AC, Turrentine MA, Belfort MA (2022) Evidence based medicine - decades later. J Matern Fetal Neonatal Med 35(3):472–475. https://doi.org/10.1080/14767058.2020.1722997. Epub 2020 Feb 2

Vrijens B, Pironet A, Tousset E (2024) The importance of assessing drug exposure and medication adherence in evaluating investigational medications: ensuring validity and reliability of clinical trial results. Pharmaceut Med 38(1):9–18. https://doi.org/10.1007/s40290-023-00503-w

Wensing M (2015) Implementation science in healthcare: introduction and perspective. Z Evid Fortbild Qual Gesundhwes 109(2):97–102. https://doi.org/10.1016/j.zefq.2015.02.014

Willis JM, Edwards R, Anstrom KJ et al (2013) Decision support for evidence-based pharmacotherapy detects adherence problems but does not impact medication use. Stud Health Technol Inform 183:116–125

Worrall J (2007) Evidence in medicine and evidence-based medicine. Philos Compass 2:981–1022. https://doi.org/10.1111/j.1747-9991.2007.00106.x

McCulloch P, Altman DG, Campbell WB et al (2009) No surgical innovation without evaluation: the IDEAL recommendations. Lancet 374(9695):1105–1112. https://doi.org/10.1016/S0140-6736(09)61116-8

[illegible]

Medication Adherence

5

Porkodi Ayyar

Abstract

Taking the medicines as prescribed and continuing the prescription regimen as advised is defined as "medication adherence". Nonadherence is a significant hurdle to improve patient health outcomes and also has negative repercussions on the healthcare systems, clinicians and other stakeholders involved in healthcare. Estimating the magnitude of medication nonadherence is a crucial step to improve adherence. Though there are many measures, none of them can completely capture nonadherence in its entirety because of inherent drawbacks of each measure. While 'subjective' measures help to understand the barriers to adherence, 'objective' measures can provide a precise measure of patient's medication-taking behaviour. Hence, a multi-measure approach is currently recommended to provide a better measure of nonadherence.

Keywords

Medication adherence · Medication compliance · Medication nonadherence

"*Keep a watch…on the faults of the patients, which often make them lie about the taking of things prescribed. For through not taking disagreeable drinks, purgative or other, they sometimes die.*"

– Hippocrates, Decorum

P. Ayyar (✉)
Department of Pharmacology, SRM Medical College Hospital and Research Centre, SRM Institute of Science and Technology, Chennai, Tamilnadu, India
e-mail: porkodi.ayyar17@gmail.com

A. Arivazhahan et al. (eds.), *Introduction to Basics of Pharmacology and Toxicology*,
https://doi.org/10.1007/978-981-95-1920-0_5

5.1 Introduction

- The WHO defines adherence as “the extent to which the persons’ behaviour (including medication-taking) corresponds with agreed recommendations from a healthcare provider”.
- Nonadherence is defined as “deviation from the prescribed medication regimen sufficient to adversely influence the regimen’s intended effect”.
- Medication nonadherence is associated with adverse health outcomes and higher healthcare costs for the patients, and it also adversely impacts the healthcare systems, clinicians, and other stakeholders.
- Compliance, therapeutic alliance, and concordance are other terms used for medication adherence.
- Over compliance—Certain diseases have well-known serious consequences if left untreated such as untreated glaucoma resulting in vision loss. In situations of the patient being aware of such dire consequences, he/she may take the drugs in excess of the prescribed quantity out of fear.

5.2 Classification of Nonadherence

Nonadherence can be classified into

- Primary nonadherence—failure to take the prescribed new drugs at therapy initiation.
- Secondary nonadherence—failure to take the prescribed medications at refills.

5.3 Causes of Nonadherence

The causes of medication nonadherence are usually multifactorial, and their knowledge is essential to design interventions to improve adherence. The WHO has categorized the causes into five categories which include (Fig. 5.1).

- Patient-related factors: Adolescence, personality disorders, substance abuse and other high-risk behaviour, physical impairments such as vision defects, cognitive defects.
- Health system/healthcare team-related factors: poor healthcare provider–patient relationship, inadequate communication, poor healthcare access, poor aftercare/discharge planning.
- Disease condition-related factors: Psychiatric disorders (e.g., depression), long duration of illness, asymptomatic diseases.
- Therapy-related factors: Complex medication regimens, undesirable side effects.
- Socio-economic factors: Poor social support, low education level, higher medication costs.

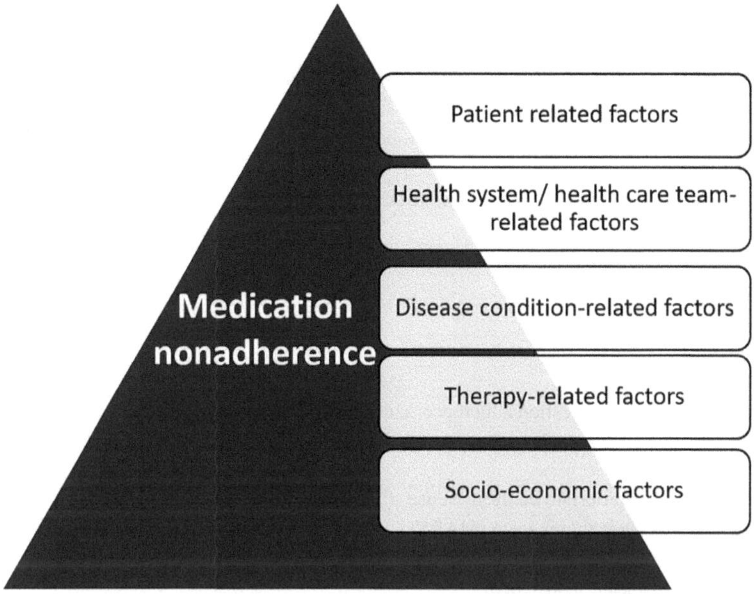

Fig. 5.1 Causes of medication nonadherence

5.4 Magnitude of the Problem of Medication Nonadherence

- Approximately 50% of patients are nonadherent to long-term medication regimens in developed countries and even higher in developing countries.
- Among kidney transplant recipients, nonadherence with immunosuppressive medications was 35.6 cases per 100 people per year which is quite high.
- Almost 50% of the patients prescribed with antihypertensive drugs ceased to take them within a year of initial prescription in one study.
- Nonadherence to statins for acute myocardial infarction in the year after hospitalization was associated with a 12–25% increased relative hazard for mortality.

5.5 Methods of Medication Adherence Assessment

Though there are numerous tools for measuring adherence, appropriate method(s) needs to be selected and tailored to individual situations and targets of the study/ setting.

The methods can be classified into either direct and indirect methods or subjective and objective methods (Table 5.1).

Table 5.1 List of methods of measuring medication adherence

Direct methods
Drug/metabolite concentration measurement in body fluids (e.g., blood or urine)
Biological marker measurement
Directly observed medication-taking behaviour
Indirect methods
Self-report and clinician assessment methods
Patient interviews by clinicians
Motivational interviews
Patient kept diaries
Questionnaires and scales
Brief medication questionnaire
Hill-Bone compliance scale
Eight-item Morisky medication adherence scale (MMAS-8)
Medication adherence questionnaire (MAQ)/ 4-item Morisky medication adherence scale (MMAS-4)
Self-efficacy for appropriate medication use scale (SEAMS)
Medication adherence report scale (MARS)
Pill count
Pharmacy data-based assessment
Medication possession ratio (MPR)
Dichotomous variable
Continuous, multiple interval measure of medication acquisition (CMA)
Continuous, multiple interval measure of medication gaps (CMG)
Continuous, single interval measure of medication acquisition (CSA)
Continuous, single interval measure of medication gaps (CSG)
Proportion of days covered (PDC)
Electronic medication packaging (EMP) devices
Medication events monitoring system (MEMS)

5.5.1 Direct Methods

Direct measures of estimating adherence include

1. Drug/metabolite concentration measurement in body fluids (e.g., blood or urine).
2. Biological marker measurement.
3. Directly observed medicationtaking behaviour.

Advantages
These methods are considered to be more robust and provide conclusive evidence that the patient has taken the prescribed medication.

Limitations
However, these methods have a number of limitations.

- Cost of analysis and technical difficulties of estimation
- Inter and intra-individual variations in drug metabolism
- Interactions with food and other drugs—unsuitable for multidrug regimens
- Anxiety and stress on patients
- White coat adherence—improved adherence around clinic visits
- Pill hiding under tongue and discarding them

The direct measures are better suited for hospitalized patients and singledose or intermittent drug regimens.

5.5.2 Indirect Methods

Indirect methods of estimating adherence include,

- Self-report and clinician assessment methods

  This assessment can be done using

- Patient interviews by clinicians
- Motivational interviews—combining estimation of adherence with intervention to improve adherence
- Patient kept diaries
- Questionnaires and scales—these validated subjective tools overcome the limitations of other self-report methods. Among the various questionnaires available, the most useful include
  - (i) Brief medication questionnaire—includes 5-item regime screen, 2-item belief screen, and 2-item recall screen.
  - (ii) Hill-Bone compliance scale—4-point Likert scale developed for anti-hypertensive medication only and includes 3 subscales of medicationtaking behaviour, appointment keeping ability and salt intake.
  - (iii) Eight-item Morisky medication adherence scale (MMAS-8)—consists of 7 dichotomous response items and a last item with 5-point Likert response with additional items assessing barriers to adherence. This scale has good validity and reliability across many chronic diseases and is the most accepted self-report measure of medication adherence.
  - (iv) Medication adherence questionnaire (MAQ)/4-item Morisky medication adherence scale (MMAS-4)—used only for assessing barriers to adherence and is the quickest to administer and score.
  - (v) Self-efficacy for appropriate medication use scale (SEAMS)—consists of 13 items ranked on 3-point Likert scale. Though validated in many chronic ailments, it is difficult to administer at the point of care due to its length.

(vi) Medication adherence report scale (MARS)—consists of 10 questions incorporating MAQ and drug attitude inventory (DAI) limited to patients with chronic psychiatric disorders.

Advantages

- Low cost and ease of administration
- Evaluate multi-drug regimens
- Assessment of barriers to adherence in addition to measuring adherence

Limitations

- Intentional or unintentional inaccurate patient reporting
- Poor patient literacy
- Bias due to negativity in questions

Pill count

- $$\left(\text{Number of dosage units dispensed} - \text{number of dosage units remained}\right) / \left(\text{prescribed number of dosage unit per day} \times \text{number of days between 2 visits}\right)$$

Advantages

- Low cost
- Simple to use

Limitations

- Pill dumping—Works on the assumption that removal of a pill is equivalent to taking the medication which may not be the case always.
- Cannot be used for medications with no discrete dosages and taken on Pro re nata (prn) ('as and when required') basis
- Adherence underestimation due to presence of surplus medication units
- Arbitrary cut-off value to differentiate adherence and nonadherence
- Does not address prescription-taking behaviour and barriers to adherence

Pharmacy data-based assessment

(i) Medication possession ratio (MPR)—(Proportion of days'' supply obtained)/(refill interval or fixed interval).

The fixed interval is used for medications used seasonally such as for asthma. Adherence overestimation occurs with this method.

(ii) Dichotomous variable—using certain criteria such as defined treatment gap, patients are categorized as compliant or not.

(iii) Continuous, Multiple Interval Measure of Medication Acquisition (CMA)—(Cumulative days'' supply obtained over a series of intervals)/(total days from the beginning to the end of the time period).

(iv) Continuous, Multiple Interval Measure of Medication Gaps (CMG)—(Cumulative days without any medication over a series of intervals)/(total days from the beginning to the end of the time period).

(v) Continuous, Single Interval Measure of Medication Acquisition (CSA)—(Days'' supply obtained in each interval)/(total days in the interval).

(vi) Continuous, Single Interval Measure of Medication Gaps (CSG)—(Number of days without any medication)/(total days in the interval).

It is suited for short-term drug use.

(vii) Proportion of days covered (PDC)—a measure of medication persistence.

Advantages

- Analysis of large population.
- Assess multiple drug medication adherence simultaneously.
- Identify patients at risk for therapy failure.

Limitations

- Can be used only in regions with centralized computer system and proper collection of complete datasets.
- Pill dumping
- Barriers to adherence cannot be completely captured.

Electronic medication packaging (EMP) devices

These devices are included in the package insert to monitor adherence of a prescription medication. These devices share few common features though not all will be present in all devices. EMP may incorporate facilities to record prescriptiontaking events, adherence performance history, drug dose reminders, digital displays and real-time monitoring.

(i). Medication Events Monitoring System (MEMS)—most used device in adherence studies. A microprocessor embedded in the container would record the time and date whenever a medication is removed. Adherence is based on the assumption that the patient takes the dose.

- Using the medication event-monitoring system to monitor monthly azathioprine adherence during a 6-month period in kidney transplant recipients demonstrated a significant correlation with adherence and rejection-free survival in the first 6 months after transplantation

Advantages

- Able to identify prescriptiontaking behaviour
- Identify whether nonadherence is sporadic or consistent and also to identify partial adherence
- Chances of patient misleading less compared to other methods

Limitations

- Accidental actuation of the container results in adherence overestimation
- Patient stress and anxiety due to surveillance
- Container difficulties—weight, high cost, incorrect usage of the cap and possibility of equipment loss

(ii). 99DOTS—mobile phone-based digital health technology for real-time remote monitoring of antituberculosis drug intake. The drug blister pack contains fixed dose combination of antituberculosis drugs with concealed phone numbers which are revealed only when the drug blister pack is opened. The patients need to make a call to the number after consuming the medication.

5.5.3 Selection of Appropriate Medication Adherence Measure

An ideal method should have the following characteristics:

- Low cost
- Reliable
- Valid
- Easy to administer
- Flexible

But none of the currently available methods have all these standards due to their inherent drawbacks.

- Direct measures are not preferred owing to their high cost and intrusiveness.
- Among the indirect methods, self-report questionnaire and patient interview are preferred in clinical settings followed by pill count method. For larger population, pharmacy refill data are the preferred measure.
- In research settings, when close to reality adherence measurement is needed, multimeasure approach balancing the advantages and limitations of one method by another is recommended. For example, in the study by Liu et al. on HIV protease inhibitors, combined use of medication event monitoring system, pill count and clinician's interview had higher predictive power to measure medication adherence compared to the separate use of each measure.
- When identification of barriers to adherence is also necessary in addition to measuring adherence, combination of a subjective and an objective measure is required.
- Cost, practicality, and complexity of analysis are potential limitations of multimeasure approach.

5.6 Consequences of Inaccurate Adherence Estimation

Faulty adherence estimation can potentially lead to adverse consequences including, but not limited to,

- Misinterpretation of drug effectiveness
- Unwarranted, potentially costly, and invasive investigations being done
- Unnecessary escalation of therapy which may be potentially dangerous
- Misleading results of clinical trials
- Wrong calculation of dose-response relationship and drug efficacy

5.7 Interventions to Improve Medication Adherence

A concise summary of interventions includes,

- Education and medical interventions
  - Patients need to be educated about their drugs name, dosage, and rationale for prescription; these points need to be emphasized during each clinic visit.
  - Patients should be made aware about the undesirable effects of their drugs.
  - Written instructions need to be provided whenever there is a change in drug frequency or dosage.
  - Patient-friendly package.
  - Number and frequency of medications to be reduced.
  - Fixed dose combinations to be used wherever possible to reduce pill burden.

  - Inexpensive drugs to be prescribed if available.
  - Overprescribing/prescribing unnecessary drugs to be avoided.
  - Adherence issues to be probed and any patient-specific issues identified need to be addressed.
  - Adherence needs to be monitored with feasible tools such as patient interview, investigations, and analysing prescription refills.
- Behavioural and psychosocial interventions
  - Patients' active participation in treatment plan needs to be ensured.
  - Patients should be made to exhibit their knowledge on medication adherence. They should also be made to demonstrate their adherence performance history on clinic visits.
  - Patient-healthcare provider communication to be strengthened.
  - Social support system needs to be identified and active involvement of the family and friends should be ensured.
  - Any underlying psychiatric disorders to be treated.
  - Discussion of adherence issues needs to be unbiased.
  - Insurance issues or workplace difficulties to be taken care of.
  - Interventions for nonadherence should be tailored to its root cause.
  - Prescriptiontaking behaviour to be made part of the daily routine.
  - Digital alarms, alerts or refill reminders can be used to assist in taking prescribed medication.
  - Continuing education, discussion, and counselling services to be provided.

Since nonadherence is multifactorial, interventions to improve adherence need to be multimodal to be successful.

5.8 Barriers to Implement Interventions

- Implementation of multimodal interventions in routine practice is difficult owing to their heterogeneity.
- Requirement of additional clinical personnel to implement interventions.
- Logistical problems may arise among various patient-care providers at different levels due to coordination issues with regard to smooth implementation of interventions.
- Lack of financial incentives to enhance medication adherence

5.9 Healthy Adherer Effect

- The observed association of good health outcomes with medication adherence might be a proxy attribute of overall healthcare-related behaviour.
- Evidence exists both for and against this phenomenon.

- In cardiovascular drug trials, drug adherent patients had better outcomes even in the placebo arm due to their healthy lifestyle behaviours with regard to diet and exercise.
- However, in the study by Rasmussen et al., better cardiovascular medications adherence was not associated with hospitalization for lung, prostate, or breast cancer

5.10 Conclusion

- Medication nonadherence is a serious underestimated threat to patient and healthcare systems and there is a clarion call to improve adherence from the clinicians and researchers.
- Measuring the quantum of problem is the first step and the measures available at present can individually measure only a few facets of this multifaceted problem and so multimeasure approach is currently recommended.
- Direct measures are seldom used due to cost limitation and intrusiveness.
- Among indirect measures, a combination of subjective methods to understand the patients' medication-taking behaviour and their barriers, and objective methods to precisely measure medication consumption are recommended to gauge the magnitude of nonadherence
- Further research is needed to improve currently available measures of adherence and/or to discover better new measures. Interventions tailored to tackle the problem more precisely are to be implemented to improve health outcomes.

Bibliography

World Health Organization (2003) In: Sabaté E (ed) Adherence to long-term therapies: evidence for action. World Health Organization. https://apps.who.int/iris/handle/10665/42682

Osterberg L, Blaschke T (2005) Adherence to medication. N Engl J Med 353(5):487–497

Fischer MA, Stedman MR, Lii J, Vogeli C, Shrank WH, Brookhart MA et al (2010) Primary medication non-adherence: analysis of 195,930 electronic prescriptions. J Gen Intern Med 25(4):284–290

Lavsa SM, Holzworth A, Ansani NT (2011) Selection of a validated scale for measuring medication adherence. J Am Pharm Assoc 51(1):90–94

Svarstad BL, Chewning BA, Sleath BL, Claesson C (1999) The brief medication questionnaire: a tool for screening patient adherence and barriers to adherence. Patient Educ Couns 37(2):113–124

Vrijens B, Vincze G, Kristanto P, Urquhart J, Burnier M (2008) Adherence to prescribed antihypertensive drug treatments: longitudinal study of electronically compiled dosing histories. BMJ 336(7653):1114–1117

Rasmussen JN, Chong A, Alter DA (2007) Relationship between adherence to evidence-based pharmacotherapy and long-term mortality after acute myocardial infarction. JAMA 297(2):177–186

Farmer KC (1999) Methods for measuring and monitoring medication regimen adherence in clinical trials and clinical practice. Clin Ther 21(6):1074–1090

Ho PM, Bryson CL, Rumsfeld JS (2009) Medication adherence: its importance in cardiovascular outcomes. Circulation 119(23):3028–3035

Jimmy B, Jose J (2011) Patient medication adherence: measures in daily practice. Oman Med J 26(3):155–159

Vermeire E, Hearnshaw H, Van Royen P, Denekens J (2001) Patient adherence to treatment: three decades of research. A comprehensive review. J Clin Pharm Ther 26(5):331–342

Tan XI, Patel I, Chang J (2014) Review of the four item Morisky medication adherence scale (MMAS-4) and eight item Morisky medication adherence scale (MMAS-8). Innov Pharm 5(3):5

Culig J, Leppée M (2014) From Morisky to hill-bone; self-reports scales for measuring adherence to medication. Coll Antropol 38(1):55–62

Thompson K, Kulkarni J, Sergejew AA (2000) Reliability and validity of a new medication adherence rating scale (MARS) for the psychoses. Schizophr Res 42(3):241–247

Nguyen TM, La Caze A, Cottrell N (2014) What are validated self-report adherence scales really measuring?: a systematic review. Br J Clin Pharmacol 77(3):427–445

Caetano PA, Lam JM, Morgan SG (2006) Toward a standard definition and measurement of persistence with drug therapy: examples from research on statin and antihypertensive utilization. Clin Ther 28(9):1411–1424

Kitahata MM, Reed SD, Dillingham PW, Van Rompaey SE, Young AA, Harrington RD et al (2004) Pharmacy-based assessment of adherence to HAART predicts virologic and immunologic treatment response and clinical progression to AIDS and death. Int J STD AIDS 15(12):803–810

Krousel-Wood M, Holt E, Joyce C, Ruiz R, Dornelles A, Webber LS et al (2015) Differences in cardiovascular disease risk when antihypertensive medication adherence is assessed by pharmacy fill versus self-report: the cohort study of medication adherence among older adults (CoSMO). J Hypertens 33(2):412–420

Checchi KD, Huybrechts KF, Avorn J, Kesselheim AS (2014) Electronic medication packaging devices and medication adherence: a systematic review. JAMA 312(12):1237–1247

Thakkar D, Piparva KG, Lakkad SG (2019) A pilot project: 99DOTS information communication technology-based approach for tuberculosis treatment in Rajkot district. Lung India 36(2):108–111

Diaz E, Levine HB, Sullivan MC, Sernyak MJ, Hawkins KA, Cramer JA et al (2001) Use of the medication event monitoring system to estimate medication compliance in patients with schizophrenia. J Psychiatry Neurosci 26(4):325–329

Liu H, Golin CE, Miller LG, Hays RD, Beck CK, Sanandaji S et al (2001) A comparison study of multiple measures of adherence to HIV protease inhibitors. Ann Intern Med 134(10):968–977

Modi AC, Lim CS, Yu N, Geller D, Wagner MH, Quittner AL (2006) A multi-method assessment of treatment adherence for children with cystic fibrosis. J Cyst Fibros 5(3):177–85

Kidney Disease: Improving Global Outcomes (KDIGO) (2009) Transplant Work Group. KDIGO clinical practice guideline for the care of kidney transplant recipients. Am J Transplant 9:S1–155

Therapeutic Drug Monitoring

6

Sushil Kiran Kunder and Avinash Arivazhahan

Abstract

Therapeutic drug monitoring is a concept that has its roots in the 1960s, and has evolved today to become a crucial tool in clinical pharmacology. Therapeutic drug monitoring is now an aspect of "personalized therapeutics". This concept uses body fluids, most commonly plasma, to measure the level of a particular drug in a person's body. This measured value then guides the clinician in making informed decisions for the betterment of individualized patient care. Therapeutic drug monitoring is particularly useful for drugs that have narrow therapeutic indices, no active metabolites, or no clinical signs of toxicity or effectiveness. This process involves a multidisciplinary team that needs to work together for screening, measuring, analyzing, and interpreting the results. Common drug classes that benefit from therapeutic drug monitoring include anti-epileptics, antipsychotics, antidepressants, etc. It is also important to consider the key limitations of this tool when interpreting the results. This chapter deals with the essentials of therapeutic drug monitoring in today's practice.

Keywords

TDM · Therapeutic range · Therapeutic window · Lithium · Personalized · Individualized

S. K. Kunder (✉)
Novo Nordisk India Ltd, Bengaluru, Karnataka, India

A. Arivazhahan
Medical Affairs & Medical Education, Novo Nordisk India Ltd., Bengaluru, Karnataka, India

A. Arivazhahan et al. (eds.), *Introduction to Basics of Pharmacology and Toxicology*,
https://doi.org/10.1007/978-981-95-1920-0_6

Fig. 6.1 Spectrum of plasma drug concentration

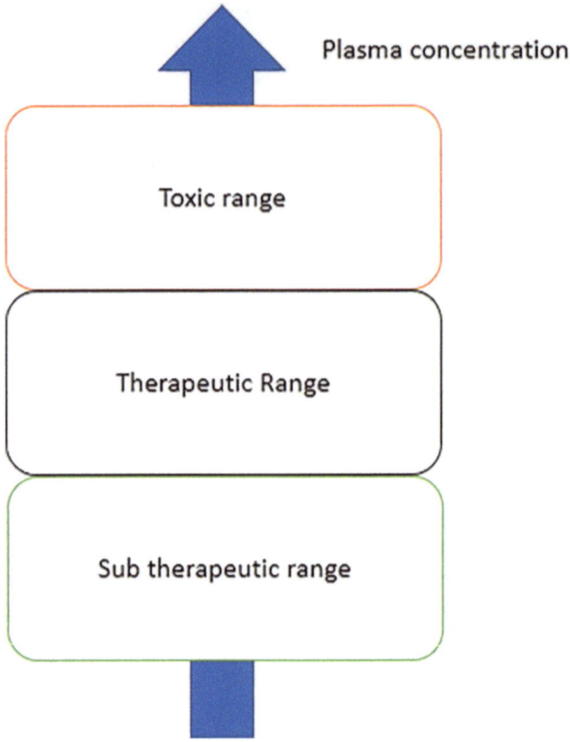

6.1 Introduction

Therapeutic drug monitoring (TDM) involves measurement of drug concentration in body fluids, with plasma being the most common fluid. TDM is usually advised and performed for drugs that have a narrow therapeutic range, or for assessing the compliance to therapy. While TDM is routinely used for drugs like anti-epileptics and aminoglycosides, it is, even today, a slowly evolving concept. The overall umbrella objective of performing TDM analysis is to ultimately individualize patient regimens and offer better safety. Clinical pharmacologists and pharmacists are considered experts in TDM analysis, the results of which are then used by clinicians to corroborate with their patients' therapeutic regimens and prescriptions. In general, concentration of drugs can have different clinical levels in a wide spectrum, as shown in Fig. 6.1.

6.2 Historical Evolution of TDM

The concept of TDM is now decades old. The earliest documentation of TDM probably starts with Buchthal in the year 1960, when he showcased an association between the extent of seizure control with the concentration of phenytoin in plasma.

The relationship between plasma concentration of lithium and its effects was then demonstrated by Baastrup and Schou in the late 1960s. The very first publication also came out in the 1960s, when Finney published a structured review on TDM. Automated analytical tools were then introduced in the 1970s, which fueled the growth and ease of performing TDM. The contributions of these evidences and the development of analytical tools ultimately have led to a better understanding of the potential benefits of TDM. The use of TDM in India began in the 1980s, following which its popularity soared to a certain extent.

6.3 Clinical Purposes of Performing TDM

While TDM may look like an isolated tool, it involves a truly multi-disciplinary approach to ensure effectiveness of its results. There is a great level of collaboration among the clinical pharmacologist or clinical pharmacist, treating clinician, nursing staff, other paramedical staff, and the patient. Although the earlier application of TDM was restricted only to the safety of drugs, today's integration has widened the scope of TDM beyond. Today, TDM is a highly useful tool to monitor various parameters or influence patient-related decisions, as listed below:

(i) To check if patients are compliant to a particular therapy that they are put on.
(ii) It acts as a guide to detect or avoid under-treatment.
(iii) It helps as a guide to detect or prevent overdosing and toxicity of therapies.
(iv) It helps in the detection of drug-drug interactions.
(v) It aids in decision to withdraw or stop or taper a particular treatment.
(vi) It is a useful tool for individualizing treatment while initiating a drug.
(vii) It is a useful tool for individualizing treatment during dose alterations.

6.4 Drugs That Can Benefit from Application of TDM

TDM may not be suitable for every drug available in the market. Many of the drugs being prescribed today may not even require TDM as a metric as the clinical picture is quite sufficient for the clinician to assess his/her patients' recovery or progress. Right from 1988, there have been several criteria developed to ensure TDM is performed only for the right drug candidates. These criteria are today more well-defined, as described below:

(i) A drug with a narrow therapeutic window: A narrow therapeutic window indicates that the drug cannot be confidently up-titrated by clinicians without the guide of TDM metrics. Hence, to ensure individualization of therapy, TDM plays a significant role here. Phenytoin would be an ideal example here.
(ii) A drug with no active metabolites: When there are active metabolites, there is no relevance of performing TDM only for the parent molecule, as there could be further therapeutic or toxic effects produced by its active metabolites. In

such cases, TDM has to then be performed for both the parent molecule and the active metabolites, which makes it tedious and complex to interpret. Opioids like tramadol or codeine can be considered as examples, wherein the active metabolites are more pharmacologically relevant than even the parent drugs.

(iii) A drug that shows good correlation with the plasma concentration and its effects: This is the core of the concept of TDM. Any drug that classically shows a direct relationship between its fluid concentration (plasma in most cases) and its therapeutic effect or its toxic effect would qualify as an ideal drug. Hence, when TDM metrics are available, the clinician can easily correlate the concentration with the expected effects, and make decisions for his/her patients. Lithium, for example, is an example for direct correlation.

(iv) A drug that does not have definite clinical signs or symptoms of toxicity or therapeutic effect: Any drug that has a pharmacodynamic indicator would not require TDM to be performed. A classical example is that of warfarin, wherein the clinician can prefer to use INR (International Normalized Ratio) to titrate the dose of warfarin. Another simple example is for insulins, which have clear clinical indicators in the form of hypoglycemia and hyperglycemia.

(v) A drug with a drug assay that is cost-effective: Beyond science, cost and affordability are important parameters to be considered, particularly in countries like India, where the medical expenses are usually paid out of pocket by our patients. Hence, there is no point in developing TDM kits for drugs for which the patients may not be able to spend. There have been studies that have shown very high contribution of TDM expense in the patients' spends during hospital stay (e.g., TDM of gentamicin was shown to contribute to 25% of patients' total medical expenses during a hospital stay), which may not be very practical and feasible in many instances.

(vi) A drug whose pharmacokinetics may vary significantly: Drugs that show significant intra-individual and inter-individual variability would also qualify for TDM analysis, since there is scope of individualization with these therapies.

While there may be no single drug that would qualify on all these criteria, Fig. 6.2 gives a non-exhaustive list of drugs that may benefit from TDM analysis.

6.5 Drug-Based Timing of TDM Analysis

Samples for analysis should be taken once the steady state (of plasma concentration) is achieved (i.e., after 4 to 5 half-lives) unless TDM is being done to predict the required dose in a patient. Drugs with long half-life should be monitored prior to attainment of steady state to prevent development of toxicity, especially in poor metabolizers (e.g., perhexiline). Drugs that are administered as a loading dose also need to be monitored to achieve an adequate dosing (e.g., phenytoin). Timing of sample collection is crucial as the plasma concentration varies with the dosing interval. Samples are usually collected prior to the next dose as the variability is usually the least during this time. This pre-dose measurement is called as the "trough"

Drugs that will benefit from TDM analysis

- Lithium
- Phenytoin
- Theophylline
- Digoxin
- Carbamazepine
- Gentamicin, tobramycin
- Cyclosporin
- Lamotrigine
- Methotrexate
- Sirolimus, tacrolimus

Drugs that may benefit from TDM analysis

- Valproate
- Phenobarbital
- Clozapine, olanzapine
- Beta blockers
- Chloramphenicol
- Amiodarone
- Protease inhibitors, NNRTIs
- Teicoplanin, vancomycin
- Tricyclic antidepressants
- Morphine, methadone

Fig. 6.2 Non-exhaustive list of drugs that would be suitable for TDM

concentration. However, sample collection can be done at any point of time for drugs like amiodarone and phenobarbitone, which have long half-lives. TDM of drugs like digoxin should not be measured prior to 6 h post dosing as they will be in the distribution phase of their pharmacokinetics. If done within 6 h, the plasma levels will falsely high, which can result in clinical decision-making fallacies. At times, the peak concentrations are measured to detect toxicity associated with the drug (e.g., lithium, carbamazepine). Once-daily dosing of aminoglycosides is monitored about 6–14 h post dosing of the drug. However, when they are administered in multiple doses, trough concentrations are measured.

6.6 Choice of TDM Techniques

TDM is regularly performed using the following two techniques, although there are other techniques available too.

(i) Immunoassay: Immunoassay (isotopic and optical) has been in use for a long time. However, this technique suffers with the drawback that there may be interference from metabolite and related compounds.

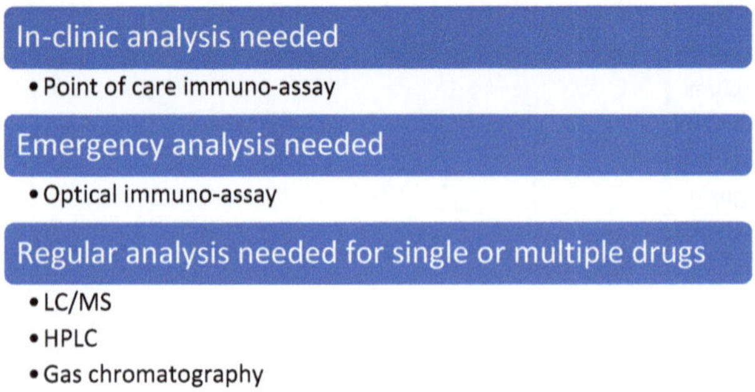

Fig. 6.3 TDM techniques as per need or request—a clinical guide

(ii) Liquid chromatography—mass spectrometry (LCMS): LCMS is now being used quite commonly for TDM. Compared to immunoassays, LCMS has improved indices of sensitivity and specificity. The major limitation with LCMS is that it is expensive due to greater instrument cost. In addition, it is also a complex technique. Due to these drawbacks, LCMS is available only in a few high-end specialized centers. LSCMS is usually performed for certain drugs for which immunoassays may not be possible.

While there is no single correct or appropriate method that is available, the choice can be guided by the type and need of TDM request, as depicted in Fig. 6.3.

6.6.1 TDM of Common Anti-epileptic Drugs

TDM is an important tool for managing patients on anti-epileptic drugs. However, it is not routinely advised for all patients, and should be reserved to specific situations. Importance of monitoring the plasma concentrations of anti-epileptic drugs has been stressed for many decades. This is mainly because anti-epileptic drugs show broad inter-individual variability and a narrow therapeutic window. In addition, anti-epileptic agents are frequently combined with each other, which adds to the complexity. Patient-specific ranges termed as "therapeutic ranges" should be set, and drug concentration should be assessed every 6–12 months or whenever clinically warranted.

Unlike first- and second-generation anti-epileptic agents, requirement of TDM in the newer third-generation anti-epileptic drugs is not well established.

Therapeutic ranges of the commonly used anti-epileptic drugs are listed in Table 6.1.

Table 6.1 Recommended therapeutic ranges for commonly used anti-epileptic drugs

Anti-epileptic drug	Recommended therapeutic range (μg/mL)
1. First-generation anti-epileptic drugs	
Phenytoin	10–20
Carbamazepine	4–12
Valproic acid	50–100
Phenobarbital	15–40
2. Second-generation anti-epileptic drugs	
Gabapentin	12–20
Lamotrigine	3–15
Topiramate	5–20
Levetiracetam	10–60
Pregabalin	2–5
3. Third-generation anti-epileptic drugs	
Rufinamide	5–30
Eslicarbazepine	3–35
Clobazam	0.03–0.3

6.6.2 TDM of Antipsychotics

Recent times have seen a significant increase in the evidences showcasing the need for use of TDM during antipsychotic therapy. A positive correlation has been observed between the therapeutic ranges of clozapine and haloperidol and their corresponding serum levels than with the daily dose of these drugs. For example, the benefit of haloperidol is lost when serum concentration is more than 10 ng/mL.

When it concerns clozapine, its metabolite is measured (i.e., norclozapine). Norclozapine levels have no relation to the efficacy of clozapine treatment. However, clozapine-to-norclozapine ratio gives a hint about patients' adherence to clozapine (i.e., 1.5 to 2 is the optimal ratio; non-adherence when the ratio falls below 0.5; ratio greater than 2 is suggestive of reduced clearance of the drug).

Risperidone, an atypical antipsychotic, has an active metabolite, 9-hydroxy risperidone. The plasma concentrations of risperidone and 9-hydroxy risperidone show inter- and intra-individual variations. 9-hydroxy risperidone has similar pharmacological properties as those of risperidone. Since both contribute to antipsychotic efficacy, monitoring plasma concentration of risperidone (parent compound) alone may lead to inaccurate interpretations.

TDM of anti-psychotics is a robust tool for tailoring treatment to the needs of specific patients. It helps in adjustment of doses, reducing toxicity, and in monitoring treatment adherence.

The therapeutic ranges of the commonly used antipsychotic agents are shown in Table 6.2.

Table 6.2 Therapeutic ranges of commonly used antipsychotic agents

Drug	Therapeutic range (ng/mL)
Haloperidol	1–10
Aripiprazole	150–500
Amisulpiride	100–320
Clozapine	350–600
Olanzapine	20–80
Paliperidone	20–60
Quetiapine	100–500
Risperidone +9-hydroxy risperidone	20–60

Table 6.3 Therapeutic ranges of immunosuppressants

Drug	Therapeutic range (trough concentration)
Tacrolimus	5–20 g/L
Sirolimus	5–15 g/L
Mycophenolate mofetil	1–3.5 mg/L
Cyclosporine	150–400 mcg/L

6.6.3 TDM of Immunosuppressants

Optimizing cyclosporine therapy is a challenge faced by transplant physicians due to high inter- and intra-subject variability and narrow therapeutic window of the drug. Measuring cyclosporine exposure is vital to prevent acute rejection and at the same time, avoid nephrotoxic adverse effects. Ideal time to collect the sample is 2 h after cyclosporine dose.

Mycophenolate mofetil is a prodrug and mycophenolic acid is its active metabolite. Pharmacokinetics of mycophenolic acid demonstrate large variability, both inter- and intra-individual. It is extensively plasma protein-bound in patients with normally functioning liver and kidneys. In patients with hyperbilirubinemia or renal compromise, there are changes seen in albumin concentration, which may lead to a change in the free and bound concentrations. Therefore, measuring the unbound mycophenolic acid concentrations might be considered.

Similar to cyclosporine, tacolimus also has a narrow therapeutic window and exhibits extensive variability. In addition, it is prone to drug interactions that are cytochrome P450-mediated. Therefore, it is ideal to dose the patient with this agent guided by the trough concentration from whole blood sample.

Therapeutic ranges of these immunosuppressants are shown in Table 6.3.

6.6.4 TDM of Antidepressants

TDM is an established tool for dose optimization in patients on tricyclic antidepressants (TCAs). TCAs can cause sedation, orthostatic hypotension, anti-cholinergic effects, and arrythmias. Thus employing TDM improves safety, efficacy, and in addition, cost-effectiveness.

Selective serotonin reuptake inhibitors (SSRIs) like paroxetine, sertraline, and fluoxetine are highly plasma protein-bound. On the other hand, fluvoxamine and citalopram are relatively less plasma protein-bound. Fluvoxamine, paroxetine, and fluoxetine have non-linear pharmacokinetics. As a result, at higher doses, their plasma concentrations increase disproportionately (more so in the elderly population). Therefore, it is difficult to guess the dose required to reach a particular plasma concentration. On the other hand, sertraline and citalopram have linear kinetics. Plasma concentration is obtained after a steady state. Fluoxetine has a half-life of 16 days and norfluoxetine, its active metabolite has a half-life of 16 hours. Therefore, norfluoxetine steady state is achieved 3 months post starting fluoxetine.

Therapeutic ranges of a few of the antidepressants can be obtained from Table 6.4.

6.6.5 TDM of Aminoglycosides

TDM has increased the safety of aminoglycosides by optimizing and individualizing dose regimens. Multiple doses of aminoglycosides are usually associated with higher nephrotoxicity rates (10–20%). However, once daily dosing aided by TDM has led to lower nephrotoxicity rates (0–14%). Once daily aminoglycosides along with TDM is now broadly accepted and is now the standard of care for multiple infection types. The concentrations are ideally measured 6 h post dosing. This is to ensure that the clearance is reasonable. In individuals with renal compromise who are dosed once in 36–48 h, monitoring trough concentration is usually advised.

6.6.6 TDM of Digoxin

Digoxin has a therapeutic range of 0.5–2 ng/mL. However, the therapeutic and toxic range overlaps to a significant extent. A patient in optimal therapeutic range can still develop signs of toxicity. TDM for digoxin is done using immunoassays (enzyme immune assays, fluorescence polarization immune assays). However, these methods may not differentiate digoxin from other drugs like spironolactone. DIGIBIND

Table 6.4 Recommended therapeutic ranges of antidepressants

Drug	Therapeutic range (ng/ml)
Fluoxetine + Norfluoxetine	120–500
Fluvoxamine	60–230
Paroxetine	30–120
Sertraline	10–150
Citalopram	50–110
Duloxetine	30–120
Venlafaxine + O-desmethylvenlafaxine	100–400

Table 6.5 Therapeutic ranges for lithium therapy

Drug	Indication	Therapeutic range (mmol/L)
Lithium	(a) Acute mania (b) Maintenance	0.8–1.2 0.4–1.0 mmol/L

(digoxin antibody), which is used during overdosage of digoxin, also renders the assays unreliable. Furthermore, digoxin-like immunoreactive factors (DLIF), which are endogenous substances can also lead to responses like digoxin, resulting in false-high values. The specificity of assessment can be improved by using newer assays like monoclonal antibody assay. Quinidine increases plasma digoxin levels by reducing renal clearance (P-glycoprotein inhibition) and also displaces digoxin from its binding site. Other drugs increasing digoxin concentration are diltiazem, amiodarone, and verapamil.

6.6.7 TDM of Lithium

The standard time to collect samples for detecting serum concentration of lithium is 10–12 h post evening dose when lithium is administered twice in a day. Based on these concentrations, the lithium dose should be tailored. Once the symptoms improve and steady state is achieved, monitoring is done once in 1–3 months.

The optimal therapeutic ranges for lithium can be found in Table 6.5.

6.7 Essentials for the Ideal TDM Assessment and Interpretation

As mentioned earlier, TDM assessment is a multi-disciplinary approach and involves multiple experts and resources.

(i) Experts: There is a bare minimal need for a clinical pharmacologist or clinical pharmacist, laboratory staff, treating clinician, nursing, and other paramedical staff. While this may be possible at hospital level, smaller clinics and labs may not be fully equipped.
(ii) Laboratory facilities: Laboratory facilities with proper quality assurance are needed for any TDM analysis.
(iii) Point-of-care analysis: While sending samples to labs is needed in many cases, some scenarios would require urgent or immediate analysis and interpretation. In such cases, point-of-care testing kits would be needed, which can greatly improve patient care.
(iv) Time taken for reporting and analysis: While TDM is time-consuming, it is ideal that the reporting and analysis are done before the patient's next dose of the drug, so that quick decisions can be arrived at.

(v) Education and awareness: There is still a great need of education and awareness amongst all stakeholders involved. The clinical pharmacologist can take up this responsibility to conduct regular scientific sessions.

6.8 Key Limitations of TDM

- The assays used may not be very accurate (measurement errors).
- Lab resources may be limited (analytical errors).
- Clinicians may not be fully equipped with the knowledge of TDM (sampling and interpretation errors).
- Assays are currently available only for a few drugs.
- Availability and access in suburban and rural areas are limited.
- The therapeutic response may be due to an active metabolite, which is not measured routinely.
- Cost is also a major limitation of TDM.

6.9 Conclusion

TDM is required for individualizing treatment for patients in order to make it safe and effective. In addition, it also aids in detecting patients who are not compliant to treatment. Time of dosing, time of sample collection, desired targets, and patients' response should be kept in mind while interpreting the assessed concentration of the drug. Based on this information, the correct regimen can be identified to reach an optimal response devoid of toxicity.

Bibliography

Adaway JE, Keevil BG (2012) Therapeutic drug monitoring and LC–MS/MS. J Chromatogr B 883:33–49

Basalingappa S, Sharma A, Amarnath S (2014) Basic concepts of therapeutic drug monitoring. Int J Curr Pharm Rev Res 5(4):70–75

Campbell TJ, Williams KM (1998) Therapeutic drug monitoring: antiarrhythmic drugs. Br J Clin Pharmacol 46:307–319

Citterio F (2004) Evolution of the therapeutic drug monitoring of cyclosporine. Transplant Proc 36(2):S420–S425

Dadiamov D (2020) Therapeutic drug monitoring of antipsychotics. Curr Psychiatr Ther 19(2):40–46

Ghiculescu RA (2008) Therapeutic drug monitoring: which drugs, why, when and how to do it. Aust Prescr 31:42–44

Grundmann M, Kacirova I, Urinovska R (2014) Therapeutic drug monitoring of atypical antipsychotic drugs. Acta Pharma 64(4):387–401

Grundmann M, Kacirova I, Urinovska R (2015) Therapeutic monitoring of psychoactive drugs - antidepressants: a review. Biomed Pap Med Fac Univ Palacky Olomouc Czech Repub 159(1):35–43

Kang JS, Lee MH (2009) Overview of therapeutic drug monitoring. Korean J Intern Med 24(1):1–10

Knezevic CE, Marzinke MA (2018) Clinical use and monitoring of antiepileptic drugs. ZALM 03(01):115–127

Krause KM, Serio AW, Kane TR, Connolly LE (2016) Aminoglycosides: an overview. Cold Spring Harb Perspect Med 6:a027029

Linder MW, Keck PE (1998) Standards of laboratory practice: antidepressant drug monitoring. Clin Chem 44(5):1073–1084

Roberts JA, Norris R, Paterson D, Martins JH (2012) Therapeutic drug monitoring of antimicrobials. Br J Clin Pharmacol 73(1):27–36

Tiwari SP (2007) Therapeutic drug monitoring of immunosuppressants: an overview. Indian J Pharmacol 39(2):66–70

Medication Errors

7

Arup Kumar Misra

Abstract

Medication error (ME) might be a complicated and unwelcome topic, but it is an unfavourable preventable occurrence that occurs when a medication is used inappropriately, leading to patient morbidity and/or mortality. Medication errors can be caused by a variety of factors, including drug-related factors (e.g., similar-sounding names, low therapeutic index), patient-related factors (e.g., poor renal or hepatic function, impaired cognition, polypharmacy), and healthcare professional-related factors (e.g., cognitive biases, use of abbreviations in prescriptions and other communications). A significant ME is one that causes mortality, shifting to an intensive care unit, or lasting damage. Medical board-governed corrective actions, legal lawsuits, criminal charges, and a loss of patient trust are some of the repercussions that doctors may experience following pharmaceutical errors. There has been mixed effectiveness in preventing prescription errors through the use of information technology, improved drug labelling, and medication reconciliation, among other strategies. For every significant ME, a root cause investigation must be performed. Acquiring knowledge regarding drug errors could potentially improve the ability of medical practitioners to treat patients safely.

Keywords

Medication error · Adverse events · Monitoring · Technology · Communication · Education

A. K. Misra (✉)
Department of Pharmacology, All India Institute of Medical Sciences,
Mangalagiri, Andhra Pradesh, India
e-mail: arup.pharma@aiimsmangalagiri.edu.in

A. Arivazhahan et al. (eds.), *Introduction to Basics of Pharmacology and Toxicology*,
https://doi.org/10.1007/978-981-95-1920-0_7

7.1 Introduction

The healthcare system is an intricate and multifaceted system that relies heavily on improvised and revolutionised technology, entails the collaboration of numerous specialists, and involves various institutions. The intricacies of India's healthcare system may put the populace at a great risk, which could exacerbate or worsen the complications brought on by these errors. Every government and healthcare regulatory agency in the world has an absolute obligation to provide the resources and medical personnel necessary to deliver healthcare to everyone. In ev,ery country, the main form of intervention offered by health services in healthcare settings is medication. The use of medication for early relief is on the rise in today's modern world, which could significantly increase medication errors (ME) and raise risks for the general public. Patient safety, according to the World Health Organisation (WHO), is defined as minimising unwarranted injury or possible risk related to medical treatment. In a nationwide poll conducted in the USA, 81% of participants reported taking a medicine in the week before the poll, and 50% reported taking one or more prescription medications at a given point in time. Modern pharmacotherapy is complicated, which can lead to mistakes made by medical experts as well as confusion among patients.

In a poll of hospitalised patients, just 27.9% of respondents could name the prescriptions they were discharged with, and even fewer could specify how they were supposed to be used. Furthermore, research has shown a correlation between medication errors and adverse outcomes, with rates of medication errors in hospital in-patients ranging from 4.8% to 5.3%.

Medication errors represent a significant clinical problem. On the other hand, even at the most basic level, these errors might have unclear definitions, and their effects on people and society may not be fully understood. "Any avoidable event that may cause or lead to inappropriate medication use or patient harm while the medication is in the control of the health-care professional, patient, or consumer" is the definition of a medication error. Medication errors can include (amongst others) prescribing the incorrect medication, delivering the wrong dosage, failing to prescribe a recommended treatment, ordering the incorrect patient, or forgetting to give a prescription when it was due. Medicine errors are typically only discovered when a patient experiences clinical repercussions, such as the development of symptoms after the medicine is administered, alerting medical personnel to the problem.

7.2 Incidence of Medication Errors

Globally, MEs are not reported unless they result in a substantial causal relationship. The different global rates of error prevalence could be a reflection of these problems. The Institute of Medicine has estimated that the annual healthcare cost associated with MEs in the United States is almost $37.6 billion, of which approximately $17 billion is attributed to avoidable errors. According to a different study, 66 million of the estimated 237 million pharmaceutical errors that occur in a single nation each year may have therapeutic significance. An estimated £98.5 million is spent annually by the government on preventable adverse drug reactions. This includes adverse drug events (ADEs) in primary care that result in hospital admission (costing £83.7 million and contributing to 627 deaths) and ADEs in secondary care that result in prolonged hospital stays (costing £14.8 million and causing or contributing to 1081 fatalities). In hospitals, the percentage of medication errors varies from 1.6% to 2.1% during the dispensing stage and from 0.3% to 9.1% for prescriptions.

Avery et al. revealed that almost 38% of patients over 75 had either a prescription error or a monitoring error, making up over 10% of patients in primary care in the UK. Patients (30%) taking multiple medications had a higher frequency of MEs. In a study conducted in Sweden, Claesson et al. discovered a high rate of MEs (42%). The majority of these mistakes were caused by incorrectly filled prescriptions, however some also resulted from patients taking the wrong dosage. Khoja et al. conducted a study in Saudi Arabia and discovered that about 20% of primary care prescriptions resulted in MEs, but not all of them were severe. In a study conducted in Mexico, Zavaleta-Bustos et al. discovered that roughly 28% of prescription errors were due to incorrect dosage regimen. Because there are several classification methods and criteria for MEs, it is very challenging to quantify their prevalence within the healthcare system. Usually, it is determined by the denominator that is being utilised, such as the patient, prescription, or particular drug. According to the state governments of Karnataka and Uttarakhand in India, there have been 14% and 26% cases of ME respectively. In a Prospective study in Indore, India, out of the total 457 errors identified, medication errors were 313 (68.5%). Majority were dosing errors (45.5%). Morbidity was absent in 375 (82%), mild in 49 (10.7%), moderate in 22 (4.8%), and severe in 11 (2.4%) errors.

Research has also been done on the frequency of injury in relation to pharmaceutical errors. In an analysis of over 10,000 prescriptions, Bates et al. found 5.3 mistakes for every 100 prescriptions. These authors did conclude, nevertheless, that adverse medication events were only caused by 0.9% of the errors. In another study involving 36 institutions, Barker et al. reported that 19% of the doses were found to be incorrect, however only 7% were thought to have the potential to cause adverse effects.

7.3 Impact of Medication Errors

MEs negatively affect both the economy of the healthcare system and the individual. It comprises unfavourable adverse drug reactions, drug-drug interactions, loss of medication efficacy, and non-compliance with therapy, all of which lower the patient's quality of life and experience. These unfavourable occurrences could then have a major impact on people's health and also worsen the financial state of the healthcare industry. Adverse events have the potential to escalate the utilisation of healthcare services, elevate hospital admissions linked to medicines, and in certain instances, result in fatalities. In certain nations, it accounts for 6–7% of admissions,

7.4.6 Dispensing Errors

Dispensing errors can happen at any point during the dispensing procedure, from the pharmacy receiving the prescription to giving the patients their medications. Errors in dispensing, which range from 1% to 24%, may involve choosing the incorrect product or strength. This may mostly happen with medications that share the same name or look. Examples of proprietary names that appear identical when handwritten are Losec® (omeprazole) and Lasix® (frusemide), underscoring the importance of prescribing generically. Numerous fatalities linked to this error have prompted the US-FDA to demand that Losec® trademarked name be altered. The lack of electronic labelling has resulted in transposition and typing errors, which are among the most frequent causes of dispensing error. Other potential dispensing errors include the wrong dose, medicine, or patient.

7.4.7 Administration Errors

These happen when there is a mismatch between the medication that the patient takes and the medication regimen that the physician has in mind. The "five rights"—administering the right medication to the right patient at the right time in the right dose via the right route—are the cornerstone of drug prescription administration. Errors in drug administration mostly relate to omissions, in which the medication is not provided for a number of reasons. Incorrect administration techniques and the use of outdated or inaccurate preparations are two more categories of drug administration problems.

7.5 Causes of Medication Errors

The "treatment process" involves all medications, as defined above. The causes of MEs are described in Fig. 7.1. Some of the examples of inappropriate prescription process that leads to medication errors are as follows.

7.5.1 Selecting a Prescription

The errors in prescription writing may lead to medication errors which may include the physicians taking an inaccurate medication history, he/she may prescribe inappropriately or ineffectively, writing the wrong drug name, and directing too little or too much of the drug.

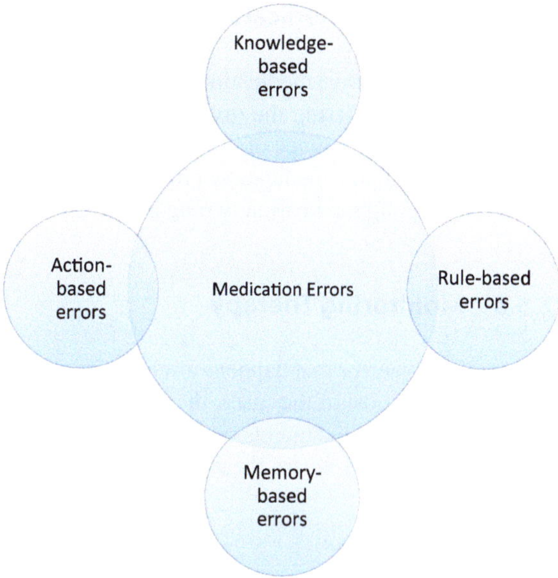

Fig. 7.1 Types and causes of medication errors as per psychological classification

7.5.2 Illegible Prescription

Illegible prescription is one of the most common medication errors. The physicians may use illegible handwriting, sometimes use improper decimal point, wrong abbreviations, and verbal orders while writing the prescription may lead to prescription errors.

7.5.3 Manufacturing the Formulation

The pharmaceutical industry may sometimes lead to medication error while manufacturing the drugs. Some of the examples of medication errors related to pharmaceutical industries are giving incorrect medication, incorrect strength of the drug, adulterants or impurities, incorrect or deceptive labelling and packaging.

7.5.4 Faulty Pharmacy

Faulty Pharmacy in the hospital may lead to medication error related to dispensing. Some of the errors seen in the pharmacy of the hospitals are dispensing the incorrect medicine, wrong formulation, or absence of safe dispensing technique when dispensing the formulation.

7.5.5 Incorrect Medication

This is one of the grave medication errors seen in the hospital wards. It is commonly seen while administering the drug to the patients. The absence of trained nursing professional or the absence of double check system may lead to this error. Some of the examples of the medication errors are giving or consuming the medication incorrectly, wrong medication, wrong dosage, wrong frequency, or wrong duration.

7.5.6 Monitoring Therapy

The medication error that happens after administering the drug are quite common in the hospital. In most of the cases, the effects of the drugs are not monitored by making the necessary adjustments or making the incorrect adjustments. This error will be seen in the wards where there is crowding, inefficient nursing professional, and lack of time.

7.6 Factors Associated with Medication Errors

The important factors which lead to ME are as follows and given in Fig. 7.2.

7.6.1 Patients

MEs are more common in-patient populations that are vulnerable. These patients' personalities, literacy levels, language hurdles, many comorbid diseases, and polypharmacy are the causes of MEs. Discordant medications can be classified as either an error of commission (the patient is taking a medication that is not on the prescription) or an error of omission (the patient is not taking a medication that was on the prescription).

7.6.2 Workplace

A crucial component of healthcare systems is the workplace. MEs may result from an inefficient and inadequate working environment. The factors at play include the healthcare professionals' increased workload or time constraints, the disruptions caused by patients and staff at work, the absence of standard protocols and procedures, a lack of resources, and problems with the working area's lighting, temperature, and ventilation.

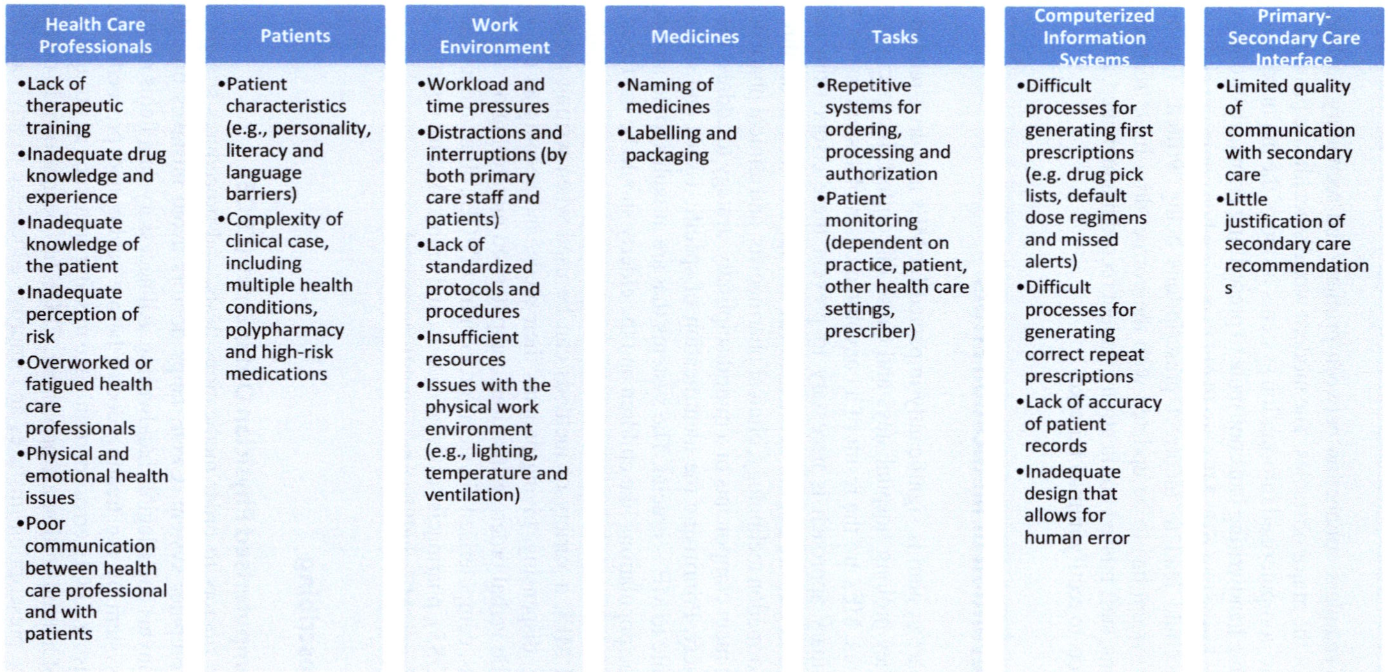

Fig. 7.2 Factors affecting Medication Errors. (Reproduced from Ambwani et al. 2019)

7.6.3 Information Technology

The lack of seamless connection between primary and secondary healthcare systems is one of the major obstacles. The modern world's healthcare providers' inability to adapt to computerised information systems is one of the major causes of MEs. While illegible handwriting can contribute to prescribing errors, electronic prescribing may help lower that risk. MEs are likely to occur when computer skills are lacking, as this could lead to incorrect prescriptions being written. The hospital's information system has to be updated with the correct drug lists, treatment-based dose regimens, staff missed notifications, patient record maintenance, and corrected system defects to rectify human mistake.

7.7 Prevention of Medication Errors

The healthcare system is significantly impacted by MEs and drug-related adverse events, as they prolong hospital stays and cause discomfort, incapacity, or higher mortality rates. MEs are the result of a convoluted chain of system issues. Often, a multidisciplinary approach is necessary to prevent these errors from occurring. Numerous strategies are put out in the medical literature to combat the threat posed by MEs. Information technology, clinical pharmacists, and clinical pharmacologists are the three main components of a multidisciplinary strategy to address the issue of MEs in society. Prioritising the identification of specific issues and shortcomings that contribute to ME is crucial. The systems that are at fault should also be examined. Specific populations like children and the elderly should be the focus of these strategies.

To avoid MEs, a variety of methods can be used when writing prescriptions, transcribing, dispensing, giving patients their meds, and keeping an eye on them. These include verbal order verification, computerised monitoring of adverse medication events, computerised physician order entry (CPOE), clinical decision support systems (CDSS), pharmacist-assisted rounds, and high-risk drug regimes. By using these techniques, MEs will be considerably decreased.

7.7.1 Prescribing

7.7.1.1 Computerised Physician Order Entry (CPOE)

By enabling doctors to order medications, tests, and procedures straight into the hospital's computer system, CPOE helps doctors avoid mistakes brought on by unclear acronyms and illegible handwriting. All necessary data fields must be filled out in the system by the treating doctor before saving and proceeding with the orders. By using CPOE, errors pertaining to missing data, such as dosage, route, and frequency of administration are prevented. CPOE has been shown in numerous trials to reduce prescription mistakes and improve adherence to advised prescribing practices. Alert functionalities are also available in the system to draw attention to important information including drug-specific allergies.

CPOE requires a large initial investment but it offers substantial financial returns in addition to improvements in resource efficiency and lower testing and imaging costs. CPOE will especially enhance communication efforts when patients are being transferred from one setting to another.

7.7.1.2 Computerised Decision Support Systems (CDSS)

Clinical decision support systems (CDSS) can be routinely used in hospitals to review orders as they are written, compare new and existing orders, check for drug-drug interactions, allergies, appropriate dosing schedules, as well as to notify physicians of relevant laboratory results that affect their decisions and the patient's plan of care. Moreover, CDSS can suggest less costly substitute drugs, which can help in settings with resource constraints. Duplications involving medication, testing, and imaging can be found and avoided using this technique.

7.7.1.3 Clinical Pharmacologist-Assisted Rounds

The most accessible resource for choosing a medicine is a clinical pharmacologist. Clinical pharmacologists are knowledgeable about the institution's formulary and can help doctors choose medications for their patients both during their hospital stay and at the time that they are discharged by addressing medication discrepancies in discharge documents, addressing polypharmacy, and emphasising the prudent use of drugs to reduce risks to patient health. They should also regularly update the list and review prescriptions written by clinicians. Clinical pharmacologists should check order sets for adherence to the formulary medicine list and avoid the use of unwarranted prescription drugs.

7.7.1.4 Handwriting

Adopting computerised systems as detailed earlier will aid in the elimination of handwritten errors and unfavourable patient outcomes. In order to reduce multiple interpretations of the same abbreviation, hospitals should implement and display a set of abbreviations in accordance with healthcare standards. The pharmacist or other relevant staff should check that the handwritten orders are complete and readable at the nursing station to make sure the intended transcription and interpretation are made. The prescription should be thoroughly checked to ensure that the medication's name, dosage form, dose, route, and frequency are all correct. It should have the doctor's signature and printed name on it for easy verifications and back-tracing as needed.

7.7.1.5 Abbreviations

Errors related to measurement units, such as utilising milligrams instead of millilitres, are frequently observed in the healthcare sector. For handwritten, patient-specific communications, the Institute for Safe Medication Practices (ISMP) has produced a list of potentially harmful acronyms, symbols, and abbreviations, which are shown in Table 7.1. While electronic prescriptions are widely recognised as a

Table 7.1 List of some examples of dangerous abbreviations, acronyms, and symbols for handwritten, patient-specific communications. (According to Institute for Safe Medication Practices (ISMP))

Abbreviation	Intended meaning	Possible mis-interpretation
U	Units	Mistaken as a zero or 4 (four) resulting in overdose
IU	International units	Mistaken as IV (intravenous) or 10 (ten)
μg	Micrograms	Mistaken for "milligram"
cc	Cubic centimetres	Mistaken as "u" (units)
IN	Intranasal	Mistaken as "IM" or "IV"
HS	Half-strength	Mistaken as bedtime
hs	At bedtime, hours of sleep	Mistaken as half-strength
SC or SQ	Subcutaneous	Mistaken as "SL" (sublingual)
SSRI	Sliding scale regular insulin	Mistaken as selective-serotonin reuptake inhibitor
AZT	Zidovudine (Retrovir)	Mistaken as azathioprine or Aztreonam
CPZ	Compazine (prochlorperazine)	Mistaken as chlorpromazine
NoAC	Novel/new oral anticoagulant	No anticoagulant

safe and reasonable means of obtaining medication, improper usage of these devices can result in MEs relating to abbreviations.

7.7.1.6 Decimal Points

The physician could reduce ten-fold dosing errors by using a zero to the left of a dose less than one (e.g., 0.1 instead of 0.1) and refrain from using a terminal zero to the right of the decimal point (e.g., 5 instead of 5.0).

7.7.1.7 Standardised Order Sets

Standardised order sets reduce variation among physicians and have been shown in some trials to shorten hospital stays and increase service quality. Doctors in a particular speciality should ideally employ a small number of agreed-upon order sets that are updated at least annually and approved by chemists.

7.7.2 Transcribing

Electronic order transcription, such as CPOE, improves transcription speed and accuracy. Additionally, using this strategy produces less MEs. It is also observed that using standardised order speeds up order transcription.

7.7.2.1 Verbal Order Verification

Wherever possible, doctors should refrain from giving verbal orders. Verbal orders pertaining to prescription orders and tests are permissible only in emergency cases. Verbal commands require a "read-back" or "repeat-back" confirmation of the entire order by the individual receiving it in order to guarantee safety. The individual providing the order will verbally acknowledge that the repeated order is correct, and the recipient will repeat the verbal order back to the ordering physician. Certain verbal pronunciation protocols should be applied. As an example, both parties should say "one two" rather than "12" to avoid the chances of mishearing and misinterpretation.

7.7.3 Dispensing

7.7.3.1 Automated Dispensing

Use of automated dispensing systems will result in fewer MEs. Commonly used automated dispensing cabinets can assist in preventing dosage errors as well as "look-alike" and "sound-alike" medication, a few of which are listed in Tables 7.2 and 7.3.

7.7.3.2 High-Risk Drug Protocols/Policies

High alert/high-risk medications are those that carry the highest risk of causing harm when misused. Some of these include heparin, warfarin, insulin, lidocaine, magnesium, muscle relaxants, chemotherapeutic agents, dextrose, narcotics, adrenergic agents, immunoglobulin, etc. (Table 7.4). These prescriptions must be kept in inventory and kept under lock and key, along with labels identifying them as high-risk drugs.

7.7.3.3 Barcoding

Healthcare systems must implement bar code technology in hospitals. Barcode systems help with better medication scheduling, fewer missed medicine doses, more effective drug monitoring, better prescription record-keeping, and enhanced staff communication. Certain barcode medication systems may also result in cost savings. Identification of the appropriate patient, medication, and dosage is made easier with the use of barcodes.

Table 7.2 Examples of some look-alike drugs (According to FDA and ISMP)

acetaZOLAMIDE	acetoHEXAMIDE
buPROPion	busPIRone
chlorproMAZINE	chlorproPAMIDE
dimenhyDRINATE	diphenhydrAMINE
glipiZIDE	glyBURIDE
hydrALAZINE	hydrOXYzine—HYDROmorphone
NIFEdipine	niCARdipine
rOPINIRole	risperiDONE
sulfiSOXAZOLE	sulfADIAZINE
TOLBUTamide	TOLAZamide
vinBLAStine	vinCRIStine

Table 7.3 Examples of some sound—alike drugs (According to FDA and ISMP)

Avanza (mirtazapine)	Avandia (rosiglitazone)
Losec (omeprazole)	Lasix (frusemide)
Quelicin (succinilcolina)	Keflin (cefalotina)
Celebrex (celecoxib)	Cerebyx (fosphenytoin)
Fluoxétine	Fluvoxamine
Reminyl (galantamine hydrobromide)	Amarel (glimepiride)
Morphine	Hydromorphone
Diamox (acetazolamide)	Zimox (amoxicillina triidrato)
Flomax (morniflumato)	Volmax (salbutamolo solfato)
Almarl (arotinolol)	Amaryl (glimepiride)
Taxotere (docetaxel)	Taxol (paclitaxel)
Dianben (metformin)	Diovan (valsartan)
Ecazide (captopril/hydrochlorothiazide)	Eskazine (trifluoperazine)
Avastin (bvacizumab)	Avaxim (hepatitis A vaccine)
Lantus (insulin glargine)	Lanvis (toguanine)

Table 7.4 List of high-risk medicine

1.	Narcotics (controlled drugs, stored under double lock): Morphine, fentanyl and pethidine
2.	Opiates: Pentazocin, tramadol
3.	Sedatives and hypnotics: Alprazolam, Chlordiazepoxide, clonazepam, diazepam, lorazepam, midazolam, zolpidem, Phenobarbitone, Dexmedetomidine
4.	Neuromuscular blocking agents: Atracurium, Pancuronium, Rocuronium, Vecuronium, and succinylcholine
5.	Intravenous Anaesthetic drugs: Ketamine and Propofol
6.	Chemotherapeutic drugs (anti-cancer): all the drugs: Parental and oral
7.	Antithrombotic agents: Warfarin, LMW heparin, Fondaparinux, Apixaban, rivaroxaban, Alteplase, Reteplase, Tenecteplase and Eptifibatide
8.	Specific medications: Insulin, injection potassium chloride, injection magnesium sulphate, injection Nitroprusside, Injection potassium phosphates, injection vasopressin, Injection Oxytocin, sodium chloride-hypertonic greater than 0.9% concentration Methotrexate (oral non-oncologic use). Epoprostenol IV
9.	Adrenergic agonist: Epinephrine, norepinephrine and phenylephrine
10.	Antiarrhythmics IV: Amiodarone and lidocaine
11.	Inotropic medications: Digoxin and Milrinone
12.	Radiocontrast agents, IV
13.	Dialysis solutions, peritoneal and hemodialysis
14.	Oral hypoglycemics

According to Institute for Safe Medication Practices (ISMP). (Reproduced from Ambwani et al. 2019)

7.7.3.4 Unit Dose Packaging

The unit dose packaging definition is "a dose of medicine prepared in an individual packet for convenience, safety, and monitoring." When combined with barcode readers and computer systems, unit dose pharmaceutical packaging improves the accuracy of the medication and dosage given to the right patient.

7.7.4 Administering/Monitoring

Errors in the drug delivery process during administration can be reduced with the use of technologies like barcoding, automated drug dispensing, and unit dose packaging. Hospitals can perform routine audits of patient charts, which aid in identifying the ineffective drug management practices there and provide guidelines to reduce errors and increase safety.

Medication errors can also be reduced with patient education. Fostering a culture of safety requires giving patients the freedom to inquire about all aspects of their care, including prescription drugs, diagnostics, and procedures. Patients who are knowledgeable can take a more active role in their own care and help achieve better results.

7.7.4.1 Medication Administration Record (MAR)

Medication administration records are systems that document the identification of the prescribing healthcare professional along with the time, date, and method of administering drugs. For the management of MEs, MAR can be used as a preventative and intervention technique. Error risk is reduced by typing orders and administration data when MAR is integrated into a computerised system. It is possible to configure the system to demand a co-signer for prescriptions (clinical pharmacologist can play a vital role here) that carry a significant risk, including opioids or anticoagulants.

7.7.4.2 Environmental Factors

MEs can largely be caused by environmental variables like noise, interruptions, and bad illumination, as well as fatigue and an overwhelming workload, as elucidated earlier in the chapter. To make sure that distractions are minimised and the workflow is optimised for the healthcare professional, hospitals should assess and monitor environmental conditions. Regardless of the degree of injury, hospital administration and doctors should look into the contributing factors when an ME occurs. MEs ought to be examined for patterns, and existing procedures ought to be enhanced and modified.

7.7.4.3 Medication Reconciliation

Medication reconciliation is a formal process that compares a patient's current medications to their medical records or medication orders to create an accurate list of their medications. This process is important to avoid medication errors like duplications, omissions, dosing errors, or drug interactions. Medication reconciliation aims to minimise adverse drug events at transition points throughout the continuum of care while precisely and fully reconciling medication to maximise drug therapy. This practice will support the sensible administration of pharmaceuticals. Medication tracking and reconciliation are made easier and more effective with the use of electronic records.

7.7.4.4 Electronic Medical Records (EMRs)

For certain hospital systems, the expenses of certain technologies might be prohibitive. In the absence of more technologically sophisticated possibilities, low-cost, low-tech instruments like EMRs should be utilised to guarantee the safest treatment practices. The adoption of EMRs is supported by several factors, including the possibility of reduced medication-related adverse events, improved health, and cost savings for healthcare. They make patient histories and records easily accessible to physicians and other healthcare providers.

7.8 Conclusion

Despite the fact that CPOE, EMRs, CDSS, barcoding and other technical advancements in medicine have demonstrated a reduction in medication errors, research has shown that malfunctioning computer interfaces, erroneous system communications, and insufficient decision assistance have all contributed to errors. In the era of electronic prescription, pharmaceutical-related adverse events include incorrect drug lists, out-of-date medication renewals, and inappropriate medication placement on electronic order sets. It is important to take faults or malfunctions into account when using this equipment or adhering to procedures. We need to accept that any scenario still carries the possibility of an error happening, and we are still evolving. Technology in the medical field will likely continue to progress in an effort to enhance patient safety and care, but it is important to understand that every new solution comes with an unexpected risk.

Safety depends on an ever-changing knowledge of how new risks are presented (mostly through non-punitive event reporting) as well as how new policies, procedures, and technological advancements affect workflow. For the institution to guarantee that all stakeholders in the varied interventions are included, spontaneous reporting of ME necessitates the implementation of a systematic procedure. Monitoring and preventing MEs on a timely basis will increase the quality of healthcare products, help healthcare professionals use drugs more rationally, and streamline system processes like prescription, order communication, product labelling, packaging, and nomenclature, compounding, dispensing, administration, distribution, and monitoring.

Bibliography

Agrawal A, Wu W, Khachewatsky I (2007) Evaluation of an electronic medication reconciliation system in inpatient setting in an acute care hospital. Stud Health Technol Inform 129:1027–1031

Alexopoulou A, Dourakis SP, Mantzoukis D, Pitsariotis T, Kandyli A, Deutsch M et al (2008) Adverse drug reactions as a cause of hospital admissions: a 6-month experience in a single center in Greece. Eur J Intern Med 19:505–510

Alldred DP, Raynor DK, Hughes C, Barber N, Chen TF, Spoor P (2013) Interventions to optimise prescribing for older people in care homes. Cochrane Database Syst Rev 2:CD009095

Ambwani S, Misra AK, Kumar R (2019) Medication errors: is it the hidden part of the submerged iceberg in our health-care system? Int J Appl Basic Med Res 9(3):135–142
Aronson JK (2004) Medication errors resulting from the confusion of drug names. Expert Opin Drug Saf 3:167–172
Aronson JK (2009) Medication errors: definitions and classification. Br J Clin Pharmacol 67:599–604
Avery A, Barber N, Ghaleb M, Franklin BD, Armstrong S, Crowe S et al (2012) Investigating the prevalence and causes of prescribing errors in general practice: the PRACtICe study. General Medical Council, London
Barker KN, Flynn EA, Pepper GA, Bates DW, Mikeal RL (2002) Medication errors observed in 36 health care facilities. Arch Intern Med 162(16):1897–1903
Bates DW, Gawande AA (2003) Improving safety with information technology. N Engl J Med 348:2526–2534
Bates DW, Boyle DL, Vander Vliet MB, Schneider J, Leape L (1995a) Relationship between medication errors and adverse drug events. J Gen Intern Med 10(4):199–205
Bates DW, Cullen DJ, Laird N, Petersen LA, Small SD, Servi D (1995b) Incidence of adverse drug events and potential adverse drug events. Implications for prevention. ADE prevention study group. JAMA 274:29–34
Bates DW, Leape LL, Cullen DJ, Laird N, Petersen LA, Teich JM et al (1998) Effect of computerized physician order entry and a team intervention on prevention of serious medication errors. JAMA 280(15):1311–1316
Bates DW, Teich JM, Lee J, Seger D, Kuperman GJ, Ma'Luf N et al (1999) The impact of computerized physician order entry on medication error prevention. J Am Med Inform Assoc 6(4):313–321
Blendon RJ, DesRoches CM, Brodie M, Benson JM, Rosen AB, Schneider E et al (2002) Views of practicing physicians and the public on medical errors. N Engl J Med 347(24):1933–1940
Briggs B (2003) CPOE order from chaos. Health Data Manag 11:44–48
Carvalho VT, Cassiani SHDB (2002) Erros na medicaçao e consequencias para profissionais de enfermagem e clientes: um estudo exploratório. Rev Latino-Am Enfermagem 10(4):523–529
Chan M, Nicklason F, Vial JH (2001) Adverse drug events as a cause of hospital admission in the elderly. Intern Med J 31:199–205
Choi JS, Lee WB, Rhee PL (2013) Cost-benefit analysis of electronic medical record system at a tertiary care hospital. Healthc Inform Res 19:205–214
Claesson CB, Burman K, Nilsson JL, Vinge E (1995) Prescription errors detected by Swedish pharmacists. Int J Pharm Pract 3:151–156
Classen DC, Bates DW (2011) Finding the meaning in meaningful use. N Engl J Med 365:855–858
de Vries EN, Ramrattan MA, Smorenburg SM, Gouma DJ, Boermeester MA (2008) The incidence and nature of in-hospital adverse events: a systematic review. Qual Saf Health Care 17:216–223
Duerden M, Avery AJ, Payne RA (2013) Polypharmacy and medicines optimisation: making it safe and sound. King's Fund, London, pp 17–25
Elliott RA, Camacho E, Jancovic D, Sculpher MJ, Faria R (2021) Economic analysis of the prevalence and clinical and economic burden of medication error in England. BMJ Qual Saf 30:96–105
European Collaborative Action on Medication Errors and Traceability (ECAMET) (2022) The urgent need to reduce medication errors in hospitals to prevent patient and second victim harm. https://ecamet.eu/wp-content/uploads/2022/03/ECAMET-White-Paper-Call-to-Action-March-2022-v2.pdf. Accessed 12 Apr 2024
Filik R, Purdy K, Gale A, Gerrett D (2006) Labeling of medicines and patient safety: evaluating methods of reducing drug name confusion. Hum Factors 48:39–47
Frush K, Hohenhaus S, Luo X, Gerardi M, Wiebe RA (2006) Evaluation of a web-based education program on reducing medication dosing error: a multicenter, randomized controlled trial. Pediatr Emerg Care 22:62–70
Gandhi TK, Weingart SN, Borus J, Seger AC, Peterson J, Burdick E et al (2003) Adverse drug events in ambulatory care. N Engl J Med 348:1556–1564

Gaur S, Sinha A, Srivastava B (2012) Medication errors in medicine wards in a tertiary care teaching hospital of a hill state in India. Asian J Pharm Life Sci 2:56–63

Hu SH, Capezuti E, Foust JB, Boltz MP, Kim H (2012) Medication discrepancy and potentially inappropriate medication in older Chinese-American home-care patients after hospital discharge. Am J Geriatr Pharmacother 10:284–295

Institute of Medicine (1999) To err is human: building a safer health system, 1st edn. National Academy Press, Washington

Jimenez Munioz AB, Muino Miguez A, Rodriguez Perez MP, Escribano MD, Duran Garcia ME, Sanjurjo SM (2010) Medication error prevalence. Int J Health Care Qual Assur 23(3):328–338

Kaufman DW, Kelly JP, Rosenberg L, Anderson TE, Mitchell AA (2002) Recent patterns of medication use in the ambulatory adult population of the United States: the Slone survey. JAMA 287(3):337–344

Khoja T, Neyaz Y, Qureshi NA, Magzoub MA, Haycox A, Walley T (2011) Medication errors in primary care in Riyadh city, Saudi Arabia. East Mediterr Health J 17:156–159

Kohn LT, Corrigan JM, Donaldson MD (eds) (2000) To err is human: building a safer health system. National Academy Press, Washington

Kumar KS, Venkateswarlu K, Ramesh A (2011) A study of medication administration errors in a tertiary care hospital. Indian J Pharm Pract 4:37–42

Kuperman GJ, Gibson RF (2003) Computer physician order entry: benefits, costs, and issues. Ann Intern Med 139:31–39

Lainer M, Mann E, Sonnichsen A (2013) Information technology interventions to improve medication safety in primary care: a systematic review. Int J Qual Health Care 25:590–598

Makaryus AN, Friedman EA (2005) Patients' understanding of their treatment plans and diagnosis at discharge. Mayo Clin Proc 80(8):991–994

Masotti P, McColl MA, Green M (2010) Adverse events experienced by homecare patients: a scoping review of the literature. Int J Qual Health Care 22:115–125

Mixon AS, Myers AP, Leak CL, Lou Jacobsen JM, Cawthon C, Goggins KM et al (2014 Aug) Characteristics associated with postdischarge medication errors. Mayo Clin Proc 89(8):1042–1051

National Coordinating Council for Medication Error Reporting and Prevention (2024) What is a medication error? https://www.nccmerp.org/about-medication-errors. Accessed 12 Apr 2024

Nichols P, Copeland TS, Craib IA, Hopkins P, Bruce DG (2008) Learning from error: identifying contributory causes of medication errors in an Australian hospital. Med J Aust 188:276–279

Norman DA (1981) Categorization of action slips. Psychol Rev 88:1–15

Parihar M, Passi GPR (2008) Medical errors in pediatric practice. Ind Pediatrics 45:586–589

Pedersen JS, Brereton L, Newbould J, Nolte E (2013) The puzzle of changing relationships. Does changing relationships between healthcare service users and providers improve the quality of care. The Health Foundation, London

Petersen LA, Brennan TA, O'Neil AC, Cook EF, Lee TH (1994) Does house staff discontinuity of care increase the risk for preventable adverse events? Ann Intern Med 121:866–872

Pirmohamed M, James S, Meakin S, Green C, Scott AK, Walley TJ et al (2004) Adverse drug reactions as cause of admission to hospital: prospective analysis of 18820 patients. BMJ 329:15–19

Reason JT (1990) Human Error. Cambridge University Press, Cambridge

Reason JT (2001) Understanding adverse events: human factors. In: Clinical risk management: enhancing patient safety. BMJ Publications, London, pp 9–30

Roque F, Herdeiro MT, Soares S, Teixeira Rodrigues A, Breitenfeld L, Figueiras A (2014) Educational interventions to improve prescription and dispensing of antibiotics: a systematic review. BMC Public Health 14:1276

Slight SP, Howard R, Ghaleb M, Barber N, Franklin BD, Avery AJ (2013) The causes of prescribing errors in English general practices: a qualitative study. Br J Gen Pract 63:e713–e720

Teich JM, Merchia PR, Schmiz JL, Kuperman GJ, Spurr CD, Bates DW (2000) Effects of computerized physician order entry on prescribing practices. Arch Intern Med 160:2741–2747

The Leapfrog Group's Patient Safety Practices (2004) The potential benefits of universal adoption. https://citeseerx.ist.psu.edu/document?repid=rep1&type=pdf&doi=197d47c73d8b0b3b092aad5393776f36cf41ae4d. Accessed on 12 Apr 2024

Westbrook JI, Woods A, Rob MI, Dunsmuir WT, Day RO (2010) Association of interruptions with an increased risk and severity of medication administration errors. Arch Intern Med 170(8):683–690

World Health Organization (2009) The conceptual framework for the international classification for patient safety. https://www.who.int/publications/i/item/WHO-IER-PSP-2010.2. Accessed 12 Apr 2024

Zavaleta-Bustos M, Castro-Pastrana LI, Reyes-Hernandez I, Lopez-Luna MA, Bermudez-Camps IB (2008) Prescription errors in a primary care university unit: urgency of pharmaceutical care in Mexico. Rev Bras Cienc Farm 44:115–125

Drug Use in Pregnancy and Lactation (Perinatal Pharmacology)

8

Vinothini Anandabaskar, Nishanthi Anandabaskar, and M. Shanthi

Abstract

Clinical pharmacology deals with the pharmacokinetics and pharmacodynamics of various drugs acting in the human system. In pregnancy and lactation, marked physiological variations affect the drug response with a special concern on fetal teratogenesis. Thus, the drugs must be used cautiously in pregnancy, lactation, and in women with childbearing potential. A considerable challenge is faced due to the paucity of available data, as pregnant and lactating women are excluded from most drug trials. The medications must be prescribed keeping in mind the risk vs benefit of the drug administration to the women. Also, the drugs should not be withheld due to their teratogenic effect, during life-threatening emergencies or serious illness to the mother. Hence, the art of drug prescribing in the perinatal period needs careful clinical discretion and a complete understanding of perinatal pharmacology. This chapter gives a bird's eye view of drug use in pregnancy and lactation.

Keywords

Teratogens · Placental barrier · Organogenesis · Embryopathy · Thalidomide

V. Anandabaskar
Department of Obstetrics and Gynaecology, Sri Ramachandra Institute of Higher Education and Research (SRIHER), Chennai, Tamil Nadu, India

N. Anandabaskar (✉) · M. Shanthi
Department of Pharmacology, Sri Manakula Vinayagar Medical College and Hospital, Puducherry, Puducherry, India

A. Arivazhahan et al. (eds.), *Introduction to Basics of Pharmacology and Toxicology*,
https://doi.org/10.1007/978-981-95-1920-0_8

8.1 Introduction

The drugs administered to pregnant and lactating mothers can cause significant fetal and neonatal risks, hence they must be used with caution. They are given taking into consideration the risk vs. benefit of the drug administration. Moreover, the safety profile of certain drugs in pregnancy and lactation is not completely studied, further limiting the use of these drugs. The drugs are given in their minimum effective dose to reduce their adverse effects. At the same time, in women with severe medical and surgical disorders, treatment should not be delayed or denied just considering the fetal risk.

8.1.1 Historical Background

The importance of drug labelling and its effects on the fetus was realized after the thalidomide disaster in 1957. The drug was used for the treatment of morning sickness and insomnia in pregnant women. This was soon followed by multiple reports of severe limb deformity called *phocomelia*, and hence the drug was withdrawn from the market in 1961. This led to the formulation of several government regulations restricting drug use in pregnancy.

8.2 Effect of Drugs in Pregnancy

The possible effects of drugs in pregnancy include the following:

(a) *Teratogenicity*: The teratogenic effect is detected at birth or in the postnatal period. For example, the limb abnormality caused by thalidomide.
(b) *Long-term latency*: The teratogenic effect is detected following a long latency period postnatally. For example, vaginal adenocarcinoma is seen in female fetuses exposed to diethylstilbesterol (DES) in-utero. This malignancy is not detected until after puberty.
(c) *Impaired intellectual or social development*: For example, in-utero exposure to phenobarbital or sodium valproate can cause cognitive impairment, intellectual disability, or maladaptive behavior in childhood.

8.3 Teratogenesis

A teratogen is an agent which acts irreversibly to alter the growth, structure, or function of the embryo or the fetus.

Teratogens can be of various types, which include:

- Viruses (e.g., Rubella, Cytomegalovirus, Varicella).
- Parasites (e.g., Toxoplasmosis).

- Spirochetes.
- Environmental factors (e.g., Radiation).
- Chemicals and heavy metals.
- Therapeutic agents (e.g., Lithium, Isotretinoin, Phenytoin, Warfarin).

The teratogenic effect depends on various factors like duration of exposure, quantity, concentration of the drug or chemical agent, and the timing of its exposure. Among them, the timing of exposure plays a significant role in deciding the extent of fetopathic or embryopathic effect (Fig. 8.1 and Table 8.1).

For instance, NSAIDs like indomethacin cause vascular disruptions if exposed in the early trimester, whereas the same drug causes premature closure of ductus arteriosus or renal failure if exposed after 32 weeks of gestation. Similarly, warfarin causes embryopathy in first trimester and causes hemorrhagic complications if exposed in the later trimesters.

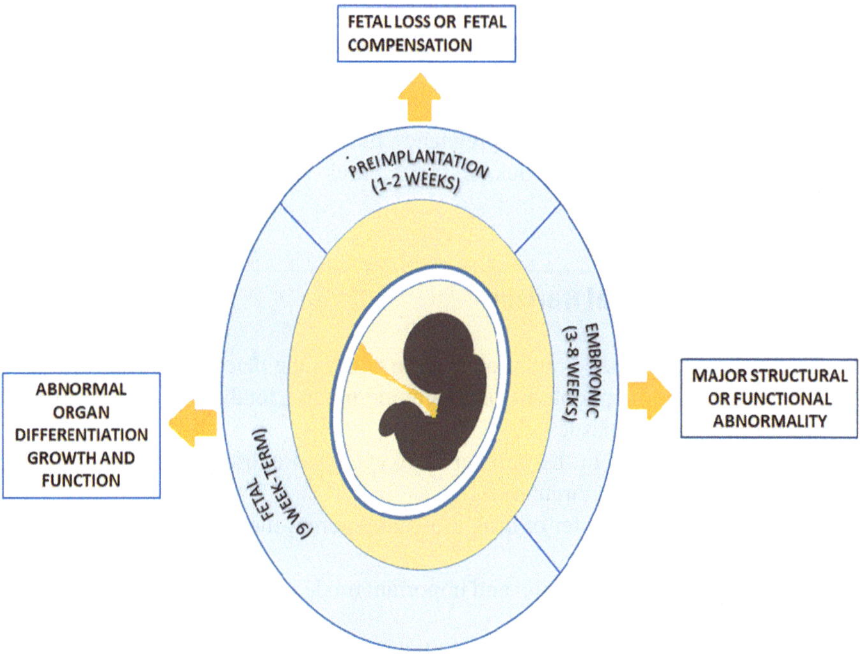

Fig. 8.1 Critical periods of fetal/embryonic development and the effects of teratogens

Table 8.1 Timing of teratogen exposure and its fetopathic/embryopathic effects

Periods of fetal/embryonic development	Effect in the fetus/embryo
Pre-implantation phase	"*All or none phenomenon*" Any insult to the embryo in the implantation phase depends on the number of cells damaged If large number of cells are affected, the insult will cause embryonic loss If few cells are disrupted, the embryo is protected through a phenomenon called "compensation", thus the fetus survives without any birth defects
Embryonic period/ period of organogenesis	This is the period of *maximal vulnerability* Any damage to fetus at this period results in structural or functional congenital abnormalities
Fetal period	This period is characterized by continued maturation and functional development Even during this period certain organs remain vulnerable

8.4 Physiological Pregnancy Changes and Their Impact on Drug Pharmacokinetics

Various physiological changes in pregnancy have been found to cause significant changes in the pharmacokinetics of drugs, thus altering their efficacy (Refer Table 8.2).

8.5 The Placental Barrier

- The maternal and fetal circulation is separated by the placental barrier.
- It is composed of trophoblasts, basement membrane, fetal capillary wall, and the intervening stromal tissue.
- It plays a major role in the transfer of oxygen and nutrients from the maternal circulation to the fetal circulation.
- It also permits the transfer of drug molecules across the barrier producing undesirable effects.
- Diffusion is the most common and important mode of transfer of drugs across the placental barrier.
- Most of the drugs cross the placental barrier to some extent except heparin and insulin.

8.5.1 Factors Influencing Trans-Placental Transfer of Drugs

The various factors that influence the trans-placental transfer of drugs include the following:

Table 8.2 The influence of physiological pregnancy changes on drug pharmacokinetics

Sl. no.	Physiological changes in pregnancy	Changes in drug pharmacokinetics
1.	**Cardiovascular system/hemodynamic changes**	
	Increased plasma volume	Volume of distribution of all drugs increases
	Increased cardiac output	Increased intramuscular drug absorption
	Decreased albumin and α_1-acid glycoprotein concentration	Increased free drug concentration of drugs that are normally highly plasma protein bound Shortening of their elimination half-life
2.	**Gastrointestinal system**	
	Delayed gastric emptying and prolonged small bowel transit time	Decrease in Cmax and increase in Tmax of rapidly acting orally administered drugs
	Increased gastric pH (due to decreased gastric acid production and increased mucous secretion)	Decreased absorption of weak acids (e.g., aspirin) since they will be predominantly ionized Increased absorption of weak bases (e.g., caffeine) since they will be predominantly unionized
	Nausea and vomiting in early pregnancy	Decreased drug absorption due to vomiting
3.	**Renal system**	
	Increased renal blood flow	Enhanced renal clearance of drugs
	A glomerular filtration rate (GFR) increases by 50% in pregnancy	
4.	**Respiratory system**	
	Increased alveolar ventilation	Enhanced alveolar drug absorption.
5.	Changes in the placental cytochrome P450 enzyme activity	Causes changes in the drug metabolism. For example, the enzyme CYP3A4 activity is increased, resulting in rapid clearance of its substrate
6.	Increased maternal body fat	Increased volume of distribution of lipophilic drugs

Cmax maximum serum concentration, *Tmax* time to maximum concentration

1. Molecular weight: Drugs with molecular weight less than 600 Daltons readily cross the placenta.
2. The drug concentration gradient across the placenta.
3. Placental thickness, surface area, and uteroplacental blood flow alter the rate of diffusion of drugs.
4. Placental drug metabolism: Placental enzymes contribute to metabolism of some drugs limiting their transfer to the fetus.
5. The presence of placental drug transporters facilitates influx and efflux of drugs across the placental barrier.
6. Protein binding of the drugs: The drugs which are unbound readily cross the placental membrane.
7. Lipid-soluble drugs are readily transferred across the placenta.
8. Fetal plasma is more acidic and hence it leads to anion trapping of basic drugs.
9. Variations in placentation: Responsible for interspecies variability in response to a particular drug or chemical agent. This explains why some drugs act as terato-

gens in humans but not in animals and vice versa. For example, thalidomide was not found to be a teratogen in rats and mice, but it is a potent human teratogen.

8.6 Risk Stratification of Drugs Used in Pregnancy

- FDA (US Food and Drug Administration) formulated guidelines for risk stratification of drugs used in pregnancy and lactation.
- This serves as a therapeutic guide for prescribing medications in pregnancy and lactation.

8.6.1 Food and Drug Administration (FDA) Classification for Drug Use in Pregnancy

The letters A-X summarized the available evidence of fetal risk associated with drug use in pregnancy, based on human and animal studies (Refer Table 8.3).

8.6.2 Pregnancy and Lactation Labeling Rule (PLLR)

The pregnancy letter categories (A-X) were replaced by the pregnancy and lactation labelling rule, which came into effect from 2015. The drugs of the same letter category had different risks associated, hence the information about the drugs was considered inadequate and oversimplified.

Table 8.3 FDA classification for drug use in pregnancy

FDA Category (USA) (was in effect from 1979–2015)	Definitions
A—controlled studies show no risk	Adequate, well-controlled studies in pregnant women have not shown any risk to the fetus in the first 3 months of pregnancy, and there is no evidence of later risk either
B—no evidence of risk in humans	There have been no adequate or well-controlled studies in women, but studies using animals have not found any risk to the fetus Or Animal studies have found risk that was not confirmed by adequate studies in pregnant women.
C—risks cannot be ruled out	No adequate, well-controlled studies in women, but studies using animals have shown a harmful effect on the fetus Or There have not been any studies in either women or animals
D—positive evidence of risk	There is clear evidence of risk to the human fetus but the benefits may outweigh the risk for pregnant women who have the serious condition that cannot be treated effectively with the safer drug
X—contraindicated in pregnancy	There is clear evidence that the medication causes abnormalities in the fetus. The risks outweigh any potential benefits for women who are pregnant

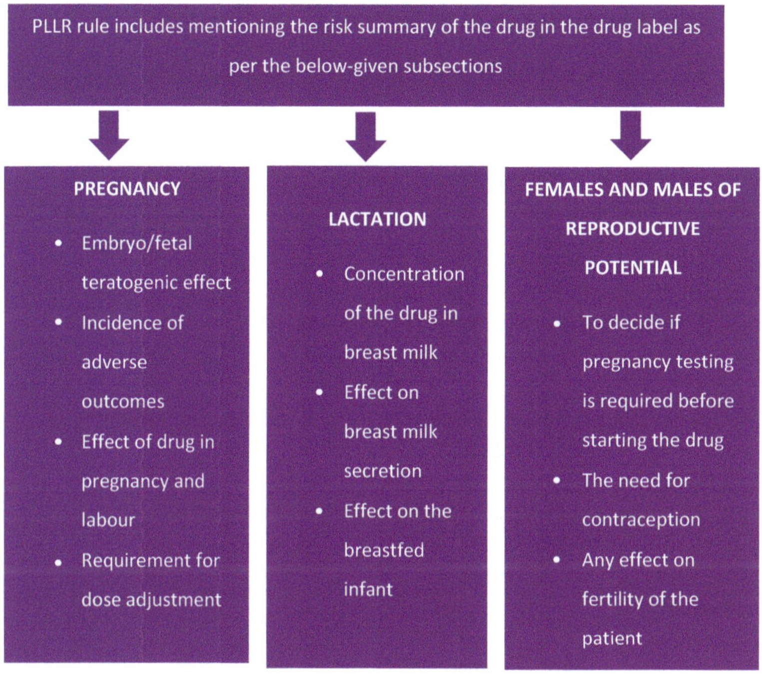

Fig. 8.2 Pregnancy and lactation labeling rule

The labeling rule includes a detailed description about the drug risks and other relevant information required by the physician to assess the risk vs. benefit ratio (Refer Fig. 8.2).

8.7 Drug Use in Lactation

- The rate of excretion of drug in breast milk depends on the following factors:
  - Lipid solubility.
  - Molecular weight.
  - Degree of protein binding.
  - Degree of ionization of the drug.
- Highly lipid-soluble drugs, drugs with low molecular weight, low protein binding, and non-ionized molecules are excreted more in the breast milk. The concentration of the drug in breast milk is proportional to the maternal serum drug concentrations.
- The major concern is the slow elimination of drugs in the infant due to immature enzyme system. Hence, the benefits of breastfeeding should be weighed against the risk of drug exposure to the infant.

8.7.1 Drugs Contraindicated During Breastfeeding

1. Cytotoxic drugs: Drugs like cyclosporine, cyclophosphamide, methotrexate, and doxorubicin have cytotoxic effect in the infants causing suppression of their immune system.
2. Drugs of abuse like cocaine, amphetamines.
3. Radioactive substances.

   (a) Iodine (^{131}I)—breastfeeding to be withheld for 2 to 14 days.
   (b) Radioactive sodium—breastfeeding to be withheld for 4 days.
   (c) Gallium-67—breastfeeding to be withheld for 2 weeks.
   (d) Technetium-99—breastfeeding to be withheld for 15 hours to 3 days.

A comprehensive list of some commonly known drugs, their effects in pregnancy and lactation are given in Table 8.4.

Table 8.4 List of some common drugs and their effects in pregnancy and lactation

Sl. no.	Drug name	Pregnancy risk	Lactation risk
Antimicrobials			
1.	**Penicillin**	Very low risk of teratogenesis in human studies	Penicillin and its derivatives are safe in nursing mothers No adverse effects noted with the therapeutic doses
2.	**Ampicillin/Sulbactam**	Risk of cleft lip and palate in the first trimester	Compatible
3.	**Amoxicillin/ clavulanate**	Amoxicillin associated with oral clefts Some reports of necrotizing enterocolitis with clavulanic acid	Mostly safe in lactation
4.	**Cephalosporins**	Very low risk in human studies	Compatible
5.	**Tetracyclines**	Contraindicated in the first and second trimester due to interference with bone mineralization They bind firmly by chelation in developing teeth and bones, cause greyish brown discoloration of deciduous teeth and inhibition of bone growth	Tetracycline has high affinity to calcium and protein, limiting its absorption from breast milk Compatible
6.	**Erythromycin**	Low embryo-fetal risk. Esolate salt causes hepatotoxicity in pregnancy	Compatible
7.	**Azithromycin**	Very low risk of teratogenesis in human studies	Compatible
8.	**Aminoglycosides**	Ototoxicity and nephrotoxicity Amikacin has less nephrotoxic effect compared to gentamycin	They have poor oral absorption, risk is minimal

(continued)

Table 8.4 (continued)

Sl. no.	Drug name	Pregnancy risk	Lactation risk
9.	**Sulfonamides**	It displaces bilirubin from its protein binding sites, hence can worsen neonatal hyperbilirubinemia if given near the time of preterm delivery Avoided in glucose-6-phosphate dehydrogenase (G6PD)-deficient mothers as they cause dose-related hemolysis in neonates. Fetus is not affected as the free bile acids are cleared by the placenta	Avoided in preterm, glucose-6-phosphate dehydrogenase-deficient infants
10.	**Nitrofurantoin**	First-trimester exposure increases the risk of cleft lip by two-fold Third trimester—Risk of hemolytic anemia in exposed newborns	Limited human studies. Probably compatible
11.	**Fluroquinolones**	Cartilage damage They cross the placenta and have a high affinity for bone tissue and cartilage	Ciprofloxacin causes neonatal clostridium difficile pseudomembranous colitis
12.	**Chloramphenicol**	Causes Grey baby syndrome They manifest as abdominal distension, respiratory abnormality, vascular collapse with ashen grey color	Has a potential for idiosyncratic bone marrow toxicity Safe to be avoided in lactation
13.	***Antimycobacterial drugs*** (isoniazid, rifampin, pyrazinamide, ethambutol)	Limited data available. Low risk of teratogenesis. Can be given as the benefit exceeds the risk	Probably compatible
14.	**Fluconazole**	Associated with a pattern of congenital malformations resembling the autosomal recessive *Antley-bixler syndrome* The abnormalities are oral clefts, abnormal facies, cardiac, skull, and long bone abnormalities noted with high dose treatment of 400-800 mg daily Lower doses are associated with only a small increase in rates of cardiac malformations	Compatible
15.	**Amphotericin B**	Very low risk of teratogenesis in animal studies	No established studies in lactation
16.	**Acyclovir**	Very low risk of teratogenesis in human data	Compatible

(continued)

Table 8.4 (continued)

Sl. no.	Drug name	Pregnancy risk	Lactation risk
17.	***Anti-retroviral drugs*** (zidovudine, Nevirapine)	Limited human pregnancy data Should be used based on risk vs benefit ratio	Contraindicated
18.	***Efavirenz***	Reports of increased incidence of neural tube defects and ocular abnormalities noted in animal study	Contraindicated
19.	***Antimalarials:*** (Hydroxychloroquine, Mefloquine, Proguanil Artemether/ Lumefantrine)	Limited pregnancy data Should be used based on risk vs benefit ratio	Limited human studies. Probably compatible
20.	**Primaquine**	Causes acute hemolytic anemia in G6PD-deficient fetus Contraindicated	Potential toxic effects observed
21.	**Metronidazole**	Use with caution in the first trimester	Excreted in breast milk. Discontinue breastfeeding for 12–24 hours following drug therapy
22.	**Albendazole**	Very low risk in pregnancy studies	Limited human studies. Probably compatible
NSAIDS			
1.	**Aspirin**	Doses for antiplatelet activity (60-150 mg/day): No evidence of fetal harm Doses for anti-inflammatory effect (325-650 mg/day): Risk of intrauterine growth restriction (IUGR) if used in the third trimester Depressed platelet function and purpura in newborn Excessive intrapartum and postpartum bleeding if taken within a week of delivery Causes fetal vascular disruption, gastroschisis, small intestinal atresia, premature closure of ductus arteriosus	Use cautiously in patients on high dose of aspirin
2.	**Diclofenac**	Avoid in first and third trimesters due to risk of pulmonary hypertension and congenital malformations	Limited human studies. Probably compatible

(continued)

Table 8.4 (continued)

Sl. no.	Drug name	Pregnancy risk	Lactation risk
3.	**Ibuprofen**	Avoid in first and third trimesters due to risk of Persistent pulmonary hypertension Congenital malformations like oral clefts and cardiac anomalies	Compatible
4.	**Indomethacin**	Causes spontaneous abortions Constriction of ductus arteriosus and oligohydramnios in third trimester Neonatal pulmonary artery hypertension with chronic use Causes reduced fetal urine production and eventually oligohydramnios Increased risk of bronchopulmonary dysplasia, severe intraventricular hemorrhage, and necrotizing enterocolitis noted	Limited human studies. Probably compatible
5.	**Acetaminophen**	Human data shows low risk. Few reports show increased risk of autism, milestone delay, hence regular use to be avoided	Compatible with breastfeeding
Drugs acting on cardiovascular system			
1.	**Angiotensin-converting enzyme inhibitors** (ACEIs) And **angiotensin receptor blockers** (ARBs)	The drug crosses the placenta, hence they cause fetal renal tubular dysplasia, resulting in irreversible renal damage and oligohydramnios The fetus eventually develops renal failure, anemia, hypocalvaria, fetal limb contractures, patent ductus arteriosus, aortic arch obstruction, hypoplastic lung development, and finally fetal death The above features are called ACE inhibitor embryopathy	Trace quantities excreted in breast milk, hence lowest effective dose should be used Compatible with breastfeeding
2.	**Atenolol**	Crosses the placenta. Some reports suggest risk of intrauterine growth restriction (IUGR)	To be avoided. Can cause neonatal bradycardia
3.	**Amlodipine**	No evidence of teratogenicity in animal studies	No well-controlled studies. Probable compatibility

(continued)

Table 8.4 (continued)

Sl. no.	Drug name	Pregnancy risk	Lactation risk
4.	**Labetalol**	Large doses cause fetal bradycardia, hypoglycemia, pericardial effusion, and myocardial hypertrophy	Compatible
5.	**Amiodarone**	Reports of fetal hypothyroidism and neurodevelopmental abnormalities	Neonatal hypothyroidism reported. Contraindicated
6.	**Digoxin**	No significant teratogenic effect	Even though digoxin is excreted in a small amount into breast milk, significant adverse effect is not noted in nursing infants
7.	**Acetazolamide**	No well-controlled studies in humans. Few studies in rodents show skeletal abnormalities	Compatible Neonatal exposure is less than 0.5% of maternal serum levels
8.	**Furosemide**	Human data shows low risk	Probable compatibility
9.	**Atorvastatin**	No adequate human studies. Reports of fetal limb abnormalities and growth restriction present	No well-controlled studies
Insulin			
1.	**Regular insulin**	Doesn't cross the placenta. Hence it is the drug of choice for diabetes in pregnancy	Compatible
Oral hypoglycemic drugs			
1.	**Metformin**	Can be given in pregnancy. No teratogenic defects reported	Compatible
2.	**Acarbose**	Animal studies show no teratogenic effect. No well-controlled studies in pregnant women	Limited human studies. Probably compatible as <2% drug is systemically absorbed
3.	**Glyburide (Glibenclamide)**	No fetal toxicity noted	Probable compatibility
Anti-histaminics			
1.	**Terfenadine:**	Increased risk of polydactyly	Compatible with breastfeeding
2.	**Pseudoephedrine**	Increased risk of gastroschisis in the first trimester	Compatible with breastfeeding
3.	**Diphenhydramine**	Causes neonatal depression if administered in labor Hence, the use of these drugs for trivial reasons is discouraged in pregnancy	Limited human data Probably compatible
4.	**Cetirizine**	Limited human studies. Animal studies suggest low risk	Limited human studies. Probably compatible

(continued)

Table 8.4 (continued)

Sl. no.	Drug name	Pregnancy risk	Lactation risk
5.	**Chlorpheniramine**	Compatible	Limited human studies. Probably compatible
6.	**Doxylamine**	Drug of choice for vomiting in pregnancy	Probable compatibility
Bronchodilators			
1.	**Terbutaline**	Few reports of cardiac defect noted. Avoided in first trimester	Probably compatible
2.	**Salmeterol**	Limited human studies No teratogenic effect identified	Probably compatible
3.	**Theophylline**	Compatible	Compatible
Anti-emetics			
1.	**Ondansetron**	Low risk of teratogenesis	Very few human studies, probably compatible
Proton pump inhibitor/H2 blocker			
1.	**Omeprazole**	Animal studies show low risk	Potential neonatal toxicity noted
2.	**Famotidine**	Compatible	Limited human studies. Probably compatible
Anticonvulsants			
1.	**Sodium valproate**	Causes fetal valproate syndrome, characterized by a distinct craniofacial appearance, limb abnormalities, neural tube defects, heart defects, central nervous system dysfunction Exposure in utero can cause poor cognitive development and a low intelligent quotient in school children	The neonatal serum concentration is less than 10% of maternal levels
2.	**Carbamazepine**	Causes facial dysmorphism, developmental delay, spina bifida, distal phalange, and finger nail hypoplasia In breastfed infants, rare reports of cholestatic hepatitis are reported	Compatible
3.	**Phenytoin**	Causes reduced folate absorption and hence lowers the serum folate levels Causes microcephaly, developmental delay, mental retardation, dysmorphic cranial features, hypoplasia of the distal phalanges and nails, and hypertelorism These features comprise the fetal hydantoin syndrome	Phenytoin is excreted in a minimal quantity in breast milk; thus, they are considered safe in lactating mothers

(continued)

Table 8.4 (continued)

Sl. no.	Drug name	Pregnancy risk	Lactation risk
4.	**Levetiracetam**	The newer agents like levetiracetam confer no fetal risk. But the reported data is less and requires long-term studies	Probably compatible
Anticoagulant drugs			
1.	**Heparin**	Does not cross the placenta, the drug of choice for patients requiring anti-coagulation	Excreted in breast milk and is not active orally
2.	**Warfarin**	It can readily cross the placenta Exposure from 6–10 weeks is associated with embryopathy—Fetal warfarin syndrome characterized by nasal hypoplasia, stippled epiphysis, depressed nasal bridge, choanal atresia, microphthalmia, optic atrophic, hypoplasia of extremities, heart disease, scoliosis, deafness and mental retardation, dandy walker malformation characterized by agenesis of corpus callosum and cerebellar vermian agenesis	Excreted only in an insignificant amount in breast milk
3.	**Enoxaparin**	Compatible	Compatible
Anti-thyroid drugs			
1.	**Propylthiouracil and methimazole**	Propylthiouracil (PTU) and methimazole induce fetal goiter in a dose-dependent manner The goal of treatment is to keep the mother slightly hyperthyroid There is an increased risk of agranulocytosis with methimazole and an increased risk of hepatotoxicity with propylthiouracil PTU is preferred to methimazole as methimazole is associated with scalp defects, aplasia cutis, esophageal atresia, and choanal atresia In 2009, FDA issued a black box warning stating that propylthiouracil causes serious liver toxicity Thus, the patients can be treated with PTU in the first trimester, which can later be switched to methimazole	Propylthiouracil avoided due to risk of liver failure Methimazole- compatible

(continued)

Table 8.4 (continued)

Sl. no.	Drug name	Pregnancy risk	Lactation risk
Anti-depressants			
1.	**Fluoxetine**	Anomalies like pulmonary valve stenosis, ventricular septal defect, and hypospadias noted	Potential toxic effect noted
2.	**Sertraline**	No adequate studies are present for sertraline	Not contraindicated
3.	**Paroxetine**	Associated with major teratogenic effects They have a two-fold increase in congenital cardiac malformations like atrial and ventricular septal defects with first-trimester exposures Late exposure is associated with neonatal behavioral syndrome characterized by transient neonatal complications like jitteriness, mild respiratory distress, transient tachypnea of newborn, weak cry, poor tone, feeding abnormalities, vomiting, hypoglycemia, and thermoregulatory instability	Breastfeeding is not contraindicated
4.	**Escitalopram**	Associated with neonatal serotonin syndrome, persistent pulmonary artery hypertension	Potential toxicity
Anxiolytics			
1.	**Benzodiazepines**	No significant risk of teratogenesis Alprazolam is rarely indicated in pregnancy. Abrupt cessation of treatment is associated with discontinuation emergent syndrome, characterized by neuropsychiatric, gastrointestinal, visual, and cardiovascular symptoms	Excreted into breast milk Causes neonatal lethargy, lethargy, and weight loss Hence better to avoid in lactating mothers due to its potential to alter the neurodevelopment
2.	**Diazepam**	Rarely cross the placenta Increased risk of oral clefts in first-trimester exposure but no long-term follow-up studies are present Prolonged CNS depression is noted in neonates exposed in utero Other symptoms are mild sedation, hypotonia, reluctance to suck, cyanosis, neonatal withdrawal symptoms, and floppy infant syndrome	Sedation effects observed in the infants

(continued)

Table 8.4 (continued)

Sl. no.	Drug name	Pregnancy risk	Lactation risk
3.	**Alprazolam**	No adequate reports. Neonatal withdrawal may be noted. No teratogenic effects observed	To be avoided due to the risk of neonatal withdrawal
Anti-psychotics			
1.	**Lithium**	Causes cardiac arrhythmias, hypoglycemia, nephrogenic diabetes insipidus, premature delivery, and floppy infant syndrome. Associated with Ebstein anomaly, with features of apical displacement of tricuspid valve resulting in severe tricuspid regurgitation and marked right atrial enlargement Neonatal lithium toxicity seen in exposure near term. Characterized by neonatal hypothyroidism, diabetes insipidus, cardiomegaly, bradycardia, cyanosis, hypotonia, and ECG abnormalities Hence, lithium dosage is to be decreased or the drug must be discontinued 2–3 days before delivery	Excreted in breast milk, the use in breastfeeding mothers is controversial
Retinoids			
1.	**Isotretinoin**	Contraindicated during pregnancy as they are potent teratogens. They are characterized by a characteristic pattern of craniofacial, cardiac, thymic, CNS anomalies, microtia, micrognathia, cleft palate, heart defects, retinal and optic nerve anomalies This is a pattern of neural crest defects called retinoic acid embryopathy Contraception must be advised 1 month before, during, and 1 month after the use of isotretinoin	Potential toxic effects observed
2.	**Acitretin (Vitamin A derivative)**	A potent teratogen. Contraindicated in pregnancy	Potential for toxicity. Better to be avoided

(continued)

Table 8.4 (continued)

Sl. no.	Drug name	Pregnancy risk	Lactation risk
Corticosteroid			
1.	**Prednisolone**	Human placenta metabolizes prednisone, reducing fetal exposure to less than 10% of maternal exposure Associated with cleft lip and palate in animal studies	Compatible
2.	**Betamethasone**	Improves fetal lung maturity. Improved perinatal outcome in preterm births	Limited human studies. Probably compatible
Antineoplastic drugs			
1.	**Cyclophosphamides**	They are alkylating agents causing damage to the developing fetal tissues They result in heritable DNA alterations in surviving cells Associated with high pregnancy loss rates The congenital malformation associated include skeletal abnormalities, limb defects, cleft palate, and eye abnormalities	Contraindicated
2.	**Methotrexate**	Can cause congenital malformations like craniofacial, axial skeletal/limb abnormalities, cardiopulmonary, developmental delay, and gastrointestinal abnormalities The craniofacial features are clover leaf-shaped skull, wide nasal bridge, low set ears, and micrognathia	It is contraindicated in breastfeeding mothers
3.	**Fluorouracil**	Structural anomalies noted in first-trimester exposures	No well-controlled studies in lactation
4.	**Azathioprine**	No adequate reports in human fetuses. Some reports show isolated skeletal defects	Probably compatible. No documented neonatal effects
5.	**Carboplatin**	Contraindicated (especially in the first trimester)	Contraindicated
Miscellaneous			
1.	**Folic acid**	Mandatory supplement in the first trimester to prevent neural tube defects	Compatible

(continued)

Table 8.4 (continued)

Sl. no.	Drug name	Pregnancy risk	Lactation risk
2.	**Caffeine**	A high dose of caffeine (equivalent to 6–8 cups of coffee/day) is associated with spontaneous abortions and low birth weight infants	Irritability and poor sleeping pattern may be observed in breastfed infants, if high dose is ingested
3.	**Ergotamine**	Contraindicated	Contraindicated
4.	**Calcitriol (Vitamin D)**	Compatible	Compatible
5.	**Diethylstilbestrol (DES)**	A known teratogen that causes vaginal clear cell adenocarcinoma, hypoplastic T-shaped uterine cavity, and withered fallopian tubes in female offspring.	Contraindicated
6.	**Thalidomide**	Causes phocomelia, characterized by the absence of one or more long bones, cardiac malformations, gastrointestinal abnormalities, eye anomalies, external ear malformations, and limb reduction defects The hands and feet are attached to the trunk occasionally by small rudimentary bones	Lack of adequate data in lactation

Bibliography

Al-Zidan RN (2021) Drugs in pregnancy: a handbook for pharmacists and physicians. Apple Academic Press, Burlington

Briggs GG, Freeman RK (2015) A reference guide to fetal and neonatal risk. Drugs in pregnancy and lactation, 10th edn. Wolters Kluwer Health, Philadelphia

Costantine MM (2014) Physiologic and pharmacokinetic changes in pregnancy. Front Pharmacol 5:65. https://doi.org/10.3389/fphar.2014.00065

Cunningham FG, Leveno KJ, Dashe JS, Hoffman BL, Spong CY, Casey BM (eds) (2022) Williams obstetrics, 26th edn. McGraw Hill, New York

Feghali M, Venkataramanan R, Caritis S (2015) Pharmacokinetics of drugs in pregnancy. Semin Perinatol 39(7):512–519. https://doi.org/10.1053/j.semperi.2015.08.003

Gabbe SG, Niebyl JR, Simpson JL, Landon MB, Galan HL, Jauniaux ERM et al (2012) Obstetrics: normal and problem pregnancies, 6th edn. Elsevier Saunders, Philadelphia

James D, Steer PJ, Weiner CP, Gonik B, Crowther CA, Robson SC (eds) (2011) High-risk pregnancy: management options, 4th edn. St Louis, Missouri, Elsevier Saunders

U.S Food & Drug Administration (FDA) (2021) Pregnancy and lactation labeling (Drugs) Final rule (PLLR) [modified 2021 May 3; Cited 2023 June 14]. Available from: https://www.fda.gov/drugs/labeling-information-drug-products/pregnancy-and-lactation-labeling-drugs-final-rule

Weiner CP, Mason C (2019) Drugs for pregnant and lactating women, 3rd edn. Elsevier, Phildelphia

Pediatric Pharmacology

9

Mirunalini Ravichandran and J. Arifunhera

Abstract

The pediatric age group includes a varied population, which does not express a linear change in body composition and function when progressing from birth into adolescence. Thus, there is an urgent need for lucidity in pediatric pharmacology. It is interesting to note that in infants and toddlers, orally administered drugs have varied absorption kinetics; while the gastric pH and emptying hinder the absorption, the immature intestinal mucosa hastens the process. Furthermore, it is observed that for children to attain complete adult homeostasis, it would take 10–12 years; thus, the larger vascular space, lower plasma protein concentrations, immature metabolism enzymes, and poor elimination process render drugs ineffective and, at times, expose them to adverse drug effects. The immature physiology of the age group makes it difficult to define the molecular soundness of the known drug mechanism in the population. This inability to understand the pharmacokinetics and pharmacodynamics stems from the lack of inclusivity of pediatric age groups in research. Further looking into the receptor physiology shows drastic variation in the expression of receptors in various tissues. For example, higher CNS expression of GABA A receptors in infants compared to older children and adults. In identifying these drawbacks, it is essential for one to understand the importance of flexible formulation options, the inclusion of a wide dose range, and a vigilant lookout for adverse drug events at every possible encounter.

M. Ravichandran (✉)
Department of Pharmacology, Jawaharlal Institute of Postgraduate Medical Education and Research (JIPMER), Puducherry, Puducherry, India

J. Arifunhera
Department of Pharmacology, Chettinad Hospital & Research Institute, Chennai, Tamil Nadu, India

A. Arivazhahan et al. (eds.), *Introduction to Basics of Pharmacology and Toxicology*,
https://doi.org/10.1007/978-981-95-1920-0_9

Keywords

Pediatric pharmacokinetics · Pharmacodynamics · Formulation · Pediatric dosing

9.1 Introduction

It is a widely accepted and debated fact that children are not miniature adults, hence the need for age-appropriate pharmacotherapy. The current pediatric therapy involves off-label prescribing with dose adjustment concerning weight and other pharmacokinetic properties. In addition, during the first decade of life, growth is not a linear process because changes in body composition and the function of the organs are dynamic and discordant, which calls for the individualization of drug doses for children.

9.2 Pediatric Pharmacology

If rational drug use and evidence-based treatment are expected, clinical trials should be conducted in pediatric subpopulations. Unfortunately, the lack of such studies over the past century has led to an incomplete understanding of the pharmacotherapeutic diaspora in the pediatric age group, leaving them devoid of the benefits of complete knowledge of the kinetic and dynamic study of drugs would provide and expose them to harm which is difficult to avoid due to lack in the same thereof.

9.3 Ontogeny and Pharmacology

It is a well-known fact that most developmental changes occur during the first year of life; hence, ontogeny plays a crucial role in deciding the pharmacotherapy of young children. The efficacy or safety or any other characteristics of a drug majorly depend on the two most critical pharmacological parameters the Pharmacokinetic and the Pharmacodynamics parameters of the drug, which will be discussed in the following sections.

9.3.1 Pharmacokinetics

Researchers have extensively studied to understand the pharmacokinetics of drugs in the pediatric population. Because the physiology of a pediatric human being is unique and ever so changing with development, hence what happens to a drug in a young child is drastically different from that in an adult (Fig. 9.1). In this section, pharmacokinetics relevant to pediatric age group will be dealt under the following headings.

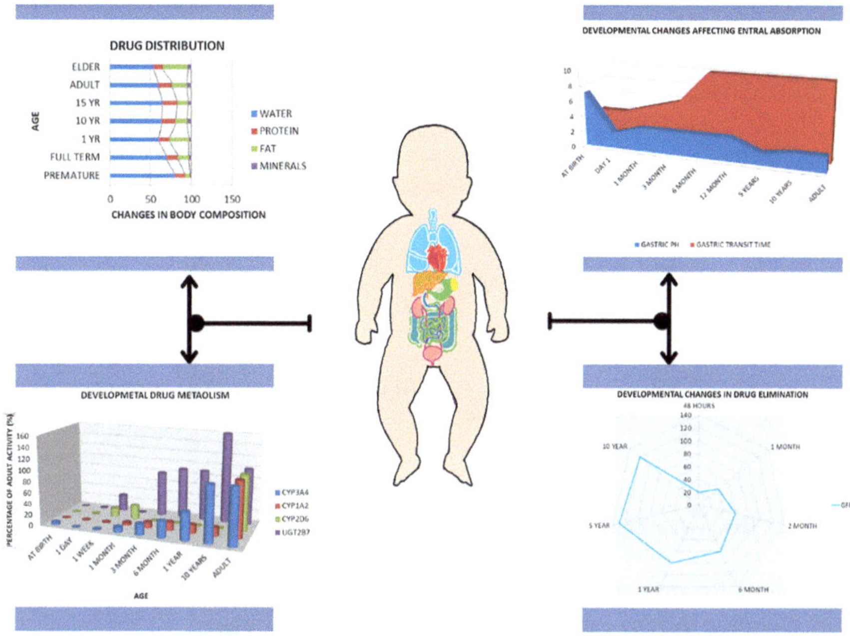

Fig. 9.1 Pediatric ontogeny changes: body composition changes, changes in enteral absorption, drug metabolism changes, and changes in drug elimination

1. Absorption
2. Distribution
3. Metabolism
4. Excretion

9.3.1.1 Absorption

Of the pharmacokinetic parameters, absorption is a vital and readily modifiable, hence given a higher weightage pertaining to pediatric drug disposition. For better understanding, absorption is classified based on the route of administration (Fig. 9.2 classifies absorption) and discussed in the same order.

9.3.1.2 Enteral Absorption

The most crucial route of absorption in the pediatric population is the enteral route of absorption (primarily oral) because most of the formulations for drugs for this age group are palatable tablets and syrups. In addition, developmental changes affect both the rate and extent of oral drug absorption.

The factors that play a vital role in enteral absorption are

- Gastric and intestinal pH
- Gastric and intestinal transit time
- Intestinal drug-metabolizing enzymes and transporters

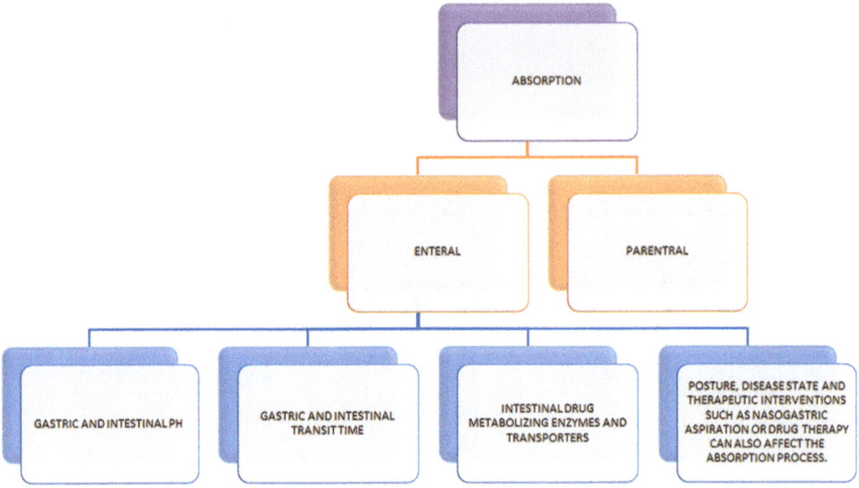

Fig. 9.2 Classification of the absorption process and factors governing it

- Posture, disease state, and therapeutic interventions such as nasogastric aspiration or drug therapy can also affect the absorption process.

9.3.1.3 Gastric and Intestinal pH

Adult values of gastric pH (1.5 to 2) are reached by 3 to 7 years of age. When the baby is born, the gastric pH is the highest (neutral pH range 6 to 8) but drops to the acidic range within a few hours, then gradually rises to typical adult values. The majority of the marketed drugs are weak bases; hence low pH of the stomach favors easy drug dissolution. A better determinant of gastric pH is the timing of meals rather than the age-related alterations in basal HCL secretion, as an exponential increase in pH is observed postprandially.

Clinical importance:

1. Phenytoin and phenobarbital (weak acid, narrow therapeutic index)—to achieve sufficient therapeutic levels, frequent dosing is required in young children
2. Beta-lactam antibiotics, e.g., benzylpenicillin (acid labile drugs)—due to the increased acidic pH observed in neonates, there warrants a dosage titration as increased absorption is observed

   * smaller stomach volumes—impaired drug dissolution

Changes in biliary functions in a growing child affect the absorption of lipophilic drugs. Even though blood levels of bile acids and *Glutathione (GSH)* conjugation exceed those of the adult values, due to immature conjugation and bile acid transport in the pediatric age group, low intra-intestinal levels are observed, thereby affecting the absorption of the drug.

9.3.1.4 Gastric and Intestinal Transit Time

The average adult gastric emptying time is 20 min for liquids. Gastric and intestinal transit time regulates the amount and duration of drug exposure to gastrointestinal mucosa and its absorption.

In neonates, gastric emptying time (GET) is delayed, delaying the absorption of orally administered drugs that are majorly absorbed in the small intestine, therefore waiting for peak concentration in blood. By 6–8 months of age, GET becomes faster and on par with the adult GET. Another critical factor is the maturity of the gastric and intestinal mucosa, which is fully attained only by 4 months of age, and the fully functional intestinal enzyme and transporter system, which matures by 6–12 months. At times, as the drug absorptive and restrictive processes of the small intestine are saturable, the GET delay in the pediatric age group prevents the overwhelming of intestinal absorption processes (Table 9.1).

9.3.1.5 Intestinal Drug-Metabolizing Enzymes and Transporters

Regarding intestinal drug-metabolizing enzymes and transporters, the CYP3A and P-glycoprotein are the most commonly found and studied enzyme and transporter per se. Studies on pediatric developmental differences in the same are very scarcely found. Other intestinal drug metabolizing enzymes are CYP1A, N-acetyltransferase, xanthine oxidase, and glutathione-S-transferase. The major enzyme CYP3A protein which accounts for 70% of the enzyme content in intestine gradually increases in

Table 9.1 Anatomical and functional changes in absorption and their significance in pediatric ontogeny

Parameter	Changes	Significance
Villi	Maturation—20 weeks After birth, first few weeks increase in surface area and density	One of the primary contributing parameters of intestinal absorption
Enterocyte height	14% increase from infancy to adulthood	No significance as microvilli and brush border density show no changes
Perfusion	First few weeks of life- mesenteric blood flow decreased	Affects absorption of acidic drugs, which already struggle due to the unfavorable pH of small intestine
Small intestine transit time	Impaired in preterm neonates	Evidence is insufficient
Bile acids	Rapid mutation of the process governing bile acid synthesis—Most evident in neonates and preterm infants	Below critical micelle concentrations—Reduced absorption of lipophilic drugs Bile acids present in breast milk
Gut microbiota	Maturation of intestinal microbiome—Responsible for bile acid deconjugation and the formation of secondary bile acids Oral bioavailability—Through direct drug metabolism	Rapid changes after birth

the first few months of life and gradually decreases to adult levels. P-gp is detected as early as 11–14 weeks in liver but only by 1 month in the intestine and adult levels are reached only by 6–12 months. As the CYP3A and P-gp share common substrates, they play a vital role in compromising bioavailability of orally administered drugs.

9.3.2 Parenteral Absorption

9.3.2.1 Intravenous Absorption

Most drugs are given intravenously to ensure maximum bioavailability, but the invasiveness of the administration makes it a less desirable route of administration.

9.3.2.2 Extravascular Absorption

- Topical route:

  Due to the immature nature of the integumentary system, topical absorption is known to have higher toxicity rates. In preterm neonates, a thinner stratum corneum enhances the absorption of drugs. Throughout childhood, cutaneous perfusion and hydration are higher than in adults, increasing the topical absorption of drugs. This risk increases on par with diseases like eczema.
- Body Surface Area:

  In pediatrics, medication is dosed very frequently based on body surface area (BSA). BSA correlates with physiological processes such as cardiac output, blood volume, and organ development. During development and growth, even though the volume of the body increases, the body surface area does not increase at the same rate. Infants have relatively larger BSA as compared to adults. This difference serves to maximize the topical dose of a drug in newborns. A newborn adult proportion of 1:9 is seen with respect to BSA. This principle does not apply to dose topical medications in infants clinically.
- Intramuscular absorption:

  Absorption through this route has a bimodal response *that is* due to immature contraction of muscles and decreased blood supply in neonates drug absorption is hampered, but the increased density of blood vessels in infant muscles as compared to children offsets the influence of the above-mentioned factors on bioavailability.
- Rectal absorption:

  In young children amplitude of rectal contraction is increased; hence easy expulsion of the suppository is seen. But certain drugs like diazepam are absorbed readily from the rectum and reach therapeutic concentration faster in blood. Bioavailability of rectally absorbed drugs is higher in young children than in older children.
- Inhalational route:

  Developmental changes in respiratory parameters play a vital role in determining the amount of drug reaching the absorption site and drug absorption per se.

But in children maximum amount of drug is found accumulated in the oral cavity; hence the amount of drug reaching the respiratory absorption surface is compromised.

9.3.3 Distribution

Factors like vascular perfusion, body composition, tissue binding characteristics, and the extent of plasma protein binding play a vital role in determining the distribution of the drug. For example, regarding body composition, in preterm neonates, neonates, and infants, larger extracellular and interstitial spaces are seen in comparison with children >12 years of age and adults. This physiological difference forms the basis for lower plasma concentrations of hydrophilic drugs, which tend to distribute in these spaces (for lipophilic drugs show the opposite characteristics) especially when administered in weight-based dosage.

Fo example, in neonates and young children (< 10 years as defined by WHO), hydrophilic drugs like aminoglycosides and paracetamol exhibit a larger volume of distribution in comparison to lipophilic medications like diazepam and propofol.

9.3.3.1 Protein Binding

In pediatric age group, the essential plasma drug binding proteins—albumin, alpha 1 glycoprotein, and plasma globulin—are found in concentrations much lower than in adults; hence plasma protein binding of drugs is also reduced in comparison. However, the protein binding reaches adult levels within the third year of life for acidic drugs. Thus, altered drug kinetics may be due to lower concentrations of plasma proteins or the immaturity of the available proteins.

Clinical implication:

In instances of impaired renal function, there is an exponential increase in the free drug plasma concentration in adults, but in neonates, even when the concentrations are within therapeutic levels, adverse drug reactions are seen. For example, CNS adverse effects are seen with phenytoin within its therapeutic range in neonates.

9.3.3.2 Drug Transporters

Drug transporter proteins play a vital role in drug distribution and elimination. In neonates and infants, drug transporter proteins follow developmental patterns and are expressed differently in various tissues and sites. The most relevant transporter proteins seen in the pediatric age group are glycoprotein P and Multidrug-Resistant protein 1 (MRP1).

9.3.4 Metabolism

Enzymatic biotransformation caters to elimination of 75% of the drugs, hence is the primary route of systemic elimination. There are two phases of metabolization

Table 9.2 Developmental classes of drug-metabolizing enzymes

Class 1	Most abundant in fetus and decline after birth	CYP3A7
Class 2	Relatively constant expression from gestation to adulthood	CYP2B6, CYP2C19, CYP3A5
Class 3	Relatively low expression in fetal liver but increase after birth	CYP1A2, CYP2C9, CYP2D6, CYP2E1, CYP3A4

reactions. Phase 1 enzymes metabolize drug through oxidation, reduction, or hydrolysis processes. Whereas phase 2 processes conjugate drug substrates.

Phase 1 and phase 2 drug-metabolizing enzymes are classified into three developmental classes as depicted in Table 9.2.

9.3.4.1 Phase 1

The primary organ involved with drug metabolism, the liver, undergoes significant development during early infancy and childhood; hence metabolism shows a higher dependence on development. Enzymes responsible for drug metabolism are either immature or present in a reduced concentration compared to an adult. Another important fact is that evidence indicates that the various systems do not mature at the same time. When metabolism is discussed, the two honorable mentions with relevant developmental changes are the Cytochrome P450 enzyme family and the phase 2 biotransformation reaction enzymes (Fig. 9.3).

CYP450 enzyme family:

9.3.4.2 Phase 2

Phase 2 biotransformation enzymes include:

1. UDP glucuronosyltransferase (UGT)
2. Glutathione-S-transferase (GST)
3. N-acetyltransferase (NAT)
4. Epoxide hydroxylase
5. Sulfotransferases (SLUT)

Pertaining to phase 2 metabolism, though the above-mentioned process is involved, UDP glucuronosyltransferase (UGT) metabolism is involved in pediatric age group predominantly.

UDP glucuronosyltransferase (UGT):

Over the years, catastrophic events among the pediatric population are a recurring and inevitable scenario. Failure to account for the developmental differences in the metabolic enzyme concentration and activity leads to untoward adverse effects in this unique population, e.g., grey baby syndrome-Chloramphenicol.

9.3.4.3 Elimination

When speaking about drug elimination, we tend to focus more on the renal elimination of drugs. But elimination always occurs through multiple routes, including exhalation, biliary secretion, and renal clearance. However, it is impossible to be

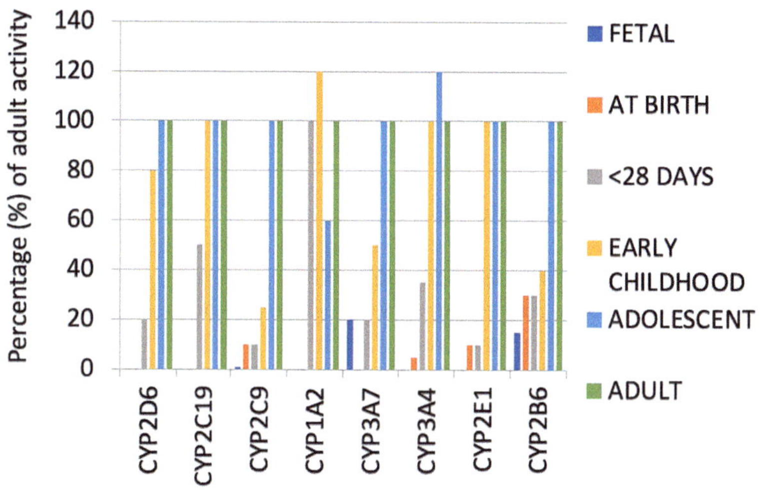

Fig. 9.3 Developmental changes in CYP450 enzyme family

Table 9.3 Age-dependent structural and functional changes of the renal system

Kidney components	Changes
Nephrons	Development completed by 36 weeks of gestation Maturation process extends into childhood Same number of nephron at birth (1 lakh per kidney) as in adult Preterm infants (continue to form nephrons after birth) do not achieve similar number of nephrons in comparison with term infants
Glomerular filtration rate	Abrupt increase after birth, till growth of the child is complete increase in GFR is seen Allometric power model—GFR at 1 year age is 90% of adult values (121.2 mL/min) In premature newborns, GFR increase follows a different trajectory
Tubular reabsorption	Very low for newborn (600 mOsm/kg), increases to 900 mosm/kg by 1 month and reaches 1200 mOsm/kg by adolescence
Renal clearance	Preterm infants' renal clearance is very low For example, clearance of the following compounds can stand as proxy for ontogeny Flucanozole, vancomycin, and amikacin (reduced in premature infants and increase with postnatal age attainment) Age-dependent clearance of PAH (p-amino hippurate)-prototypical marker of renal clearance Low at birth but comparable to adult values by 2 years
Transporters	Basolateral uptake (OAT1, OAT3, and OCT2) and apical efflux (P-gp) transporters significantly low in newborn and infants

indifferent to the renal system's importance in eliminating drugs, because it is the only organ system where the gross developmental variations in elimination process are well characterized. Surprisingly, the well-observed age-related changes in kidney structure do not extrapolate to the changes in function (Table 9.3).

Renal clearance is governed by three major processes, viz.:

1. Glomerular filtration
2. Tubular secretion
3. Tubular reabsorption

9.3.4.4 Glomerular Filtration Rate

1. Development begins from the early fetal stage to early childhood
2. Dependent on gestational age and post-natal adaptations
3. GFR is dependent on the process of nephrogenesis, which completes by 34 gestational weeks, and also a post-natal adaptation of the renal system is seen
4. Variability in the GFR range is seen with development: term neonates- 2 to 4 mL/min/1.73 m2, preterm –0.6 to 0.8 mL/min/1.73 m2 with a rapid increase during the first 2 weeks of life. This then gradually rises till 8–12 months when adult values are reached.

9.3.4.5 Tubular Secretion

Tubular secretion is immature at birth and only reaches adult values by the first year of life. Hence the developmental difference in the renal system failed to account for drug dosing regimen, increases systemic exposure, and risk of adverse drug reactions; thus, for drugs with substantial renal clearance, the kidney is a major determinant of the age-specific drug dosing regimen, e.g., Digoxin and gentamicin.

9.4 Pharmacodynamics (PD)

"Is the pharmacokinetic data enough to predict the nature of drug and its regimen?"—is a much pondered question. Animal studies and only a few studies conducted on children have proven the importance of development on the drug action. Even though some insight has been gained regarding the same, the rarity of such studies especially on children and thereby the scarcity of data on PD developmental differences, is the largest challenge to overcome in pediatric pharmacology.

9.4.1 Drug Receptor

Factors associated with drug-receptor response, as mentioned below, have been found to have relevant developmental changes.

1. Receptor number
2. Density
3. Distribution
4. Function
5. Ligand binding affinity

For example, receptors for g-aminobutyric acid (GABA), the most prevalent inhibitory neurotransmitter is reduced early in infancy in animals. Study in humans found that the GABA A receptor, which binds benzodiazepines and barbiturates, has significantly higher CNS expression levels in children at the age of 2 years as compared to older children and adults. These data suggest that the expression of GABA receptors increases rapidly early in infancy, then subsequently declines with age.

Another example for receptor showing changes with development in the CNS is the m-opioid receptor, the numbers of which are markedly reduced (i.e., > 50%) in newborn as compared to adult rats. Regional opioid receptor distribution in the brain also exhibits developmental differences. Neonates, receptor density is lower in the areas of the brain responsible for analgesic effect (e.g., cortex, thalamus, hippocampus) as compared to those areas of the brain responsible for autonomic side effects (e.g., pons, medulla, hypothalamus), where receptor density approximates that observed in adults.

9.4.2 Pharmacodynamics Biomarkers

Why are studies on PD not done routinely?

The reason behind this lies with the difficulty in validation of PD endpoints in pediatric population. Hence comes the need for PD biomarkers. Characteristics of a PD biomarker to study the pediatric population should have the following attributes to enable assessment of drug exposure and response over the different developmental stages.

1. Non-invasive
2. Robust

Some of the PK biomarkers studied and used for the PD studies in pediatric population are:

1. Gastric pH monitoring and stable isotope breath tests (13 C acetate and 13 C octanoate) which are used to assess acid-modifying and prokinetic agents
2. Histamine skin-prick test—pharmacodynamics properties of antihistamines
3. Spirometry—effect of drugs on pulmonary function in children with asthma and other chronic lung diseases
4. Hemoglobin A1c plasma—efficacy of hypoglycemic agents
5. Drug minimal inhibitory (MIC) and minimal bactericidal concentrations (MBC)—assess antibiotic and antimycobacterial drug regimens
6. Urinary excretion of 6-b hydroxy cortisol—to assess induction of CYP3A4.

9.5 Therapeutic Considerations

9.5.1 Formulation

Even though oral formulations are the most common type of formulation prescribed in children and adults, feasibility to the conventional solid formulation used extensively in adults is impractical, as current standards of dosing are based in pediatric population. Hence introduction of age-appropriate oral formulations as listed below is widely used in this population as they can be used flexibly and accuracy of dosage is achieved. As the primary deciding factor for any successful oral drug administration, especially in this population, is the palatability of the formulation, formulating a dosage form that ensures stability of the drug, accurate dosing and does not add to the adverse effect profile of the active agent is a challenge in itself.

Most common formulations used:

1. Solutions
2. Suspensions
3. Chewable tablets
4. Rapidly disintegrating oral tablets

Challenges faced while formulating newer dosage forms:

1. Minute dose difference to ensure precise dosing
2. Lower dose due to PK variability
3. Limited swallowability
4. Limited palatability decreasing adherence
5. Sub population may show adverse drug reactions and toxicity

9.5.2 Adverse Drug Reactions

1. Greater off-label use of drugs in pediatric patients
2. An under-appreciation for ADRs that appear to have a predilection for infants and children (e.g., hepatotoxicity associated with valproic acid, weight gain from the use of psychoactive medications, paradoxical CNS responses to commonly used drugs) and cannot always be reliably predicted from adult ADR profiles
3. The relative inability of young children (especially those that are non-verbal) to report symptoms that may be associated with an ADR
4. The fact that available reporting systems are largely designed to capture ADRs in adults

9.5.2.1 Pediatric Dosing

The age-old practice of calculating pediatric dose from the weight of the child relative to the adult has failed to consider the developmental differences in the ontogeny and hence producing ineffective systemic exposure of the drug in comparison with adults. This prevents the use of simple formulas based on the allometry of pediatric age group to determine drug dosing.

Even though the weight-based dosing practices may achieve the clinical target in young children and adolescents, this does not hold true for neonates and infants. Hence more than 20 newer techniques have been devised, because even patient-specific PK data obtained from TDM monitoring is unable to individualize drug dosing. The most common methods are using total body weight (TBW) or body surface area (BSA). Though TBW and BSA have shown to achieve similar plasma concentration in their respective dosing, drugs like warfarin with high plasma protein binding (i.e., V_d equates ECF) BSA is the preferred method. Wherein for drugs with high tissue distribution (i.e., V_d exceeds ECF), TBW is an apt parameter to determine the initial dosing (Fig. 9.4).

In cases of developmental immaturity, it's important to know the apparent elimination t-half of the drug and to estimate the apparent V_d for that individual.

Calculation by age: Young's rule

$$\text{Dose} = \text{Adult dose} \times \frac{Age(years)}{Age+12}$$

Calculation by weight: Clark's rule

$$\text{Dose} = \text{Adult dose} \times \frac{Weight(kg)}{70}$$

$$\text{Dose} = \text{Adult dose} \times \frac{Weight(lb)}{150}$$

Assumption:

1. Child's weight, height and body composition are age appropriate and normal
2. Reference normal adult has TBW and BSA of 70 kg and 1.73 m^2

Child dose ($V_d < 0.3$ L/kg) = (Child BSA in $m^2/1.73\ m^2$) x Adult dose

Infant dose ($V_d > 0.3$ L/kg) = (Infant BW in $m^2/70$ kg) x Adult dose

Fig. 9.4 Pediatric dosage calculation formulae

Bibliography

Conklin LS, Hoffman EP, van den Anker J (2019) Developmental pharmacodynamics and modeling in pediatric drug development. J Clin Pharmacol 59:S87–S94

Kearns GL, Abdel-Rahman SM, Alander SW, Blowey DL, Leeder JS, Kauffman RE (2003) Developmental pharmacology – drug disposition, action, and therapy in infants and children. N Engl J Med 349:1157–1167

Thabet Y, Klingmann V, Breitkreutz J (2018) Drug formulations: standards and novel strategies for drug administration in pediatrics. J Clin Pharmacol 58:S26–S35

van den Anker J, Reed MD, Allegaert K, Kearns GL (2018) Developmental changes in pharmacokinetics and pharmacodynamics. J Clin Pharmacol 58:S10–S25

Ward R, Sherwin CMT (2015) Ethics of drug studies in the newborn. Pediatr Drugs 17:37–42

Geriatric Pharmacology

10

Priyadharsini Raman Palanisamy

Abstract

Irrational drug use, a major problem in health care, can be resolved by implementing the concept of evidence-based medicine, rational prescription of drugs and ensuring good prescribing practices. The elderly population, being the high drug-consuming age group, needs special attention in their drug intake and drug effects encountered. Geriatric pharmacology promotes rational prescribing through a combined approach of considering the patients' health status, drugs prescribed, and appropriateness of drugs among the elderly patients. The change in body parameters in the elderly population results in altered pharmacokinetics and pharmacodynamics and a detailed knowledge about the changes will help individualizing the drug therapy. An age-related decline in the physiological function, high prevalence of comorbidities along with polypharmacy can lead to adverse drug reactions and drug interactions. The appropriateness of the drugs prescribed for the elderly population can be evaluated using explicit and implicit methods. American Beers criteria is one of the most commonly accepted explicit tools and it summarizes the list of inappropriate medications in the elderly, drugs to be used with caution in the elderly, drugs to be avoided in the elderly, and clinically important drug-drug interactions. The review focuses on the points to be considered on various aspects while prescribing to an elderly patient.

Keywords

Geriatric · Polypharmacy · Deprescribing · Elderly · Beer's criteria

P. R. Palanisamy (✉)
Department of Pharmacology, Jawaharlal Institute of Postgraduate Medical Education and Research (JIPMER), Karaikal, Puducherry, India
e-mail: kd0017@jipmer.ac.in

A. Arivazhahan et al. (eds.), *Introduction to Basics of Pharmacology and Toxicology*,
https://doi.org/10.1007/978-981-95-1920-0_10

10.1 Introduction

Geriatric population includes the people aged ≥65 years and geriatric pharmacology deals with the effect of ageing process on drug pharmacokinetics, drug effects in the elderly population. There are several changes at the molecular and cellular levels that happen with ageing. The homeostatic mechanisms are blunted due to increased physiological stress, and the functional units of every organ are reduced with time. The increased incidence of various diseases in the elderly population also makes them prone to polypharmacy. These anatomical and physiological changes, along with the increased use of the drugs, warrant a careful watch in elderly patients. The term "Special Populations" applies to the geriatric age group (apart from others) due to the presence of comorbidities, polypharmacy, age-related physiological changes influencing the drug pharmacokinetics, and high vulnerability to adverse drug reactions.

10.2 Physiological Changes and Their Pharmacological Implications

10.2.1 Absorption of Drugs

The absorption of a few drugs may be impaired due to physiological changes in the gastrointestinal tract, as listed in Table 10.1.

DOPA decarboxylase in the gastric mucosa is reduced, which also hastens the absorption of the drugs like levodopa.

Table 10.1 Changes in body parameters and their pharmacological implications

S. no.	Gastrointestinal organ	Change in body parameter	Pharmacological implication
1.	Stomach	Decreased gastric parietal cells Decreased gastric acid secretion Increased pH of the gastric environment Decreased GI motility Decreased blood flow	Basic drugs are better unionized in the alkaline medium and hence, absorption may be increased
2.	Small intestine	No change in motility	–
3.	Colon	Decreased colonic transit	–
4.	Pancreas	Reduced lipase and trypsin levels	–

Table 10.2 Changes in body parameters and their pharmacological implications

S. no.	Change in body parameter	Pharmacological implication
1.	Reduced lean body mass Reduced body water	Hydrophilic drugs: Volume of distribution is decreased Plasma concentration of hydrophilic drugs increases E.g., digoxin, lithium, gentamicin
	Increased body fat	Lipophilic drugs: Volume of distribution increases E.g., morphine, benzodiazepines
2.	Plasma protein binding: Less albumin levels Increased alpha glycoprotein levels	Acidic drugs bind to albumin (ex: Warfarin, acetylsalicylic acid) Basic drugs bind to alpha glycoprotein (ex: Propranolol, lidocaine) The effects of highly protein-bound drugs are increased Ex: Sulfonylureas group of drugs causes hypoglycemia Warfarin causes risk of bleeding Drug-drug interactions Adverse drug reactions

10.2.2 Distribution of Drugs

Changes in the body mass, body fat, and plasma protein levels alter the distribution of both lipid-soluble and water-soluble drugs (Table 10.2).

The free drug concentration increases and thus, geriatric patients are more prone to encounter acute effects of drugs, particularly when highly protein-bound drugs are prescribed. The ratio of the bound drug to free drug is altered. The loading dose may need to be adjusted accordingly in such scenarios.

10.2.3 Metabolism of Drugs

Decreased cardiac output in the elderly leads to less perfusion of organs like liver and kidney, which will reduce the overall metabolism. Based on the hepatic extraction ratio (ratio of hepatic clearance of the drug to the hepatic blood flow), the drugs are classified into high, intermediate and low categories. The clearance of the drugs with the high extraction ratio is mainly dependent on the blood flow, which in turn is affected in older age groups. Phase I reactions mediated by CYP450 enzymes are also affected and reduced with increasing age. There are no major alterations with phase II reactions (conjugation). Liver disease in the elderly demands dose adjustments, particularly with drugs that are metabolized in liver.

Table 10.3 Changes in body parameters and their pharmacological implications

S. no.	Change in body parameter	Pharmacological implication
1.	Decreased liver mass	First pass metabolism of drugs decreases; bioavailability increases E.g., opioids, metoclopramide
2.	Decreased blood flow to the liver	Drugs with the high extraction ratio are affected E.g., pethidine, propranolol
3.	Decreased number of nephrons Decreased renal mass Decreased glomerular filtration rate	Renal clearance of drugs is reduced Dosing to be adjusted according to the reduced creatinine clearance

10.2.4 Excretion of Drugs

Renal blood flow, creatinine clearance, and tubular clearance are usually decreased, resulting in reduced elimination of drugs and prolonged half-life of drugs. Renal function can be monitored by serum creatinine levels (Table 10.3).

10.3 Pharmacodynamic Alterations

The functional reserve alters with increasing age, leading to increase in the sensitivity to certain drugs. The conformational change in receptors, upregulation or downregulation of receptors, and the physiological changes in the elderly may also affect the responsiveness to certain drugs. Examples include increased anticoagulant effect with warfarin, increased antihypertensive effect with verapamil, and decreased antagonistic effect with propranolol, among others.

10.3.1 Effects of Ageing on Different Drug Groups

The most commonly prescribed drug groups in the elderly population include antidiabetics, antihypertensives, diuretics, anticoagulants, non-steroidal anti-inflammatory drugs (NSAIDs), drugs for urinary incontinence, drugs for Alzheimer's disease, anti-Parkinsonian drugs, anticancer drugs, etc. The most common over-the-counter (OTC) drugs used are paracetamol, proton pump inhibitors and H_2 blockers.

10.3.2 Analgesics and Anti-inflammatory Drugs

The most common indication of analgesic and anti-inflammatory drugs in the elderly patients is for the management of osteoarthritis. NSAIDs cause adverse effects like gastrointestinal ulcers and irreversible renal toxicity. Chronic use of

NSAIDs and concomitant use of NSAIDs with antiplatelet drugs or corticosteroids are to be avoided. Prophylactic use of proton pump inhibitors and H_2 blockers may reduce the risk of developing gastrointestinal ulcers.

10.3.3 Drugs Acting on Blood System

There is increased inhibition of vitamin K-dependent clotting factors when warfarin is prescribed to elderly patients. The mechanism for the increased inhibition of vitamin K-dependent clotting factors is still unclear yet the factors like debility, liver disease with increase in age could be the reasons, because the supply of vitamin K to the liver and the synthesis of clotting factors is reduced. The adverse effects of warfarin (such as bleeding) can be prevented by careful monitoring of INR values.

10.3.4 Drugs Acting on the Cardiovascular System

10.3.4.1 Drugs for Angina

β-receptor downregulation, reduction in the affinity towards receptors, and conformational change in receptors are seen in the elderly. Though β-adrenoreceptors are desensitized, and the efficacy of beta-blockers is decreased in the elderly, β-blockers have many advantages like reducing the episodes of angina, risk of cardiovascular disease and death. The preferred β-blockers in the elderly are metoprolol, bisoprolol, and the efficacy, tolerance of β blockers is well established in clinical trials. Among the nitrates, short-acting nitrates are preferred. The plasma half-life and the volume of distribution of the nitrates are higher with elderly and so nitrate-induced hypotension and bradycardia is frequent in this population. The initial dose of nitrates should be less in elderly patients compared to young patients. Calcium channel blockers are the alternatives if β blockers are not well tolerated in stable angina.

10.3.4.2 Drugs for Arrhythmias

Clearance of antiarrhythmic drugs like quinidine, lignocaine and procainamide decreases with age, thus prolonging their half-lives. Disopyramide is to be avoided in the elderly due to its anti-cholinergic side effects.

10.3.4.3 Drugs for Heart Failure

The prevalence of heart failure is high in old age, which demands use of digoxin. The clearance and volume of distribution of digoxin are increased, which necessitates assessment of kidney functions before administering the drug. Factors that lead to increased toxicity of digoxin in the geriatric population are hypokalemia, hypoxemia and hypomagnesemia. The diuretic response with the use of furosemide is reduced due to the reduction in renal plasma volume and tubular secretion of the drug.

10.3.4.4 Drugs for Hypertension

In old age, the sensitivity to the calcium channel blockers is increased, which is manifested as fall in BP and heart rate. There is no significant change in the number and sensitivity to α-receptors with age. The antihypertensive medication is the major aggravating factor for orthostatic hypotension in elderly which indicates the need for careful monitoring while treating hypertension. Thiazide diuretics may cause hyperuricemia, hypokalemia and hyperglycemia, which tend to aggravate concomitant diseases like gout, cardiac arrhythmias and diabetes mellitus respectively. This can be prevented by starting therapy with low doses. Excretion of thiazides and other diuretics also increases with increasing age. The selection of antihypertensive in geriatric age group should be done after considering the factors like comorbidities, compliance, renal parameters, and electrolyte levels. The antihypertensive drug groups which had shown benefit in cardiovascular disease outcome are thiazide diuretics, ACE inhibitors, angiotensin receptor blockers and calcium channel blockers. The antihypertensive medication should be started at low dose after assessment of orthostatic hypotension and gradually titrated considering the tolerance. The renal function and the serum potassium levels should also be monitored.

10.3.5 Drugs Acting on the Central Nervous System

The geriatric population is highly vulnerable to the adverse effects of drugs acting on the CNS. Geriatric disorders related to the CNS include Parkinsonism, Alzheimer's disease, schizophrenia, depression, senile dementia, etc.

Benzodiazepines are possibly the most commonly prescribed group of drugs and the incidence of their adverse effects increases with increasing age. The vulnerability of the elderly population to these adverse effects is due to high sensitivity to these drugs, increased half-life of the drugs, age-related decline in renal or liver function and chronic use of these drugs. In the elderly, drugs get accumulated in lipid tissues, prolonging their half-lives. Long-term usage of benzodiazepines may lead to adverse effects like dementia, ataxia, withdrawal symptoms and higher incidence of falls and fractures. As per Beers criteria, short-acting benzodiazepines are to be preferred over their long-acting and intermediate-acting counterparts.

Depression in the elderly is mostly unnoticed, undiagnosed or may even be confused with other CNS-related conditions. Metabolism of drugs used for management of depression is slower in the elderly population and hence, the adverse effects tend to be higher. Anticholinergic adverse effects of tricyclic antidepressants may worsen pre-existing Alzheimer's disease. Other side effects include sedation and orthostatic hypotension. SSRIs (selective serotonin reuptake inhibitors) may be preferred over TCAs (tricyclic antidepressants). Alternatively, TCAs with low antimuscarinic effects may be considered. Use of lithium causes renal toxicity in the elderly, and the concomitant use of thiazide diuretics can aggravate toxicity of lithium.

The usage of antipsychotics is high in the old age for managing schizophrenia, delirium and dementia. These drugs typically result in extrapyramidal symptoms as their adverse effects (more common with typical antipsychotics). Doses of these drugs should not be increased to the maximum limit. Phenothiazines may be preferred when sedation is required. Haloperidol or atypical antipsychotics are preferred if sedation is not needed. Haloperidol should be used cautiously as it can cause extrapyramidal symptoms. Chlorpromazine is prone to cause orthostatic hypotension due to its alpha-blocking property, which can be prevented by starting the drug at low doses. Drugs like thioridazine, olanzapine, risperidone, ziprasidone and aripiprazole are relatively safer drugs.

Centrally acting anticholinergic drugs may cause confusion, constipation, dry mouth and thus are not recommended for drug-induced Parkinsonism that is caused by antipsychotic use.

Elderly patients are sensitive to the adverse effects of drugs used to manage Alzheimer's disease (CNS-related symptoms and anticholinergic adverse effects). Drugs like donepezil, rivastigmine, galantamine and memantine are safer compared to tacrine.

10.3.6 Other Drugs

Drugs belonging to antihistaminic and antispasmodic groups of drugs cause anticholinergic adverse effects. The diabetes in elderly is treated with metformin because the drug has various advantages like low incidence of hypoglycemia, low cost, good tolerance and the drug can be started if the GFR (glomerular filtration rate) is greater than 30 mL/min. Antidiabetic drugs like short-acting sulfonylureas (Ex: Glipizide) are recommended in metformin intolerance. A dose of 2.5 mg glipizide, a short-acting drug is started and then increased to 5–10 mg if adequate glycemic control is not achieved. Long-acting drugs like glibenclamide, glyburide have increased half-lives, thus increasing the risk of hypoglycemia. The antiemetic drug, metoclopramide, may be avoided due to the risk of causing extrapyramidal adverse effects. Instead, domperidone or ondansetron may be used. Estrogens and androgens have high carcinogenic potential and should be used with caution in old patients.

10.4 Drug-Related Problems in the Elderly

10.4.1 Polypharmacy

The presence of multiple comorbidities in an elderly patient leads to polypharmacy (prescription of several groups of drugs). Elderly age is an important risk factor for non-communicable diseases like diabetes mellitus, hypertension, heart failure, and cancers. Polypharmacy is the routine and concurrent use of more than five drugs. The consequences of polypharmacy in the elderly are increased adverse drug reactions, increased health care costs, higher risk of drug interactions, reduced patient compliance and poor health outcomes. Polypharmacy and irrational drug use are also directly related to increased readmission of patients.

10.4.2 Appropriateness/Inappropriateness of Drugs

Polypharmacy can be appropriate or inappropriate based on the correlation with evidence-based medicine. Appropriate polypharmacy is the justified usage of multiple medicines based on patients' clinical morbidities and standard treatment guidelines. Inappropriate drugs are those that are better avoided in people aged 65 years or older for several reasons (ineffectiveness or increased risk of adverse effects or availability of better alternatives). Appropriateness of drugs can be assessed using two methods—implicit and explicit. The implicit method is specific, patient-oriented and can be modified based on the clinical condition and comorbidities. The disadvantages of this method include requirement of high knowledge to decide specific therapies and increased time to decide on the therapy. Explicit screening tools give a generalized list of inappropriate drugs and contraindications which are based on expert opinions and available literature. A comparison of explicit tools that include Beers criteria, START/STOPP criteria, and FORTA is summarized in Table 10.4.

The American Beers criteria, being the mostly widely used tool, summarizes potentially inappropriate medications in the elderly, drugs to be used with caution and drugs to be avoided or dose to be reduced in patients with reduced kidney function. The first-generation antihistamines, the centrally-acting anticholinergics for drug-induced Parkinsonism, antispasmodics are better avoided in the elderly due to their anticholinergic side effects. The potentially inappropriate medications and the drugs to be used with caution are listed below (as per American Geriatric Society Beer Criteria, 2019).

1. The risk of bleeding complications with aspirin increases with age. The benefit of the drug is less for primary prevention of cardiovascular diseases whereas it is clearly indicated for secondary prevention.
2. Antipsychotics, SSRIs, SNRIs and TCAs may cause SIADH and hyponatremia. The sodium level should be strictly monitored while prescribing these drugs in old age.
3. Quinidine and dextromethorphan may cause falls and are to be prescribed with caution.
4. Anticoagulants like dabigatran and rivaroxaban may cause GI bleeds. They should be used with caution when used for the treatment of venous thromboembolism and atrial fibrillation in people aged more than 75 years.
5. Cotrimoxazole should be used cautiously in patients taking ACE inhibitors and ARBs as the reduced creatinine clearance may elevate the risk of hyperkalaemia.

Table 10.4 Comparison of explicit screening tools

	Beers criteria 2019 (American Geriatric Society)—the most widely used criteria	START/STOPP [Screening tool of older persons potentially inappropriate prescriptions (STOPP) and the screening tool to alert doctors to the right treatment (START)]	FORTA (fit fOR the aged)
Origin	1991; Updated four times since then; Last update 2019	2008 (version 1); 2015 (version 2)	2008 by Professor Martin Wehling
Aim	To identify inappropriate medication use among the elderly (> 65 years of age)	To identify potentially inappropriate medications (STOPP) and identify potential prescribing omissions (START)	To categorize the drugs into those that are beneficial and those that are contraindicated in the elderly
Development method	13-member expert team; Delphi method; 88 drugs classified under 5 categories	19 experts from 13 European countries reviewed proposed criteria; After Delphi validation method, 114 criteria finalized—80 STOPP criteria and 34 START criteria	47 experts in Delphi consensus method; 264 drugs classified under 26 categories
Drug categories	1. Drugs to be avoided in the elderly 2. Drugs to be avoided in the elderly with certain diseases 3. Drugs to be used with caution 4. Drugs to be avoided or adjusted in patients with renal disease 5. Drug-drug interactions to be avoided in the elderly	Prescription of drugs 1. For not a clinically approved or evidence-based indications 2. For long duration exceeding the recommended time 3. With interaction between other drugs 4. With interaction in diseases 5. In irrational dosages	1. Absolutely: Complete benefit in patients 2. Beneficial: Has benefit with limited safety issues 3. Caution: To be used carefully; to identify better alternatives 4. Don't: To be completely avoided
Pros	1. Summarizes the drugs to be avoided completely and those that can be used with caution 2. Includes evidence-based recommendations	1. The effectiveness of START/STOPP as intervention in RCT proved	1. Prescribers are guided to use the most beneficial drugs in common conditions like diabetes mellitus, hypertension 2. Potentially dangerous drugs are highlighted 3. Safer alternative drugs are recommended 4. Supported by RCT evidence

(continued)

Table 10.4 (continued)

	Beers criteria 2019 (American Geriatric Society)—the most widely used criteria	START/STOPP [Screening tool of older persons potentially inappropriate prescriptions (STOPP) and the screening tool to alert doctors to the right treatment (START)]	FORTA (fit fOR the aged)
Cons	Clinical benefit is not proven by RCTs; no recommendation of safer alternative drugs	No recommendation of safer alternatives	Drug-disease and drug-drug interactions are not mentioned

10.4.3 Drug-Drug Interactions

Drug-drug interactions, being a consequence of polypharmacy, may be pharmacokinetic or pharmacodynamic in nature. The factors that influence drug-drug interactions include the age of the patient and the number of drugs prescribed to the patient (Table 10.5).

On the other hand, pharmacodynamic interactions are due to enhanced effects of two drugs due to increased sensitivity or interaction between drugs having low therapeutic index. Herbal medications can also cause interactions. For example, the anticoagulant effect of warfarin is increased with the concomitant use of *Gingko biloba*. Also, increased symptoms of serotonin syndrome are seen with the use of SSRIs along with St. John's wort.

A list of clinically important drug interactions that are better avoided in the elderly population is given below (as per Beers criteria, 2019).

- Concomitant use of ACE inhibitor with a potassium-sparing diuretic is to be avoided due to the risk of causing dangerous hyperkalemia
- Concomitant use of two anticholinergics is to be avoided to prevent cognitive dysfunction in the elderly
- Use of more than 3 CNS-related drugs may increase the risk of falls and fractures
- Combining corticosteroids and NSAIDs may aggravate peptic ulcer and is better avoided
- Use of lithium with ACE inhibitors or loop diuretics is to be avoided to prevent lithium toxicity
- Use of theophylline with cimetidine or ciprofloxacin is preferably to be avoided to prevent theophylline toxicity
- Concomitant use of warfarin with amiodaraone, ciprofloxacin or macrolides is to be avoided to prevent bleeding (INR to be monitored strictly, if used)
- The concomitant use of peripheral α-1 blockers with loop diuretics causes urinary incontinence
- The concomitant use of cotrimoxazole with phenytoin can increase phenytoin toxicity

Table 10.5 Examples of pharmacokinetic drug-drug interactions in the elderly

Level of pharmacokinetic disruption	Drug A	Drug B	Interaction
Absorption	Ketoconazole/ salicylates	H_2 blockers/proton pump inhibitors/ antacids	Antiulcer drugs prevent the absorption of ketoconazole and salicylates, as they are best absorbed in acidic environment
	Levodopa	Anticholinergic drugs	The absorption of levodopa is reduced by delaying the gastric emptying
	Bisphosphonates	Calcium	Calcium has increased binding capacity with bisphosphonates
Distribution	Digoxin	Quinidine	Drugs with high plasma protein binding may displace one drug from albumin. Quinidine causes digoxin toxicity by reducing digoxin binding to plasma proteins
Metabolism	Simvastatin	Phenytoin	Enzyme induction results in reduced response Phenytion is an enzyme inducer and may increase the metabolism of simvastatin
	Cisapride	Erythromycin	Erythromycin inhibits the metabolism of cisapride Enzyme inhibition results in increased response
Excretion	Lithium	ACE inhibitors	ACE inhibitors increase the tubular reabsorption of lithium causing drug toxicity With reduced renal function toxicity increases

10.4.4 Adverse Drug Reactions

The geriatric population in both the outpatient department and the intensive care units is typically associated with a very high number of prescribed drugs. The incidence of drug reactions in the elderly is on the higher side compared to younger patients. This may be due to errors on the prescriber's end or on the patient's end.

Prescribers may be ignorant towards the age-related pharmacokinetic changes and their impact on drug therapy. From the patient's angle, errors can happen due to non-documented use of drugs without the knowledge of prescriber and abuse of drugs. Recognition of adverse drug reactions is difficult as the symptoms may mimic other diseases that are highly prevalent in this age group.

A few methods to prevent adverse drug reactions in the elderly are listed below:

- Listing of prescribed, OTC drugs and herbal medications used by every patient and recording the maintenance of drugs.
- Adverse drug reactions should be considered a possibility when any new symptom is identified in an elderly patient.
- Brown bag analysis is to be performed—Analysis of the bag of medications, including routine treatment drugs, OTC drugs, nutritional supplements of every elderly patient.
- Identifying the rationale and need for every drug and avoiding drugs with major adverse effects.
- Initiating drug therapies at low doses for drugs that have increased sensitivity in elderly patients.
- Introducing a simple regimen and reducing the dosing frequency of drugs.
- Sensitizing the patients about the adverse effects and drug interactions when using multiple drugs.
- Application of clinical monitoring and therapeutic drug monitoring, whenever required.

10.5 Deprescribing in the Elderly

Deprescribing is the process of stopping drugs that are considered to be "not indicated" or "not appropriate" in elderly patients. The steps in the process of deprescribing in the elderly include the following:

- Listing the medications prescribed to the patient.
- Assessing the patient's adherence to the drugs.
- Recognizing the medications that have no clinical benefit or tend to cause adverse drug reactions or lower patient adherence.
- Identifying a strategy to deprescribe drugs.
- Monitoring and reviewing the patients after implementing the deprescription strategy for any withdrawal reactions, adverse effects and therapeutic benefits.

10.6 Conclusion

In old age, there occur several structural and functional changes, which disturb homeostasis. It is mandatory that a prescriber should have sound knowledge of the age-related pharmacokinetic and pharmacodynamic changes, comorbidities, concomitant drug interactions, adverse drug reactions, contraindicated drugs in the elderly, and the drugs to be used with caution while individualizing the drug therapy for elderly patients.

Bibliography

Baldoni AO, Chequer FM, Ferraz ER, Oliveira DP, Pereira LRL, Dorta DJ (2010) Elderly and drugs: risks and necessity of rational use. Braz J Pharm Sci 46:617–632
Brahma DK, Wahlang JB, Marak MD, Sangma M (2013) Adverse drug reactions in the elderly. J Pharmacol Pharmacother 4(2):91–94
By the 2019 American Geriatrics Society Beers Criteria Update Expert Panel (2019) American Geriatrics Society 2019 updated AGS beers criteria for potentially inappropriate medication use in older adults. J Am Geriatr Soc 67(4):674–694
Curtin D, Gallagher PF, O'Mahony. (2019) Explicit criteria as clinical tools to minimize inappropriate medication use and its consequences. Ther Adv Drug Saf 10:1–10
Davies EA, O'Mahony MS (2015) Adverse drug reactions in special populations-the elderly. Br J Clin Pharmacol 80(4):796–807
Frank C, Weir E (2014) Deprescribing for older patients. CMAJ 186(18):1369–1376
Gujjarlamudi HB (2016) Polytherapy and drug interactions in elderly. J-Life health 7(3):105–107
Jansen PAF, Brouwers JRBJ (2012) Clinical pharmacology in old persons. Scientifica 2012:723678
Katzung BG (2018) Special aspects of geriatric pharmacology. In: Katzung BG (ed) Basic and clinical pharmacology. McGraw-Hill Medical, New Delhi
Malgoni AA, Jackson SHD (2004) Age related changes in pharmacokinetics and pharmacodynamics: basic principles and practical applications. Br J Clin Pharmacol 57(1):6–14
O'Mahony D, O'Sullivan D, Byrne S et al (2014) STOPP/START criteria for potentially inappropriate prescribing in older people: version 2. Age Ageing 44:213–218
Vogele A, Johansson T, Renom-Guiteras A, Reeves D, Rieckert A, Schlender L, Teichmann AL, Sönnichsen A, Martinez YV (2017) Effectiveness and safety of beta blockers in the management of hypertension in older adults: a systematic review to help reduce inappropriate prescribing. BMC Geriatr 17:224
Yakaryılmaz FD, Öztürk ZA (2017) Treatment of type 2 diabetes mellitus in the elderly. World J Diabetes 8(6):278–285

Bibliography

11 Usage of Drugs in Various Pathological States

Shravan Venkatraman

Abstract

The pharmacokinetics of the commonly used drugs in kidney and liver dysfunction is to be known to all treating physicians. Most of the drugs are eliminated via urine or bile. Drugs causing toxicity to these eliminating organs (kidney, liver) require dosage adjustment. Some effects of the drug are measured by their plasma drug levels and this will give a hint regarding the patient compliance and also the toxicity. This chapter will highlight the important changes in sepsis, liver and kidney dysfunction, and drug dose adjustment required in liver and kidney diseases.

Keywords

Kidney disease · Clearance · Liver toxicity · Sepsis · Antibiotics

11.1 Introduction

Individualized dosing also known as precision dosing takes into account of the drug attributes [e.g., narrow therapeutic index (NTI), pharmacokinetic/pharmacodynamic (PK/PD) variability], characteristics of the disease state, and patient-specific factors (e.g., organ function, gene variants), to maximize drug therapy. The right drug should reach the right patient at the right dose. In case of hepatic, kidney dysfunction, drug dose has to be modified in order to avoid adverse effects. Aminoglycosides like amikacin and gentamicin require dose modification in patients with renal dysfunction since these groups of drugs are nephrotoxic and also fall in narrow therapeutic range.

S. Venkatraman (✉)
Department of Clinical Pharmacology, Jawaharlal Institute of Postgraduate Medical Education and Research (JIPMER), Puducherry, India

A. Arivazhahan et al. (eds.), *Introduction to Basics of Pharmacology and Toxicology*,
https://doi.org/10.1007/978-981-95-1920-0_11

11.2 Drug Use in Kidney Diseases

The effect of drugs is altered in renal disease resulting in toxicity which is reduced by mitigating the drug doses. There are three basic ways that renal illness and drugs interact.

- Patient susceptibility
- Pharmacodynamic change
- Pharmacokinetic change

GFR is estimated to diagnose renal disease and also in estimating the drug clearance by kidney. Estimated GFR (eGFR) can be measured because drug moieties are cleared from body by means of kidney. Glomerular filtration rate (GFR) less than 60 ml/min and albumin more than 30 mg/g of creatinine with altered anatomical and physiological function of kidney for 3 months means chronic kidney disease.

11.2.1 Estimation of Creatinine Clearance

Dosage of the drug should be adjusted according to the drug clearance.

$$\text{The Cockroft Gault formula : GFR}$$
$$= \{((140 - \text{age}) \times \text{weight}) / (72 \times \text{Creatinine})\} \times 0.85 \ (\text{if female})$$

Estimation of creatinine clearance based on age, weight, serum creatinine, and gender (15% less in women) is done using the above formula.

11.2.2 Factors and Conditions That May Worsen the Renal Injury

- Nephrotoxic drugs (NSAIDs, aminoglycosides, iodinated contrast)
- Uncontrolled diabetes
- Systemic hypertension
- Proteinuria
- Dehydration
- Smoking
- Hyperlipidemia
- Hyperphosphatemia

11.2.3 Therapeutic Index

It is calculated by the formula

$$\text{Therapeutic index} = \text{Minimum toxic dose} / \text{Minimum effective dose}$$

- Drug dosing is very important in drugs having narrow therapeutic range like lithium, digoxin, aminoglycosides, and antiseizure drugs.
- They require monitoring of plasma drug levels and they are used to provide accurate assessment of dosing requirements.
- There can be recommended biomarkers for dose titration, e.g., International Normalized Ratio (INR) for warfarin dosage.

The mechanisms behind nephrotoxic potential of antineoplastic drugs are

- Intravascular volume depletion.
- Urinary tract obstruction secondary to malignancy.
- Example: Methotrexate, when given through intravenous route, at doses less than 0.5–1 g/m^2 is not associated with toxicity to kidneys. At a high dose of 1–15 g/m^2 it damages the renal tubules. This is minimized by alkalinization of urine and maintaining adequate urine output.

11.2.4 Clinical Implications

- Dose adjustments for patients with renal function can be done by.
  - Reducing the drug dose.
  - Lengthening the dosing interval. This is usually preferred in drugs having narrow therapeutic range.
  - Aminoglycoside regimens can be tailored to each patient using drug concentrations and PK-guided dosing has been shown to decrease length of hospital stay without increasing nephrotoxicity. Once daily therapy is found to minimize nephrotoxicity since the drug exhibits concentration-dependent killing.
  - Kidney has a role in clearance of 50% insulin from the circulation In patients with impaired renal function, renal metabolism of insulin is affected and hence requirements of insulin are reduced markedly. The insulin requirement is increased in diabetic patients.
  - Imipenem is always given with cilastatin, a dehydropeptidase inhibitor, to enhance the effectiveness of the antibiotic.
  - Measuring drug levels with narrow therapeutic range will be different in case of patients who are anephric.
  - For example, Phenytoin, an antiseizure drug, has restrictive elimination which is shown in the drug distribution and excretion. Restrictive elimination means the clearance of phenytoin is not dependent on blood flow but depends on enzymatic activity and binding to blood.
  - In patients with normal renal function, phenytoin binding to plasma protein is 92% in comparison with 84% in case of anephric patients. In case of uremia, volume of distribution is increased which is reflected by decrease in binding of phenytoin to the plasma proteins. This is seen by decreased total (protein

bound + free) drug levels which can mislead the physicians to increase the dose of the drug inappropriately.
  - To prevent this, rapid ultrafiltration procedures are done to measure free drug levels in the patients with uremia for dose adjustment.

11.2.5 Dosing in Patients Requiring Renal Replacement Therapy

- Supplementation of dose is required for patients requiring renal replacement therapy only if extracorporeal clearance (CL_{EC}) is more than 30% of renal and non-renal clearance($CL_R + CL_{NR}$).
- Patients undergoing sustained low efficiency dialysis (dialysis which lasts only for 6–12 hours and is preferred in acute renal failure), doses should be adjusted for creatinine clearance of about 10–50 ml/min.
- The drug lost in hemodialysis can be calculated by measuring plasma drug levels and this helps in refining supplemental dose (D_{sup}) estimates.

$$D_{sup} = \left(C_{target} - C_{measured}\right) V_d$$

- Maintenance dose multiplication factor (MDMF) is to be calculated in augmenting the dose in case of renal replacement therapy. Increasing the dosing interval and reducing the drug dose is essential. Increased dosing interval can be measured by dividing the maintenance dosing interval by MDMF.
- Drugs which are tightly bound to plasma proteins (e.g., phenytoin, cyclosporine) need not require alteration in the dose.

11.3 Drug Use in Liver Diseases

Presence of hepatic dysfunction changes the pharmacokinetics of the drug including the absorption and disposition of the drug. The problem with hepatic dysfunction is that there is no clear indicator to find out the degree of hepatic dysfunction. Liver function tests can only detect liver cell damage rather than the physiological function of the liver. Chronic liver disease can alter the pharmacokinetics of the drug.

Hepatic dysfunction can occur due to

1. Alcoholic liver disease (cirrhosis).
2. Chronic infection of liver—Hepatitis B and C.
3. Primary Sclerosing cholangitis.
4. Drug-induced hepatotoxicity.

11.3.1 Factors Guiding Dose Adjustment

- Pharmacokinetics of the medication (e.g., hepatic metabolism, excretion).
- Safety of alternative medications.
- Coexisting conditions (e.g., renal impairment).
- Concurrent medications (i.e., risk of drug-drug interaction).
- Severity of liver disease.

11.3.2 Absorption

- Amount of absorption is not reduced whereas the rate of absorption is decreased in patients with cirrhosis.
- The reason for cirrhotic patients who take furosemide having decreased rate of absorption is impaired gastrointestinal motility. There can also be increased gastrointestinal motility when patients take prokinetic agents like erythromycin and the reason for differential nature of motility is functional and not organic.

11.3.3 Distribution

Hydrophilic drugs like β-lactam antibacterials and digoxin require increased loading dose for rapid action since the volume of distribution is increased in patients having ascites/edema.

11.3.4 Metabolism

High extraction depends on hepatic blood flow whereas low extraction is capacity-limited. Commonly used drugs like sumatriptan, morphine, and isosorbide dinitrate undergo high extraction and are clinically relevant. In cirrhotic patients, clearance of these drugs is reduced due to decreased hepatic blood supply. This is the reason to start on low dose (Table 11.1).

11.3.5 Clearance

- In patients with cirrhosis, there is decreased renal plasma flow and glomerular filtration rates. The low creatinine level can be due to impaired synthesis of creatine and decreased skeletal muscle mass.
- Estimating the creatinine clearance by Cockcroft formula may overestimate the rate of glomerular filtration. Serum cystatin C level, an endogenous marker for kidney function, more accurately reflects glomerular filtration in patients with cirrhosis.

Table 11.1 Impact of cirrhosis on pharmacokinetics

Impact	Inference
Alteration in hepatic blood flow	Increase in bioavailability and higher concentration of drugs in serum
Portosystemic shunting	Allow cardioactive substances to bypass liver and affect the normal heart physiology
Changes in cytochrome P450 activity	Loss of function of cytochrome P450 results in lower first-pass drug extraction, e.g., clarithromycin
Hypoalbuminemia	High binding profile to albumin results in more unbound drug in serum
Cholestasis	Affects drug clearance resulting in toxicity

- Aminopyrine breath test is a broad measure of hepatic microsomal metabolism of the drug since aminopyrine is metabolized by 6 cytochrome P450 enzymes.

11.3.6 Clinical Implications

- Empiric dose reduction with monitoring clinically is a commonly used method to reduce the risk of the adverse drug reactions.
- Drugs with high rate of hepatic extraction have higher drug levels in serum thereby necessitating dose reduction.
- Drugs with low rate of hepatic extraction and narrow therapeutic range should be given with caution are the most dangerous drugs. If these drugs are given, both initial and maintenance doses should be reduced by ≥50% of the normal dose in patients with chronic liver disease.
- In patients with liver disease requiring morphine, lower doses of the drug should be given at regular intervals. Low doses of fentanyl are used through intravenous route and hydromorphone can be given orally or IV.
- The sedative effects of benzodiazepines are more in cirrhotic patients and their effects can be reversed by administration of flumazenil.
- Antipsychotics can cause neurological adverse reactions in cirrhotic patients since the metabolism of the drug is prolonged and it is advisable to discontinue antipsychotics since their effects cannot be reversed by antidote.
- **Pugh Modification of Child's Classification** of liver disease severity is commonly used to formulate dosing recommendations of the drug in patients with liver disease. They can be used as a guide to reduce normal maintenance dose by 50% in patients with mild disease and to reduce by 75% in moderate liver disease. Depending on the safety, the drug's use is considered in severe hepatic disease.
- ACE Inhibitors and NSAIDs should be avoided since they can precipitate renal failure.
- Beta-lactam antibiotics that contain N-methyl thiotetrazole side chain (e.g., Cefotetan) should be used for patients with advanced cirrhosis with coagulation

disorders. The rationale of using cefotetan is that it inhibits γ carboxylation of vitamin K-dependent clotting factors.

- Formation of active metabolite should also be considered, e.g., Losartan is metabolized to EXP3174 which is responsible for the drug's prolonged action. In trials, the standard dose of losartan produces 5 times increase in plasma drug concentrations in cirrhotic patients whereas the plasma levels of EXP3174 are increased two-fold. This is the rationale to start at a lower dose of losartan in cirrhotic patients.
- Dose of sedatives will precipitate confusion, disorientation and coma that look like hepatic encephalopathy. In experiments, hepatic encephalopathy is shown to have increase in neurotransmission of GABA which can be antagonized by flumazenil (Decrease in GABA level is the rationale).
- Reduced responsiveness of loop diuretics to treat ascites in cirrhotic patients is present that cannot be overcome by larger doses. The reason may be due to presence of sodium retention having a role in the development of ascites.
- In hepatorenal syndrome, if the drug is eliminated primarily by kidneys (e.g., Carbenicillin for Pseudomonas infection) with biliary excretion contributing up to 20%. It is essential to start the drug with low doses in cirrhotic patients who are given carbenicillin which is excreted primarily via kidneys.
- Alcoholic patients are more prone to hepatotoxic effects of paracetamol. Since there occurs induction of CYP2E1 by taking alcohol, this further increases the generation of N-acetyl-p-benzoquinone imine.

11.4 Pharmacokinetics in Sepsis

- Sepsis is a syndrome manifested by dysregulated host response to systemic infection.
- The balance between pro- and anti-inflammatory processes in tissue injury, organ dysfunction is not controlled.
- It is difficult to predict the pharmacokinetics since the factors responsible for causing sepsis are both dynamic and interacting (Table 11.2).

11.4.1 Clinical Implications in Sepsis

1. **Intravenous Anesthetic Agents:**

   - Ketamine is metabolized in the liver by cytochrome P450 enzymes to active metabolite norketamine and clinical effect is prolonged in hepatic impairment.
   - Normally, ketamine stimulates the release of endogenous catecholamines offsetting its myocardial depressant activity.
   - Ketamine produces sympathetic stimulation through release of endogenous catecholamines offsetting the depressant action on myocardium. In septic shock, there is domination of intrinsic depressant activity resulting in cardio-

Table 11.2 Pharmacokinetics in sepsis

Properties	Inference
Absorption	There occurs delay in absorption with respect to all routes of administration. Factors responsible include hypoperfusion, mucosal edema, venous congestion, motility dysfunction, alteration of intraluminal pH
Distribution	Volume of distribution of hydrophilic drugs is increased in case of liver cirrhosis and heart failure. In case of lipophilic drugs, Vd is decreased, e.g., midazolam can have more rapid onset due to decreased protein binding in hypoalbuminemia
Metabolism	Drug metabolism in liver depends on 3 factors which include Hepatic blood flow Free unbound fraction of the drug Intrinsic enzymatic capacity of hepatocytes Based on hepatic extraction ratio, drugs may be classified as high (>0.7), intermediate (0.3–0.7), or low (<0.3).
Elimination	Reduced in acute kidney injury since renal blood flow is decreased which is essential for active tubular secretion of the drugs, e.g., Beta-lactam antibiotics, digoxin, and furosemide

vascular collapse. **This makes ketamine to be given at a lower dose for induction of anesthesia.**

2. **Benzodiazepines:**
    - They are lipophilic and more than 95% of the drug is bound to albumin. In case of hypoalbuminemia, there is increase in volume of distribution resulting in increased half-life and its action.
    - Lorazepam is metabolized into an inactive compound and clinical effects are prolonged in liver and renal failure.
    - It is to be noted that doses of benzodiazepines should be reduced in sepsis, titrated to clinical effect, and given as boluses rather than continuous infusion.
3. **Non-depolarizing Neuromuscular Blocking Agents:**
    - Benzylisoquinolinium and aminosteroid non-depolarizing neuromuscular blocking agents are positively charged with small volumes of distribution, which tends to increase in cases of hepatic dysfunction.
    - Atracurium is exception which is not affected by hepatic and renal dysfunction and it is an advantage in critically ill patients having sepsis.
    - Atracurium is metabolized by non-specific plasma esterases and Hofmann elimination which is a spontaneous, non-enzymatic process.
4. **Opioids:**
    - Absorption and distribution of opioids depend on the degree of ionization.
    - Weak bases (opioids) bind to alpha-acid glycoprotein whose level increases in sepsis and this leads to decrease in volume of distribution and clearance resulting in prolonged duration of action.
    - Transdermal preparations of opioids are avoided in sepsis because of the unpredictable skin blood flow and absorption are unpredictable.

5. **Vasoactive Substances:**

 - Patients having sepsis and acidemia (metabolic disorder characterized by accumulation of acid with low pH) require increased concentrations of exogenous and endogenous catecholamines to produce the same increase in arterial pressure in comparison with patients without sepsis and this phenomenon is referred to as vascular hyporesponsiveness.
 - Vascular hyporesponsiveness occurs due to downregulation of catecholamine receptors, increased nitric oxide production, and generation of oxygen-free radicals resulting in vasodilatation.
 - Vasoactive agents affect the pharmacokinetics of other drugs since they have impact on cardiac output and blood flow.

6. **Antimicrobials:**

 - Antimicrobials which are hydrophilic have low volume of distribution and are eliminated by kidneys. In case of sepsis, there occurs endothelial dysfunction, altered protein binding and large volume of IV fluids administration results in increased volume of distribution and subtherapeutic plasma concentration.
 - This becomes a problem in case of drugs which exhibit time-dependent killing like beta-lactams.
 - Since the volume of distribution is increased, there occurs a sub-therapeutic concentration and in turn leads to inappropriate microbial clearance.
 - It is justifiable to give maximum amount of loading dose followed by maintenance dose.
 - Lipophilic antimicrobials may require dose adjustment in cases of hepatic failure. For example, metronidazole should be reduced to one-third of the normal dose and administered once daily.
 - In case of acute kidney injury, further dose modification is required to counteract the risk of toxicity due to defective renal clearance (Boxs 11.1 and 11.2).

Box 11.1: Examples of Hydrophilic Drugs

Class of hydrophilic antimicrobials	Examples
Aminoglycosides	Gentamicin, tobramycin, amikacin

Class of hydrophilic antimicrobials	Examples
Beta-lactams	Carbapenem: Meropenem, ertapenem Penicillins: Amoxicillin, piperacillin Cephalosporins: Cefuroxime, ceftriaxone, ceftazidime
Glycopeptides	Vancomycin, teicoplanin

Box 11.2: Examples of Lipophilic Antimicrobials

Classes of lipophilic antimicrobials	Examples
Nitroimidazoles	Metronidazole
Fluoroquinolones	Ciprofloxacin, moxifloxacin, levofloxacin
Oxazolidinones	Linezolid
Macrolides	Clarithromycin, erythromycin, azithromycin
Lincosamides	Clindamycin
Tetracyclines	Doxycycline, tigecycline, minocycline

11.5 Pharmacokinetics in Other Organ Dysfunction

- In congestive heart failure, the pathophysiological changes may result in alterations in drug pharmacokinetics. Drugs that exhibit narrow therapeutic range like digoxin, antiarrhythmics are monitored by measuring the serum concentrations to avoid toxicity.
- Due to compensatory peripheral vasoconstriction, the volume of distribution of drugs is reduced in heart failure. This is the reason for smaller loading doses for drugs like lignocaine, quinidine, and disopyramide.
- Cardiac output is reduced in case of congestive heart failure and so the blood flow to organs of elimination is reduced.
- Hypoperfusion to liver and kidneys results in impairment of clearance of drugs.
- Depending on the elimination half-life, titration should involve smaller dose increments and monitoring of plasma drug concentrations is essential.
- Adverse drug reactions occur commonly in the elderly.
- Patients treated with target dose of ACE inhibitors and Beta-blockers in clinical practice were few in contrast to the dose in trials (COPERNICUS, MERIT-HF, and Val-HeFT).
- Chronic obstructive pulmonary disease is associated with polypharmacy. Patients with severe pulmonary disease have decreased clearance of the drug resulting in toxicity. The rationale is to start the drug low and go slow to prevent unintended exposure.

11.6 Conclusion

Drug use in various pathological states like renal, liver, and heart dysfunction is to be known for the clinicians for dose adjustment. The pharmacokinetics of the commonly used drugs should be known since the effect of the drugs with narrow therapeutic range can be known by measuring the plasma drug levels in order to avoid toxicity. This will also give a clue regarding the patient compliance since some patients avoid taking drugs due to fear of toxicity.

Bibliography

Atkinson SGM (2002) Pharmacokinetics in patients requiring renal replacement therapy. A. Atkinson, G. Susla. National Institutes of Health Clinical Center
Charlton M, Thompson JP (2019) Pharmacokinetics in sepsis. BJA Educ 19(1):7–13
Delcò F, Tchambaz L, Schlienger R, Drewe J, Krähenbühl S (2005) Dose adjustment in patients with liver disease. Drug Saf 28(6):529–545
Doogue MP, Polasek TM (2011) Drug dosing in renal disease. Clin Biochem Rev 32(2):69–73
Franz CC, Hildbrand C, Born C et al (2013) Dose adjustment in patients with liver cirrhosis: impact on adverse drug reactions and hospitalizations. Eu r J Clin Pharmacol 69:1565
Hendrayana T, Wilmer A, Kurth V, Schmidt-Wolf IG, Jaehde U (2017) Anticancer dose adjustment for patients with renal and hepatic dysfunction: from scientific evidence to clinical application. Sci Pharm 85(1):8
Lewis JH, Stine JG (2013) Review article: prescribing medications in patients with cirrhosis – a practical guide. Aliment Pharmacol Ther 37:1132
Mangoni AA, Jarmuzewska EA (2019) The influence of heart failure on the pharmacokinetics of cardiovascular and non-cardiovascular drugs: a critical appraisal of the evidence. Br J Clin Pharmacol 85(1):20–36
Marti CN, Fonarow GC, Anker SD, Yancy C, Vaduganathan M, Greene SJ, Ahmed A, Januzzi JL, Gheorghiade M, Filippatos G, Butler J (2019 Mar) Medication dosing for heart failure with reduced ejection fraction – opportunities and challenges. Eur J Heart Fail 21(3):286–296
McNeill RP, Zhang M, Epton MJ, Doogue MP (2021) Drug metabolism in severe chronic obstructive pulmonary disease: a phenotyping cocktail study. Br J Clin Pharmacol 87(11):4397–4307
Nau R, Sörgel F, Eiffert H (2010) Penetration of drugs through the blood-cerebrospinal fluid/blood-brain barrier for treatment of central nervous system infections. Clin Microbiol Rev 23(4):858–883
Shammas FV, Dickstein K (1988) Clinical pharmacokinetics in heart failure. An updated review. Clin Pharmacokinet 15(2):94–113
Soleimanpour H, Safari S, Shahsavari Nia K, Sanaie S, Alavian SM (2016) Opioid drugs in patients with liver disease: a systematic review. Hepat Mon 16(4):e32636
Srinivas N, Maffuid K, Kashuba ADM (2018) Clinical pharmacokinetics and pharmacodynamics of drugs in the central nervous system. Clin Pharmacokinet 57(9):1059–1074
Sullins AK, Abdel-Rahman SM (2013) Pharmacokinetics of antibacterial agents in the CSF of children and adolescents. Paediatr Drugs 15(2):93–117
Tegeder I, Lötsch J, Geisslinger G (1999) Pharmacokinetics of opioids in liver disease. Clin Pharmacokinet 37:17–40
Tyson RJ, Park CC, Powell JR, Patterson JH, Weiner D, Watkins PB, Gonzalez D (2020) Precision dosing priority criteria: drug, disease, and patient population variables. Front Pharmacol 11:420
Williams RL, Benet LZ (1980) Drug pharmacokinetics in cardiac and hepatic disease. Annu Rev Pharmacol Toxicol 20(1):389–413

toxicity. This may also have a negative effect regarding patient compliance since some patients avoid taking drugs due to fear of toxicity.

Bibliography

Part II

Drug Discovery and Development

High-Throughput Screening and Computer-Aided Drug Designing

12

Mageshwaran Lakshmanan

Abstract

The term high-throughput screening (HTS) was unknown to the scientific literature until the mid-1980s, but it has undergone rapid evolution in the past 30 years. The HTS enables pharmaceutical companies to compete in the 'new-drug invention race' in the current era, as HTS provides screening of >1,00,000 compounds per day using microplates and various automated robotic systems. The core step involved in the development of a successful HTS campaign involves the implementation of the correct 'assay'. HTS assays can be functional or non-functional assays. Another aspect of HTS is the development and maintenance of compound libraries. Compound libraries are growing steadily now by acquiring data on all the medicinal chemistry molecules, using combinatory-chemistry methods, and purchasing compound collections from library vendors, academia, etc. The main technical aspects of HTS involve automation mode, plate storage systems, robotic arms, and detection assays. Similar to HTS, the computer-aided drug design (CADD) field has also grown significantly and is employed parallelly with HTS in the early phases of drug development. CADD utilizes both structure and ligand-based drug design methods. Various commercial computational codes are available for these CADD approaches. This chapter reviews the various technical aspects of HTS and CADD in detail.

Keywords

HTS · High-throughput screening · Computer-aided drug design · CADD · LBDD · SBDD

M. Lakshmanan (✉)
Department of Pharmacology, Thanjavur Medical College, Thanjavur, Tamilnadu, India

A. Arivazhahan et al. (eds.), *Introduction to Basics of Pharmacology and Toxicology*,
https://doi.org/10.1007/978-981-95-1920-0_12

12.1 Introduction to High-throughput Screening

In the modern pharmaceutical drug invention process, high-throughput screening (HTS) has a central function as it has effectively minimized the duration of screening time for identification of potential 'hits'. The term 'HTS' was unknown to the scientific literature until the mid-1980s, but it has undergone rapid evolution in the past 30 years. In the traditional drug screening process, the compounds are synthesized in large quantities (up to grams) for testing on animals/isolated tissues/whole cells leading to 'low throughput'. On the contrary, a common assay is used in HTS for iterative testing of various molecules for quick screening. HTS requires only compounds in nanogram quantity and it screens directly using target molecules. The present pharmaceutical screening assay has a screening throughput of >10,000 wells per day (HTS) to >1,00,000 wells per day (ultra HTS). Thus, HTS enables pharmaceutical companies to compete in the 'new-drug invention race' in the current era.

12.2 Certain Terminologies Related to HTS

- **Assay**: In terms of HTS, the 'assay' is defined as an 'experimental step' that is designed precisely and effectively to measure the test molecule's effect on certain cellular/biochemical processes.
- **Active molecule**: During the HTS process, when there is biochemical activity occurs in one well at a particular concentration of test substance, that test substance is termed 'active'.
- **Confirmed active molecule**: When the same activity is reproduced by retesting, the 'active' molecule becomes 'confirmed active'.
- **Hit molecule**: Using certain 'deselection assays' the possible presence of artifacts in the 'confirmed active' molecule is removed and upon retesting, if biochemical activity still occurs, then the molecule is now called a 'hit' molecule.
- **Confirmed hit molecule**: The 'hit' becomes 'confirmed hit' after establishing structure confirmation, purity testing (using LCMS), and dose-response curve.
- **Lead molecule**: Finally, a series of similar molecules is developed from the 'confirmed hit' by altering its chemical structure and a member of this series that shows promising chemical optimization is called a 'lead molecule'.
- Thus, HTS provides a starting point of chemical structure/analogs for the scientific team involved in drug invention to initiate further steps to convert the starting chemical structure into active confirmed active hit confirmed hit lead 'molecule'.

12.3 Components of HTS

12.3.1 Assay

- The core step involved in the development of a successful HTS campaign involves the implementation of the correct 'assay'.
- **Characteristics of an assay in HTS**:
  - Should be free from bias.
  - Should be simple for the automation requirements.
  - Should produce more reliable results.
  - Should reduce cost and time.
  - Should consume fewer reagents.
  - Should require a minimal volume of test molecule for screening.
  - Should have consistent reproducibility.
- **Type of assay**:
  - Functional assay: This type of assay measures the activity of the test molecule to modify the function of certain target protein (e.g., modulation of sodium influx across sodium ion channels).
  - Non-functional assay: This type of assay measures mainly the binding capacity of the test molecule to the target protein.
  - In general, functional assays are more reliable than non-functional assays in the development of the lead molecule. The non-functional assays are done in primitive steps of drug development and help to identify potential active molecules.

12.3.2 Compound Libraries

- Another important component of HTS is the development of compound libraries. Before the 1990s, only a few thousand molecules have been archived by pharmaceutical companies. Later, in the mid-1990s, up to 100,000 compounds have been collected. The count reached 0.5 million compounds at the end of the 1990s and the compound library count became >1.5 million in the mid-2000s. It is growing steadily now by acquiring data on all the medicinal chemistry molecules, using combinatory-chemistry methods, and purchasing compound collections from library vendors, academia, etc.
- The following are the key aspects of assembling and developing the distinguished HTS library.
  - Involvement of cheminformatics tools to collect data on compounds regarding.
    - Chemical property (complexity, molecular weight, reactivity, uniqueness, etc.
    - Physical property (melting point, boiling point, density, etc.)
    - Physiochemical property (aggregation, solubility, etc.)

    - Predicted characteristics (toxicology, preliminary pharmacokinetic data, etc.)
  - Incorporating the current experiences/lessons learned with the molecules in HTS into the existing compound library data and refining them.
  - Adherence to the structural-design-characteristics guidelines published by various regulatory authorities.

- **Lipinski's rule of five:** This rule was developed to predict the 'drugability' of the new molecular entity for a particular target (except active transporters). With the help of Lipinski's rule of five and other cheminformatics tools, the classification of molecules in the evolving compound library is fine-tuned. Lipinski's rule states that a compound will have poor absorption by the oral route when it has.
  - More than 5 hydrogen bond donors.
  - More than 10 hydrogen bond acceptors.
  - >500 Dalton molecular weight
  - and its calculated Log P (cLop P) >5; Log P is Log_{10} (partition coefficient of the particular compound). Lipinski's rule of five applies only to the drug developed for the oral route and only 50—55% of drugs developed obey this rule. Nevertheless, this rule helps to fine-tune the compound library in HTS.

- **Considerations of the compound library**:
  - **Storage format**: A suitable solvent is a must while storing the compounds at -20 °C to -80 °C. Dimethyl-sulfoxide (DMSO) is one of the most commonly used solvents for storing compounds as it has minimal interference while doing an assay. The major disadvantage of using DMSO is its hygroscopic nature. When left open, DMSO can draw water as much as 50% of its volume. Peptides and other high molecular-weight compounds may require alternative solvents.
  - **Purity and integrity:** When the stored sample is thawed for analysis, it should maintain purity and integrity. Thus, too many freezing and thawing cycle should be avoided while performing primary screening in HTS. Repeated freezing-thawing of a small-sized molecule can lead to precipitation and thus integrity is affected. Hence, a part of the sample thawed should be subjected to quantitative analysis to have data about the purity and integrity of the testing compound every time.

12.3.3 Technical Aspects of HTS

12.3.3.1 Automation Modes

- Automation is vital in testing millions of compounds per day in HTS. Three modes of automation are commonly employed in HTS.
- **Batch mode**: In this mode, assays of smaller volumes are performed by the machine and the scientists manually move plates (in stacks) from one point to the other during each step of screening. The main advantage of batch mode is lower cost and the significant disadvantage is the increase in variability in results.

- **Semi-automated mode**: In this mode, most of the parts of assay steps are automated and manual involvement is very limited. This mode can improve the variability in results of batch mode to a certain extent. This mode is commonly involved in low-medium HTS that handles less than 50,000 compounds per day.
- **Integrated mode:** This mode is also called a 'robotic system' wherein scheduling software controls the multiple conveyor systems/articulating arm that performs all the steps of assays. This mode is very costly and has the least variability in the results. The key differences between batch, semi-automated, and integrated mode of automation in HTS are given in Table 12.1.

12.3.3.2 Plate Storage

- Storing the microplates during the assay process is a vital step in HTS. Two types of storing are utilized (stackers and shelf-based).
- **Shelf-based storing**: In this method, microplates are stored either as open racks or in incubators. Humidity, temperature, and gaseous exchange are controlled very precisely. The microplates in the top and bottom shelf are exposed to the same conditions which minimize the variability in results. Robotic incubators can accommodate hundreds of plates at the same time and the rocking (gentle shaking) option is also available to improve the output. Integrated automation

Table 12.1 Differences between the three modes of automation in the HTS

S. no	Property	Batch mode	Semi-automated mode	Integrated mode
1	Type of operation	Manual for significant steps	Most of the steps are automated with limited manual input	All the steps are automated (robotic system)
2	Flexibility for use	Very limited	Moderate flexibility	High flexibility
3	Requirement of scheduling software	No	Limited	Compulsory
4	Size of the system	Benchtop	Benchtop/custom tables	Room size with dedicated UPS
5	Power requirement	Operates on home power	Operates on home power	Requires high-voltage AC power
6	Plates used	96 or 384 wells	96 or 384 wells	384 or 1536 wells
7	Plate movement logic	Loaded manually (attached plate stackers)	Arm with limited axis movement range (pick and place type)	Robot arm with full articulation
8	Walkaway processing capacity	25 microplates	75 microplates	1000 microplates
9	Primary use	Low HTS (<25 plates/day)	Low medium (<50,000 compounds/day)	High and ultra HTS volume HTS (>50,000 compounds/day)
10	Example	Thermo Combi CyBio SELMA	CyBio FeliX Tecan Freedom EVO	Microstar HighRes Biosystems

mode adapts the shelf-based storing method and utilizes a multi-axil robotic arm to perform all the functions.

- **Stackers:** In this method, microplates are stacked (up to 50 microplates) over the other in a cassette holder and this setup is linked with a detection device or plate washer. The major disadvantage of this system is high variability in the assay as temperature, humidity, and other parameters vary highly between the first and last microplate. Stackers are commonly employed in 'batch' automation mode.

12.3.3.3 Robotic Arms

- In HTS, the robotic arms are used to transfer/move the consumables/reagents from one point to another in a timed manner for the smooth and efficient running of assays. The robotic arm maintains consistency and reduces the variability in the results. Various types of robotic arms are used in HTS and are explained as follows:
- **Simple plate movers**: These types of robotic arms are the least in design complex. It shifts the microplates from 'stacker' to other associated devices like plate washers/detection devices. The command sets of simple plate mover type of robotic arm are condensed and are under the control of the associated device's software.
- **Limited access arm**: These types of robotic arms have 2-4 degrees of freedom and the movement can be linear or circular. Limited access robotic arm can present consumables, shift stackers, and deliver reagents. The gripping capacity limits the functions of this type of robotic arm.
- **Fully articulate robotic arm:** This type of robotic arm has 5–6 degrees of freedom. It uses rotatory joints and supports a wide range of applications. They are also called 'industrial robots' and are located in the center of the working station in a fixed position. The software commands are highly complex and require multiple programs to control the function. For the safety of humans, fully articulate robotic arms are often guarded with physical barriers.
- **Challenges and hurdles:**
  - Robotic arms are required to be 'taught' and 'retaught' regarding the positions to maintain the alignment of microplates and peripherals regularly.
  - Special training in 'teaching' robotic arm is required and it is a tedious and time-consuming process.
  - Provision of a safe working place around the robotic arm is challenging owing to the complexity of functions performed by the arm.
  - Implementation of physical guarding barriers and measures adds to the cost of maintaining the robotic arms.

12.3.3.4 Liquid Handling

- Another important technical aspect of HTS is dispensing the reagents and liquids during the assay. The primary goal is to maintain the constant volume for each step of the assay and reduce the wastage at the same time. Liquid transfer variation accounts for a major proportion of variability observed in the assay results.

Thus, various methods of liquid dispensing mechanisms have been developed and used.

- **Air displacement dispenser**: In this technique, a plunger inside the cylindrical structure aspirates or dispenses the liquid. The aspirated liquid and the plunger are separated and not allowed to interact by a small air gap. Disposable tips are used in this method and can aspirate or dispense the liquid as low as 0.25 μL. It is compatible with 96-well, 384-well, and 1536-well microplates.
- **Positive displacement dispenser**: The set is similar to the air displacement dispenser but without the presence of an air gap. This method uses fixed tips instead of disposable ones. The fixed tips are made of stainless steel to minimize the adsorption of compounds during aspiration/dispensing. This dispenser can aspirate as low as 25 nL. However, this type of dispenser is often not compatible with 1536-well microplates due to space constraints.
- **Acoustic transfer dispenser**: In this method, sound waves are sent through the liquid phase by the transducers to create droplets of a specific size to dispense. This is one of the methods for a non-contact dispensing system. It is used frequently in steps involving compound addition during the assay. The advantages are the absence of cross-contamination and minimal waste of liquids. However, it requires a specific compatible source plate which adds to the cost of the assay. Also, aspiration cannot be done with this method; only dispensing can be performed. The dispensing range is 1 nL to 100 μL.
- **Peristaltic pumps:** This is another non-contact dispensing system (which cannot be used for aspiration) that utilizes peristaltic pumps and flexible tubing to move liquids to the microplates from the reservoir. Dispensing speed can be adjusted based on the reagent used. The dispensing range is 50 nL to 3 mL.
- **Recent methods of dispensing:** Various recent methods like solenoid-syringe, solenoid-pressure bottle system, and Piezo-stack-actuator-based liquid handling, are also employed in the industry commonly. These techniques have minimal dead volume (the volume that remains after aspiration in the container) and have high accuracy. The dispensing volume ranges from 200 pL to 50 μL.

12.3.4 Detection Technologies in HTS

- Various detection technologies are employed by the industry in HTS to quantify or measure the physical phenomenon, chemical reaction, or biological changes that occur in the screening assays. The following are commonly used detection techniques.
- **Absorbance**: By measuring the amount of light with a particular wavelength that is absorbed when the light passes through the contents in the microplate, it is possible to quantify the concentration of the content. Absorbance can be photometric or colorimetric absorbance.
- **Fluorescence intensity (FI)**: Fluorophore is a compound with fluorescence property (i.e., emitting light upon excitation by light of a particular wavelength). In FI assays, the concentration of fluorophore can be estimated by using a par-

ticular wavelength to excite and measure the intensity of light (higher wavelength) emitted. Since the linear correlation is observed between the emitted light intensity and concentration of fluorophore, quantification of assay content can be performed.

- **Time-resolved fluorescence (TRF):** In the conventional FI method, the excitation and emission occur at the same time and can cause high background noise. Moreover, a high false positive rate in HTS is observed with the FI method as a certain chemical used in HTS also has fluorescence properties. In the TRF method, the lanthanide chelate (Europium ion—Eu^{3+}) is used as a label and the emitted light intensity of the Eu^{3+} ion is measured only after a particular time. The fluorescence lifetime of the Eu^{3+} ion is relatively long (μs—ms) with higher emission intensity than other noise signals. Thus after a particular time, decay of the background fluorescence emission occurs while the fluorescence emission of the Eu^{3+} ion persists. Thus improved accuracy in the quantification of the assay content and higher assay sensitivity is achieved in TRF.
- **Fluorescence resonance energy transfer (FRET):** This technique is mainly used for molecular interaction assay. Two fluorophores are used in this method—donor and acceptor fluorophore. In FRET, as a first step, the donor fluorophore absorbs energy and transfers it (radiationless transmission) to the acceptor fluorophore. This results in a reduction in the FI of donor fluorophore and an increase of the same in acceptor fluorophore. The transmission of energy occurs only when both fluorophores are located very close (10—100 Å) indicating the biological interaction between the molecule.
- **Time-resolved FRET (TR-FRET)**: It is also called homogenous TR-FRET (HTRF). This technique combines both the FRET and TRF principles. The Eu^{3+} ion and terbium cryptate are used in the first- and second-generation HTRF respectively. Using lanthanide labels as fluorophores in the HTRF technique increases the accuracy and sensitivity more than traditional FRET. Miniaturization of HTRF is possible up to 1536 wells and hence HTRF is frequently used in interaction assays in HTS.
- **Fluorescence polarization (FP):** This method is based on the principle that the rate of molecular rotation is inversely proportional to the degree of polarization of emitted light by the molecule. Thus when a small molecule ligand (<1500 Da) is attached to a fluorophore and excited with polarized light, it emits mostly depolarized light. Inversely, when a large molecule is attached to a fluorophore and excited with polarized light, it emits significantly polarized light. Thus the degree of polarization changes according to the size of the molecule. This is because the large molecule-fluorophore complex undergoes only a minimal rotation speed and hence the emitted light will be still polarized to a significant degree. This property can be used to quantify/measure the interactions of biomolecules of varying sizes (peptides and oligonucleotides) at a higher rate of accuracy. FP method is also used in the competitive binding assay in HTS wherein reduction in FP signal is noted in presence of inhibitors. The major advantages of FP are that non-radioactive, separation of the free and bound

ligand is not required, and can be carried out in the solution phase of the lowest volume (10 μL).

- **Fluorescence correlation spectroscopy (FCS):** FCS is based on the principle that when a molecule labeled with fluorophore is allowed to diffuse in and out of a minute observatory volume of a sample under a 'confocal system' setup, the fluctuation in the fluorescence emitted is captured and correlated with time. Using a hardware correlator or computer-based software; a correlation curve can be derived. From this curve, various parameters of the molecule like local concentration, diffusion coefficient, the interaction between molecules, and hydrodynamic radius can be derived. The sensitivity of FCS is very high (detect even up to one molecule in the sample).
- **Fluorescence-lifetime-correlation spectroscopy (FLCS).** This technique combines the principles of both FCS and time-correlated single photon counting (TCSPC). This technique is more accurate than FCS as it can eliminate the background noise and cross-talk better than FCS.
- **Chemiluminescence:** It is similar to fluorescence but it does not require an external light source to excite the photons; excitation occurs by chemical reaction. When biomolecules (like luciferin and luciferase) are used, then the technique becomes bioluminescence. Background interference is low in the luminescence method than fluorescence as an external light source is not used. However, luminescence requires absolute darkness and photon multiplier tubes (PMT) to detect the photons generated by chemical reactions. Various modalities of luminescence like ALPHA (amplified-luminescence-proximal-homogenous assay), BiLC (biomolecular luciferase complementation), BRET (bioluminescence-resonance-energy transfer), and electro-chemiluminescence are commonly employed in HTS assays.
- **Radiometric assays:** These use radioisotopes (^{3}H, ^{33}P, ^{125}I, ^{14}C, and ^{35}S) to evaluate/monitor the kinetics/activity of specific enzymes or receptors in HTS. A popular radiometric assay method used is scintillation-proximity assay (SPA). SPA is commonly used in CAM (cellular adhesion molecule) binding assays, protein-peptide interaction assays, DNA-protein interaction assays, receptor binding assays, radioimmunoassays, and enzyme assays. In SPA, the radioactive decay is converted to light energy when a radionuclide and a bead that contains scintillant (a molecule that emits UV/visible light upon excitation by high-energy rays) are in close proximity. The biomolecule of interest (e.g., receptor/enzyme/DNA) is tagged with SPA beads and a radionuclide is attached to its ligand (forming radioligand). A blue light will be emitted when both the SPA bead and radioligand are in close proximity indicating the interaction between the ligand and the biomolecule of interest. Similar to luminescence, this method also requires PMT detectors. Alternatively, CCD (charged-coupled device) camera detector can also be used. Commercially SPA-flash plates of 96—384 wells are available and being used in HTS screening.

12.4 Quality Control in HTS

- The degree of confidence in the HTS results depends upon the type of assay, primary screen replication, and determination of various quality control (QC) parameters (like signal/noise ratio, repeatability, etc.). A high degree of false positive results are seen in fluorescence intensity assays and reporter gene assay techniques and thus without an effective QC, the results are highly unreliable.
- One method to reduce the false positive rate is performing independent replications of the primary screening assay. Occasionally, it can also reduce the false negative rate for some assay techniques.
- QC is very significant for assays with very minimal difference between positive and negative control (small window). Moreover, when a good positive control for the assay does not exist and hence the difference between negative and positive control is unknown (unknown window), then QC plays an important role in this situation.
- 'Artifacts' in the assays with high false positive rates can be identified by comparing the primary screen with the historical screens. Similarly, the 'missed hits' in the assays with false negative rates can be identified by analyzing the primary screen along with bioactivity profile information and the compound structure of the interested target.

12.5 Computer-Aided Drug Design

12.5.1 Definition

Computational approaches that are used in pharmaceuticals to invent/discover a molecule (often a series of a molecule with similar biochemical nature) and develop them into a potential 'hit' or lead molecule is called 'computer-aided drug design' (CADD). CADD is used for the identification of ligand/hit and also for optimization of those ligand/hit molecules.

12.5.2 Types of CADD

- CADD comprises various computational approaches in which two or more are used during the preclinical phases of drug development. CADD approaches can be broadly divided into three groups.
- **Structure-based methods**: (The 3D structure of the target is known).
  - Molecular docking.
  - Homology modeling.
  - Fragment-based screening.
  - De-novo modeling design.
- **Ligand-based methods**: (The 3D structure of the target is unknown).
  - Quantitative structure-activity relationship (Q-SAR).

  - Molecular similarity.

- **Hybrid methods** (Both the structure of the target and ligand are known. These methods are based on end-points).
  - 3D pharmacophore modeling.

12.5.3 Molecular Docking (MD)

- Using virtual simulation programs, protein, and small molecule interactions can be modeled and studied at the atomic level. This data is then used to predict the behavior of that particular small molecule at the target binding site.
- Using the MD method, the conformational changes that can occur in ligand and target protein can be visualized and the binding affinity of the molecule with the target protein is also estimated. The data generated from this method is utilized for fine-tuning (optimization) of small molecule series.
- Docking can be done in three ways.
  - Rigid MD: Target and ligand are rigid entities.
  - Flexible MD: Target and ligand are flexible entities.
  - Flexible ligand MD: Ligand is flexible while the target is a rigid entity.
- Various simulation MD codes are available commercially. Codes like NAMD, GROMACS, CHARM, AMBER, and OpenMM are often used in pharmaceuticals.

12.5.4 Homology Modeling

- Homology modeling involves the generation of unknown protein structures based on the information from the known protein structure of similar biological activity.
- Homology modeling is performed in four steps: template selection and target-template alignment (usually performed together) followed by model construction and finally 'model assessment'.
- The simplest approach of template identification in homology modeling is done by 'serial-pairwise-sequence-alignment' using 'search techniques' in databases like BLAST, FASTA, and PSI-BLAST. Hence it is evident that the first two steps of homology modeling—template selection and target-template alignment—are often performed together.
- Using the information generated in the selected template and target alignment, a 3D structure model of the target is constructed (model construction). It can be done in one of the three methods—fragment assembly, segment matching, or spatial restraint satisfaction method.
- Finally, the constructed target's 3D structure model can be assessed using various computation codes like ProQres, Verify3D, Prosall, and Errat.

- The overall accuracy of homology modeling-based 3D structure construction highly depends upon the 'sequence identity' between the template and target protein. The model tends to be reliable when the sequence identity is above 50%.

12.5.5 Fragment-Based Screening

- Fragment-based screening in CADD is another SBDD approach in which a fragment of a molecule is identified in HTS during the 'hit-finding phase' and subsequently grown, merged, or linked with larger lead molecules.
- The success of fragment-based screening relies mainly on two factors: the low complexity and low molecular weight (less than 300 Da) of the 'fragments' that are being selected. Typically in the drug development process from fragment to lead molecule, the potency is improved up to 100 times.
- Sotorasib (Ras GTPase inhibitor) used in non-small cell lung carcinoma and asciminib (tyrosine kinase inhibitor) used in CML were invented using this approach.

12.5.6 De-Novo Drug Modeling

- When a drug is developed without a 'starting template' using computational growth algorithms, then the approach is called de-novo drug modeling.
- Advantages:
  - Explores wider chemical entities.
  - Molecules with novel properties can be designed.
  - Time and cost-efficient drug development.
- Often this approach adapts both SBDD and LBDD methods during the developmental steps. Tools for structure-based de-novo drug design include LUDI, HIPPO, PRO_LIGAND, and MCSS (multiple-copy simultaneous search). For ligand-based de-novo drug design, tools like SYNOPSIS, DOGS, and TOPAS are often used.

12.5.7 Q-SAR

- It is one of the most popular LBDD approaches in CADD. QSAR is based on the fact that the molecular structure determines a biological activity of a ligand and therefore minor variations alter its biological activities.
- QSAR is a mathematical/computational model which aims to identify the significant correlations between a series of structurally similar molecules and their functions.
- The first step of QSAR is the creation of a library of the lead molecule that shows the desired biological activity. This is followed by a model generation that pre-

dicts the 'quantitative relation' between the structure and biological activities of these molecules.
- Based on the data generated, the existing lead molecule is structurally modified to increase the chances of becoming a new drug.

12.5.8 Pharmacophore Modeling

- Pharmacophore: It represents the 3D arrangements of features (steric and electronic configuration) that are required for optimal supra-molecular interactions between a ligand and target protein so that a particular biological activity can be stimulated or inhibited. Pharmacophore does not represent the actual connection (bond formation in the functional group) between the target and ligand. It denotes the vital features that are required for such interactions.
- Lead molecules can be quickly identified using the pharmacophore modeling method.
- Using computational codes and tools like PHASE, LigandScout, Catalyst, and Discovery studio are available commercially for 3D pharmacophore modeling.

12.5.9 Drugs Discovered Using CADD

- Oxymorphone (Opioid receptor antagonist)—using molecular docking method.
- Saquinavir (HIV protease inhibitor)—using the Pharmacophore method.
- Zanamivir (Antiinfluenza drug)—using de-novo modeling design.
- Dorzolamide (Antiglaucoma drug), Sotorasib (anticancer), and asciminib (anticancer)—using the fragment-based screening method.
- Norfloxacin (Fluoroquinolone antibiotic)—using the QSAR method.
- Other drugs like Captopril, Indinavir, Ritonavir, Tirofiban, Aliskiren, and oseltamivir have also been discovered using CADD methods.

Bibliography

1. Yu W, Weber DJ, MacKerell AD (2023) Computer-aided drug design: an update. Methods Mol Biol 2601:123–152
2. Yu W, Alexander D, MacKerell J (2017) Computer-aided drug design methods. Methods Mol Biol (Clifton, NJ) 1520:85
3. Wildey MJ, Haunso A, Tudor M, Webb M, Connick JH (2017) Chapter Five – High-throughput screening. In: Goodnow RA (ed) Annual reports in medicinal chemistry. Academic Press, Amsterdam, pp 149–195
4. Veselovsky AV, Ivanov AS (2003) Strategy of computer-aided drug design. Curr Drug Targets Infect Disord 3(1):33–40
5. Szymański P, Markowicz M, Mikiciuk-Olasik E (2011) Adaptation of high-throughput screening in drug discovery—toxicological screening tests. Int J Mol Sci 13(1):427–452

6. Sabe VT, Ntombela T, Jhamba LA, Maguire GEM, Govender T, Naicker T et al (2021) Current trends in computer aided drug design and a highlight of drugs discovered via computational techniques: a review. Eur J Med Chem 224:113705
7. Mayr LM, Bojanic D (2009) Novel trends in high-throughput screening. Curr Opin Pharmacol 9(5):580–588

Phase 0 Clinical Trials

13

Avinash Arivazhahan

Abstract

Clinical trials are essential to ensure that the drugs, devices and related entities that come into use by the general population are safe and efficacious for utility. The drug development process is a lengthy, regulated and streamlined process that starts in the laboratory, moving into animal studies and then finally into human trials. These human trials, also called clinical trials are divided into 5 phases—0, 1, 2, 3 and 4. Phases 1 to 4 are performed for all drugs and devices (without waivers), while Phase 0 is more of an exploratory trial, which is not routinely conducted. However, Phase 0 is very important in a few therapeutic areas and clinical populations. Phase 0 trials are sometimes interchangeably known as "micro-dosing studies". The most common application of Phase 0 trials is in the area of oncology. This chapter details the intricacies of Phase 0 trials in full length.

Keywords

Micro-dosing · Clinical trials · Oncology · Clinical studies · Drug development

13.1 Introduction

The complex and complicated process of drug development and testing happens over several years across a set of trials or studies, starting with pre-clinical (no human subjects) to clinical trials (involving human subjects or volunteers or sometimes, patients). The very first clinical trial that has been clearly reported in documented literature is the famous "James Lind scurvy experiment". This widely cited

A. Arivazhahan (✉)
Medical Affairs & Medical Education, Novo Nordisk India Ltd., Bengaluru, Karnataka, India

A. Arivazhahan et al. (eds.), *Introduction to Basics of Pharmacology and Toxicology*,
https://doi.org/10.1007/978-981-95-1920-0_13

clinical trial involved randomization of sailors into multiple groups, with varying interventions being done for scurvy. At the end of this trial, citrus fruits were found to have the most beneficial effects on the sick sailors. Since then, there have been multiple trials involving human volunteers and subjects. As times have evolved, the rules and restrictions surrounding clinical trials have also evolved, today keeping the volunteer safety and choice central.

13.2 Phases of Clinical Trials

Clinical trials, as the name suggests, are the first ever instance where a drug is properly studied in humans. Prior to this, there would have been animal studies, lab studies and sometimes PK/PD studies, depending on the type of drug being developed. All new drugs coming into the market go through at least three clinical trial phases before launch—Phases 1, 2 and 3. Phase 0 does not occur for all drugs, but selectively. Phase 4 happens after the launch of a product in the market (hence, also known as "post-marketing studies").

13.3 Phase 0 Trials

Phase 0 clinical trial is technically the first instance where an investigational drug or product is tested for the first time in human volunteers or patients. As mentioned earlier, this phase is not a routine part of the clinical trial process. Hence, in many cases, the first instance of human volunteer testing happens in Phase 1 studies, wherein the Phase 0 study is skipped.

The Phase 0 trials are also sometimes interchangeably known as "pilot trials", "pre-Phase 1 trials", "proof-of-concept clinical trials" or "exploratory IND (ExpIND) studies".

13.3.1 Objectives of Phase 0 Trials

There have been several situations where a drug looks extremely promising in the pre-clinical testing, but fails miserably in the human testing, due to various reasons, thus keeping the success rates of the first human testing very low (as shown in Fig. 13.1). The key objective of doing a Phase 0 study is to assess if the investigational drug or product really does what it is expected to do. This gives the researchers an idea of whether it would make sense to continue testing this drug or product in further phases of clinical trials. This could potentially help in making an informed decision on continued exploration of the said drug or product.

As an example, in oncology Phase 0 trials, the investigators would get a fair picture of the actual mechanism of action of the drug or product, its target sites, its pharmacokinetics and pharmacodynamics, etc. In addition, the adverse event profiling of the drug can be done to a certain extent. However, an important point to

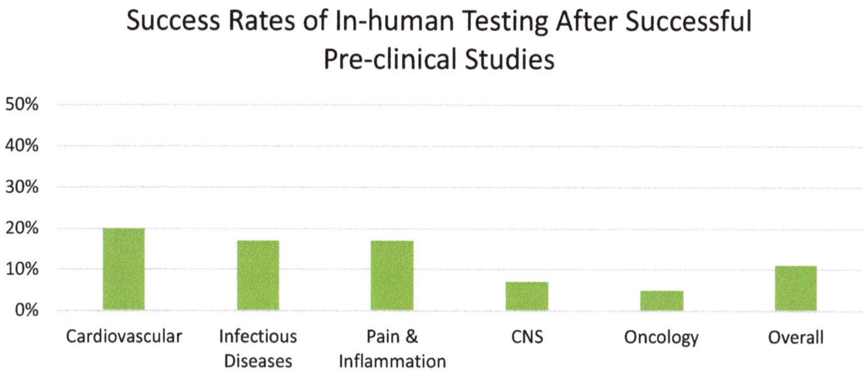

Fig. 13.1 Success rates across therapy areas in human trials. (Data from 1991 to 2000)

remember is that the dose of the drug or product used in Phase 0 may be very low (micro-dosing Phase 0 trials) to produce either the complete effects or the adverse effects at full therapeutic doses of the same.

Hence, on the whole, the objectives of performing Phase 0 trials are as follows:

- Helping in making informed research decisions on further development of the new drug or product.
- Helping in enhancing the efficiency of the development program of the new drug or product.
- Helping in raising the chances of successful approval and marketing of the new drug or product.

13.3.2 Methodology of Phase 0 Trials

As these are exploratory studies, the sample size is usually kept very low. The number of human volunteers (or clinically diagnosed patients, as the case may be) is minuscule in Phase 0 studies, usually averaging just 10 to 12, with many studies having an upper cap at 15. The trial duration is also extremely short in most cases, averaging less than 7 days in most cases, with many studies setting an upper cap of 7 to 10 days.

It is crucial to understand clearly that while the researcher may not get the exact therapeutic effect of the drug or product, he/she can get preliminary data of the intended mechanism of action. As an example, for an oncology drug, the research will know if the drug is able to enter the bloodstream and successfully target the end organ or site. Data from Phase 0 trials cannot be used to interpret a drug's clinical efficacy or safety.

13.4 Types of Phase 0 Trials

13.4.1 Types Based on the Dosing Used

Based on the dosing that is used in the trial, Phase 0 trials are broadly divided into 2 types: micro-dosing studies and pharmacological-dosing studies. As the names suggest, the former group intends to use sub-therapeutic doses of the drug or product while the latter uses the full clinical dose. The former requires minimal testing in the pre-clinical stages, whereas the latter requires extensive evaluation in the pre-clinical stages to ensure a wide therapeutic window. US-FDA defines "micro-dosing" as 1/100th of the pharmacologically effective dose that was calculated during pre-clinical animal studies. The upper cap of dosing is set at 100 mg for non-protein agents and 30 nmol for protein agents.

While the majority of the oncology Phase 0 trials are micro-dosing studies, there is a key exception. Agents being developed for neuro-oncological conditions may not suit for this design. This is due to the fact that sub-therapeutic doses may not be sufficient enough to penetrate the blood-brain barrier in many scenarios. Hence, there is a subset of pharmacological-dosing studies being used in the domain of neuro-oncology called the "window of opportunity Phase 0 trials". These trials involved patient volunteers who are scheduled for tumour resection, wherein the patients are administered therapeutic doses prior to the surgery. The biopsy is then used to check for penetration of the drug being tested.

13.4.2 Types Based on the Trial Objectives

Basis the objectives of the trial design, we can group Phase 0 studies into 2 categories: those that intend to study only the human pharmacokinetics (PK), and those that would study both PK and pharmacodynamics (PD). PK studies might be less invasive for the participants, compared to the PK/PD studies. In most cases, the PK studies are usually micro-dosing studies, and the PK/PD studies are pharmacological-dosing studies.

Between the two types, the PK/PD studies offer better insights to the researchers in terms of further vision for development. There could be two broad outcomes of these studies, if the trial fails:

(a) Pharmaceutical failure: the tissue biopsy fails to show adequate levels of the drug being present.
(b) Pharmacological failure: the tissue biopsy shows adequate levels of the drug but the target or receptor is not affected.

In the instance of a pharmaceutical failure, the researcher can either try another Phase 0 trial with an escalated dose or revisit the pre-clinical program. If it is a pharmacological failure, the researcher would have to either revisit the preclinical program or abort further development.

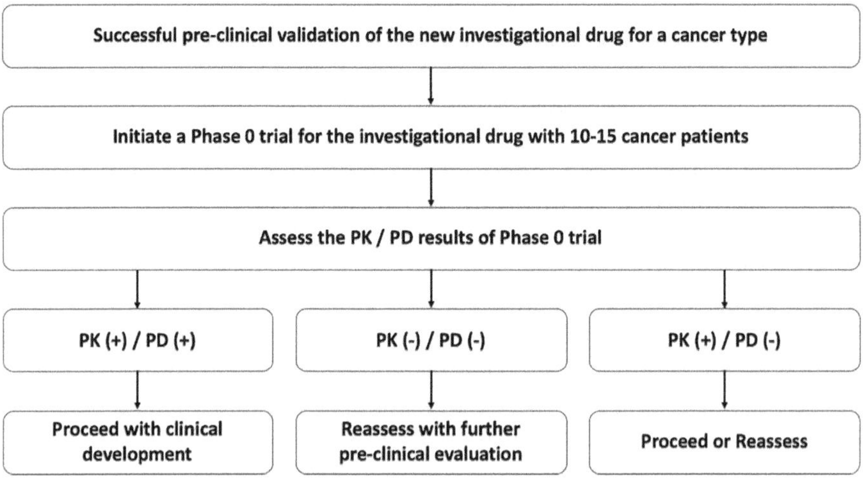

Fig. 13.2 Decision-making model for Phase 0 trials

13.5 Decision-Making Process in Phase 0 Trials

Clearly, the most important objective of Phase 0 trials is to guide in decision-making process of subsequent development of the said product or drug. A decision model is indicated in Fig. 13.2, with the example of an investigational drug developed in oncology.

13.6 Ethical Issues in Phase 0 Trials

While Phase 0 trials sound quite important from a research perspective, there are ethical issues surrounding these. The most important concern is the uncertainty of any clinical benefit with the investigational drug or product at this point of time. Since the dosing is usually sub-therapeutic in the majority of Phase 0 trials, the volunteer or the participating patient may not receive any tangible benefit by taking part. Further, the duration of these studies is extremely short to guarantee positive results. On the other end of the spectrum, there could be potential adverse events that can arise even at these low doses and with this short duration course.

In addition, once a volunteer or a patient consents to participate in Phase 0, he/she loses the opportunity to participate in other exploratory studies for a certain buffer or washout period (of at least 2 weeks minimally). Also, there could potentially be involvement of invasive procedures (including tissue biopsies) in the majority of oncology Phase 0 trials.

Having mentioned these ethical issues, there are clear guidelines and ways to overcome these limitations: clear explanation to the volunteers or patients, and receipt of documented informed consent for participation. The crux remains that the patient volunteer should clearly understand that this is a Phase 0 trial, and hence he/

she may not receive any clinical benefit at the end of the trial period. At the same time, there are recommendations that the participants in such Phase 0 trial should be given preference to participate in further phases of clinical development of the agent, if found to be successful.

13.7 Regulatory Standpoint for Phase 0 Trials

While there have been regulatory guidelines in place for clinical trials of Phases 1 to 4 for very long, guidance for Phase 0 trials was introduced only in January 2006 by the US-FDA. The official terminology for Phase 0 trials as used by the US-FDA in its guidance document is "explorational investigational new drug (IND) study". The goal, as per the regulatory authority, is to understand the new drug without exposing the study participants to its full effects.

In its guidance document, US-FDA states that these exploratory IND studies may be considered for drugs intended for any clinical indication, but urges the manufacturers and researchers to particularly consider these studies when working on drugs that are intended to be used in clinically serious indications (related to targeted therapies in the fields of oncology, immunology, etc.).

Following the release of this guidance in 2006, the first documented Phase 0 trial was conducted in 2007 to evaluate the preliminary effects of a poly-ADP ribose polymerase inhibitor, named ABT-888 at that point in time. Following a successful validation in this Phase 0 trial, the new drug candidate moved into further phases of clinical trials, ultimately being named veliparib, which currently holds an orphan drug status (awarded by the US-FDA in November 2016) for the management of non-small cell lung carcinoma.

13.8 Conclusion

Drug development is a lengthy and expensive process, at the end of which many drugs may not even see the light of the day. While traditionally human testing has begun with Phase 1 trials, the advent of Phase 0 trials in 2006 has its fair share of advantages. When used judiciously, Phase 0 trials offer the researchers in the industry to gauge the agent's PK and PD properties, and make an informed decision to continue or discontinue further development, thereby saving plenty of resources, which can then be diverted to research in other directions. Phase 0 trials also come with inherent limitations and ethical issues, which are subdued to a certain by the guidance from regulatory authorities and field experts.

Bibliography

Burt T, Yoshida K, Lappin G, Vuong L, John C, de Wildt SN et al (2016 Apr) Microdosing and other phase 0 clinical trials: facilitating translation in drug development. Clin Transl Sci 9(2):74–88

Doroshow JH, Kummar S (2009) Role of phase 0 trials in drug development. Future Med Chem 1(8):1375–1380

Fromer MJ (2006) FDA introduces new phase 0 for clinical trials: some enthusiastic, some Skeptical. Oncol Times 28(15):18–19

Gawai AA, Shaikh F, Gadekar M, Deokar N, Kolhe S, Biyani KR (2017) A review on: phase '0' clinical trials or exploratory investigational new drug. Turk J Pharm Sci 14(1):84–89

Gupta UC, Bhatia S, Garg A, Sharma A, Choudhary V (2011) Phase 0 clinical trials in oncology new drug development. Perspect Clin Res 2(1):13–22

Kummar S, Rubinstein L, Kinders R, Parchment RE, Gutierrez ME, Murgo AJ et al (2008) Phase 0 clinical trials: conceptions and misconceptions. Cancer J 14(3):133–137

Kummar S, Doroshow JH, Tomaszewski JE, Calvert AH, Lobbezoo M, Giaccone G (2009) Task force on methodology for the development of innovative cancer therapies (MDICT). Phase 0 clinical trials: recommendations from the task force on methodology for the development of innovative cancer therapies. Eur J Cancer 45(5):741–746

LoRusso PM (2009) Phase 0 clinical trials: an answer to drug development stagnation? J Clin Oncol 27(16):2586–2588

Rani PU, Naidu MU (2008) Phase 0 – microdosing strategy in clinical trials. Indian J Pharmacol 40(6):240–242

Phase 1 Clinical Trials

14

Ashwini Patil

Abstract

Any new drug or entity that comes into market needs approval from regulatory agencies of the respective geography. For these approvals, there is a standardized flow of events that includes multiple phases of clinical trials, wherein the testing is performed in human volunteers or patients. While Phase 0 clinical trials are not mandatory for every drug or candidate, Phase 1 is invariably the starting point for the vast majority of drugs. In Phase 1 trials, the pool of testing is limited to a very small number of trial participants—healthy participants or patients. This phase of clinical trials focuses on "dose ranging", wherein the ideal doses that would be safe for the end users or patients can be determined. Hence, determination of safety and the adverse effects at different doses is a priority in this phase. This chapter will elucidate the must-knows of Phase 1 clinical trials.

Keywords

Dose ranging · Clinical trials · Drug safety · Clinical studies · Drug development

14.1 Clinical Trial Phases

New drugs are developed through a series of procedures, where findings from small preliminary clinical studies inform the design of larger subsequent studies. During the development of a new drug, it is crucial to identify its properties in the early stages and then develop a research proposal tailored to these characteristics.

Different stages involved in clinical trials are quickly summarized in Table 14.1.

A. Patil (✉)
Sanofi India Ltd., Pune, India

A. Arivazhahan et al. (eds.), *Introduction to Basics of Pharmacology and Toxicology*,
https://doi.org/10.1007/978-981-95-1920-0_14

Table 14.1 Clinical trials: Overview of various phases

Phases	Phase 0	Phase 1a/1b	Phase 2a/2b	Phase 3a/3b	Phase 4
Dosing	Sub-therapeutic	Ascending doses	Therapeutic dose	Therapeutic dose	Therapeutic dose
Number of subjects	About 10	20–100	100–300	1000–2000	Anyone seeking treatment
Main goal of clinical phase	Pharmacokinetics and pharmacodynamics	Dose ranging	Drug efficacy	Therapeutic effect	Long-term effects

14.2 Introduction to Phase 1 Trials

According to the International Conference on Harmonization, Phase I studies generally have one or a combination of the following objectives:

- To estimate safety and tolerability of the predicted dose range and identify the nature of any potential adverse drug reactions.
- To characterize the drug's pharmacokinetic parameters, which include A (absorption), D (distribution), M (metabolism), and E (excretion), as well as evaluate its clearance and anticipate any potential accumulation that could inform dosage and dosing regimens.
- To provide preliminary estimates of the drug's activity and potential effectiveness, which may influence dosage and dosing regimens in subsequent studies.
- To provide an early assessment of drug activity, particularly when it can be easily measured with short-duration drug exposure in patients at this initial stage.

14.3 Phase 1 Clinical Trials

Phase 1 trials are subject to more rigorous monitoring than other phases of drug development because they represent the first time a new drug is being tested in humans (since Phase 0 trials do not happen for all new drugs, Phase 1 is usually the first human exposure for most new drugs in investigation). Furthermore, they are generally planned for healthy participants to evaluate the safety of the new drug, even though newer therapies for certain ailments like as HIV infection or Cancer are reasonably often first investigated in patients. Phase 1 clinical trial determines the best way to administer a drug, its frequency, maximum tolerated dose (MTD), and side effects. During this phase, factors such as pharmacokinetics, tolerability, and pharmacodynamics are assessed. Most critically, these studies establish the safety of the drug for human use.

The chief desired outcome of Phase 1 trials is mainly to prevent unnecessary exposure of participants to ineffective doses while ensuring safety. Initial studies of a new drug assess short-term toxicity in humans to determine the maximum tolerated dose (MTD). Long-term and cumulative toxicities are beyond the clinical scope of this phase. Another key objective of this phase of clinical trials is to determine a dose range appropriate for testing efficacy in further trials, namely the Phase 2 clinical trials. Typically, Phase 1 studies are conducted via "open label" study design, which means that they are not controlled, randomized, or blinded. Without utilizing these strategies to reduce bias, it is difficult to ensure that treatment groups are comparable in all aspects other than the treatment they receive. Efficacy cannot be accurately assessed if treatment arms are not directly comparable.

In this phase, as subjects are usually healthy volunteers, there are several advantages due to their participation. Their recruitment can be more rapid (in comparison to other phases). Also, participants do not have coexisting diseases, and also not on concomitant drugs that would be confounding factor for the outcome of the clinical trial. These studies have a lower risk of toxicity but do not fully reflect the drug's effects on patients. For drugs with high toxicity risks, such as cancer treatments or immunosuppressants, Phase 1 trials are usually conducted with appropriate patient populations.

Phase 1 trials aim to characterize the pharmacokinetic properties of a drug by analyzing its absorption, distribution, metabolism, and excretion. These studies measure drug concentrations in bodily fluids or tissues over time, following single or multiple doses. They also examine bioavailability, food effects on drug concentration, and genetic impacts on metabolism, such as variations in cytochrome P450 enzymes. To ensure data represents the broader population, these trials should include diverse participants of different ages, races, and genders. Typically, Phase 1 trials use young male volunteers, which may not fully reflect the target population's pharmacokinetic profile. Including diverse ethnic and racial backgrounds helps identify differences in drug metabolism due to genetic polymorphism.

Although drug efficacy is not the main focus of a Phase 1 trial, pharmacodynamic evaluations are usually included to provide an early estimate of potential effectiveness. Pharmacodynamic studies show the relationship between drug dose and clinical response through various laboratory tests, non-invasive tests, vital signs, or clinical assessments of disease. The initial pharmacodynamic data, alongside pharmacokinetic data, inform recommendations for Phase 2 trial drug doses and dosage regimens. However, these data have limitations due to the small number of participants, and the absence of randomization, control, and blinding.

Phase 1 trials have limited capacity to evaluate efficacy. For instance, a drug curing 5% of patients might seem ineffective if no responsive patients are in the trial. Human trials mark Phase 1, but further phases better establish a drug's effectiveness with more data. Only 25–30% of drugs in Phase 1 reach Phase 3, proving both safety and efficacy.

To conserve financial resources, pharmaceutical companies frequently decide to delay additional pharmacokinetic studies, such as assessing pharmacokinetics in patients with hepatic or renal impairment or evaluating drug-drug interactions, until Phase 2 or Phase 3 trials. As a result, this crucial information, which could be highly pertinent to the target population, is often absent from Phase 1 trial data. Consequently, the efficacy data from Phase 1 trials may present an overly optimistic view of a treatment's practical utility. It is important to note that the primary objective of Phase 1 trials is human pharmacology, with only minimal emphasis on potential efficacy.

In the context of dermatologic diseases, Phase 1 studies of drugs may take a tangential from traditional models when the medications under investigation have already been tested in humans for other indications. For instance, drugs that are being evaluated for psoriasis may have previously undergone clinical trials for oncology or organ transplantation. Some medications studied for onychomycosis may also be assessed for systemic mycoses. While much is known about their pharmacokinetics, safety, and tolerability, Phase 1 studies in dermatology confirm or refine these data for skin-related conditions. Such studies focus on drug distribution in nails, skin, sebum, or sweat, which are more relevant than serum or plasma levels. Additionally, Phase 1 trials often explore new administration routes, especially if a systemic drug shows potential for topical use. A notable example is minoxidil, originally an oral antihypertensive, which was subsequently tested as a topical treatment for alopecia.

Dermatologic studies often rely on direct visual assessments of the disease state to evaluate initial efficacy, rather than using blood tests or radiologic studies as surrogate endpoints. Although this approach appears to offer a more straightforward and accurate method for determining efficacy, significant variability in the data can arise, especially when different investigators conduct assessments for the same patient throughout the trial. One advantage of clinical studies in dermatology is the ease with which skin biopsies can be obtained. These biopsies serve to examine cell kinetics or various cell markers, thereby contributing to a better understanding of the drug's mechanism of action. Conversely, in oncology trials, obtaining repeated tumor biopsies throughout the study is often impractical, making it challenging to facilitate direct histopathological evaluation of the drug's effects.

Given the availability of substantial human pharmacologic data, many dermatologic studies may occur as a combination of Phase 1 and Phase 2 trials. In these Phase 1/2 trials, greater emphasis is placed on preliminary evidence of efficacy in a randomized and controlled manner, alongside dose-response assessments across various dosages within a carefully defined subset of patients. The broader efficacy data generated from this design enhances the likelihood of extrapolating initial findings from a limited number of patients to a broader target population. Nevertheless, the target population may encompass a wider range of disease characteristics than the study population, which is defined by strict inclusion and exclusion criteria.

Phase I trials generally involve 20–100 participants, who are overseen by clinical researchers. If no significant adverse effects are observed, doses are gradually increased, and patients are evaluated to see how they respond to the treatment. These dose escalation studies aim to identify the optimal and safest dose for administration, while also reviewing the dose fraction that could potentially cause harm based on findings from animal studies. These trials are typically conducted by contract research organizations (CROs). In this phase, testing is usually done in a chronological manner, with data being analyzed following each patient or small group of patients.

14.4 Estimation of Initial Dose in Phase 1 Clinical Trial

It is important to ensure appropriate drug dosing for any administration purpose. Selecting the initial drug dose for clinical trials in both animals and humans is a significant consideration. It is essential to recognize that dose scaling should not be based solely on body weight, as this approach is not suitable. This is mainly because different species have varying biochemical and functional systems, affecting pharmacokinetics. Thus, to enhance the safety of clinical trials, it is essential to take into account body surface area, physiological time, and pharmacokinetics when extrapolating doses from animals to humans. There are several ways to calculate doses: factor-based, similar drug, pharmacokinetic guidance, and comparative methods. The dose by factor method is an approach that uses no observed adverse effect levels (NOAEL) from preclinical toxicological studies to estimate the human equivalent dose (HED). The NOAEL is transformed into the HED using suitable scaling factors to adjust for body surface area differences among species. This method focuses on selecting a dose that minimizes the risk of toxicity rather than one that has minimal pharmacological activity in humans. The similar drug method leverages existing pharmacokinetic data from another drug with comparable pharmacological properties. In contrast, the pharmacokinetically guided approach emphasizes drug activity over dose scaling between species. The comparative approach employs various techniques to determine the initial dose, followed by data comparison and optimization to identify an appropriate starting dose. Regulatory guidance from the US Food and Drug Administration (FDA) places significant emphasis on the NOAEL obtained from preclinical toxicology studies. The European Medicines Agency (EMA) recommends the minimal anticipated biological effect level (MABEL) approach, considering all available in vivo and in vitro data. Both NOAEL- and MABEL-derived HEDs can be further adjusted by applying safety factors to increase the likelihood that the initial dose will not lead to toxicity in humans. The disadvantage of NOEL is its conservative approach due to arbitrary safety factor. It also neglects the interspecies differences in pharmacology. The limitation of MABEL is that it requires extensive mechanistic data.

14.5 Dose Administration Regimen in Phase 1 Study

Single- and multiple-dose administration regimens are incorporated in initial safety and tolerability studies. Data from Phase 1 trials are frequently published for cytotoxic drugs used in oncology, where established dose escalation protocols provide models for evaluating these trials critically. The preliminary dose is generally determined based on previous animal studies, with the lowest dose selected as outlined earlier. For instance, in clinical trials for new oncology drugs, this dose is often set at 1/10th of lethal dose for 10% mice (mouse LD10), unless other toxicology findings in different species warrant a lower dose. A dose escalation model is traditionally used to rapidly increase dosage in initial study groups to quickly find low toxicity levels. This is typically followed by smaller increases in dosage, under the assumption that therapeutic effects may emerge at doses close to toxic levels. Very few patients (fewer than 10) receive a specific dose and are monitored for toxicity before subsequent groups are treated at the next higher dose. The conventional dose escalation strategy frequently leads to numerous participants in Phase 1 trials receiving sub-therapeutic doses of the investigational drug, consequently offering no clinical benefit. Alternative dose escalation methods, informed by preclinical pharmacokinetic and pharmacodynamic data, may be employed to minimize the number of patients administered doses below the therapeutic threshold. During Phase I, both dose-toxicity and dose-efficacy curves are established.

It includes the following studies:

1. Single ascending dose trials (Phase IA)
2. Multiple ascending dose trials (Phase IB)
3. Food effect studies

1. **Single ascending dose trials (Phase IA):**
   - Phase IA trials consist of small subject groups.
   - In these trials, participants receive a single dose of the medication while being closely monitored over a defined time frame.
   - If no significant adverse effects are observed and the pharmacokinetic data aligns closely with the anticipated safety profiles, the dose is increased.
   - Subsequently, a different group of subjects is tested with the higher dosage.
   - This process continues until predetermined safety thresholds for the drug are reached or until toxic adverse events, known as the maximum tolerated dose (MTD), occur.
2. **Multiple Ascending Dose Trials (Phase IB):**
   - These studies aim to deepen the knowledge of the pharmacokinetics and pharmacodynamics related to multiple doses of the medication.
   - In these studies, a cohort of patients receives several small doses of the drug, while samples of blood, urine, and other bodily fluids are collected at various intervals.
   - Later, these are evaluated to understand pharmacokinetics and pharmacodynamic profile of drug.
   - The dosage is then increased in subsequent groups, up to a predetermined limit.
3. **Food Effect Studies:**
   - The bioavailability studies of food effect are generally carried out for new medications as part of the investigational new drug application process to assess how food influences the absorption rate and extent of a new drug when taken shortly after eating (under fed conditions), compared to administration in a fasting state.

- Food can change a drug's bioavailability and affect bioequivalence between test and reference products.
- Food affects bioavailability significantly, with clinical implications, by:
  - Delay of gastric emptying.
  - Stimulation of bile secretion.
  - Alteration of gastrointestinal pH levels.
  - Increase of splanchnic blood flow.
  - Modification of drug metabolism in the intestines.
  - Physical or chemical interaction with the dosage form or drug.
- Food influences drug bioavailability most when taken shortly after a meal.
- The caloric and nutrient composition, volume, and temperature of the meal can change gastrointestinal physiology, affecting transit time, permeability, dissolution, and systemic availability.
- High-calorie, high-fat meals are more likely to disrupt gastrointestinal function and affect drug bioavailability.
- High-calorie and high-fat meals are recommended for fed bioequivalence and food effect bioavailability studies.
- Guidelines suggest a two-treatment (fed vs. fasting), two-sequence, two-period crossover study design.
- The formulation is administered on an empty stomach in the first period and after a test meal in the second period, with a washout period between treatments.
- The test meal should contain 800–1000 calories, with 50% from fats. It should include approximately 250 calories from carbohydrates, 150 from proteins, and 500–600 from fats.

14.6 Dose Escalation Methods

1. **Rule-Based Method**
2. **Model-Based Method**

1. **Rule-Based Method:**
   - Rule-based designs eliminate the need for any prior assumptions regarding the dose-toxicity relationship, allowing for both dose escalation and de-escalation based on the occurrence or absence of toxicity, including smaller fractions of the previous dose.
   - These techniques are simple to execute and do not necessitate the use of specialized software.

(a) **Conventional 3 + 3 design:**

- The process continues with groups of three patients. The initial dosage is determined based on extrapolated toxicological data from animal studies.
- Predefined increasing dose levels typically follow a modified Fibonacci sequence, where the increments in dosage decrease as the dose rises. For instance, the first dose may be doubled compared to the previous one, followed by increases of 67%, 50%, 40%, and so on, in accordance with the modified Fibonacci pattern.
- In the event that no patients within the cohort experience dose-limiting toxicity, an additional three patients will be administered the next higher dose.
- Should one patient encounter dose-limiting toxicity, the same dosage will be given to an additional three patients.
- This dose escalation process will proceed until at least two patients in a cohort of three to six exhibit dose-limiting toxicities.
- The recommended dosage for Phase II trials will be established as the maximum dose that remains below the toxic level.

- Other rule-based dose escalation methods include "2 + 4," "3 + 3 + 3," "3 + 1 + 1" (best of five), Accelerated Titration Design, Isotonic Regression Model, Rolling Six Designs, and Biased Coin Up-and-Down Design Rules.

(b) **"2 + 4" design:**

- If one dose-limiting toxicity occurs in the first two patients, four more will be added.
- However, the stopping criteria remain consistent with those used in "3 + 3" studies.

(c) **"3 + 3 + 3" design:**

- Introduce a third cohort if two of the first six patients report dose-limiting toxicity.
- Halt the study if three out of nine patients experience dose-limiting toxicity.

(d) **"3 + 1 + 1" (best of five) design:**

- Include an additional patient if one or two dose-limiting toxicities occur among the first three patients.
- Add another patient if two dose-limiting toxicities are noted among the four treated patients.
- Continue dose escalation if no toxicities are detected in three patients, one in four, or two in five.
- Halt the trial if three or more toxicities are reported.

(e) **Accelerated Titration Design:**

- This method combines aspects of both the 3 + 3 design and model-based design.
- Patients are assigned to various doses according to established protocols.

- Pharmacologically guided dose escalation enhances the traditional 3 + 3 design, based on the premise that animal model studies can accurately predict dose-limiting toxicities associated with plasma drug concentrations.
- Initially, plasma exposure is estimated from preclinical data, and pharmacokinetic information is subsequently collected for each patient to inform future dosing.

(f) **Isotonic Regression Model:**

- This model operates under the assumption that toxicity does not diminish with increasing dose, and thus applies isotonic regression to the collected data.
- The dose administered is estimated to approach the maximum tolerable toxicity level.

(g) **Rolling Six Designs:**

- This design allows adding 2 to 6 patients at a dose level, considering enrolled and evaluable patients, those with dose-limiting toxicity, and those still at risk.
- It aims to shorten the study duration when dose range information is available, especially in pediatric populations.

(h) **Biased Coin Up-and-Down Design:**

- This approach requires prompt reporting of treatment responses or toxicity assessments.
- In this method, each patient's dose is determined based on the toxicity data from the most recently completed subject, allowing for the simultaneous study of multiple patients.

- Another rule-based design enables the allocation of subsequent patients to doses according to the toxicity outcomes observed at the current dose by estimating the toxicity probability interval using the beta-binomial model.

2. **Model-Based Method:**

- These designs use statistical models to identify dose levels leading to toxicity by analyzing patient data, creating a precise dose-toxicity curve.
- Bayesian models are frequently used, estimating Θ to shape the dose-toxicity curve, modified by toxicity per Bayes' theorem.
- Traditionally, these designs provide a confidence interval for recommended doses in Phase II trials.
- The first Bayesian model-based method was the "continual reassessment method," which was implemented in early Phase I clinical trial designs. Early estimates of Θ are obtained from experts familiar with preclinical data or knowledgeable about similar drugs.
- Patients are administered doses believed to be nearest to the maximum tolerated dose (MTD).

- The probability of dose-limiting toxicity is evaluated for each new patient until a specific condition halts the trial.
- Modifications include starting at the lowest dose, incrementally increasing doses, stopping dose escalation if toxicity occurs, treating multiple patients at the same dose, and expanding the cohort.
- An alternative Bayesian method, called escalation with overdose control, helps avoid exposing patients to excessively toxic doses.

Additional model-based designs incorporate time-to-event endpoints as well as efficacy and toxicity assessment methods. These designs accurately predict the target probability of dose-limiting toxicity for Phase II trials, avoiding excessive patient exposure to suboptimal doses. Strategies for dose-escalation in clinical trials that involve drug combinations include alternating escalations across different dose levels, concurrent increases for both drugs, escalating one drug to the recommended Phase II dose while keeping the other at a fixed level, and raising one drug to the recommended Phase II dose while maintaining the other at a low dose.

In a review article on dose escalation methods, the authors reported that 88% of Phase I clinical trials employed either a traditional or modified 3 + 3 dose escalation approach. They observed an estimated median rate of dose-limiting toxicity of 6%. The authors advised that initial dosing, dose levels, and dose-escalation steps should prioritize patient safety, minimize the number of patients exposed to subtherapeutic doses, and optimize drug combinations for subsequent studies. Nevertheless, there are no established clinical trial designs specifically tailored for molecularly targeted drugs with a well-defined relevant target and a validated system for evaluating target inhibition.

14.7 What Additional Factors Should Be Taken into Account in Phase I Trials?

Phase I trials traditionally involve single ascending dose (SAD) studies, with staggered multiple ascending dose (MAD) studies following. Since adaptive clinical trial designs emerged in 2004, combining SAD/MAD studies has been planned to potentially shorten timelines by 12 months compared to conducting separate trials.

This design allows for concurrent SAD and MAD studies, exploring new doses in adaptive cohorts, with established start and stop criteria for safety. First-in-human studies can evaluate food and formulation effects, integrating them into adaptive designs to guide clinical development. These assessments align with the SAD arm once dose escalation reaches a relevant level, crucial for drugs with nonlinear pharmacokinetics. Ideally, evaluations should use a crossover design for better insights.

The FDA has also provided guidance for first-in-human trials regarding the assessment of immunogenicity for therapeutic protein products. Phase I trials offer the first chance to assess the immunogenic potential of a new biologic drug, impacting clinical safety and efficacy, since animal studies cannot reliably predict human immune responses.

14.8 Challenges Associated with Phase 1 Trial's Study Designs

Many molecularly targeted or biological agents are given as continuous oral or repetitive intravenous doses, leading to chronic or delayed toxicities. These cumulative effects must be considered in Phase II dose determination. Early assessment of dose-limiting toxicities may miss late or cumulative adverse events. Study designs like the "Time-to-Event Continuous Reassessment Model" (TiTE-CRM) and others aim to address these issues but are not widely used in clinical trials.

The TiTE-CRM, compared to the traditional 3 + 3 design, resulted in shorter trials and more patients treated near the maximum tolerated dose. However, its application in two Phase I chemoradiotherapy studies did not confirm these advantages, highlighting the need for real-world testing to validate such models.

14.9 Global Considerations for Phase I Trial

Numerous factors collectively influence the selection of study sites or countries for first-in-human trials, including the sponsors' operational regions, the ease of patient enrollment, regulatory obligations, and the distribution of the target patient population. Once these factors are established, early engagement and well-timed communication with local health authorities are essential for the success of the studies. Prior to initiating such interactions, gaining a thorough understanding of regulatory agency expectations is advantageous. Available guidance documents can aid sponsors in preparing for and facilitating more effective discussions. In situations where clear guidance is absent, collaborating with experienced local contract clinical research organizations and key opinion leaders can be beneficial for coordinating and supporting the studies.

Bibliography

1. National Library of Medicine. Medical subjects headings. Available: http://www.nlm.nih.gov/mesh/MBrowser.html
2. Food and Drug Administration (1997) International conference on harmonization: guidance on general considerations for clinical trials. Docket number 97D–0188. Washington (D.C.): Food and Drug Administration Department of Health and Human Services. Fed Regist 62:66113–66119. Available: http://www.fda.gov/Cder/Guidance/1857fnl.pdf
3. Storer BE (1989) Design and analysis of phase I clinical trials. Biometrics 45:795–798. https://doi.org/10.2307/2531693
4. Rogatko A, Schoeneck D, Jonas W, Tighiouart M, Khuri FR, Porter A (2007) Translation of innovative designs into phase I trials. J Clin Oncol 25:4982–4986. https://doi.org/10.1200/JCO.2007.12.1012
5. Storer BE (2001) An evaluation of phase I clinical trial designs in the continuous dose-response setting. Stat Med 20:2399–2408. https://doi.org/10.1002/sim.903

6. Graham MA, Workman P (1992) The impact of pharmacokinetically guided dose escalation strategies in phase I clinical trials: critical evaluation and recommendations for future studies. Ann Oncol 3:339–347
7. Leung DH, Wang Y (2001) Isotonic designs for phase I trials. Control Clin Trials 22:126–138. https://doi.org/10.1016/S0197-2456(00)00132-X
8. Skolnick JM, Barrett JS, Jayaraman B, Patel D, Adamson PC (2008) Shortening the timeline of pediatric phase I trials: the rolling six design. J Clin Oncol 26:190–195. https://doi.org/10.1200/JCO.2007.12.7712
9. Durham SD, Flournoy N, Rosenberger WF (1997) A random walk rule for phase I clinical trials. Biometrics 53:745–760. https://doi.org/10.2307/2533975
10. Ivanova A, Montazer-Haghighi A, Mohanty SG, Durham SD (2003) Improved up-and-down designs for phase I trials. Stat Med 22:69–82. https://doi.org/10.1002/sim.1336
11. Stylianou M, Follmann DA (2004) The accelerated biased coin up-and-down design in phase I trials. J Biopharm Stat 14:249–260. https://doi.org/10.1081/BIP-120028518
12. Ji Y, Li Y, Nebiyou Bekele B (2007) Dose-finding in phase I clinical trials based on toxicity probability intervals. Clin Trials 4:235–244. https://doi.org/10.1177/1740774507079442
13. O'Quigley J, Pepe M, Fisher L (1990) Continual reassessment method: a practical design for phase I clinical trials in cancer. Biometrics 46:33–48. https://doi.org/10.2307/2531628
14. Faries D (1994) Practical modifications of the continual reassessment method for phase I cancer clinical trials. J Biopharm Stat 4:147–164. https://doi.org/10.1080/10543409408835079
15. Goodman SN, Zahurk ML, Piantadosi S (1995) Some practical improvements in the continual reassessment method for phase I studies. Stat Med 14:1149–1161. https://doi.org/10.1002/sim.4780141102
16. Moller S (1995) An extension of the continual reassessment methods using a preliminary up-and-down design in a dose finding study in cancer patients in order to investigate a greater range of doses. Stat Med 14:911–922. https://doi.org/10.1002/sim.4780140909
17. Piantadosi S, Fisher JD, Grossman S (1998) Practical implementation of a modified continual reassessment method for dose-finding trials. Cancer Chemother Pharmacol 41:429–436. https://doi.org/10.1007/s002800050763
18. Rogatko A, Babb JS, Tighiouart M, Khuri FR, Hudes G (2005) New paradigm in dose-finding trials: patient-specific dosing and beyond phase I. Clin Cancer Res 11:5342–5346. https://doi.org/10.1158/1078-0432.CCR-05-0458
19. Riviere MK, Le Tourneau C, Paoletti X, Dubois F, Zohar S (2014) Designs of drug-combination phase I trials in oncology: a systematic review of the literature. Ann Oncol. https://doi.org/10.1093/annonc/mdu516
20. https://www.fda.gov/files/drugs/published/Food-Effect-Bioavailability-and-Fed-Bioequivalence-Studies.pdf
21. Muglia JJ, DiGiovanna JJ (1998) Phase 1 clinical trials. J Cutan Med Surg 2(4):236–241. https://doi.org/10.1177/120347549800200413
22. Hansen AR, Graham DM, Pond GR, Siu LL (2014) Phase 1 trial design: is 3 + 3 the best? Cancer Control 21(3):200–208. https://doi.org/10.1177/107327481402100304
23. Shen J, Swift B, Mamelok R, Pine S, Sinclair J, Attar M (2019) Design and conduct considerations for first-in-human trials. Clin Transl Sci 12(1):6–19. https://doi.org/10.1111/cts.12582. Epub 2018 Aug 24. PMID: 30048046; PMCID: PMC6342261
24. Mahan V (2014) Clinical trial phases. Int J Clin Med 5:1374–1383. https://doi.org/10.4236/ijcm.2014.521175
25. Muller PY, Milton M, Lloyd P, Sims J, Brennan FR (2009) The minimum anticipated biological effect level (MABEL) for selection of first human dose in clinical trials with monoclonal antibodies. Curr Opin Biotechnol 20(6):722–729. https://doi.org/10.1016/j.copbio.2009.10.013

Phase 2 Clinical Trials

15

Sarjana Atal

Abstract

Drug development is lengthy and costly, with few candidates progressing from Phase 1 to Phase 2 trials. Phase 1 assesses dosing and side effects, while Phase 2 involves more participants, providing broader data on dosing, safety, and some efficacy. Phase 2 acts as a bridge to large-scale Phase 3 trials, which determine the drug's final outcome. This chapter provides an overview of Phase 2 clinical trials.

Keywords

Drug efficacy · Clinical trials · Drug safety · Clinical studies · Drug development

15.1 Introduction to Phase 2 Trials

Phase 2 clinical trials, or "therapeutic exploratory trials," assess a treatment's efficacy and safety in several hundred participants. These trials help determine optimal doses, dosing schedules, administration methods, and endpoints to inform Phase 3 planning. Preliminary drug efficacy is evaluated by:

1. Comparing results with historical controls from established therapies.
2. Testing different dosing groups.
3. Randomizing subjects into trial arms.

S. Atal (✉)
Sanofi India Ltd., Bhopal, India

A. Arivazhahan et al. (eds.), *Introduction to Basics of Pharmacology and Toxicology*,
https://doi.org/10.1007/978-981-95-1920-0_15

Subdivisions of Phase 2 Trials
Phase 2 trials include:

- Phase 2a: Pilot "proof of concept" studies to show efficacy or biological activity.
- Phase 2b: Dose-finding studies to identify the effective dose with minimal side effects.
- Phase 2c: Assess intermediate efficacy, safety, and tolerability to guide Phase 3 decisions.

Key considerations for evaluating Phase 2 Trials
Key considerations for evaluating a Phase 2 study include:

1. Study design.
2. Predefined endpoints (response rate, time-to-event analysis).
3. Selection criteria.
4. Statistical aspects (Type 1/2 errors, sample size, stopping rules).
5. Additional factors (patients enrolled/analysed, expected endpoint results, methods for estimating results, and use of comparison groups).

15.2 Different Phase 2 Trial Designs

Phase 2 trials can use single-stage, multi-stage, randomized control, or randomized selection designs. All aim for simplicity, rapid completion, and limiting patient exposure to inferior treatments. Trial design mainly depends on three statistical parameters:

1. α (type I error/false positive rate).
2. β (type II error/false negative rate).
3. δ (targeted effect size).

The sample size is calculated to detect δ at a significance level of α with a power of $(1 - \beta) \times 100\%$. Phase 2 studies are typically powered to reduce the risk of incorrectly dismissing a potentially effective treatment (i.e., $\beta \leq 0.2$, and often set at 0.1, ensuring less than a 20% probability of wrongly rejecting a promising therapy). Likewise, these studies frequently allow for a higher-than-normal probability of type I error, as reflected by an α value of 0.05 or greater. Study designs may involve a single arm with an external comparator sourced from published literature or historical controls, or they may include multiple arms assigned through randomization. The following section provides a brief overview of the key features of these trial designs:

1. **Single-Stage Phase 2 Trial Design**

Single-stage designs are the most straightforward approach, employing a predetermined sample size and lacking provisions for interim analysis. All participants receive the same intervention, and outcomes are evaluated upon completion of accrual. This design is particularly suitable for estimating response rates with a defined endpoint. However, its principal limitation lies in potential confounding between outcome and trial effects, as it does not allow separation of factors such as patient selection, eligibility criteria, imaging techniques, assessment schedules, and treatment settings from the actual impact of the intervention on clinical results.

2. **Multi-Stage Phase 2 Trial Design**

To address ethical and economic considerations, clinical trials are often structured with multiple stages. Phase 2 studies typically involve a limited number of patients, generally resulting in no more than two stages. Two-stage designs incorporate interim statistical analyses after initial enrolment. If efficacy does not reach a predefined threshold in the first stage, further enrolment is discontinued; conversely, if the threshold is achieved, additional participants are recruited in the second stage to enhance the precision of efficacy estimates. Recent modifications allow simultaneous evaluation of toxicity and efficacy within two-stage frameworks, facilitating early termination for safety or futility but not for overwhelming success. These designs are advantageous when rapid assessment of primary endpoints (e.g., response at 3 months) enables timely interim analysis. A potential drawback is that ongoing accrual may need to pause during interim evaluations, although Bayesian approaches offer alternatives by permitting continuous monitoring of success probability as data accumulate.

Given the inherent limitations and biases associated with single-arm or multi-arm study designs, innovative adaptive methodologies have been developed to enable seamless trial progression and minimize the risk of false positives.

3. **Randomized Phase 2 Trial Design**

The use of randomization mitigates the influence of unknown and known prognostic factors by allocating them evenly across treatment groups. Randomized Phase 2 trial designs can be classified into the following categories:

- Parallel non-comparative single-arm experimental arms, each governed by an independent decision rule.
- Randomized selection ("pick the winner") designs aimed at identifying the most promising regimen among several comparable experimental interventions.
- Randomized screening designs intended to compare an experimental regimen with the current standard of care.

The salient features of each of these designs are summarized below.

4. **Randomization to Parallel Noncomparative Regimens**

This design incorporates randomization into two or more experimental treatment arms primarily to minimize bias, including patient selection bias, and to control for both known and unknown baseline imbalances between arms. Each treatment arm functions as an independent Phase 2 study, with "promising activity" determined via comparison to historical controls and defined thresholds for α (usually 0.1) and β (typically 0.1). Such an approach is advantageous when comparing multiple experimental regimens concurrently without direct comparisons; each regimen that satisfies pre-specified success criteria may progress to further evaluation in larger trials.

While this method is not widely employed across most disease areas, it remains particularly appealing in early Phase 2 contexts where a reliable early endpoint—such as tumour response—can be directly attributed to the intervention under investigation (i.e., a single-agent trial). Success typically necessitates comprehensive subsequent assessment of promising regimens in a Phase 2b setting that includes direct comparative analysis of safety and efficacy outcomes among the randomized arms.

5. **Randomized Selection Designs**

Randomized selection designs were first introduced by Simon et al. to identify the most promising experimental regimen among several candidates using a ranking and selection methodology. The regimen deemed most promising is subsequently compared to standard of care within a larger Phase 3 trial.

These designs are particularly relevant when comparing different administration methods, dosing schedules, or combination regimens involving a novel experimental agent alongside a common core regimen. The principal aim is to prioritize among "experimental" regimens in cases lacking prior data favouring one over another. Participants are randomized to two or more competing regimens or agents, after which results are ranked and the highest-performing arm selected for further research. Sample size is calculated to ensure a high probability of selecting the superior arm, provided its expected outcome exceeds others by a clinically meaningful margin (e.g., at least 15%). Notably, this design does not evaluate the null hypothesis of equivalency and thus does not elucidate relative efficacy between similar regimens. For instance, Lustberg et al. utilized this approach to compare two doses of Mitomycin C followed by irinotecan in advanced oesophageal and gastro-esophageal junction adenocarcinomas, employing a two-stage Simon design with distinct efficacy decision rules for each arm (α and β set at 0.1). Follow-up rankings recommended the low-dose arm as both well tolerated and effective.

Selection within screening designs can also consider factors such as safety profiles, cost, convenience, or quality of life, aligning these approaches closely with routine clinical practice.

6. **Randomized Screening Designs**

This category of study design facilitates a nondefinitive comparison of one or more experimental regimens against standard-of-care treatments within a Phase 2 framework. For example, the evaluation of two bevacizumab doses combined with carboplatin and paclitaxel versus carboplatin and paclitaxel alone (as a concurrent control) in chemotherapy-naïve patients with non-small cell lung cancer exemplifies this approach. Results from this randomized Phase 2 trial supported advancement to a pivotal Phase 3 trial, establishing the efficacy of high-dose bevacizumab plus carboplatin and paclitaxel.

Rubinstein et al. formally advocated for preliminary, nondefinitive experimental-to-standard-of-care comparisons through deliberate selection of statistical parameters—α, β, and δ—optimized to distinguish non-promising regimens while advancing those warranting further investigation. These studies are not substitutes for definitive Phase 3 trials but function as tools to prioritize regimens meriting additional evaluation.

Careful selection of statistical parameters is essential: sample size should remain practical (typically about 100 patients), and outcomes must be robust. Excessively high false-positive rates ($\alpha > 0.20$) risk an increase in unsuccessful Phase 3 studies; conversely, a high false-negative rate ($\beta > 0.20$) may result in discontinuing promising therapies prematurely. Similarly, setting a large targeted difference (δ) increases the likelihood of discarding potentially beneficial regimens.

7. **Phase 2/3 Trial Design**

Phase 2/3 randomized designs efficiently compare experimental and standard therapies by using similar eligibility criteria in both phases. An interim analysis after Phase 2 checks efficacy and toxicity before moving to Phase 3. Patient data from Phase 2 contribute to the final analysis, reducing study time and patient numbers. Table 15.1 outlines the main advantages and disadvantages of leading recommended Phase 2 trial designs.

Table 15.1 Key points of primary Phase 2 trial designs

Designs	Advantages	Disadvantages
One-stage one-arm design	Compare with historical control Smallest sample size Simple design	Delay the evaluation of effectiveness Historical control may not be valid Subject to population differences, time trends, evaluation bias, etc.
Gehan's two-stage design	With interim monitoring Rule out ineffective drug with minimized sample size	No testing on agents showing some promise Only suitable for binary outcome The endpoint is different from that in following Phase 3 trial

(continued)

Table 15.1 (continued)

Designs	Advantages	Disadvantages
Simon's two-stage design	The samples in two stages are optimized Quickly screen out agents without effectiveness while testing further agents with some promise Two choices: optimal versus minimax	Only suitable for binary outcome The endpoint is different from that in the following Phase 3 trial
Bayesian Phase II design	Flexible monitoring schedule More efficient and robust	Intensive computation Relies heavily on statistician during trial
Randomized Phase 2 design	Use of randomization Reliable control and less bias More similar to Phase 3 trial	Sample size increases Length of trial increases Cost increases
Phase 2 pick the winner design	Efficient and effective way of comparing Two or multiple experimental regimens Each experimental regimen compared with historical controls	Not appropriate for comparison of adding an experimental agent to standard regimen
Phase 2 screening design	Limits the sample size required for a randomized Phase 2 comparison Good for comparison of the addition of an experimental agent to standard regimen	No statistical comparison between the selected arms
Phase 2 randomized discontinuation design	Good when significant continued benefit after initial benefit implies significant benefit overall, and vice versa, or when benefit is restricted to a nonidentifiable subgroup of patients	May need a large number of patients treated at a treatment not effective for them
Phase 2/3 design	Use of Phase 2 data in Phase 3 trial Minimize delay in starting up Phase III study Use of concurrent control Useful for new drugs showing efficacy	Large sample sizes Needs Phase 3 infrastructure developed even if it stops early

15.3 Phase 2 Clinical Trial Protocol Template

The NIH provides a Clinical Trial Protocol Template (https://osp.od.nih.gov/policies/clinical-research#tab1/), recommended for Phase 2 or 3 trials conducted under FDA IND or IDE. This template helps investigators create protocols that comply with ICH E6 Good Clinical Practice.

At this stage, sponsors, investigators, and the FDA typically meet to review preliminary data, evaluate the IND, and discuss moving to Phase 3. Topics include trial design, outcomes, safety, data collection, case report forms, and manufacturing issues. Figure 15.1 outlines this process.

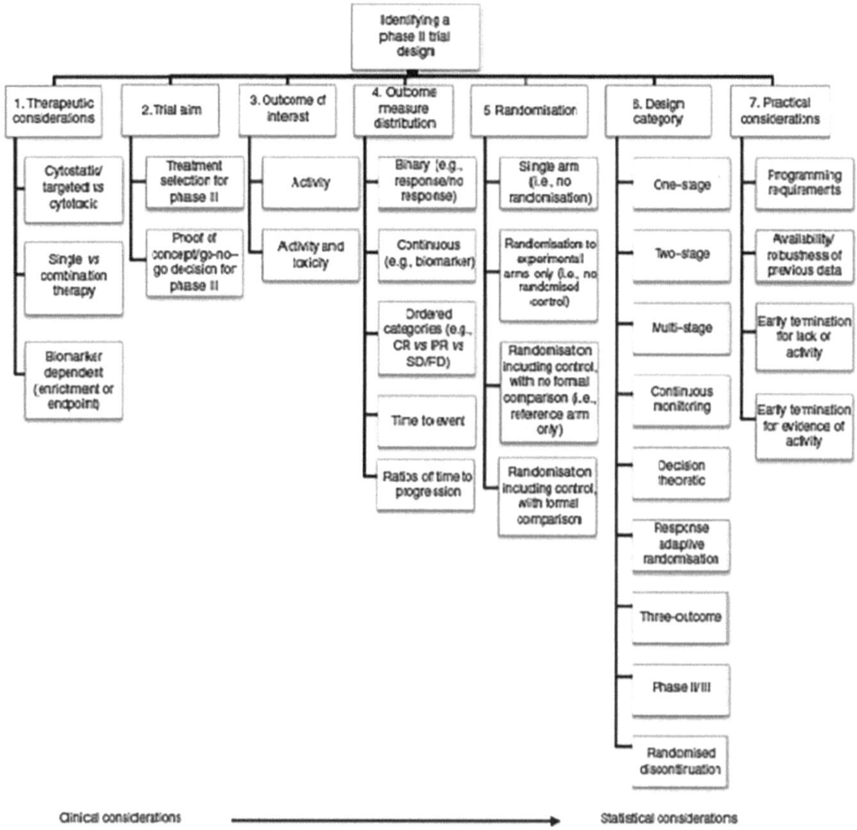

Fig. 15.1 Flow diagram of Phase 2 design trial process

15.4 Potential Failure Rates and Cost Burden

Concerns regarding Phase 2 predictivity—both for effective pipeline screening (i.e., negative predictivity) and reducing Phase 3 failures (i.e., positive predictivity)—have led to several innovations in Phase 2 trial design. The success rate for transition from Phase 2 has been reported at 30.7%, which is substantially lower than that of other phases. Recent studies on drug development success rates indicate that Phase 2 success percentages range from a high of 56.6% (Haematology) to a low of 23.7% (Psychiatry). At this stage, sponsors must determine whether to invest in large, costly Phase 3 studies or discontinue development based on various factors including commercial considerations.

Adaptations in trial design have emerged in response to these challenges. In March 2004, the FDA noted a slowdown in the approval of innovative medical therapies and increased interest in novel trial designs through initiatives such as the critical pathway initiative. The passage of the 21st Century Cures Act by Congress in December 2016 dedicated $500 million for an "innovation account" intended to support NIH funding and accelerate regulatory approval for medical therapies.

Adaptive study designs have contributed to reduced false positives in Phase 2 data, but they often involve additional costs and participant burdens. For instance, randomization in Phase 2 may require a larger patient cohort due to the need for comparator arms. Enrichment strategies, pharmacodynamics, and real-time pharmacokinetic assessments may necessitate more frequent and sometimes invasive sample collection.

The financial and social costs introduced during Phase 2 differ from those in Phase 3. Ethical justification for risk exposure in Phase 3 stems from clinical equipoise, reflecting uncertainty between experimental and standard treatments, and supporting potential therapeutic benefit. In contrast, clinical equipoise is less established in early efficacy tests, where direct evidence is limited and the likelihood of identifying a beneficial intervention remains low.

It is necessary for investigators, funding agencies, sponsors, and stakeholders to define an optimal threshold for false positives in Phase 2—balancing the benefits of preventing negative Phase 3 trials against added costs—and to implement policies guiding trialists toward this balance. Phase 2 trial designs should aim to optimize both positive predictivity and efficient progression of candidate therapies.

15.5 Application of Phase 2 Results in Clinical Practice

Phase 2 studies are exploratory, and results should be interpreted with caution. These studies are typically not designed to deliver definitive efficacy comparisons and may be susceptible to biases such as selection, surveillance, and publication bias. However, there are circumstances, particularly in rare diseases or when Phase 3 research is impractical, in which clinicians rely on Phase 2 data alone. Understanding these limitations allows for appropriate application of Phase 2 findings to clinical decision-making, provided the drug receives subsequent approval after Phase 3 studies.

Phase 2 data may offer clinical insights into rare conditions where insufficient patient numbers prevent randomized trials. For example, treatments for T-cell Chronic Lymphocytic Leukaemia may rely on case reports, series, or robust Phase 2 studies instead of randomized controlled Phase 3 designs. In contrast, for common malignancies like B Cell Chronic Lymphocytic Leukaemia, higher incidence rates make it feasible to conduct comprehensive Phase 3 trials. While Phase 2 findings can inform treatment recommendations, their provisional status should be acknowledged, and conclusions may change following Phase 3 results.

15.6 Conclusion

The frequency of Phase 2 clinical trials is increasing, yet these studies are not substitutes for randomized, controlled Phase 3 trials. Well-constructed Phase 2 trials, featuring transparent reporting of design, eligibility, endpoints, and statistical analyses, can provide useful evidence in select circumstances, assuming subsequent market approval post-Phase 3. Adaptive trial designs have been proposed to expedite clinical testing, decrease required enrolment, improve predictions of treatment success, and reduce drug development costs. Implementation of these designs remains limited, attributed to gaps in information on completed adaptive trials, practical understanding of their conduct, and concerns regarding regulatory scrutiny. Further data are required to assess whether adaptive Phase 2 designs enhance prediction of Phase 3 outcomes and reduce overall development costs.

Bibliography

1. Tomblyn MR, Rizzo JD (2007) Are there circumstances in which phase 2 study results should be practice-changing? Hematology Am Soc Hematol Educ Program 2007:489–492
2. BiomedTracker. Clinical development success rates 2006–2015. Available at https://www.bio.org
3. Brown S, Gregory W, Twelves C et al (2011) Designing phase II trials in cancer: a systematic review and guidance. Br J Cancer 105:194–199
4. Chen Z, Zhao Y, Cui Y, Kowalski J (2012) Methodology and application of adaptive and sequential approaches in contemporary clinical trials. J Probab Stat 2012:Article ID 527351, 20 pages
5. Hey SP, Kimmelman J (2013) Ethics, error, and initial trials of efficacy. Sci Transl Med 5(184):184fs16
6. Sharma MR, Stadler WM, Ratain MJ (2011) Randomized phase II trials: a long-term investment with promising returns. J Natl Cancer Inst 103(14):1093–1100
7. Umscheid CA, Margolis DJ, Grossman CE (2011) Key concepts of clinical trials: a narrative review. Postgrad Med 123(5):194–204
8. Mandrekar SJ, Sargent DJ (2010) Randomized phase II trials: time for a new era in clinical trial design. J Thorac Oncol 5(7):932–934
9. Van Norman GA (2019) Phase II trials in drug development and adaptive trial design. JACC Basic Transl Sci 4(3):428–437

Phase 3 Clinical Trials

16

Anuhya Vinayaka

Abstract

Drug development process flows seamlessly from Phase 0 to Phase 2 clinical trials, post which eligible drug candidates ultimately move into large-scale Phase 3 clinical trials. Phase 3 trials involve many more patients or volunteers than the earlier phases, and are considered the cornerstone in the human testing journey. The added benefit with Phase 3 trials is that there is also head-to-head comparison that is performed against existing standard therapy. Additionally, Phase 3 trials are also randomized in order to avoid bias. Blinding is also performed in many of the Phase 3 studies. Once a drug's safety and efficacy are ascertained in large Phase 3 trials, the drug would be given marketing approval by the country's regulatory body. Among the various phases of clinical trials, this phase is considered to be the most expensive as well as the most expansive. This chapter provides information on the various aspects involved in Phase 3 clinical trials.

Keywords

Drug efficacy · Clinical trials · Drug safety · Randomization · Blinding · Drug development

16.1 Introduction

There are three actions of a drug: the one we want, the one we don't want, and the one we don't know about. Clinical trials in drug development not only aid in understanding the parameters that we seek but it opens up a new dimension of possibilities that can happen over the course and the ultimate aim is patient benefit. Phase 3

A. Vinayaka (✉)
Novartis Healthcare Pvt. Ltd., Hyderabad, India

A. Arivazhahan et al. (eds.), *Introduction to Basics of Pharmacology and Toxicology*,
https://doi.org/10.1007/978-981-95-1920-0_16

trials involve the most extensive testing of the drug to fully assess its efficacy and safety in a large group of target population. This is the phase, where the chemical turns into a drug.

16.2 Timeline of Phase 3 Trials

- After a proof-of-concept is established in Phase 2 that the investigational medicinal product elicits a pathophysiological signal which produces an expected response in healthy volunteers, therapeutic confirmation is performed in patient population. The efficacy of the product and safety is confirmed in this phase.
- Trials are conducted in large groups (several hundreds to tens of thousands) across diverse population (multi-centric and multi-country) that reflect the patients for whom the drug is ultimately intended. The investigational product is evaluated in the same manner the drug is expected to be used by health care professionals after marketing.
- These trials often take at least 2–5 years to complete.
- Comparisons are made between the new treatment and standard of care. Placebos maybe used but they're never used alone if there is a treatment available. Sometimes, a patient who is randomly assigned to the placebo for part of the study will at some point be offered the standard of care as well.
- Observation of other specific characteristics of the drug.
- Approval for drug registration is sought after Phase-3—New Drug Application (NDA) submission.

16.3 Concept of "Investigational New Drug" (IND)

In the U.S. setting, IND Application is made by the sponsor to U.S. Food and Drug Administration (FDA) after the pre-clinical research is complete. In the pre-clinical development, the sponsor's primary goal is to determine if the product is reasonably safe for initial use in humans and if the product exhibits pharmacological activity that justifies commercial development. Based on the pre-clinical study data, the application is made to warrant a study in human subjects for the purposes of clinical treatment when no approved therapies are available.

IND allows the use of investigational medicinal product in next phase drug development, i.e., an approval to begin the clinical trials. The IND application is used for both drugs and biologicals. The FDA has 30 days to review the submission. IND application is exempted for studies with approved marketed drugs, bioavailability, and bioequivalence studies. After an IND application is approved, Phases 1 and 2 are conducted in healthy volunteers to understand the human pharmacology and safety, and therapeutic exploration with dose range finding studies are performed. Once the proof-of-concept is proven, starting dose, maintenance dose, and optimal doses are selected for therapeutic confirmation and comparison.

16.4 Types of Phase 3 Clinical Trials

(i) **Phase 3a:** Sufficient and significant data is collected in this phase to confirm the efficacy and safety. FDA requires two pivotal studies per indication for approval. These studies are done prior to New Drug Application (NDA) submission.

(ii) **Phase 3b:** Also called as Label expansion studies. Studies are done in special populations like elderly age, children, pregnancy and lactation, patients with diabetes mellitus, hypertension, and renal impairment. These studies are done after NDA submission and are usually done to check for safety in other populations. These studies allow patients to continue on treatment who continue to derive clinical benefit.

16.5 Non-inferiority and Superiority Trials

Hypotheses in clinical trials can be stated in terms of differences in the mean response of an outcome of interest. A well-designed clinical trial would specify the kind of hypothesis to be tested and procedures to be used for analysis of primary outcomes. For example, depending on the purpose of trial, studies are designed to test the superiority and non-inferiority between different treatments. In Table 16.1, Drug A is an anti-hypertensive which is the reference product and Drug B is the investigational product whose anti-hypertensive effect is compared to the reference Drug A.

It is preset or it is specified prior to the start of the study by the sponsor that the drug would be superior or non-inferior for which the primary objective of the study is considered. This primary objective would later translate as the approved indication in the product label when the drug is marketed. The sponsor may also choose a placebo as a reference product in superiority trials when the standard of care is not available.

16.6 Randomized Trials

Randomized controlled trials (RCT) is an experimental methodology for impact evaluation in which the population receiving the treatments or intervention (intervention group) is chosen at random and the control group is also chosen at random

Table 16.1 Comparison of outcomes of Drug A with Drug B

	Superiority	Non-inferiority
Outcome of drug A	10 ± 2 mm of Hg	10 ± 2 mm of Hg
Outcome of drug B	15 ± 2 mm of Hg	8 ± 4 mm of Hg
Interpretation	Drug B has better reduction than Drug A	Drug B produces same effect or not worse than that of Drug A

from the same patient population. Patients are assigned randomly to either intervention or control group. By randomization, selection or allocation bias and confounding can be avoided that can distort the results. Advantages of randomization are that the procedure is performed in a valid manner and the allocation cannot be predicted, characteristics of patient population will be comparable evenly balanced between the groups at baseline, i.e., prior to the start of the study, and permits use of probability theory to check for difference in outcome between groups.

Randomization allocation is usually categorized under fixed and adaptive:

Fixed			Adaptive		
Simple	Block	Stratified	Baseline	Minimization	Response

(i) **Simple Randomization:** This is a simple and easy randomization method where a number or code generator is used to assign the patients. Common reference to flipping a coin (heads or tails) to assign the patients on treatment group for heads and control group for tails. However, this methodology is not suitable for small group trials where there is a high chance of imbalance. The imbalance would further reduce the statistical power leading to inappropriate data analysis.

(ii) **Block Randomization:** Patients are segregated into blocks with specified block size. For example, the study may specify four patients in one block, then the block size is called four and possible sequences of the blocks can be made. For example, in a study, the patients are grouped in blocks of four and assigned to treatment arms A and B. The block size of four can make six possible sequences AABB, BBAA, ABAB, BABA, BAAB, and ABBA. The disadvantage of block randomization is that it can be predicted by alteration of the sequences. To counter this bias the allocator must hide the block size and use randomly mixed block sizes.

(iii) **Stratified Randomization:** Patient population is divided into desirable number of strata or subgroups based on similar characteristics or attributes like age, gender, nationality, education level, etc. Within the subgroups, a simple random or block randomization is performed. Stratification cannot be performed if the complete population cannot be assigned into strata. Often, the strata maybe overlapping if the patients meet the criteria for inclusion into multiple strata which ultimately results in misinterpretation of the population. Hence, the characteristics to consider the subgroups should be minimal to avoid multiple stratified variables which would be difficult to place samples in both groups with equally same numbers. Baseline measurements are essential prior to randomization. Advantages of this type of randomization are that a subgroup analysis can be performed and the outcomes can accurately reflect the general population. [https://doi.org/10.4055%2Fcios.2014.6.1.103] Large multicentric randomized trials do not usually use stratification as the chance of arriving at an imbalance is less in the patient population.

For example, hypertensive patients may be segregated into strata based on age group (<40 years, 40-60 years, >60 years) and gender (male, female).

(iv) **Baseline Adaptive Randomization:** Adaptive randomization strategies change the allocation probabilities as enrollment progresses. The process of enrollment of patients into a study does not necessarily happen in few days but may take months. During enrollment, if an imbalance is noticed where the difference in the number of patients in a study group is greater than a pre-specified value the allocation probability is adjusted so that it is higher for the group with fewer patient study group. Common methods used to make patients in each study groups equal or nearly equal are "biased coin randomization" and "urn randomization". Biased coin randomization attempts to balance the allocation based on the previous allocation and it does not take patient's response into consideration.

(v) **Minimization Adaptive Randomization:** In general, adaptive stratification methods incorporate several prognostic factors in making an "overall assessment" of the group balance or lack of balance. Participants are then assigned to a group in a manner which will tend to correct an existing imbalance or cause the least imbalance in prognostic factors. Various methods can be used as the measure of imbalance in prognostic factors. Minimization gives unbiased estimates of treatment effect and slightly increased power relative to stratified randomization. These methods are being used, especially in clinical trials of cancer where several prognostic factors need to be balanced, and the sample size is typically 100–200 participants [Lawrence, p. 135].

(vi) **Response Adaptive Randomization:** Response adaptive randomization uses information on participant response to intervention during the course of the trial to determine the allocation of the next participant. The next participant is assigned to the same group as the first participant if the response to the intervention was a success; otherwise, the participant is assigned to the other group. These methods do maximize the number of participants on the "superior" intervention, the possible imbalance will almost certainly result in some loss of power and require more participants to be enrolled into the study than would a fixed allocation with equal assignment probability.

16.7 RCT Study Designs

RCTs are conducted based on the guidelines provided in the CONSORT (CONsolidated Standards of Reporting Trials) Statement, enabling readers to understand the study design, conduct, analysis, and interpretation of results data.

Major categories of RCT study designs include:

1. Parallel group.
2. Crossover.
3. Cluster.
4. Factorial.

1. **Parallel group:** Study is designed with 2 treatment arms wherein the patients are randomly assigned between treatment arms. One of the arms will serve as a comparator or reference control.
2. **Crossover:** Study is designed with 2 treatment arms wherein the patients receive both treatments. The patients would initially receive one treatment for certain duration and after a washout period these patients would move to other arm and receive another treatment. Every patient will act her or his own control. A Latin square design variation is used for crossover models. In Latin square design, each patient received each intervention once.

	Period 1	Period 2
Group 1	A	B
Group 2	B	A

3. **Cluster:** Patients are allocated into treatment arms in clusters (e.g., population from hospitals, villages, schools). These designs have one or more factors imbedded within one or more factors. For example, to study the different interventions in Heart failure patients from randomly selected hospitals.
4. **Factorial:** Patients of the same group will be tested for 2 or more interventions at the same time period. The design consists of two or more interventions (factors), with each intervention having two or more levels. By testing multiple interventions at the same time, the number of patients or the sample sized required is reduced. Below is an example of a 2 × 2 factorial design wherein 2 treatment interventions at different dose levels are studied in 4 groups (ac, ad, bc, bd).

		Treatment I	
		Dose c	Dose d
Treatment II	Dose a	ac	ad
	Dose b	bc	bd

16.8 Blinding in Clinical Trials

During the clinical trials, bias in determining the treatment effects is a concern. Bias is a systematic error or "difference between the true value and that actually obtained due to all causes other than sampling variability" [Lawrence, p. 147]. The factors that influence the bias can be done with intention or without intention or both. Bias is a significant aspect starting from designing the trial, study conduct, analysis of data, and reporting of data to different stakeholders involved.

- Blinding in clinical trials is one of the methods used to reduce or avoid the bias. In the blinded clinical trials, the patient does not know the treatment they are receiving. Placebos are usually used when the trials are blinded.
- Allocation concealment is done for blinding in which the investigational products are administered in number/color-coded containers and a central randomization in computer is performed. Only the Pharmacist has a control over allocation and randomization.
- Having a large sample size does not necessarily reduce the bias.

(i) **Open/Unblinded:** No blinding is done. Both the patient and all investigators know the treatment the patient has been assigned to.
(ii) **Single:** Only the patient does not know the treatment received.
(iii) **Double:** Both patient and treating healthcare professional do not know the treatment received.
(iv) **Triple:** Patient, treating healthcare professional, and the sponsor (individuals who assess the outcome) do not know the treatment received.

A clinical trial should ideally have a double-blind design in order to limit potential problems of bias during data collection and assessment. In studies where such a design is impossible, other measures to reduce potential bias are advocated [Lawrence, p. 148].

Protocol design of the clinical trials is done according to the Standard Protocol Items: Recommendations for Interventional Trials (SPIRIT) Statement. This statement provides guidance on the minimum content of a clinical trial protocol. It has a 33-item checklist that applies to all clinical trials and focuses on content rather than format. Adherence to the guideline enhances transparency, completeness of trial protocols for benefit of patients, investigations, institutional review boards, peer reviewers, journals, trial registries, policy makers, regulators, and other key stakeholders.

Below is an example of the flow of events in a phase 3 trial:

1. Enrollment.
2. Allocation.
3. Follow-up.
4. Analysis.

16.9 Patient Selection: Inclusion and Exclusion Criteria

Defining the study population is primarily based on the unmet need in the disease area for which the study drug is being investigated. And before designing the population, defining the disease is important based on the significant features including the age, gender, clinical presentation with course and its natural progression, anatomical features, risk/trigger factors, incubation period/transmission in infectious diseases, supportive laboratory investigations, and relevant medical history, etc. and finally response to already available treatments for the disease condition should be evaluated.

16.10 Categories to Consider for Selection Criteria Categories

(i) Demographics: Age, gender, race, geographical area, socio-economic status. For example, sickle cell anemia and malaria are endemic in tropical regions and people who are of African descent.
(ii) Disease of interest: Diagnostic tests, staging, seriousness, severity, and available treatment modalities.
(iii) Allergies: To previous medications or other ingredients apart from the active.
(iv) Screening: To check for acceptable laboratory values of different organ functions, other supportive imaging, cardiac profile, and metabolic panel considering the pharmacokinetics and pharmacodynamics of the investigational product. Baseline investigations are performed to check inclusion into the study and also serve for comparative analysis during the study course or at the end of study.
(v) Concurrent disease conditions and concomitant medications used: To check for any confounding factors or may threaten the safety of patient. For example, history of cardiac disease may exclude a patient from receiving a drug with potential cardiotoxicity, history of hemorrhagic stroke may exclude a patient from receiving a drug that alters the coagulation profile. High-risk patients who have a probability of suffering side effects or less life expectancy are excluded. Concomitant medications and study drug can have drug interactions.
(vi) Pregnancy/lactation and fertility status: Patients should be put on birth control or post-menopausal patients will be included for a drug whose embryo-fetal toxicity is unknown.
(vii) Ability to consent and comply: Consent to take part in the study and compliance to the treatment medications and also attend the visits are important for ethical reasons and favorable study outcomes.

16.11 Sampling

Sample should be representative of the study population and should not be biased. It is important to understand the theoretical and accessible study populations. If a study is intended to be conducted in female diabetes patients above 60 years of age, not all patients can be accessed and willing to be part of the study. Hence, it is convenient to identify the accessible population with no bias and are representative of the general population.

(i) Simple random sampling: All patients will have an equal chance of being selected for the sample.

(ii) Stratified random sampling: Population is divided into groups or strata based on specific preset characteristics. For example, systolic heart failure patients having ejection fraction less than 45% or cardiac failure patients who are class II and above based on NHYA classification.
(iii) Proportionate sampling: This type of sampling is a variation of stratified sampling, wherein the proportions in strata are relative to the population size. For example, in the population size, there are 70% female patients with systolic heart failure having ejection fraction less than 45% then the sample size of 100 patients should include 70 females and 30 males.
(iv) Systematic sampling: Patients are selected symptomatically as n^{th} patient (e.g., every fifth patient) in the population.
(v) Cluster sampling: Patients are grouped into clusters randomly. For example, cardiac failure patients of a group of hospitals or primary school children who are anemic from a geographical region.
(vi) Quota sampling: Another variation of stratified sampling where the selection is non-random. After dividing the population into groups or strata, patients are selected based on a specified number from each stratum.
(vii) Convenience sampling: Patients are chosen arbitrarily for studying diseases like STDs in sex workers or surgical and orthopedic interventions in the population of the army.
(viii) Snowball sampling: Patients are recruited from patients who are already recruited or part of study, e.g., from friends or family members or office colleagues.

16.12 Endpoints

An endpoint is an overall outcome that the clinical trial aims to measure. Phase-3 trial outcomes are usually in terms of efficacy parameters for a disease characteristic like decrease in signs or symptoms (clinical benefit) or complete recovery or achieving remission or changes in test results like laboratory and radiological findings. These endpoints are extrapolated to entire population of patients based on similarities to the patients in clinical trials. When the intervention achieves the endpoint, the trial is determined as a success depending on which the regulatory approvals are sought. Characteristics of endpoint include:

- Clinically relevant.
- Closely and comprehensively reflects overall disease being treated.
- Sensitive and has good discrimination.
- Reliable (precise, low variability, and reproducible across all studies).
- Robust to dropouts and missing data.
- Does not influence treatment response or have biological.
- Practical (implementable at different geographies and economical).

(i) Primary endpoint: These endpoints define the disease outcomes that the clinical trial answers the most important question, if the treatment intervention is efficacious as compared to the existing treatments or in diseases where there is no treatment available. Primary endpoints are usually powered.
(ii) Co-Primary endpoint: Regulatory authorities have advised to consider more than one primary endpoint for determining the success of intervention and strengthening evidence for the effect.
(iii) Secondary endpoint: They answer the relevant questions about drug's effect on the primary endpoint and they further demonstrate the additional effects on the disease condition.
(iv) Surrogate endpoint: They measure the effect of a specific intervention that is relevant and correlates with the primary clinical endpoint. In a few studies, biomarkers are used as substitute to the clinical endpoint which are also called as surrogate biomarkers, e.g., HbA1C reduction is a surrogate biomarker in studies on Diabetes. Surrogate endpoints also help in early approval of drugs which are intended to be used in serious or life-threatening diseases like cancers and diseases of public health concern like pandemic. For example, antibody titers, decreased hospitalization, and recovery rates are considered as surrogate endpoints for the development of antiviral therapy of COVID-19 and COVID-19 vaccines.
(v) Oncology endpoints: Disease-free survival, progression-free survival are the common endpoints considered in cancer trials. Disease-free survival is the length of time until the cancer recurs after treatment with the study drug or until the patient dies whichever comes first. Progression-free survival is the length of time until the cancer progresses or until the patient dies whichever comes first. Clinical differentiation of these end points is often difficult and is dependent on radiological imaging for assessing the status of underlying malignancy. RECIST (Response Evaluation Criteria in Solid Tumors) Criteria is one of the common criteria for measuring cancer based on the lesions as target and non-target lesions. Response criteria are further characterized as complete response (CR), partial response (PR), progressive disease (PD), and stable disease (SD).
(vi) Safety endpoint: Although primary and secondary endpoints are specified before the start of the study, safety endpoints do not necessarily require to be identified prior. For example, in studies of diabetes, reduction in HbA1C is a primary endpoint and decreased hospitalizations are a safety end point.

Characteristics of Safety Endpoints

- Detrimental to the patient.
- Not always pre-specified.
- Not always validated.
- Not always randomized or stratified in advance.
- Do not necessarily have to be statistically significant.

Safety Reporting in Clinical Trials

- Adverse event (AE) and serious adverse event (SAE) reporting in clinical trials are regulatory requirements and they are important for safety monitoring of interventional products.
- All serious, unexpected events require expedited reporting.
- Fatal and life-threatening, unexpected events should be reported no later than 7 calendar days after first knowledge by the sponsor.
- Other Serious (hospitalization, prolonged hospitalization, significant disability, congenital birth defect, medically significant), unexpected events should be reported no later than 15 calendar days after first knowledge by the sponsor.
- Reporting of events occurs through conventional CRFs (case record forms) which would be faxed or mailed to the sponsor or the investigators may directly report in electronic data capture (EDC) system to the sponsor.
- Reports are usually in specific formats that are preferred by the regulatory authorities.
- For example, MedWatch forms to FDA, CIOMS-I as per ICH E2B.
- Special considerations to blinded studies are given before submitting the reports to health authorities, blind is broken/unblinded.
- Events that occur after the study has ended will also be reported provided the events occurred within five half-lives of the drug or within 30 days.
- Relatedness of events with the study drug is usually performed based on Bradford Hill criteria and different scales or scoring methodology is used to classify the relatedness by different sponsors. For example, causality assessment scales like WHO classification, Naranjo's algorithm, Karch and Lasagna's scale, Kramer scale, Yale algorithm, European ABO system, and Spanish imputation system.
- Signal detection activities are performed by the sponsor on a real-time basis to detect and report to regulators.

16.13 Clinical Trial Facilitation Group (CTFG) and Its Activities

CTFG acts as a forum for discussion to agree on common principles and processes to be applied throughout the European medicines regulatory network.

- CTFG promotes harmonization of clinical trial assessment decisions and administrative processes across the national competent authorities (NCAs).
- Annual safety update reports (DSURs) and SUSARs (suspected unexpected serious adverse reactions) are monitored with exchange of opinions or assessment of critical topics.
- Recommendations to special scenarios like contraception and pregnancy testing in clinical trials and guidance on performing clinical trials during the COVID-19 pandemic.
- Investigator brochures (IB) and reference safety information sections of IB are prepared in compliance with the CTFG Q&A.

16.14 New Drug Application (NDA), Biologics License Application (BLA), and Abbreviated New Drug Application (ANDA)

- New drug application is a collection of all the information during the drug development process for allowing FDA review. The data gathered during the animal studies and human clinical trials of an IND become part of the NDA. An approval is granted based on the.

  1. Analysis of the target condition and available treatments.
  2. Assessment of benefits and risks from clinical data.
  3. Strategies for managing risks.

- Proposed labelling (package insert) summarizes the important aspects of the development program and provides information on the usage of the product.
- Risk mitigation strategies (REMS—Risk management and mitigation strategies) should also be included as part of the NDA submission.
- ICH conferences have harmonized the content of all the sections of the US NDA and the EU dossier as a Common Technical Document (CTD).
- BLA is the counterpart of NDA and it includes products like monoclonal antibodies, cytokines, growth factors, enzymes, immunomodulators, thrombolytics, proteins extracted from animals or microorganisms including recombinants (except clotting factors), and other non-vaccine immunotherapies.
- ANDA is made for the review and potential approval of generic products. Generic applicants must scientifically demonstrate that their product performs in the same manner as the innovator drug.

16.15 Various Regulatory Approvals by US-FDA

(i) Accelerated approval: FDA grants an accelerated approval status for products that are intended to treat serious or life-threatening conditions and provide therapeutic benefit over available therapies. Surrogate endpoints play a major role in seeking accelerated approval.

(ii) Fast Track designation: Fast Track is a process designed to facilitate the development and advance the review of drugs that treat serious conditions, and fill an unmet medical need, based on promising animal or human data. Fast tracking can get important new drugs to the patient earlier, e.g., Branaplam for the treatment of Huntington's disease.

(iii) Breakthrough Therapy: This designation expedites the development and review of drugs that are intended to treat a serious condition, and preliminary clinical evidence indicates that the drug may demonstrate substantial improvement over available therapy.

(iv) Priority Review: Priority review means that FDA aims to take action on an application within 6 months, compared to 10 months under standard review. A Priority Review designation directs attention and resources to evaluate drugs that would significantly improve the treatment, diagnosis, or prevention of serious conditions.

(v) Regenerative Medicine Advanced Therapy (RMAT): RMAT designation is given for cell therapies, therapeutic tissue engineering product, human cell and tissue product or any combination product using such therapies, e.g., Tisagenlecleucel for follicular lymphoma.

Bibliography

1. Umscheid CA, Margolis DJ, Grossman CE (2011) Key concepts of clinical trials: a narrative review. Postgrad Med 123(5):194–204
2. El-Hagrassy MM, Duarte DGG, Thibaut A, Lucena MFG, Fregni F (2018) Principles of designing a clinical trial: optimizing chances of trial success. Curr Behav Neurosci Rep 5(2):143–152
3. Follmann D, Proschan M (2020) Two stage designs for phase III trials. medRxiv [Preprint]. 2020.07.29.20164525
4. Buyse M (2016) Phase III design: principles. Chin Clin Oncol 5(1):10
5. Fogel DB (2018) Factors associated with clinical trials that fail and opportunities for improving the likelihood of success: a review. Contemp Clin Trials Commun 11:156–164
6. Dilts DM, Cheng SK, Crites JS, Sandler AB, Doroshow JH (2010) Phase III clinical trial development: a process of chutes and ladders. Clin Cancer Res 16(22):5381–5389
7. Shen C, Tannenbaum D, Horn R, Rogers J, Eng C, Zhou S et al (2022) Overall survival in phase 3 clinical trials and the surveillance, epidemiology, and end results database in patients with metastatic colorectal cancer, 1986–2016: a systematic review. JAMA Netw Open 5(5):e2213588
8. Clinical NB, Designs T (2019) Indian. Dermatol Online J 10(2):193–201
9. Saw SM, Lim SG (2000) Clinical drug trials: practical problems of phase III. Ann Acad Med Singap 29(5):598–605
10. Takebe T, Imai R, Ono S (2018) The current status of drug discovery and development as originated in United States academia: the influence of industrial and academic collaboration on drug discovery and development. Clin Transl Sci 11(6):597–606. https://doi.org/10.1111/cts.12577
11. Akhondzadeh S (2016) The importance of clinical trials in drug development. Avicenna J Med Biotechnol 8(4):151

that would significantly improve the treatment, diagnosis, or prevention of serious conditions.

vii) Regenerative Medicine Advanced Therapy (RMAT): RMAT designation is [illegible]

Phase 4 Clinical Trials

17

Akila Srinivasan, Vimala Ananthy, and Santhosh Shivabasappa

Abstract

Phase 4 studies, also known as post-marketing surveillance (PMS) studies, are a crucial step of drug development and are carried out after marketing approval of the drug. The objective is to obtain detailed information on the safety and effectiveness in a real-world setting of the newly approved drug or device. Since Phase 3 trials are carried out for a shorter duration in a population of few hundreds to few thousands, they may not be able to detect all adverse effects, especially those that are rare or those that occur on chronic use of the drug or device. The methodology for post-marketing surveillance is chosen based on the objectives of the study and each comes with its own share of advantages and limitations. A major proportion of Phase 4 studies are observational in nature; however, there are some clinical trial-based designs, which are performed depending on the requirements. Periodic submission of aggregate safety reports is a regulatory requirement during Phase 4 of drug development. This chapter seeks to provide an overview of post-marketing surveillance studies and their importance in drug development.

Keywords

Post-marketing surveillance · Phase 4 study · Effectiveness · Large simple trials

A. Srinivasan (✉) · V. Ananthy
Department of Pharmacology, Mahatma Gandhi Medical College and Research Institute (MGMCRI), Sri Balaji Vidyapeeth, Pondicherry, India
e-mail: akilasrinivas@gmail.com

S. Shivabasappa
Senior Clinical Research Scientist, Qure.ai, Bengaluru, Karnataka, India

A. Arivazhahan et al. (eds.), *Introduction to Basics of Pharmacology and Toxicology*,
https://doi.org/10.1007/978-981-95-1920-0_17

17.1 Introduction and Definition

The US-FDA states that "post-marketing studies are carried out following FDA approval of a treatment, offering more details including the treatment's risks, benefits, and best use." Phase 4 studies are a crucial step of drug research, which offer detailed data on the safety and real-world effectiveness of the licensed medicine, and are evaluated in a non-experimental setting. All studies conducted after the marketing authorization or approval has been obtained for the medicinal product are referred to as phase 4 studies. PMS studies are these studies that, in compliance with the label, must be conducted as observational studies in a naturalistic environment as mandated by the regulatory agency. Research on cost-effectiveness and more extensive outcome indicators such as functioning and standard of life could be undertaken during phase 4.

17.2 Need for Phase 4 Studies

- It is crucial to conduct a phase 4 study following drug approval due to the low sample numbers, brief duration, and strict inclusion and exclusion criteria in the phases of clinical trials conducted prior to approval.
- As per reports, 20% of drugs have had further black box warnings after having been on sale, and 4% of drugs were eventually taken off the market due to safety concerns, although these signals were not picked up during the earlier phases of clinical trials.
- Phase 4 trials provide reliable information and warnings to healthcare facilities to promote awareness on the proper use of new medications.
- They also help to minimize adverse outcomes by implementing the necessary safety measures and quickly compiling data on significant adverse reactions.
- Doctors may find new information about a drug by happenstance when they use it in a wide range of patients with various ethnicities, underlying illnesses, and concurrent medications.
- Vulnerable populations that are usually excluded during the previous phases of clinical trials are exposed to the newly approved treatment during Phase 4, offering data and evidence of its effectiveness and safety.

17.3 Phase 4 Study Designs

The study design of Phase 4 clinical trials depends on the objectives (safety evaluation, assessment of effectiveness, optimization of use, etc.). Safety evaluation and submission of aggregate safety reports is a regulatory requirement in Phase 4 studies. Some of the commonly used study designs have been explained below.

17.4 Post-authorization Safety Study (PASS)

A post-authorization safety study (PASS) is defined as "*any study relating to an authorised medicinal product conducted with the aim of identifying, characterising or quantifying a safety hazard, confirming the safety profile of the medicinal product, or of measuring the effectiveness of risk management measures.*"

A PASS is carried out to assess the safety and benefit-risk profile of a product and thereby aid in regulatory decision-making. PASS can be either imposed or voluntary: imposed by a regulatory authority or voluntarily carried by the Market Authorization Holder (MAH).

The following are a few of the study designs which may be selected for performing Phase 4 studies:

- Active surveillance studies.
- Observational studies.
- Clinical trials (large simple trials).
- Drug utilization studies.

17.4.1 Active Surveillance Studies

- In active surveillance, patients exposed to a particular medicinal product are actively monitored for adverse events through an ongoing organized process.
- For instance, all patients prescribed with a particular medicinal product are followed up through a risk management system, where they may be asked to participate in a brief survey and if required, can be contacted at a later stage with their permission.
- This helps in generating comprehensive clinical data (especially on adverse events) and laboratory data of patients taking a particular product. This may provide more information on safety profile of a drug.
- Some of the methods by which active surveillance can be carried out include: review of medical records specially focusing on major expected adverse events (e.g., in hematological disorders) and other events. Intensive monitoring of case records and patients' interviews is carried out at sentinel sites.
- Other methods are Prescription Event Monitoring (PEM), where patient records from prescription data as well as from health insurance claims may be followed up to assess outcomes.
- Details such as patient demographics, details of the medicinal product, indication for its use, duration of therapy, adverse events, clinical course, and outcome can be obtained through PEM.
- The treating physicians could be requested to fill questionnaires on patient outcomes at regular intervals.
- However, this method also has a few limitations. Only a few medicines prescribed in hospitals can be monitored by PEM. There are chances of loss of patient follow-up, selective sampling bias, and reporting bias.

- **Another method is to conduct registry studies.** Registries can be maintained for patients with specific diseases or conditions and for patients taking a particular medicinal product.
- The choice of registry for performing the observational study will be governed by the objectives, comparator groups, and outcomes to be assessed. It must be kept in mind that observational registries should not be used to evaluate efficacy.
- However, data on clinical conditions, medicine utilization patterns, patient-reported outcomes, safety, and effect modifiers (dose of medication, age of patients, concomitant disease or drugs) can be studied for medicinal products where efficacy has already been estimated in RCTs.
- Registries are more commonly used in post-marketing surveillance of orphan diseases. Further details are provided in the section relating to PMS of orphan drugs.

17.4.2 Observational or Non-interventional Studies

A significant proportion of the Phase 4 studies are observational in nature.

17.4.2.1 Cross-sectional Observational Design

- A cross-sectional study uses information gathered on a group of patients at one particular point in time, independent of their exposure history or state of illness.
- The main purpose of these types of studies is to collect data for surveys and ecological analysis.
- The inability to explicitly address the temporal connection between exposure and outcome is a limitation of cross-sectional studies.

17.4.2.2 Cohort Study

- A cohort study monitors a group at risk of an event that is important, to see if it appears over a time period.
- Since incidence rates can be computed, the population exposures during follow-up are known. Many cohort studies that involve exposure to therapeutic product select and track comparative cohorts of interest based on medication use throughout time.
- When it is necessary to understand not only the relative risks of adverse events but also their incidence rates, cohort studies come in assistance.
- They are also helpful for assessing several adverse events that occur during a single research study/period.
- It could be challenging to find enough patients who are exposed to the medication of interest (such as an orphan drug) or to conduct research on extremely uncommon outcomes.
- Patients for cohort research can be identified using data gathered especially for the study at hand or from sizable automated databases.
- Cohort studies can also be used to investigate safety issues in specific populations (pregnant women, pediatric age, patients with concurrent illnesses, and the

elderly) by stratifying the cohort if there are enough patients in it or by oversampling these patients.

17.4.2.3 Case-Control Study

- Case-control studies are structured to evaluate potential correlations between an exposure which is the drug and their uncommon adverse effects
- Case-control studies are carried out, for example, in response to concerns that the use of oral contraceptives may be associated with an increased risk of thromboembolism and thrombophlebitis.
- The patients are compared to age-matched controls that do not have thromboembolism but are as comparable as possible to a group of cases.

17.4.2.4 Post-marketing Surveillance from Spontaneous Reporting Databases

- Pharmacovigilance and pharmaco-epidemiological studies constitute a major part of PMS studies since Phase 3 clinical trials may not be powered to detect uncommon, rare adverse events and adverse events that occur after chronic use, as mentioned earlier.
- Pharmacovigilance systems of many countries are largely dependent on spontaneous reporting systems (voluntary reporting) for PMS.
- Physicians, other healthcare professionals, and consumers can directly report ADRs to these Spontaneous Reporting Systems (SRS). This is beneficial in detecting novel ADRs, hypothesis generation as well as signal detection.
- For example, MedWatch is a voluntary adverse event reporting system where adverse events detected by physicians can be reported to the FDA through an online form on the FDA website.
- The FDA reviews and analyzes these reported adverse events and based on the information, new regulatory recommendations may be generated and communicated to physicians.

17.4.3 Clinical Trials

17.4.3.1 Randomized Controlled Trials (RCT)

A Phase 4 randomized controlled trial is a type of clinical trial that, once a medication or technology has been approved for use in the general public, randomly allocates participants to a group receiving treatment and a control group. The objectives include:

- **Safety:** To keep an eye on long-term safety and looking for any unusual or novel side effects.
- **Effectiveness:** To assess the treatment's response in a large patient population.
- **Risks and benefits:** To examine any potential hazards or additional benefits. Assessing the impact of the treatment on the patients' quality of life.
- **Cost-effectiveness:** To understand the treatment's financial viability.

- **Sub-group populations**: To learn more about how the treatment functions in various demographic groups.

17.4.3.2 Large Simple Trials

- Large simple trials include a large number of participants with broad inclusion criteria (as recommended in the approved drug label) such as those encountered in routine clinical practice. It combines the favorable aspects of RCTs with features of an observational study.
- The outcomes studied in large simple trials are clinically meaningful outcomes, which can help in improving patient care. The data collection methods employed in large simple trials are often those that minimally affect routine medical care (e.g., data collected from Electronic Health Records, administration of questionnaires, etc.).
- The similarity that large simple trials share with RCTs is that patients are allotted by randomization to the study groups based on the principle of clinical equipoise.
- The follow-up duration for patients who drop-out or discontinue treatment in a large simple trial is carried on for a longer time as compared to that in RCTs where follow-up may be only for a short duration after treatment is discontinued.
- The endpoints measure effectiveness based on clinically relevant outcomes (e.g., incidence of death, hospitalization or life-threatening events).
- General practitioners are often commonly involved in conducting large simple trials while clinical research physicians often conduct RCTs under conditions of intensive monitoring.

Pragmatic trials: These trials aim to increase the chance that the intervention rather than some other factor causes the study outcome (internal validity).

- Pragmatic trials place an emphasis on external validity while preserving as much internal validity as possible.
- Decision makers in healthcare require to know precisely what they can anticipate from the available diagnostic or therapeutic option once applied in the real-world setting (external validity).

17.4.3.3 Prospective, Randomized, Open-Label, Blinded Endpoint (PROBE) Design

- The PROBE study design was first proposed by Hansson et al. in 1992 as a cost-effective alternative to randomized, double-blind clinical trials.
- In this study design, the investigators and the participants are both aware of the treatment they are receiving. However, they are blinded with regard to the outcome assessment.
- The outcomes are assessed by an independent committee which has no knowledge of the treatment allocation, thereby ensuring lack of bias in measurement of the trial outcomes.

- This study design has been used in many studies for its advantages such as: it is more cost-effective than a traditional double-blind study design; patient compliance is usually better since patients are taking a regular prescribed medication.
- In a double-blind study, often due to the presence of anonymized bottles containing code numbers, some patients may be uncomfortable to take the medication leading to higher risk of drop-outs. The other advantage is that this study design provides a real-world scenario with the similarity to clinical practice.
- The above advantages make this study design suitable for conducting Phase 4 studies.

17.4.4 Drug Utilization Studies

- The WHO has defined drug utilization studies (DUS) as studies that assess the marketing, distribution, prescription, and use of medicinal products in a society, with special emphasis on the resulting medical and socioeconomic consequences.
- By conducting DUS, we can obtain information on use of medications in various populations including pediatric and geriatric patients, pregnant women, and those with renal or liver dysfunction.
- Data on concomitant medications may also be obtained. The denominator data from Drug Utilization studies can also be helpful in estimating rates of adverse drug reactions. Data on inappropriate prescribing can also be obtained from DUS.

17.4.5 Other Phase 4 Studies

In addition to the above study designs, drug-drug interaction studies, formulation advancement studies, and studies to assess safety in special populations are also often employed in Phase 4 trials, as described below.

17.4.5.1 Drug–Drug Interaction Studies

- Combining the use of two or more medications is a common therapeutic approach for a variety of illnesses or patient populations.
- In these circumstances, there is a chance of a drug-drug interaction.
- Drug-drug interactions, also known simply as drug interactions, pose a serious risk to the effectiveness and safety of any or all of the medications when administered together.
- Such an interaction could result in a loss of efficacy as well as serious side effects, toxicity, and rarely, even death.
- Because drug interactions have historically resulted in the withdrawal of medications from the market or at the advanced clinical stage of development, they can also seriously hurt a pharmaceutical manufacturer's portfolio.

17.4.5.2 Formulation Advancement Studies

- It is possible to alter a drug's formulation according to commercial, manufacturing, or clinical requirements after the FDA approves it.
- These adjustments could come in the form of better formulations, new therapeutic applications, or novel delivery methods.
- Modifications to the drug's composition may affect the way the body absorbs it.
- It is critical to comprehend how these modifications may impact the medication's safety and effectiveness.
- Clinical formulation studies can be avoided by using formulation bridging procedures, which can speed up medication development.
- Drugs that are modified formulations of already approved medications may be processed using the 505(b)(2) route.
- It can save money and time by enabling sponsors to leverage pre-existing clinical data.

17.4.5.3 Special Population Studies

- Pregnancy exposure registers (PERs), healthcare database research, case-control studies, reports from medical organizations or various pharmaceutical companies, spontaneous reports, reports on cases or literature, and reports from other sources are all examples of PMS.
- Throughout the whole pregnancy, the woman should be watched for negative effects using any kind of PMS.
- To evaluate pre-term and post-term births, every attempt should be made to gather the pregnancy result and the age of gestation at birth.
- Precise recording of exposure timing, dosage, and duration for pharmaceutical products is crucial.
- Compiling the date of pre-conception exposure is also crucial for medications that are long-acting or genotoxic.
- Accurate dates of medication administration and the last menstrual cycle as well as date of conception are essential for evaluating exposure timing.
- A thorough history of the mother and the child is also prudent for the investigation and comprehension of pregnancy instances.

17.5 Post-marketing Surveillance of Orphan Drugs

- An orphan drug is one that is used to treat an orphan disease. In the United States, a disease that affects fewer than 200,000 people is defined as an Orphan disease. Commonly, post-approval study designs for rare diseases are observational (both prospective and retrospective).
- A common challenge in PMS of rare diseases is that the natural history of a rare disease may not be completely understood, hence making it difficult to differentiate between ADRs and natural sequelae of the disease.
- Retrospective studies are often based on information from medical records, Electronic Health Records or data from insurance claim databases, etc. Risk fac-

tors associated with rare diseases can be identified from case-control studies where the patients with the particular rare disease are the cases and the data of non-affected controls are derived from the same region or getting treated by the same network of physicians (for other diseases).
- Original data collection from prospective studies can help in overcoming many of the limitations from retrospective studies such as missing information from secondary data sources.
- Registries often enroll a patient at diagnosis and prospective, nested studies conducted from patient population enrolled in registries may be beneficial in obtaining real-world data.
- Registries are of two types: disease registries and product-based registries. Disease registries focus on a wide range of patients with a particular rare disease while product-based registries concentrate on patients who are administered a particular medicinal product and their health outcomes. Product-based registries are often maintained by pharmaceutical companies as a part of PMS and may sometimes include a comparator group receiving standard of care.

17.6 Regulatory Aspects and Submission of Aggregate Safety Reports

17.6.1 Periodic Safety Update Reports (PSUR)

- The PMS data has to be submitted by the MAH to the regulatory authority at specified intervals.
- The ICH E2C(R1) guidelines in 1996 endorsed the format of PSUR as a common format for submission of safety data collected at specified times after approval of a medicinal product.
- In India, as per the Drugs and Cosmetics Act, 1940 and Rules, 1945 including the New Drug and Clinical Trial Rules, 2019, the timeline for submission of PSUR is once in 6 months for the first 2 years from date of approval of the new product, and once a year for the next 2 years. This may be extended if there is a need for continued pharmacovigilance for public health reasons.
- The PSUR must be submitted within 30 calendar days of the last day of reporting period. In case of occurrence of Serious Adverse Event (SAE), it must be reported to Central Licensing Authority within 15 days of initial receipt of information by the MAH.
- A single PSUR should be submitted by the MAH containing information on all approved indications, route of administration, dosage forms, and regimens. In rare cases of formulations for completely different indications, a separate PSUR may be required.
- In a CDSCO notification dated 26th February 2024, the process of PSUR submission has become fully online through Sugam portal and from 11th March 2024, the process of offline submission of PSUR has been discontinued.

17.6.2 Periodic Benefit-Risk Evaluation Report (PBRER)

- The ICHE2C (R2) guidelines prescribed the use of PBRER for post-marketing surveillance. The European Medicines Agency (EMA) requires submission of PMS data in PBRER format. This is because it has been recognized that the assessment of risk would be more relevant when the risk was considered in background with the benefits of the product, leading to concept of overall benefit-risk evaluation of the medicinal product.
- Generally, one PBRER is prepared for an investigational product with different formulations, dosage forms, regimens or indications.
- In rare cases with relevant justification, e.g., for entirely different indications, submission of separate PBRERs may be considered acceptable. In case of fixed dose combinations, the information may be submitted either as a separate PBRER or included under the PBRER of one of the individual substances.
- The PBRER should also be submitted every 6 months for the first 2 years and then annually thereafter.

17.6.3 Post-marketing Adverse Drug Experiences Report (PADER)

- PADER is one of the preferred formats for the MAH and sponsor to submit PMS data to the US-FDA after a drug obtains marketing approval.
- It should be submitted by the sponsor for NDA (for innovator compound), ANDA (generics) as well as for BLA (for biologics) according to US 21 CFR 314.80 to US FDA.
- It contains narratives for all the 15-day alerts of serious and unlisted events reported during the reporting interval.
- All the other cases (serious listed, non-serious unlisted, non-serious listed) during the reporting interval are included under non-15-day alerts.
- The timelines for PADER submission are quarterly for the first 3 years then once every year.

17.7 Ethical Aspects of Phase 4 Clinical Trials

- The vast difference between Phases 1 to 3 and Phase 4 clinical trials is that the latter use approved medications for treatment and are conducted in a clinical setting (unlike a research setting like in the other phases). Hence, the lines of distinction get indistinct between research and treatment.
- Although Phase 4 is often conducted by physicians who have less experience with clinical research as opposed to investigators who conduct Phases 1 to 3, the methodological, ethical aspects, and research integrity in clinical research during Phase 4 must be held to the same standards as the earlier phases of clinical trials.

- There should be no conflict of interest on the part of the researcher or the clinician to enroll more patients in the Phase 4 study to achieve a certain sample size for financial or professional interests.

17.7.1 Seeding Trials

- Some post-marketing trials are conducted not just to collect scientific data on the product but also to promote the prescribing and marketing of the newly approved product.
- Some features of a seeding trial include: investigators with inadequate clinical research experience, presence of too many investigators, lack of appropriate control group, broad eligibility criteria, protocol for the trial being developed by the marketing division rather than the Medical or the Research & Development division of the MAH.
- Ethically, these trials have a lot of undesirable outcomes: the participants are not fully aware of the objectives of the study from the informed consent documents, and hence, these trials are grossly discouraged.

17.8 Challenges with Post-marketing Studies

- Spontaneous ADR reporting systems constitute a major portion of post-marketing surveillance reports. However, these databases have some inherent limitations.
- Firstly, under-reporting of ADRs is a challenge to be tackled. Some of the factors leading to under-reporting include lack of time, hectic schedules of physicians as well as lack of sensitization about the significance of ADR reporting.
- Another factor in spontaneous reporting databases is different types of bias like notoriety bias (number of reported adverse events with a particular drug increases dramatically after a safety alert has been issued by the regulatory authorities as compared to number of baseline reports with the same drug before the safety alert), Weber effect (reporting of Adverse events slowly increases in the first 2 years, attaining a maximum at the end of 2 years after marketing approval of a drug and then slowly decreases over time) and higher reporting of serious events as compared to non-serious events. As discussed above, under-reporting is also a type of bias leading to errors in estimating ADR incidence rates.
- As an example, in a study conducted on the French pharmacovigilance database, the number of reported cases of valvulopathies with pergolide increased from zero to 63 after the safety alert. Similarly, the number of tuberculosis reports with infliximab were two and seven before and after the safety alert respectively.

17.9 Signal Detection, Safety Monitoring, and Benefit-Risk Assessment

- A signal is defined by WHO as "reported information on possible causal relationship between an adverse event and a drug, the relationship being unknown or incompletely documented previously".
- During PMS, signals may be detected from various sources including spontaneous reporting databases, data from PEM, through record linkage from large databases, registries, and so on. Use of data mining software engines helps in generating signals from large databases.
- Unexpected adverse effects recognized during PMS have historically led to various actions such as change in product labels, restricted use, product recalls, etc. A few examples have been given below. In 1987, a review of prescription records by the New Zealand Intensive Medicines Monitoring programme showed reports of cough being one of the most common ADRs of ACE inhibitors. Similarly, a PMS study was carried out from the FDA Adverse Event Reporting System, which detected signals of Torsades de pointes with olanzapine, amisulpride, and cyamemazine. Another example is a Prescription Event Monitoring study showing sibutramine's higher propensity of being associated with cardiovascular disease. Eventually, the drug was withdrawn due to higher risk of serious cardiovascular disease (CVD) adverse events. Further, PMS data of the prokinetic drug, cisapride showed increasing number of reports QT prolongation, tachyarrhythmias, and torsades de pointes, thereby leading to a black box warning and ultimate withdrawal of the drug in 2000.

Key Points

- The main objective of Phase 4 clinical trials is to study the long-term safety of the marketed new product.
- There can be different study designs for a Phase 4 studies, which include post-marketing surveillance studies, large simple trials, registry-based studies, and so on.
- The Marketing Authorization Holder should submit aggregate safety reports such as PSUR/PBRER or PADER to the relevant regulatory authorities during Phase 4. The timelines vary depending on the regulatory authority to whom it has to be submitted.

Bibliography

1. Alomar M, Tawfiq AM, Hassan N, Palaian S (2020) Post marketing surveillance of suspected adverse drug reactions through spontaneous reporting: current status, challenges and the future. Ther Adv Drug Saf 11:2042098620938595

2. Andre EB, Reynolds R, Caubel P, Azoulay L, Dreyer NA (2020) Trial designs using real-world data: the changing landscape of the regulatory approval process. Pharmacoepidemiol Drug Saf 29(10):1201–1212
3. Central Drugs Standard Control Organisation. PSUR submission checklist. [Internet]. Available from: https://cdsco.gov.in/opencms/export/sites/CDSCO_WEB/Pdf-documents/PSUR_PV_AEFI/PSUR-Submission-checklist.pdf. Accessed 21 Oct 2024
4. Central Drugs Standard Control Organisation. Submission of online applications of PSUR. [Internet]. Available from: https://cdsco.gov.in/opencms/resources/UploadCDSCOWeb/2018/UploadCircularFile/psur%20130.pdf. Accessed 21 Oct 2024
5. Central Drugs Standard Control Organisation. Pharmacovigilance guidance document for marketing authorization holders of pharmaceutical products version 2.0. [Internet]. Available from: https://cdsco.gov.in/opencms/opencms/system/modules/CDSCO.WEB/elements/download_file_division.jsp?num_id=MTIwMDc=. Accessed 21 Oct 2024
6. Coulter DM, Edwards IR (1987) Cough associated with captopril and enalapril. Br Med J (Clin Res Ed) 294(6586):1521–1523
7. Czernichow S, Batty GD (2010) Withdrawal of sibutramine for weight loss: where does this leave clinicians? Obes Facts 3:155–156
8. Dang A (2023) Real-world evidence: a primer. Pharmaceut Med 37(1):25–36
9. European Medicines Agency. ICH guideline E2C (R2) on periodic benefit-risk evaluation report (PBRER) 2013. [Internet]. Available from: https://www.ema.europa.eu/en/documents/regulatory-procedural-guideline/international-conference-harmonisation-technical-requirements-registration-pharmaceuticals-human-use-guideline-e2c-r2-periodic-benefit-risk-evaluation-report-step-5_en.pdf. Accessed 21 Oct 2024
10. European Medicines Agency. Guideline on good pharmacovigilance practices (GVP)—module VII–periodic safety update report. June 2012. [Internet]. Available from https://www.emwa.org/Documents/Freelancer/regulatorywriting/PSUR%20guideline_02jul12-GVP_moduleVII.pdf. Accessed 21 Oct 2024
11. European Medicines Agency. Guideline on good pharmacovigilance practices (GVP)—module VII–periodic safety update report. December 2013. [Internet]. Available from: https://www.ema.europa.eu/en/documents/scientific-guideline/guideline-good-pharmacovigilance-practices-gvp-module-vii-periodic-safety-update-report_en.pdf. Accessed 21 Oct 2024
12. European Medicines Agency. Guideline on good pharmacovigilance practices (GVP)—module VIII—post-authorisation safety studies (Rev 3). 2017. [Internet]. Available from: https://www.ema.europa.eu/en/documents/scientific-guideline/guideline-good-pharmacovigilance-practices-gvp-module-viii-post-authorisation-safety-studies-rev-3_en.pdf. Accessed 21 Oct 2024
13. European Medicines Agency. Post-authorization safety studies. [Internet]. Available from https://www.ema.europa.eu/en/human-regulatory-overview/post-authorisation/pharmacovigilance-post-authorisation/post-authorisation-safety-studies-pass. Accessed 21 Oct 2024
14. Faillie JL, Montastruc F, Montastruc JL, Pariente A (2016) Pharmacoepidemiology and its input to pharmacovigilance. Therapie 71:211–216
15. Glasser SP, Salas M, Delzell E (2007) Importance and challenges of studying marketed drugs: what is a phase IV study? Common clinical research designs, registries, and self-reporting systems. J Clin Pharmacol 47(9):1074–1086
16. Gliklich RE, Dreyer NA, Leavy MB (eds) (2014) Registries for evaluating patient outcomes: a user's guide. Agency for Healthcare research and quality (US), Rockville
17. Hansson L, Hedner T, Dahlöf B (1992) Prospective randomized open blinded end-point (PROBE) study. A novel design for intervention trials. Blood Press 1(2):113–119
18. Hill TP (2012) Conducting phase IV clinical studies: a moral imperative? ecancermedicalscience 6:276
19. Hillman D, Ryder C (2019) Applying for an EU marketing authorisation: a pharmacovigilance perspective. Regul Rapp 16:23–27

20. Hohenschurz-Schmidt DJ, Cherkin D, Rice AS, Dworkin RH, Turk DC, McDermott MP et al (2023) Research objectives and general considerations for pragmatic clinical trials of pain treatments: IMMPACT statement. Pain 164:1457–1472
21. Klein E, Bourdette D (2013) Postmarketing adverse drug reactions: a duty to report? Neurol Clin Pract 3(4):288–294
22. Klepper MJ (2004) The periodic safety update report as a pharmacovigilance tool. Drug Saf 27:569–578
23. Kohro T, Yamazaki T (2009) Cardiovascular clinical trials in Japan and controversies regarding prospective randomized open-label blinded end-point design. Hypertens Res 32(2):109–114
24. Kulkarni TN, Kulkarni NG (2019) Authoring a periodic adverse drug experience report… here's what you need to know! Perspect Clin Res 10(2):95–99
25. Lesko SM, Mitchell AA (2006) The use of randomized controlled trials for pharmacoepidemiology. In: Strom BL, Kimmel SE (eds) Textbook of pharmacoepidemiology, pp 311–320. [Internet]. Available from: https://pharmacystblog.wordpress.com/wp-content/uploads/2019/05/textbook-of-pharmacoepidemiology.pdf. Accessed 21 Oct 2024
26. Maier WC, Christensen RA, Anderson P (2017) Post-approval studies for rare disease treatments and orphan drugs. Adv Exp Med Biol 2017:197–205
27. Matsuda S, Aoki K, Kawamata T, Kimotsuki T, Kobayashi T, Kuriki H, Nakayama T, Okugawa S, Sugimura Y, Tomita M, Takahashi Y (2015) Bias in spontaneous reporting of adverse drug reactions in Japan. PLoS One 10(5):e0126413
28. Meyboom RH, Egberts AC, Edwards IR, Hekster YA, de Koning FH, Gribnau FW (1997) Principles of signal detection in pharmacovigilance. Drug Saf 16:355–365
29. National Institutes of Health (NIH). Definition of orphan drug. [Internet]. Available from: https://www.cancer.gov/publications/dictionaries/cancer-terms/def/orphan-drug. Accessed 21 Oct 2024
30. Padhy BM, Meher BR (2019) Seeding trials: marketing gimmick or credible scientific research. Indian J Anaesth 63(3):235–238
31. Pariente A, Gregoire F, Fourrier-Reglat A, Haramburu F, Moore N (2007) Impact of safety alerts on measures of disproportionality in spontaneous reporting databases the notoriety bias. Drug Saf 30:891–898
32. Perrio MJ, Wilton LV, Shakir SA (2007) The safety profiles of orlistat and sibutramine: results of prescription-event monitoring studies in England. Obesity (Silver Spring) 15(11):2712–2722
33. Poluzzi E, Raschi E, Koci A, Moretti U, Spina E, Behr ER, Sturkenboom M, De Ponti F (2013) Antipsychotics and torsadogenic risk: signals emerging from the US FDA adverse event reporting system database. Drug Saf 36:467–479
34. Quigley EM (2011) Cisapride: what can we learn from the rise and fall of a prokinetic? J Dig Dis 12(3):147–156
35. Raj N, Fernandes S, Charyulu NR, Dubey A, Ravi GS, Hebbar S (2019) Postmarket surveillance: a review on key aspects and measures on the effective functioning in the context of the United Kingdom and Canada. Ther Adv Drug Saf 10:2042098619865413
36. Reynolds RF, Lem JA, Gatto NM, Eng SM (2011) Is the large simple trial design used for comparative, post-approval safety research? A review of a clinical trials registry and the published literature. Drug Saf 34:799–820
37. Rizzo M. The ethics of phase IV clinical trials. American Academy of Neurology. [Internet]. Available from: www.aan.com/global/axon/assets/6110.pdf. Accessed 21 Oct 2024
38. Roehr B (2013) The appeal of large simple trials. Br Med J 346:f1317
39. Sands A, Van Drongelen A, Geertsma R, Roszek B, Esteve PB, Silo H. Guidance for post-market surveillance and market surveillance of medical devices, including in vitro diagnostics. [Internet]. Available from: https://rivm.openrepository.com/handle/10029/624891. Accessed 21 Oct 2024
40. Suvarna V (2010) Phase IV of drug development. Perspect Clin Res 1(2):57–60
41. US Food and Drug Administration. Providing post-market periodic safety reports in the ICH E2C (R2) format (periodic benefit-risk evaluation report). Guidance for industry 2013. [Internet]. Available from https://www.fda.gov/media/85520/download. Accessed 21 Oct 2024

42. Uppsala Monitoring Centre. World Health Organization. [Internet]. Available from: https://who-umc.org/media/164092/general-information-about-signal-published-in-who-pn.pdf. Accessed 21 Oct 2024
43. Vlahović-Palčevski V, Mentzer D (2011) Postmarketing surveillance. Handb Exp Pharmacol 205:339–351
44. Weber J (1984) Epidemiology of adverse reactions to nonsteroidal anti-inflammatory drugs. Adv Inflamm Res 6:1–7

Ethics in Clinical Trials

18

K. Mythili Bai, C. Madhavrao, Gerard Marshall Raj, Sushil Sharma, and Santenna Chenchula

Abstract

This chapter reviews the ethical structure underlying clinical testing. It describes the chronological development of this field, with the crucial milestones—the Nuremberg Code, the Declaration of Helsinki, and the Belmont Report—all of which recognize three basic principles: respect for persons, beneficence, and justice. These formative documents are required to protect participant rights and to maintain public trust in research.

The chapter underlines informed consent, confidentiality, and privacy as being critically important, while it also mentions historical violations of ethics as a justification for rigorous oversight in research practices. It also looks at various regulatory frameworks, such as ICH GCP, guidelines by CIOMS, WHO standards, and roles of national regulatory authorities like FDA, EMA, and CDSCO.

It discusses the complexities regarding informed consent, especially in vulnerable populations, ethical dilemmas around placebo use, and randomization of trials. It also addresses new trial designs, issues related to data privacy and post-trial obligations, with an emphasis on participant welfare and scientific integrity as imperatives.

K. Mythili Bai
Government Siddhartha Medical College, Vijayawada, India

C. Madhavrao (✉) · S. Sharma
All India Institute of Medical Sciences [AIIMS], Mangalagiri, India

G. M. Raj
Department of Pharmacology, All India Institute of Medical Sciences (AIIMS) Bibinagar, Hyderabad, Telangana, India

S. Chenchula
All India Institute of Medical Sciences [AIIMS], Bhopal, India

A. Arivazhahan et al. (eds.), *Introduction to Basics of Pharmacology and Toxicology*,
https://doi.org/10.1007/978-981-95-1920-0_18

The modern-day challenges also include the use of artificial intelligence and patient-centric approaches, which raise very pertinent questions related to algorithmic bias and engagement of participants. Ethics committees and CABs are highlighted for their contributions toward culturally sensitive research practices.

In the end, this chapter recommends continuous education in ethics and the elaboration of unified ethical standards internationally, while compliance with established guidelines is vital for participant protection and responsible medical knowledge acquisition.

Keywords

Ethical framework · Informed consent · Beneficence · Justice · Regulatory frameworks · Vulnerable populations · Data privacy · Algorithmic bias · Ethics education

18.1 Introduction

Clinical trials represent a crucial facet in the advancement of medical research, as they furnish the essential evidence necessary for evaluating both the safety and efficacy of novel treatments. However, the ethical dilemmas embedded within the execution of these trials demand meticulous navigation to protect participants' rights and sustain public trust in the overarching research paradigm. This chapter explores the fundamental ethical principles that underpin clinical trials; it also scrutinizes the regulatory frameworks that have been instituted to guarantee the consistent enforcement of these standards. Furthermore, it contends with the dynamic challenges that researchers and ethics committees encounter in their endeavors to uphold ethical integrity throughout the trial process. Although significant progress has been made in this arena, ongoing vigilance is imperative because the landscape of medical research is perpetually evolving.

18.2 Historical Context of Ethics in Clinical Trials

18.2.1 The Evolution of Ethical Standards

In the last 100 years, the ethical guidelines have evolved significantly in clinical research involving human experiments. In the past, the regulations for conducting clinical trials were not that stringent with compromise in the safety of study participants. As many unethical practices were highlighted involving human experimentation in the past history, which led to the development of many ethical principles and guidelines in conducting the clinical trials. The development of these standard guidelines has uplifted the dignity, rights, and safety of study participants in the clinical research.

18.2.2 The Nuremberg Code and Its Impact

First among the ethical principles and most important is the Nuremberg Code, developed following the Second World War and instrumental in developing a system to guide ethical standards in research with human participation. This was developed in response to acts committed during the war by Nazi physicians and has underlined principles such as voluntary consent-imposed duties to avoid unnecessary harm or distress in medical research.

18.2.3 The Declaration of Helsinki

It was adopted by the World Medical Association (WMA) in 1964 based on principles laid down by the Nuremberg Code. It once and for all introduced basic elements that would later be referred to as independent ethical review, distinguishing between therapeutic and non-therapeutic research. The Declaration has undergone a number of revisions since its adoption because of changing ethical positions and also recent medical scientific developments. The latest being released in October 2024 during the 75th WMA General Assembly held in Helsinki, Finland.

18.2.4 The Belmont Report

The 1979 publication of the Belmont Report represented important steps of advancement in ethical guidelines by codification in three key principles: respect for persons, beneficence, and justice. These core elements have remained part of the basic underpinning of ethical framework in clinical research and continue to influence regulatory requirements throughout the world.

18.2.5 Key Ethical Violations in Clinical Trial History

Historical incidents like the Tuskegee Syphilis Study and the Guatemala Syphilis Experiment stand as examples of how grave consequences may be perpetrated owing to ethical violations in research. The above incidents made informed consent an important aspect and further imposed the need for strict ethical vetting in research methodologies.

Common ethical issues in clinical trials in the 'history with examples' are depicted in Table 18.1.

Table 18.1 Common ethical issues in clinical trials in the 'history with examples'

Sl. No	Ethical issue(s)	Description	Example(s)
1	Informed consent	Inadequate provision of information about the trial's risks and benefits	Tuskegee syphilis study (1932–1972)
2	Coercion and undue influence	Participants pressured or unduly influenced into participation	Guatemala Syphilis Experiments (1946–1948)
3	Deception and misleading information	Providing false or misleading information about the study	Willowbrook Hepatitis Study (1956–1970)
4	Exploitation of vulnerable populations	Targeting vulnerable groups without proper safeguards	Havasupai Tribe Genetic Research Controversy (2004)
5	Lack of scientific rigor	Conducting trials without solid scientific basis or objectives	Radium Girls Cases (1920s)
6	Discriminatory participant selection	Bias in the selection of participants	Stanford Prison Experiment (1971)
7	Inadequate risk management	Insufficient assessment and management of potential risks	Thalidomide Tragedy (1950s)
8	Ethical issues with placebo use	Using placebo instead of proven treatments in trials	NIH Antiviral Study (1980s)
9	Privacy violations	Breaches of participant confidentiality and privacy	Human Radiation Experiments (1950s–1970s)
10	Post-trial access to effective treatments	Failure to provide continued treatment after the trial concludes	Argentina AIDS Trials (1990s)
11	Transparency issues	Inadequate disclosure of trial results and outcomes	Sickle Cell Anemia Trials (1970s)
12	Insufficient adverse event monitoring	Poor monitoring and reporting of adverse effects	Dalkon Shield Cases (1970s)
13	Unethical data practices	Falsification or manipulation of trial data	Andrew Wakefield's Vaccine Study (1998)
14	Consent issues with minors	Ethical concerns regarding obtaining consent from minors	Nuremberg code (post-WWII)
15	Bias toward positive outcomes	Emphasis on positive results while ignoring negative findings	Bhopal Gas Tragedy (1984)
16	Conflicts of interest	Influence of financial or personal interests on trial conduct	Merck Vioxx Controversy (2004)
17	Ethical concerns in genetic research	Issues related to genetic privacy and ethical research practices	HeLa Cells Controversy (1950s-present)
18	Cultural insensitivity	Ignoring cultural contexts and norms during trials	Nuremberg Trials (1947)

(continued)

Table 18.1 (continued)

Sl. No	Ethical issue(s)	Description	Example(s)
19	Exploitation of economically disadvantaged	Utilizing low-income populations without adequate protection	Tuskegee Syphilis Study (1932–1972)
20	Mismanagement of research funds	Improper use or allocation of research funding	Paolo Macchiarini Fraudulent Research (2010s)
21	High-risk drug trials: Ethical issues	Conducting trials with high-risk drugs without appropriate safety measures	Ischemia Trial (1990s)
22	Participant autonomy issues	Lack of respect for participants' autonomy and decision-making	Willowbrook Hepatitis Study (1956–1970)
23	Follow-up care after trials	Inadequate follow-up and care post-trial participation	Hemophilia Trials (1980s)
24	Misrepresentation of risk-benefit ratio	Misleading participants about the risk-benefit ratio of the trial	Thalidomide Disaster (1950s)
25	Institutional trust exploitation	Abusing trust placed in institutional settings for unethical practices	Johns Hopkins Neonatal Trial (1990s)

18.3 Universal Core Ethics Principles in Clinical Trials

18.3.1 Respect for Persons

This principle stresses respect for persons, including individual autonomy while protecting those with diminished autonomy. One of the ways by which respect for persons would be addressed is through informed consent which allows communication and mutual understanding between the researchers and participants.

18.3.2 Beneficence

Whereas the principle of beneficence demands that researchers maximize the possible benefits and minimize the possible risks for participants in the study, it demands no less than prudent judgments of risk-benefit ratios in advance of initiating a trial, and ongoing monitoring during the research itself to guarantee participants' safety.

18.3.3 Justice

Justice considers the fair distribution of research risks and benefits. It requires that subject selection be equitable and that the most vulnerable among the populations are not exploited in the selection process.

18.3.4 Informed Consent

Informed consent is not obtained by simply getting a signature but ensuring that the participant comprehensively understands what they are being evaluated for, the risks of the trial, and their freedom to withdraw at any time without penalty.

18.3.5 Confidentiality and Privacy

Clinical trials need to ensure, at all costs, the confidentiality and privacy of the participants. There would have to be some sort of protection for personal information, with an assurance that participant records would be used only and exclusively for the purposes declared in the consent form.

18.4 Regulatory Frameworks and Guidelines

18.4.1 International Ethical Guidelines

Most of the international guidelines provide the frameworks for ethical conduct. For example, guiding documents such as the Council for International Organizations of Medical Sciences guidelines, International Council for Harmonisation's Good Clinical Practice guidelines, and the World Health Organization guidelines enumerate areas of comprehensive ethical standards for the global execution of clinical trials.

18.4.2 National Regulatory Authorities

Most of the countries in the world have instituted a national regulatory agency for the oversight of clinical research. To name a few, leading ones among these regulatory agencies, for enforcement of ethical guidelines and protection of participants in their respective areas, include the EMA, the US FDA, and the Indian CDSCO.

18.4.3 Role of Institutional Review Boards (IRBs) and Ethics Committees

Ethics committees/IRBs have the responsibility to protect the rights and welfare of research participants. They review research proposals to ensure that they meet basic ethical requirements and limit the risks as possible to study participants.

18.4.4 Ethics in Multinational Clinical Trials

Diverse ethical issues are associated with conducting clinical trials in various countries around the world. For example, standards of informed consent will differ from country to country, as will oversight by regulatory authorities. Ethical consistency in a way must be balanced with respect for the local culture and regulations to safeguard the integrity of multinational trials.

Common ethical challenges in 'multicentric global clinical trials' are highlighted in Table 18.2.

Table 18.2 Common ethical challenges in 'multicentric global clinical trials'

Sl. No.	Ethical challenge(s)	Description
1	Culturally informed consent	Ensuring that informed consent processes are adapted to the cultural and linguistic needs of participants from diverse regions, ensuring clarity and respect
2	Equitable access to clinical trials	Guaranteeing that participants across different regions have equal access to trials, avoiding disparities and ensuring fair inclusion
3	Regulatory and ethical compliance	Adhering to the diverse regulatory standards and ethical guidelines of multiple countries while striving for a unified approach to research ethics
4	Safeguarding vulnerable groups	Implementing additional protections for vulnerable populations, such as children, elderly, or economically disadvantaged individuals in all participating locations
5	Cultural considerations in study design	Designing study protocols that respect and accommodate local cultural norms and practices, ensuring the research is relevant and respectful to all participants
6	Data security and privacy	Ensuring stringent measures to protect participant's personal and health data, adhering to international and local data protection regulations
7	Management of Adverse Events	Establishing clear and consistent procedures for identifying, reporting and managing adverse events across all trial sites to ensure participant safety
8	Fair compensation and expense reimbursement	Ensuring that all participants receive fair compensation and reimbursement for their participation, considering regional economic conditions and standards
9	Global ethical oversight	Coordinating ethical oversight across multiple regions to ensure uniform ethical standards and address region-specific ethical challenges effectively
10	Post-trial access and benefits	Providing continued access to effective treatments or interventions after the trial ends and ensuring that benefits are available to participants, particularly in underserved regions

18.5 Bioethics of Informed Consent Process in Clinical Trials

18.5.1 Components of Informed Consent

The basic elements of informed consent include disclosure, understanding, voluntariness, competence, and agreement. It is incumbent upon the researchers to ensure that these elements are instituted and that they are all understood by potential participants before they can agree to participate in the research study.

18.5.2 Challenges in Obtaining Genuine Informed Consent

Sometimes, truly informed consent is hard to obtain, in cases of vulnerable populations, when either language might act as a barrier or complex medical information is to be conveyed. Researchers have an ethical commitment in discussing any lingering issues and having the participants fully understand what they are presenting to them.

18.5.3 Special Considerations for Vulnerable Populations

Special populations include children, pregnant women, and individuals with cognitive impairments, who need special protection through consent and assent in clinical research. Ethical guidelines spell out what must be done while obtaining consent and assent with a view to protect such populations and ensuring their welfare.

18.5.4 The Role of Technology in Informed Consent

Digital technologies have made informed consent more interactive and accessible. However, these advancements have also created new challenges, such as ensuring digital literacy among participants and safeguarding electronic data.

18.6 Ethical Challenges in Clinical Trials in General

Clinical trials form a very basic foundation in the approval of new treatments and therapies and building up the medical knowledge. However, they also come along with serious ethical challenges, which must be well managed to keep participants safe and maintain the integrity of the research findings. Such challenges are faced from many aspects like related to trial design, participant selection, informed consent, and balancing scientific goals against their ethical considerations.

A list of common ethical challenges encountered in clinical trials is depicted in Table 18.3.

Table 18.3 List of common ethical challenges encountered in clinical trials

Sl. No.	Ethical challenge(s)	Description
1	Informed consent	Participants must be thoroughly informed about the trial's purpose, procedures, risks and benefits allowing them to make an educated decision
2	Voluntary participation	Participation should be entirely voluntary, with the freedom to withdraw at any stage without facing any penalties or negative consequences
3	Risk-benefit evaluation	The potential benefits of the trial should outweigh the risks and efforts must be made to minimize any possible harm to participants
4	Confidentiality and privacy	Participant's personal data must be handled with utmost care, ensuring it is kept confidential and used only for the purposes outlined in the consent
5	Protection of vulnerable groups	Extra safeguards should be in place for vulnerable populations, such as minors or the elderly, to protect their rights and Well-being
6	Ethics committee approval	All trials must receive approval from an independent ethics committee or institutional review board (IRB) to ensure participant protection
7	Equitable participant selection	Participants should be selected based on fair and scientifically sound criteria, avoiding exploitation or discrimination
8	Transparency and disclosure	Researchers must fully disclose all relevant information about the trial, including any potential conflicts of interest or funding sources
9	Scientific content	The trial should be scientifically sound, using rigorous methods to ensure reliable results and ethical conduct
10	Access to post-trial benefits	Participants should have access to beneficial treatments or interventions identified during the trial, particularly in resource-poor settings
11	Compensation for adverse effects	There should be provisions to compensate participants who experience adverse effects or harm as a result of the trial
12	Cultural considerations	The trial should be sensitive to cultural differences, particularly in international settings, to respect local customs and values
13	Managing conflicts of interest	Any potential conflicts of interest should be identified and managed to prevent bias in the trial's design, conduct, or reporting
14	Data accuracy and integrity	Ensuring the data collected is accurate, reliable, and free from fabrication or manipulation, maintaining the integrity of the research
15	Ethical use of placebos	Placebos should only be used when no proven intervention exists and participants should not be deprived of necessary treatments
16	Benefit sharing	Communities involved in the research should share in the benefits, especially when the research is conducted in low-income or developing regions
17	Dual use and misuse of research	Researchers must consider the potential for misuse of their findings, especially in fields involving sensitive or dangerous technologies

(continued)

Table 18.3 (continued)

Sl. No.	Ethical challenge(s)	Description
18	Proxy consent	Ethical issues arise when someone other than the participant provides consent, such as in the case of minors or incapacitated individuals
19	Trial registration and reporting	Trials should be registered in public databases and results should be transparently reported, regardless of whether the outcomes are positive or negative
20	Community involvement	Engaging with the community during the trial design and implementation to ensure the research aligns with local needs and values
21	Fair distribution of risks and benefits	Ensuring that the risks and benefits of the trial are fairly distributed among all participants, avoiding exploitation of any group
22	Appropriate incentives	Incentives should not be so large as to coerce participation but should fairly compensate for time and expenses incurred by participants
23	Training for research staff	All personnel involved in the trial must be properly trained in ethical research practices and the specific protocols being used
24	International ethical standards	When conducting trials internationally, researchers must adhere to ethical standards that respect the cultural and legal norms of the host country
25	Ongoing monitoring and audits	Continuous monitoring by independent bodies is crucial to ensure that the trial adheres to ethical standards and that participants' safety is prioritized

18.6.1 Informed Consent

Informed consent is one of the basic principles of ethical clinical research. The nature, aim, risks, and benefits of the trial must be fully understood by the study participants before accepting to take part in the study. Difficulty in truly obtaining informed consent exists especially when the participants have low medical knowledge, language issues, cognitive impairments, or from vulnerable groups, for example, underprivileged people, minors, or those with life-threatening diseases. Furthermore, consent forms should be complete, clear, and understandable; meanwhile, the researchers should ensure the participants clearly understand that it is their right to withdraw from the study at any time without giving any reasons and without any adverse consequences.

18.6.2 Vulnerable Populations

This serves to acknowledge that most research involving vulnerable populations such as prisoners or institutional employees, pregnant women, the geriatric population, children, individuals with mental disabilities, and economically disadvantaged individuals who are not fully capable of providing an informed decision. These groups are considered vulnerable to coercion or exploitation. Researchers should, therefore, take extra precautionary measures to protect them, obtain informed consent from legally authorized representatives, justify the necessity of such research and the inherent inability to be replicated with populations at a lesser perceived risk, and also offer support throughout the research study.

Common ethical challenges in clinical trials involving 'pregnancy and lactation' are highlighted in Table 18.4.

Common ethical challenges in clinical trials involving 'elderly population' are highlighted in Table 18.5.

18.6.3 Balancing Risk and Benefit

The underlying basic ethical principle in clinical trials is the principle of beneficence, which demands that there is maximization of possible benefits while at the same time keeping possible harm minimal to participants in the study. Assessing an acceptable risk-benefit ratio can, however, be a backbreaking process in its complexity. Researchers have to evaluate preferred risks, which are likely to occur as a result of potential physical trial harm, psychological distress, and socioeconomic consequences, cautiously against expected benefits. The latter is particularly difficult in early-phase trials, like Phase I, where risks are usually increased and benefits to participants are generally not well defined.

18.6.4 Randomization and Placebo Use

The clinical trials are characterized by randomization and the use of placebos, which reduce biases and enhance scientific rigor. On the other hand, they give rise to a number of ethical issues, particularly when there is already an existing therapy to be withheld in control group participants. This issue, however, is more serious in trials of serious or life-threatening conditions in as much as withholding treatment can lead to harm or even death. The use of placebos, according to ethical guidelines, is acceptable only in situations where established interventions do not exist and participation will not expose subjects to an unduly high risk of harm.

18.6.5 Conflicts of Interest

Conflicts of interest arise when some financial or personal interests of researchers, sponsors, or institutions may compromise objectivity or judgment in carrying out or reporting the work. Such conflicts may give rise to biased study design; manipulation of data; selective reporting of results; unethical recruitment of research participants; or other forms of malpractice. Specifically, disclosure of all possible conflicts of interest is required and efforts toward quasi-independent oversight by ethics committees or data monitoring boards are much needed.

Table 18.4 Common ethical challenges in clinical trials involving 'pregnancy and lactation'

Sl. No.	Ethical challenge(s)	Description
1	Informed consent and decision-making	Pregnant and lactating participants must be provided with clear, comprehensive information to make an informed decision, considering potential risks to themselves and their child
2	Risk-benefit assessment	The potential risks to both the mother and the fetus or infant must be carefully evaluated against the possible benefits, ensuring that risks are justified and minimized
3	Fetal and neonatal safety	Special precautions must be taken to protect fetal and neonatal health, with rigorous evaluation of any potential harm during the trial
4	Vulnerability protections	Pregnant and lactating women are a vulnerable population, requiring additional protective measures to safeguard their health and that of their child
5	Ethical rationale for inclusion	A strong ethical justification is required for including pregnant and lactating women in trials, particularly when alternative study populations are available
6	Monitoring for maternal and child health	Continuous monitoring is essential to detect and respond to any adverse effects on the mother or child during the trial
7	Minimizing teratogenic exposure	Careful management of exposure to potential teratogens is crucial to avoid harm to fetal development, with clear communication of these risks to participants
8	Long-term follow-up for participants	Ensuring long-term follow-up is crucial to track any delayed effects on both the mother and child after trial participation
9	Balancing conflicting interests	Ethical challenges may arise when the interests of the mother and fetus conflict; these must be carefully navigated to prioritize health outcomes
10	Impact on breastfeeding and infant health	Consideration must be given to the potential effects of the trial on breastfeeding and the health of the nursing infant, with efforts to minimize any negative impacts
11	Regulatory and ethical oversight	Trials involving this population must undergo stringent ethical review and comply with regulations that ensure their protection and safety
12	Access to comprehensive medical care	Participants should receive appropriate medical care during and after the trial, particularly if the study leads to complications related to pregnancy or lactation
13	Culturally sensitive communication	Researchers must communicate in a manner that is culturally sensitive and respects the values and concerns of pregnant and lactating participants
14	Transparent reporting and disclosure	Findings, including any adverse outcomes, should be transparently reported to inform future research and clinical practices, ensuring the safety of this population
15	Ensuring equitable inclusion	Pregnant and lactating women should not be unfairly excluded from clinical research, ensuring they have access to potential benefits from new treatments and therapies

Table 18.5 Common ethical challenges in clinical trials involving 'elderly population'

Sl. No.	Ethical challenge(s)	Description
1	Informed consent and cognitive function	Ensuring that elderly participants can provide informed consent, with special attention to cognitive function, which may be compromised in some individuals
2	Evaluating risk-benefit balance	The risks and benefits must be carefully assessed, taking into account the unique health challenges and comorbidities often present in elderly participants
3	Designing age-appropriate trials	Clinical trials should be specifically tailored to address the health conditions, vulnerabilities and physiological differences of elderly participants
4	Vigilant monitoring for side effects	Elderly participants require more frequent monitoring for side effects, given their increased susceptibility to adverse reactions and complications
5	Avoiding coercion and ensuring voluntary participation	Extra precautions must be taken to ensure that elderly participants are not coerced into participating, especially if they rely on others for their care
6	Ensuring access to ongoing medical care	Elderly participants should have access to continuous medical care during and after the trial, particularly if they experience negative health effects related to the study
7	Inclusive representation	Older adults should be adequately represented in clinical trials, avoiding unnecessary exclusion and ensuring they can benefit from research findings relevant to their age group
8	Respecting autonomy and personal dignity	The autonomy and dignity of elderly participants must be upheld, with their right to make decisions about their own involvement in the trial fully respected
9	Addressing frailty and increased vulnerability	Additional safeguards are necessary to protect frail and vulnerable elderly participants from potential exploitation and to ensure their Well-being during the trial
10	Ethical oversight and regulatory adherence	Clinical trials involving the elderly must undergo thorough ethical review and comply with relevant regulations to protect this population and ensure ethical conduct throughout the study

18.6.6 Globalization of Clinical Trials

Clinical trial expansion into low- and middle-income countries presents some unique ethical issues. While it facilitates conducting studies in heterogeneous populations, there's a risk of potential exploitation of vulnerable populations, discrepancies in regulatory standards, and inadequate oversight. In certain settings, access to healthcare and literacy may pose difficulties to the informed consent process. The prevailing ethical practices would assure that the research meets the needs of the host country and that the local communities are adequately involved in the research process so that they might stand a fair share of the benefits accruing to them as a result of this study.

18.6.7 Data Privacy and Confidentiality

Among the major ethical concerns in clinical trials, confidentiality and protection of privacy for study participants are critical, increasingly so with access to and usage of electronic health records and digitally captured information. Breaches of confidentiality can result in adverse discrimination, stigmatization, and emotional insults. Researchers must establish provisions whereby data is secure, anonymous, or de-identified whenever possible, and informed consent is clearly obtained concerning the use and distribution of such data from study participants.

18.6.8 Post-trial Access and Obligations

Ethical issues also arise with respect to participants in terms of access to efficacious treatments after a trial has ended. In the event of a trial showing the efficacy of a new treatment, moral compulsions could arise on the continuing availability of the intervention to participants and possibly to the community at large, especially when the trial had taken place in low-resource settings. Post-trial access should be discussed during the study design by the researchers and sponsors, who should develop pragmatic plans for continuing care with the involvement of local stakeholders.

18.6.9 Scientific Integrity and Publication Bias

Integrity is one of the important components in the proper ethical conduct of scientific research, that is, there should not be any publication bias in which positive outcomes would be emphasized, and negative results or inconclusive results are suppressed. These biases may mislead the scientific community and practitioners in health and the general public by giving opposing and falsely assuring views than what is actual concerning effectiveness and safety of an intervention. Translational research needs to ensure trials are transparent, register them in publicly accessible databases, publish all results without exception on outcomes, and adhere to guidelines on ethics in reporting.

18.6.10 Regulatory and Ethical Oversight

Excellence in ethical review is central to the protection of the rights and welfare of participants in clinical trials. This involves the responsibility for reviewing study protocols, actively monitoring trials, and enforcing ethical requirements, which falls upon regulatory agencies and ethics committees-including IRBs. In reality, the implementation of ethical oversight varies greatly depending on the region because of their wide variation in resources, human capacity, and regulatory environments. These further challenges may be addressed through expanded international collaboration, harmonization of ethical standards, and training of ethics committees.

18.7 Ethical Issues in Trial Design and Conduct

18.7.1 Risk-Benefit Analysis

One of the most defining features of an ethical trial design is careful assessment of risks versus benefits. Investigators investigate any prospective benefits that might be conferred by a study on study participants in relation to risks to which the participants would be exposed, and such risks must be measured with regard to their likelihood and seriousness.

18.7.2 Placebo Use and Ethical Considerations

Using placebos in clinical trials thus raises serious ethical issues when an intervention for a particular medical condition is already known. Researchers must, therefore, justify using placebos based on scientifically strong grounds and should ensure no harm or unnecessary risks or harms to participants occur during the process of the clinical trial.

18.7.3 Randomization and Equipoise

One of the key features of clinical trial designs is randomization, enabling nonbiased comparisons among groups that get different treatments. Ethical dilemmas arise in a situation where randomization conflicts with the obligation of an investigator to provide optimal care and the requirements for randomization. In the resolution of such ethical tension, a concept described by true doubt as to which treatment is best is referred to as equipoise.

18.7.4 Ethical Challenges in Emerging Trial Designs

Novel study designs also include adaptive designs and decentralized trials; each of these brings different ethical concerns. While they provide more flexibility and perhaps better efficiency, ethical implications must be considered with due attention to the protection of the rights and welfare of research participants.

18.7.5 Compensation and Reimbursement for Participants

Provision of compensation for time and inconvenience caused in clinical trials is not only common but also entails ethical challenges—in narrowing down on the appropriate compensation. Researchers should tend to work out ways in which the compensations would not be coercive or unduly influence a participant's decisions to enroll in the study.

Table 18.6 Common ethical challenges in clinical trials related to 'study design and statistical considerations'

Ethical issue(s)	Ethical consideration	Description
Informed consent	Comprehensive participant information	Participants must be fully informed about the study's objectives, procedures and potential risks
Study design transparency	Disclosure of design limitations	Researchers should openly acknowledge any limitations or potential weaknesses in the study design
Randomization	Fair participant allocation	Randomization helps prevent selection bias by ensuring all participants have an equal chance of receiving any intervention
Blinding	Minimizing bias	Implementing blinding for both participants and researchers to reduce biases in treatment and outcomes assessment
Statistical power	Adequate sample size	Determining an appropriate sample size to ensure the study has sufficient power to detect meaningful effects while minimizing errors
Data integrity	Honest data reporting	Ensuring all data is reported accurately and without distortion to maintain the study's validity
Risk-benefit analysis	Weighing risks against benefits	Evaluating that the benefits of the study justify any potential risks to participants
Interim analysis	Ethical criteria for early termination	Establishing criteria for early termination of the study if interim results indicate clear benefits or harms
Missing data management	Ethical imputation techniques	Employing appropriate and unbiased methods to address missing data
Conflict of interest	Disclosure of financial and personal interests	Transparent reporting of any financial or personal conflicts that could affect study outcomes

Common ethical challenges in clinical trials related to 'study design and statistical considerations' are shown in Table 18.6.

18.8 Ethical Considerations in Data Management and Reporting

18.8.1 Data Integrity and Fabrication

Data integrity is one of the most crucial issues that appear in clinical research. Manipulation in findings, selective reporting of results, and other forms of scientific misconduct are some recognized ethical concerns. Ethical practices assure transparency and accountability in the research study to maintain their trustworthiness.

18.8.2 Participant Confidentiality and Data Protection

The growth of data digitization has created two important ethical concerns-especially participant confidentiality and data security. Researchers are ought to take serious measures while protecting data of participants and to follow laws related to data protection, such as the General Data Protection Regulation in the European Union.

18.8.3 Ethical Reporting of Adverse Events

Timely reporting and accuracy account for two of the most important features of reporting adverse events in clinical trials. From an ethical perspective, all researchers have the responsibility to monitor any adverse events occurring due to their research and report these in a timely manner, primarily to contribute to protection of participants and foster future research and clinical practices.

18.8.4 Publication Ethics and Dissemination of Results

Ethical considerations go greater than execution to dissemination of results of clinical trials. Researchers are under an ethical obligation to publish honest and transparent findings regardless of the outcomes for building the scientific knowledge bank and guiding clinical practice.

Common ethical challenges in clinical trials in context to 'publication ethics' are highlighted in Table 18.7.

18.9 Ethical Challenges in Specific Types of Clinical Trials

18.9.1 Pediatric Clinical Trials

Pediatric research is rather unique, as it entails special ethical complexities. Most importantly, children cannot provide informed consent for themselves. A legal guardian will have to provide the consent for the child with the inclusion of the child's assent, based on developmental stage and the particular disease understanding of the child.

Common ethical challenges in clinical trials involving 'children' are highlighted in Table 18.8.

18.9.2 Trials in Developing Countries

Trials in underdeveloped countries raise ethical concerns about the exploitation of participants, unequal access to benefits, or even compromised regulatory oversight.

Table 18.7 Common ethical challenges in clinical trials in context to 'publication ethics'

Ethical issue(s)	Description	Challenge(s)	Proposed solution(s)
Selective reporting	Choosing to publish only certain results from a study	Can lead to a biased representation of the research findings, omitting negative results	Require the publication of all study outcomes, regardless of their nature; promote transparency in reporting
Publication bias	Favoring the publication of positive or significant results over non-significant findings	Skews the literature and may misrepresent the effectiveness or safety of interventions	Support the inclusion of all results in the literature; encourage journals to accept studies based on quality, not results
Duplicate publications	Submitting the same research or results to multiple journals	Can inflate the apparent volume of research; may mislead the scientific community	Implement checks to detect duplicate submissions; enforce policies against redundant publications
Authorship discrepancies	Disputes over who is credited as an author and the order of authors	Potential exclusion of key contributors; disputes can arise over authorship claims	Establish clear guidelines for authorship; ensure all substantial contributors are recognized
Plagiarism	Unauthorized use or replication of another's work	Undermines academic integrity and can have legal implications	Utilize plagiarism detection tools; provide training on proper citation and attribution practices
Data manipulation	Altering or falsifying data to achieve desired results	Compromises the reliability of research and can mislead subsequent studies	Enforce rigorous data integrity checks; institute penalties for data manipulation
Conflicts of interest	Financial or personal interests influencing the presentation of research	Can lead to biased findings or compromised study integrity	Mandate full disclosure of all potential conflicts; ensure transparency in study reporting
Transparency of reporting	Withholding essential information or data from publications	Leads to incomplete or misleading interpretations of the research	Ensure that all relevant data and methodology are reported; adhere to comprehensive reporting guidelines
Ethical approval disclosure	Not disclosing whether the study received ethical review and approval	Lack of transparency regarding the ethical conduct of the research	Require explicit disclosure of ethical review status in publications; confirm adherence to ethical standards
Post-publication corrections	Correcting errors or inaccuracies after the study has been published	Misinformation may persist if errors are not addressed promptly	Establish a clear process for issuing corrections; ensure that errata are promptly published and widely disseminated

Table 18.8 Common ethical challenges in clinical trials involving 'children'

Sl. No.	Ethical challenge(s)	Description
1	Parental or Guardian permission	In Pediatric trials, obtaining informed permission from parents or legal guardians is crucial, ensuring they fully understand the study's purpose and potential risks
2	Child's assent	Beyond parental consent, the child's assent should be obtained whenever possible, respecting the child's willingness to participate in the trial
3	Risk minimization	Any risks to child participants should be minimized, with only essential procedures conducted and the potential benefits must justify these risks
4	Benefit justification	The trial must demonstrate that the potential benefits to the child outweigh any risks, especially when the study involves more than minimal risk
5	Safeguarding vulnerable populations	Children, being a vulnerable group, require additional protective measures to prevent exploitation or unnecessary harm during the research
6	Fair participant selection	Children should be selected based on scientifically sound criteria, ensuring that no group is unfairly burdened or exploited
7	Child-friendly communication	Information about the trial should be presented in a way that is understandable to the child, appropriate for their age and developmental level
8	Long-term monitoring	Adequate long-term monitoring should be provided for child participants to track any delayed effects from the interventions or procedures used
9	Ongoing parental engagement	Parents should be kept informed throughout the trial, with the opportunity to withdraw their child if concerns arise, ensuring their ongoing involvement
10	Privacy and confidentiality	The personal information of child participants must be securely protected, with strict confidentiality maintained throughout the trial
11	Adherence to Pediatric regulations	The trial must comply with specific Pediatric research regulations, ensuring that ethical and legal standards are upheld throughout the study
12	Appropriate compensation	Compensation provided to children and their families should be fair, covering time and discomfort without creating undue influence to participate
13	Managing conflicts of interest	Potential conflicts of interest in pediatric research should be carefully managed to maintain the integrity of the trial and prioritize the child's welfare
14	Transparent reporting	Results of the trial, whether favorable or not, should be transparently reported, particularly regarding safety and effectiveness for the pediatric population
15	Post-trial access to benefits	If the trial identifies beneficial treatments, there should be mechanisms in place to ensure continued access to these treatments for child participants after the study concludes

Table 18.9 Common ethical challenges in clinical trials in 'low middle-income countries'

Ethical challenge(s)	Description
Informed consent and understanding	Ensuring that the consent process is adapted to the local cultural and linguistic context and that participants fully comprehend the trial's scope, risks and benefits
Equitable access to clinical trials	Making sure that trials are accessible to local populations and designed to benefit the communities where they are conducted, avoiding exploitation of participants
Protection from exploitation and vulnerability	Implementing measures to protect vulnerable groups from exploitation, ensuring that trials do not disproportionately affect economically disadvantaged individuals
Cultural sensitivity and respect	Conducting trials in a manner that is respectful of and aligned with local cultural practices and norms, ensuring cultural appropriateness in all aspects of the research
Adherence to local and international standards	Complying with both local ethical guidelines and international best practices, ensuring that trials are conducted with integrity and respect for local regulations
Data privacy and confidentiality	Ensuring that participants' personal and health data are securely protected, following rigorous data privacy protocols to safeguard against unauthorized access or breaches
Fair compensation and community benefits	Providing appropriate compensation for participant's time and expenses and ensuring that the benefits of the trial are accessible and beneficial to the local community
Access to continued care and treatment	Facilitating continued access to effective treatments post-trial and ensuring that participants receive follow-up care, especially if the trial demonstrates positive outcomes
Transparency and accountability	Maintaining transparency in the conduct and results of the trial and ensuring accountability for ethical practices and the impact of the research on the local community
Building local research capacity	Investing in and supporting local research infrastructure and expertise, fostering collaborations with local institutions to strengthen research practices and build sustainable capabilities

Researchers will have to confront issues of the respective trials so as to make sure that the trials are ethically conducted and the participants are fairly treated.

Common ethical challenges in clinical trials in 'low middle-income countries' are highlighted in Table 18.9.

18.9.3 Genetic and Genomic Research

Many genetic and genomic studies raise special ethical challenges, such as protection of genetic privacy, consent about use of samples in the future, or even genetic discrimination. The investigators should approach these ethical issues in the design of the study and through open communication with the participants.

Common ethical challenges in clinical trials with 'gene therapy products (GTP)' are highlighted in Table 18.10.

Table 18.10 Common ethical challenges in clinical trials with 'gene therapy products (GTP)'

Sl. No.	Ethical challenge(s)	Description
1	Informed consent and understanding	Participants must be thoroughly informed about the complexities and potential long-term consequences of gene therapy, ensuring they can make well-informed decisions
2	Risk-benefit evaluation in experimental therapies	Carefully weighing the potential risks and benefits is crucial, especially given the experimental nature and potential unpredictability of gene therapies
3	Ongoing safety monitoring	Implementing long-term monitoring is essential to detect any delayed or unexpected effects, given the permanent alterations often involved in gene therapy
4	Genetic privacy and data protection	Protecting participants' genetic information from unauthorized access and ensuring strict confidentiality to prevent misuse is critical
5	Germline therapy and future generations	Ethical concerns about germline gene therapy involve the potential for genetic changes to be passed on to future generations, raising significant consent and long-term impact issues
6	Equitable access and selection criteria	Ensuring fair and equitable access to gene therapy trials, avoiding discrimination and protecting vulnerable populations from exploitation
7	Managing uncertainty and potential risks	Clearly communicating the inherent uncertainties and potential risks of gene therapy to participants is essential to maintain transparency and trust
8	Ethical and regulatory compliance	Strict adherence to ethical guidelines and regulatory standards is necessary to ensure that gene therapy trials are conducted responsibly and safely
9	Balancing innovation with ethical responsibility	While pursuing innovative gene therapies, it is vital to prioritize participant safety and ethical integrity, avoiding rushed processes that could compromise standards
10	Post-trial access and continuing care	Ensuring that participants have access to ongoing care and necessary treatments after the trial, especially if the gene therapy shows effectiveness but is not yet commercially available

18.9.4 Emergency Research and Waiver of Consent

Of course, informed consent cannot be obtained in all emergency conditions. Ethical regulations indeed allow for waiver of consent in some conditions; nevertheless, researchers will have to ensure that such trials are justified, and protection for participants' rights is maximally granted.

Common ethical challenges in clinical trials with 'stem cell therapy products' are highlighted in Table 18.11.

Common ethical challenges in clinical trials involving 'end-of-life care' situations are highlighted in Table 18.12.

Table 18.11 Common ethical challenges in clinical trials with 'stem cell therapy products'

Sl. No.	Ethical challenge(s)	Description
1	Informed consent and understanding	Ensuring participants fully grasp the experimental nature of stem cell therapy, including potential risks, benefits, and uncertainties, with comprehensive education
2	Evaluating risk-benefit ratio	Carefully assessing the potential risks and benefits of stem cell interventions, considering the experimental nature and possible long-term effects
3	Ethics of stem cell sourcing	Addressing ethical considerations regarding the origins of stem cells, such as the use of embryonic stem cells, ensuring ethical sourcing and proper consent
4	Long-term monitoring for safety and efficacy	Conducting thorough long-term follow-ups to monitor for delayed or unforeseen effects, given the potential for lasting impacts from stem cell treatments
5	Ensuring fair access and inclusion	Providing equitable access to stem cell trials and ensuring fair participant selection, avoiding exploitation and ensuring representation across diverse populations
6	Protecting genetic and personal privacy	Safeguarding participant's genetic and personal data, ensuring confidentiality and preventing unauthorized use or breaches of privacy
7	Adherence to ethical and regulatory standards	Complying with strict ethical guidelines and regulatory standards to ensure responsible conduct and integrity in stem cell research and trials
8	Managing expectations and communication	Clearly communicating the experimental status of stem cell therapies and managing participant's expectations about potential outcomes and success rates
9	Ethics of placebo use	Considering the ethical implications of using placebo controls, particularly in scenarios where effective alternatives are available and participants might be deprived of benefits
10	Post-trial access to effective treatments	Providing mechanisms for participants to continue receiving the stem cell therapy if it proves effective, addressing availability issues after the trial concludes

Table 18.12 Common ethical challenges in clinical trials involving 'end-of-life care' situations

Ethical issue(s)	Description	Ethical concern	Considerations for resolution
Informed consent	Ensuring patients are fully aware of and understand the trial procedures given their terminal illness	The challenge of obtaining informed consent from patients who may be compromised by their illness	Simplify consent forms and process and ensure that patients fully understand the trial. Consider involving family members
Patient vulnerability	Addressing the increased vulnerability of patients nearing the end of life	Risk of exploiting patient's vulnerable state for research purposes	Implement additional protections and ensure comprehensive support for patients

(continued)

Table 18.11 (continued)

Ethical issue(s)	Description	Ethical concern	Considerations for resolution
Risk-benefit analysis	Weighing the potential risks of the trial against the possible benefits to patients	Ensuring that the risks are not disproportionately high compared to the benefits	Conduct a thorough risk-benefit evaluation and monitor it throughout the trial
Impact on quality of life	Assessing how participation in the trial affects the patient's quality of life	Concerns about potentially diminishing the quality of life due to trial participation	Regularly assess and address any negative impacts on the patient's quality of life
Use of placebos	Ethical implications of administering a placebo when effective treatments might be available	Possible denial of effective treatment to terminally ill patients	Ensure placebo use is scientifically justified and offer effective treatment options as needed
Respecting patient preferences	Honoring patient's wishes regarding their end-of-life care	Ethical issues regarding disregarding patient preferences in the trial context	Design the trial to align with patient preferences and provide flexibility to accommodate their wishes
Handling withdrawal	Managing the process of patients withdrawing from the trial or continuing care	Ethical considerations around the impact of withdrawal on patient care and Well-being	Provide clear guidelines for withdrawal and ensure continuity of care for patients
Impact on families and caregivers	Considering the effect of the trial on patient's families and caregivers	Ethical concerns about the emotional and physical burden placed on families and caregivers	Provide support and resources for families and caregivers throughout the trial
Transparency and honesty	Ensuring clear communication about the trial's aims, methods and outcomes	Ethical issues related to maintaining honesty and transparency with patients	Ensure all trial-related information is communicated clearly and accurately to participants
Post-trial care	Offering appropriate care and support after the trial concludes	Ethical concerns about ensuring ongoing support and care for patients who participated in the trial	Arrange for continued care and support for patients following the trial's conclusion

18.10 Contemporary Challenges and Future Directions in Clinical Trial Ethics

18.10.1 The Rise of Artificial Intelligence (AI) and Big Data

The integration of AI and big data analytics into clinical trials still raises new ethical concerns: algorithmic bias, data protection, and clarity of AI-driven decisions. According to ethics, these technologies must be used responsibly by the researchers in a manner respectful of rights in the logic of participants.

18.10.2 Patient-Centric Trials and Ethical Implications

New focus is being directed toward patient-centric trials, designed to maximize both participant engagement and contribution throughout the research process. Although this does bring a number of ethical advantages in improving informed consent and participant retention, there will be some concerns regarding what exactly would be the level of involvement of a given patient in the study design, and potential sources of bias. The capability of fostering thoughtful participant involvement without sacrificing scientific integrity is of importance to all researchers.

18.10.3 The Ethics of Compassionate Use and Expanded Access Programs

Compassionate use and expanded access programs are designed to provide availability to investigational treatments outside of a clinical trial when alternative therapies are unavailable. Whereas such programs may be extremely important in offering critical care for people with life-threatening conditions, a number of ethical issues arise on the question of the fairness of the approach, balance of risk versus benefit, and its impact on the recruitment of participants into clinical trials.

18.10.4 Challenges of Conducting Trials During Public Health Emergencies

Public health crises, like those caused by pandemics, create special ethical demands on clinical trials. The urgent need for speedy development of treatment may place pressure on researchers to compromise ethical standards that places the safety of study participants at risk. Ethical frameworks must evolve to address such situations and ensure that trials are responsibly conducted with considerations for urgent public health needs.

Common ethical challenges in clinical trials during 'public health emergencies' are highlighted in Table 18.13.

18.10.5 Transparency and Public Trust in Clinical Trials

It is thus of utmost importance to maintain the same level of trust and confidence in clinical research from the general public for continued participation and support of clinical trials. Moral problems related to transparency are from the top, including selectivity in reporting results, conflict of interest, and poor disclosure of funding sources, which can thus easily jeopardize the confidence of the public. This calls for openness by researchers and institutions as they promote free flow in communication to establish a relationship based on trust and credibility.

Common ethical challenges in clinical trials 'sponsored by pharmaceutical industries' are highlighted in Table 18.14.

Common ethical 'challenges and solutions' in clinical trials are highlighted in Table 18.15.

Table 18.13 Common ethical challenges in clinical trials during 'public health emergencies'

Ethical challenge(s)	Description	Example
Informed consent challenges	Difficulties in ensuring fully informed consent due to the urgency and limited information available	COVID-19 Vaccine Development (2020–2021)
Risk-benefit assessment	Struggles with accurately assessing and balancing risks versus benefits in crisis situations	Ebola Vaccine Trials (2014–2016)
Ensuring equity in recruitment	Ensuring fair and inclusive participant selection, especially for vulnerable or marginalized groups	Zika Virus Research (2016)
Privacy and data protection	Maintaining participant confidentiality and safeguarding data privacy amidst accelerated data collection	H1N1 Influenza Studies (2009)
Ethical use of placebos	Concerns over using placebos when effective treatments might be critically needed	SARS Research Trials (2003)
Continued access to treatment	Providing ongoing access to effective treatments for participants after trial completion	COVID-19 Monoclonal Antibody Studies (2021)
Transparency in reporting	Ensuring clear and open communication of trial results to the public and relevant stakeholders	COVID-19 Vaccine Efficacy Reports (2020–2021)
Use of experimental treatments	Ethical considerations when administering treatments that are not yet fully approved or tested	Ebola Therapeutic Trials (2014–2016)
Avoiding coercion in participant enrolment	Preventing undue pressure or coercion in recruiting participants during emergencies	Zika Virus Vaccine Trials (2016)
Ethical oversight and regulatory compliance	Ensuring rigorous ethical review and adherence to regulatory standards throughout the trial process	COVID-19 Therapeutic Trials (2020–2021)

Table 18.14 Common ethical challenges in clinical trials 'sponsored by pharmaceutical industries'

Ethical issue(s)	Description	Challenge(s)	Recommended solution(s)
Conflict of interest	Balancing sponsor interests with the integrity of the research	Potential bias in study design, execution and reporting due to sponsor influence	Enforce strict conflict-of-interest policies; ensure transparency in research processes
Data integrity	Maintaining accuracy and honesty in reporting trial results	Pressure from sponsors to alter or suppress unfavorable results	Implement rigorous data validation procedures; conduct independent audits to ensure accuracy

(continued)

Table 18.14 (continued)

Ethical issue(s)	Description	Challenge(s)	Recommended solution(s)
Participant recruitment	Recruiting participants in an ethical manner, avoiding exploitation	Pressure to quickly recruit participants might lead to ethical compromises	Follow ethical recruitment practices; ensure informed consent is properly obtained and documented
Regulatory compliance	Adhering to all relevant regulatory requirements and guidelines	Sponsors might attempt to circumvent regulations to expedite processes or reduce costs	Conduct regular regulatory compliance checks; ensure adherence to established guidelines
Transparency of results	Ensuring that all results, both positive and negative, are publicly reported	Risk of selective reporting or withholding of negative findings	Mandate full disclosure of all results; promote open access to comprehensive study findings
Pressure to report Favorable outcomes	Managing the pressure to publish only positive results	Sponsors may exert pressure to highlight only favorable outcomes	Support the publication of all results, regardless of outcome; foster independent review mechanisms
Informed consent	Ensuring participants are fully aware of the trial's sponsor and potential biases	Participants may not be fully informed about the sponsor's role or possible biases	Clearly disclose sponsor information and potential conflicts in the consent process
Financial influence on research	Addressing the impact of financial relationships on research integrity	Financial ties might influence study design or outcomes	Require detailed disclosure of financial relationships; ensure research is conducted impartially
Ethical oversight	Ensuring robust and independent review of the research	Possible influence or delays caused by sponsors affecting the ethical review process	Ensure that ethical review boards operate independently and transparently; avoid sponsor interference
Access to post-trial care	Providing continued access to effective treatments after the trial ends	Risk of discontinuing access to successful treatments; compensation issues	Develop clear post-trial care policies; ensure transparent communication about ongoing treatment options

Table 18.15 Common ethical 'challenges and solutions' in clinical trials

Ethical issue(s)	Overview	Challenge(s)	Proposed solution(s)
Informed consent	Ensuring participants are fully aware of the trial's purpose, risks and benefits	Information may be too complex; risk of coercion or misunderstanding	Simplify consent documentation; employ interactive consent methods
Protection of vulnerable groups	Safeguarding participants who are particularly susceptible, such as children and the elderly	Risk of exploitation; ensuring valid consent and protection measures	Implement additional safeguards; adapt consent processes for specific groups

(continued)

Table 18.15 (continued)

Ethical issue(s)	Overview	Challenge(s)	Proposed solution(s)
Confidentiality and privacy	Securing participants' personal information	Risk of data breaches; challenges in managing sensitive data securely	Use robust data protection measures; enforce strict data access controls
Balancing risk and benefit	Assessing whether the potential benefits justify the risks involved	Risks might outweigh benefits, especially in early-phase trials	Conduct comprehensive risk-benefit analyses; ensure ethical justification of trials
Use of placebo controls	Administering placebos when effective treatments are available	Ethical issues with withholding effective treatment; potential harm to participants	Use placebos only when no standard treatment exists; review ethically
Cultural sensitivity	Addressing and respecting cultural differences in trial design and conduct	Risk of cultural insensitivity; potential misalignment with cultural norms	Integrate cultural competence into trial design; collaborate with cultural advisors
Financial incentives	Providing monetary compensation for participation	Risk of undue influence or coercion; exploitation of financially vulnerable individuals	Ensure compensation is fair and does not pressure participants; consider ethical oversight
Researcher dual roles	Managing the dual responsibilities of researchers as both caregivers and scientists	Potential conflicts of interest; risk of biased results	Clearly define and separate roles; maintain transparency and objectivity in research
Data integrity	Ensuring accuracy and honesty in reporting trial data	Risk of data manipulation or misrepresentation; pressure to produce favorable results	Enforce strict data integrity protocols; facilitate independent peer reviews
Access to post-trial treatments	Providing continued access to effective treatments after trial completion	Ensuring ongoing benefit for participants; potential disparities in treatment access	Plan for post-trial access strategies; establish clear policies for continued treatment access

18.11 The Role of Ethics Committees (ECs) and Institutional Review Boards (IRBs)

18.11.1 Important Responsibilities and Functions of Ethics Committees (ECs)

Ethics committees and Institutional Review Boards have the responsibility of protection of rights and welfare of participants involved in research studies. This comprises the review of study protocol, informed consent form review, and follow-up on research as a way of ensuring that the protection is according to ethical requirements.

18.11.2 Challenges Faced by Ethics Committees

Ethics committees often have to balance scientific progress with participant protection, manage conflicts of interest, and cultural differences in multinational studies. It is amidst these complexities that the committees should be very well informed on ethical principles, as well as particular contexts of studies they review.

18.11.3 Enhancing the Effectiveness of Ethics Committees

Ethics committees need regular training combined with contact with researchers and the establishment of standardized procedures for protocol review to increase the effectiveness of the same. A heterogeneous makeup of the committee will also reduce the potential for bias and enhance decision-making.

18.11.4 The Importance and Role of Community Advisory Boards

It is true that through the addition of significant community insights and perspectives into the various research initiatives, a CAB (Community Advisory Board) can strengthen the work of ethics committees. In other words, what a CAB does is ensure that clinical trials are appropriate, address community needs, and ensure public trust.

18.12 Future Perspectives and Innovations in Ethical Conduct

18.12.1 Emerging Ethical Frameworks for Clinical Trials

More modern-day requirements have led to the building of new ethical frameworks as clinical research moves forward into the future. These could include guidelines on the use of AI in research, considerations to take in decentralized trials for ethics, and standards in patient engagement. Collaboration of stakeholders is necessary to ensure that guidelines are comprehensive and adaptable to diverse unforeseen situations.

18.12.2 The Impact of Digital Health on Ethics

Digital health technologies are increasingly being integrated into clinical trials, from wearable devices and mobile health applications, including telemedicine. All these innovative technologies make research more effective, but at the same time, they create serious ethical concerns with regard to data security and unequal access. Ethical guidelines have to evolve in response to these challenges and ensure responsible use of digital health technologies in clinical research.

18.12.3 Internationalization of Clinical Trials and Alignment of Ethical Standards

The internationalization trend in clinical trials calls for harmonization in ethical standards spread across various regions of the world. It provides a clear means for international collaborations and therefore universally accepted ethical guidelines that can help fill gaps in rulings and make certain that trials conducted from anywhere around the world are pitching for high standards of ethics.

18.12.4 Building Ethical Capacity in Low- and Middle-Income Countries

Development of ethical capabilities in LMICs is critical in developing ethics in international trials. This would include training for local researchers and ethics committees, development of regulatory frameworks, and most importantly, collaboration between high-income countries and LMICs in giving importance to ethical research practices.

18.12.5 The Role of Ethics Education and Training

Education and training in research ethics are indispensable for all stakeholders in clinical trials which include researchers, ethics committee members, and study personnel. Continuous education will reassure that one is updated on all state-of-the-art ethical guidelines and the upcoming new challenges and the best practices in conducting the ethical research.

SWOT analysis of ethical issues involved in clinical trials is highlighted in Table 18.16.

Table 18.16 'SWOT' analysis of ethical issues involved in clinical trials

Ethical issue(s)	Strengths	Weaknesses	Opportunities	Threats
Informed consent	Ensures participants are fully aware of trial details and risks	Potential for misinterpretation or incomplete understanding	Opportunities to develop clearer consent materials and processes	Inadequate understanding can lead to ethical breaches
Participant autonomy	Respects individual's rights to make informed decisions about participation	Vulnerable populations may struggle with full comprehension	Improving consent methods for vulnerable groups enhances autonomy	Coercion or pressure can compromise genuine consent
Risk-benefit analysis	Balances potential risks with expected benefits to protect participants	Risk assessment can be subjective and challenging	Develop more precise risk-benefit evaluation frameworks	Misjudgment can result in undue harm or minimal benefit to participants

(continued)

Table 18.16 (continued)

Ethical issue(s)	Strengths	Weaknesses	Opportunities	Threats
Data integrity	Promotes accuracy and reliability in research data	Risks of data manipulation or selective reporting	Implement advanced data management and verification technologies	Data falsification or bias can undermine research credibility
Equity and fairness	Strives to ensure equal opportunity for all participants	Recruitment and access disparities can occur	Create initiatives to enhance diversity and inclusiveness in trials	Inequities in access may worsen existing health disparities
Confidentiality	Safeguards participants' private and sensitive information	Risk of breaches or unauthorized data access	Employ robust data protection and encryption techniques	Breaches of confidentiality can have serious ethical and legal repercussions
Ethics review	Provides oversight to ensure adherence to ethical standards	Ethics review can be slow and bureaucratic	Streamline ethics review processes for greater efficiency	Delays in review may impede trial progress and participant recruitment
Handling adverse events	Prioritizes participant safety and response to adverse events	Inconsistent identification and reporting of adverse effects	Enhance monitoring and reporting systems for adverse events	Inadequate response to adverse events can harm participants
Transparency	Ensures open communication about trial procedures and findings	Risk of incomplete or biased reporting	Foster greater transparency in research practices and results	Lack of transparency can erode public trust in clinical research
Post-trial access	Provides continued access to effective treatments after trials	Challenges in maintaining treatment access post-trial	Develop policies to ensure ongoing access to successful treatments	Insufficient post-trial access can lead to ethical and practical issues

18.13 Conclusion

Ethics in clinical trials is a constantly evolving discipline, considering new challenges and opportunities arising in medical research. It is therefore important that the deeper ethical intricacies of clinical trials are taken into consideration for the protection of the rights, safety, and well-being of study participants involved, at the same time promoting the advancement of scientific knowledge.

Ethical principles ultimately help to protect trial participants, ensure public confidence, and guarantee scientific integrity. As clinical research becomes increasingly complex and globalized, there needs to be a mutual relation of strong ethics, regulation, and development of a culture of ethical accountability from all parties involved. Such an approach will empower the research community to vouch for the highest ethics by allowing medical science contribution with respect for, and protection of, human dignity.

These ethical challenges can only be met if there is a commitment to ethical principles, rigorous oversight, transparency, and ongoing dialogue among various stakeholders which include researchers, participants, regulatory bodies, and the public. With the construction of such an environment, it would be possible for clinical trials to retain public confidence and support in the development of safe and effective medical treatments.

Bibliography and Further Reading

Anderson ML, Califf RM, Sugarman J, Participants in the NIH Health Care Systems Research Collaboratory Cluster Randomized Trial Workshop (2015) Ethical and regulatory issues of pragmatic cluster randomized trials in contemporary health systems. Clin Trials 12(3):276–286. https://doi.org/10.1177/1740774515571140. Epub 2015 Mar 1. PMID: 25733677; PMCID: PMC4498459

Arpaillange P, Dion S, Mathe G (1985) Proposal for ethical standards in therapeutic trials. Br Med J (Clin Res Ed) 291(6499):887–889. https://doi.org/10.1136/bmj.291.6499.887. PMID: 3931754; PMCID: PMC1416707

Ashcroft RE, Chadwick DW, Clark SR, Edwards RH, Frith L, Hutton JL (1997) Implications of socio-cultural contexts for the ethics of clinical trials. Health Technol Assess 1(9):i–iv. 1–65. PMID: 9483158

Barton JM, Macmillan MS, Sawyer L (1995) The compensation of patients injured in clinical trials. J Med Ethics 21(3):166–169. https://doi.org/10.1136/jme.21.3.166. PMID: 7674282; PMCID: PMC1376693

Bernstein SL, Feldman J (2015) Incentives to participate in clinical trials: practical and ethical considerations. Am J Emerg Med 33(9):1197–1200. https://doi.org/10.1016/j.ajem.2015.05.020. Epub 2015 May 29. PMID: 26095131; PMCID: PMC4562811

Blehar MC, Spong C, Grady C, Goldkind SF, Sahin L, Clayton JA (2013) Enrolling pregnant women: issues in clinical research. Womens Health Issues 23(1):e39–e45. https://doi.org/10.1016/j.whi.2012.10.003. PMID: 23312713; PMCID: PMC3547525

Bosnjak Pasic M, Vidrih B, Sarac H, Pasic H, Vujević L, Soldo Koruga A, Rajič F (2018) Clinical trials in developing countries – ethical considerations. Psychiatr Danub 30(3):285–291. https://doi.org/10.24869/psyd.2018.285. PMID: 30267519

Chattopadhyay S, De Vries R (2013) Respect for cultural diversity in bioethics is an ethical imperative. Med Health Care Philos 16(4):639–645. https://doi.org/10.1007/s11019-012-9433-5. PMID: 22955969; PMCID: PMC3562559

Clayton DG (1982) Ethically optimised designs. Br J Clin Pharmacol 13(4):469–480. https://doi.org/10.1111/j.1365-2125.1982.tb01407.x. PMID: 7066161; PMCID: PMC1402044

(2008) Clinical trials in India: ethical concerns. Bull World Health Organ 86(8):581–582. https://doi.org/10.2471/blt.08.010808. PMID: 18797610; PMCID: PMC2649459

Corrigan O (2003) Empty ethics: the problem with informed consent. Sociol Health Illn 25(7):768–792. https://doi.org/10.1046/j.1467-9566.2003.00369.x. PMID: 19780205

De Meulemeester J, Fedyk M, Jurkovic L, Reaume M, Dowlatshahi D, Stotts G, Shamy M (2018) Many randomized clinical trials may not be justified: a cross-sectional analysis of the ethics and science of randomized clinical trials. J Clin Epidemiol 97:20–25. https://doi.org/10.1016/j.jclinepi.2017.12.027. Epub 2018 Jan 3. PMID: 29306063

Erb T, Sugarman J (2000) Ethical issues on informed consent and recruitment for clinical trials. Anesthesiology 92(6):1851–1852. https://doi.org/10.1097/00000542-200006000-00063. PMID: 10839949

Ervin AM, Taylor HA, Meinert CL, Ehrhardt S (2015) Research ethics. Evidence gaps and ethical review of multicenter studies. Science 350(6261):632–633. https://doi.org/10.1126/science.aac4872. PMID: 26542556; PMCID: PMC4832919

(1970) Ethical problems in clinical research. Can Med Assoc J 102(9):983–984. PMID: 4951063; PMCID: PMC1946724

Gammelgaard A, Bisgaard H (2007) Evidence-based medicines for children: ethical aspects. Eur Respir J 29(4):821–822. https://doi.org/10.1183/09031936.00162106. Author reply 822. PMID: 17400886

Gangestad AK, Salata RA (2012) Ethical issues in microbicide clinical trials for HIV prevention. Curr HIV Res 10(1):105–112. https://doi.org/10.2174/157016212799304670. PMID: 22264052

Gennery B (2005) Academic clinical research in the new regulatory environment. Clin Med (Lond) 5(1):39–41. https://doi.org/10.7861/clinmedicine.5-1-39. PMID: 15745196; PMCID: PMC4954065

Georgiev AM, Krajnović D, Milovanović S, Ignjatović S, Djurić D, Marinković V (2013) Analysis of regulatory-ethical framework of clinical trials. Srp Arh Celok Lek 141(9–10):659–666. https://doi.org/10.2298/sarh1310659m. Serbian. PMID: 24364230

Gonorazky SE (2015) Universal ethical principles and their application in clinical drug trials. Salud Colect 11(1):49–65. https://doi.org/10.18294/sc.2015.415. English, Spanish. PMID: 25853830

Graf C, Wager E, Bowman A, Fiack S, Scott-Lichter D, Robinson A (2007) Best practice guidelines on publication ethics: a publisher's perspective. Int J Clin Pract Suppl 61(152):1–26. https://doi.org/10.1111/j.1742-1241.2006.01230.x. PMID: 17206953; PMCID: PMC1804120

Helmchen H, Müller-Oerlinghausen B (1975) The inherent paradox of clinical trials in psychiatry. J Med Ethics 1(4):168–173. https://doi.org/10.1136/jme.1.4.168. PMID: 775089; PMCID: PMC1154497

Herxheimer A (1993) Clinical trials: two neglected ethical issues. J Med Ethics 19(4):211, 218. https://doi.org/10.1136/jme.19.4.211. PMID: 8308875; PMCID: PMC1376340

Hunt A, Saenz C, Littler K (2019) The global forum on bioethics in research meeting, "ethics of alternative clinical trial designs and methods in low- and middle-income country research": emerging themes and outputs. Trials 20(Suppl 2):701. https://doi.org/10.1186/s13063-019-3840-3. PMID: 31852514; PMCID: PMC6921436

Joseph PD, Craig JC, Caldwell PH (2015) Clinical trials in children. Br J Clin Pharmacol 79(3):357–369. https://doi.org/10.1111/bcp.12305. PMID: 24325152; PMCID: PMC4345947

Kauffman RE (1994) Drug trials in children: ethical, legal, and practical issues. J Clin Pharmacol 34(4):296–299. PMID: 8006195

Kaye M (1987) Can "ethical" clinical trials be unethical? CMAJ 137(11):988. PMID: 3676954; PMCID: PMC1267411

Kon AA (2010) Ethical rules for human subjects research: a case where the "is" must inform the "ought". Am J Bioeth 10(6):14–15. https://doi.org/10.1080/15265161003728829. PMID: 20526960; PMCID: PMC2882624

Koski G (2003) Ethical issues in antiepileptic trials: old issues in a new world. Epilepsia 44(Suppl 7):16–18. https://doi.org/10.1046/j.1528-1157.44.s7.8.x. PMID: 12919334

Kottow MH (2009) Clinical and research ethics as moral strangers. Arch Immunol Ther Exp 57(3):157–164. https://doi.org/10.1007/s00005-009-0027-8. Epub 2009 May 29. PMID: 19479200

Lau JT, Mao J, Woo J (2003) Ethical issues related to the use of placebo in clinical trials. Hong Kong Med J 9(3):192–198. PMID: 12777655

Laventhal N, Tarini BA, Lantos J (2012) Ethical issues in neonatal and pediatric clinical trials. Pediatr Clin N Am 59(5):1205–1220. https://doi.org/10.1016/j.pcl.2012.07.007. Epub 2012 Aug 26. PMID: 23036252; PMCID: PMC3465563

Li RH, Wacholtz MC, Barnes M, Boggs L, Callery-D'Amico S, Davis A, Digilova A, Forster D, Heffernan K, Luthin M, Lynch HF, McNair L, Miller JE, Murphy J, Van Campen L, Wilenzick M, Wolf D, Woolston C, Aldinger C, Bierer BE (2016) Incorporating ethical principles into clinical research protocols: a tool for protocol writers and ethics committees. J Med Ethics 42(4):229–234. https://doi.org/10.1136/medethics-2014-102540. Epub 2016 Jan 25. Erratum in: J Med Ethics. 2016 Jul;42(7):449. doi: 10.1136/medethics-2014-102540corr1. PMID: 26811365; PMCID: PMC4819642

Lidz CW, Albert K, Appelbaum P, Dunn LB, Overton E, Pivovarova E (2015) Why is therapeutic misconception so prevalent? Camb Q Healthc Ethics 24(2):231–241. https://doi.org/10.1017/S096318011400053X. PMID: 25719358; PMCID: PMC9067606

Lima C (2005) Ensaios clínicos: vulnerabilidade e relativismo etico [Clinical trials: vulnerability and ethical relativism]. Acta Medica Port 18(3):221–226. Portuguese. Epub 2005 Jun 18. PMID: 16207458

Mathé G, Dion S (1985) Proposal for ethical standards in therapeutic trials. Br Med J (Clin Res Ed) 291(6510):1720. https://doi.org/10.1136/bmj.291.6510.1720-a. PMID: 3935254; PMCID: PMC1418819

McDonald PJ, Kulkarni AV, Farrokhyar F, Bhandari M (2010) Ethical issues in surgical research. Can J Surg 53(2):133–136. PMID: 20334746; PMCID: PMC2845955

McMillan JR, Conlon C, Nuffield Council on Bioethics (2004) The ethics of research related to health care in developing countries. J Med Ethics 30(2):204–206. https://doi.org/10.1136/jme.2002.001263. PMID: 15082819; PMCID: PMC1733832

Miller L, Folayan M, Allman D, Nkala B, Kasirye LM, Mingote LR, Calazans G, Mburu R, Ntombela F, Ditmore M (2010) How ethical is your clinical trial? Int J Clin Pract 64(9):1179–1182. https://doi.org/10.1111/j.1742-1241.2010.02421.x. Epub 2010 Jun 16. PMID: 20561091; PMCID: PMC2916216

Millum J, Grady C (2013) The ethics of placebo-controlled trials: methodological justifications. Contemp Clin Trials 36(2):510–514. https://doi.org/10.1016/j.cct.2013.09.003. Epub 2013 Sep 12. PMID: 24035802; PMCID: PMC3844122

Ornek Büken N, Büken E (2003) Tip etiği ve tip hukuku açisindan klinik ilaç araştirmalari [clinical drug research from medical ethics and legal perspectives]. Turk Psikiyatri Derg 14(4):289–299. Turkish. PMID: 14704931

Palmer CR (1993) Ethics and statistical methodology in clinical trials. J Med Ethics 19(4):219–222. https://doi.org/10.1136/jme.19.4.219. PMID: 8308877; PMCID: PMC1376342

Participants in 2006 Georgetown University Workshop on Ancillary-Care Obligations of Medical Researchers Working in Developing Countries (2008) The ancillary-care obligations of medical researchers working in developing countries. PLoS Med 5(5):e90. https://doi.org/10.1371/journal.pmed.0050090. PMID: 18494553; PMCID: PMC2386835

Ravinetto R, Buvé A, Halidou T, Lutumba P, Talisuna A, Juffrie M, D'Alessandro U, Boelaert M (2011) Double ethical review of north-south collaborative clinical research: hidden paternalism or real partnership? Trop Med Int Health 16(4):527–530. https://doi.org/10.1111/j.1365-3156.2011.02732.x. Epub 2011 Feb 1. PMID: 21410849

Resnik DB (2009) Re-consenting human subjects: ethical, legal and practical issues. J Med Ethics 35(11):656–657. https://doi.org/10.1136/jme.2009.030338. PMID: 19880699; PMCID: PMC3971530

Resnik DB, Tinkle SS (2007) Ethical issues in clinical trials involving nanomedicine. Contemp Clin Trials 28(4):433–441. https://doi.org/10.1016/j.cct.2006.11.001. Epub 2006 Nov 17. PMID: 17166777; PMCID: PMC2695593

Skierka AS, Michels KB (2018) Ethical principles and placebo-controlled trials – interpretation and implementation of the declaration of Helsinki's placebo paragraph in medical research. BMC Med Ethics 19(1):24. https://doi.org/10.1186/s12910-018-0262-9. PMID: 29544543; PMCID: PMC5856313

Strong C (2011) Regulatory and ethical issues for phase I in utero gene transfer studies. Hum Gene Ther 22(11):1323–1330. https://doi.org/10.1089/hum.2011.062. Epub 2011 Sep 23. PMID: 21846200; PMCID: PMC3225039

Swain TR (2014) Clinical trials for children: some concerns. Indian J Pharmacol 46(2):145–146. https://doi.org/10.4103/0253-7613.129300. PMID: 24741182; PMCID: PMC3987179

Tabbara K, Al-Kawi MZ (2006) Ethics in medical research and publication. Ann Saudi Med 26(4):257–260. https://doi.org/10.5144/0256-4947.2006.257. PMID: 16880727; PMCID: PMC6074504

Thomas G (2021) Ethical issues in randomised trials in surgery. Indian. J Med Ethics VI(1):1–5. https://doi.org/10.20529/IJME.2020.099. PMID: 34081000

Turner MA (2015) Clinical trials of medicines in neonates: the influence of ethical and practical issues on design and conduct. Br J Clin Pharmacol 79(3):370–378. https://doi.org/10.1111/bcp.12467. PMID: 25041601; PMCID: PMC4345948

Warnock GL (2004) Raising the bar for the ethical integrity of clinical trials. Can J Surg 47(5):327–328. PMID: 15540682; PMCID: PMC3211949

Weigmann K (2015) The ethics of global clinical trials: in developing countries, participation in clinical trials is sometimes the only way to access medical treatment. What should be done to avoid exploitation of disadvantaged populations? EMBO Rep 16(5):566–570. https://doi.org/10.15252/embr.201540398. Epub 2015 Apr 7. PMID: 25851646; PMCID: PMC4428044

Vaccine Clinical Trials

19

C. Madhavrao, K. Mythili Bai, Santenna Chenchula, and Sushil Sharma

Abstract

Vaccines are a cornerstone of public health and have enabled the complete eradication of human diseases such as smallpox and control of conditions such as polio. Development of vaccines involves a multi-step process from foundational research and preclinical testing through to clinical trials, regulatory review, and post-marketing surveillance. The clinical trials of vaccines are done in several phases: Phase I is a study of small groups regarding safety and immune response; Phase II will include expanded diverse populations to evaluate the safety and immunogenicity of the vaccine; Phase III will determine efficacy and safety in larger cohorts, leading to the regulatory approval of vaccines. Phase IV continues to monitor post-marketing and post-distribution vaccines for their continued safety and effectiveness.

Immunology, including innate and adaptive immunity, was identified as a key factor, so that it can interpret the immune response to vaccination with biomarkers of antibody levels and T-cell activity, providing valuable insights into its immunogenicity. Strong statistical methodologies, including randomization and careful sample size determination, help with the validity of trial results. Special populations present special ethical challenges: special considerations are made for informed consent and placebo use.

C. Madhavrao (✉) · S. Sharma
All India Institute of Medical Sciences [AIIMS], Mangalagiri, India

K. Mythili Bai
Government Siddhartha Medical College, Vijayawada, India

S. Chenchula
All India Institute of Medical Sciences [AIIMS], Bhopal, India

A. Arivazhahan et al. (eds.), *Introduction to Basics of Pharmacology and Toxicology*,
https://doi.org/10.1007/978-981-95-1920-0_19

In this respect, regulatory bodies like the FDA, EMA, and WHO are very instrumental in ensuring vaccine safety and effectiveness through expedited pathways such as Emergency Use Authorizations to help with these public health crises.

These will involve state-of-the-art approaches, such as adaptive trial designs, integration of real-world data to improve efficiency of trials, and community trust. The forward direction for vaccine research includes personalized strategies for vaccination, next-generation vaccine platforms and universal vaccines, and use of artificial intelligence-machine learning in pinpointing optimization in trial processes. Regulatory framework adaptation and fostering global harmonization are going to hold the key for improving access to vaccines for populations across the world.

Keywords

Vaccines · Public health · Clinical trials · Immunogenicity · Regulatory agencies · Phase I/II/III trials · Emergency Use Authorization (EUA) · Adaptive trial designs · Personalized vaccinology

19.1 Introduction

Vaccination is one of the most powerful tools available to public health-from the eradication of smallpox and the near eradication of polio to the control of many infectious diseases. Even as this represents such a fact, the road of vaccine development is very long and laboriously slow because a vaccine has to go through meticulous clinical trials that ensure safety, efficacy, and immune response capability.

Vaccines have been responsible for the prevention of infectious diseases, thereby reducing illness and death rates around the world. Vaccine development proceeds with very strict scientific procedures, which include clinical trials. Such trials are extremely important in determining the safety, response of the body to the vaccine, and efficiency of a vaccine before it is approved for public administration. The trials, carried out in phases, each have different goals and methods. This chapter discusses the immunizations, describes their structure and stages, ethical concerns, regulatory guidelines, and the challenges found within contemporary medical practice.

Four important pillars of vaccine development are depicted in Table 19.1.

Table 19.1 Four important pillars of vaccine development

Quality
Safety
Immunogenicity
Efficacy

A list of unique features of vaccine clinical trials is highlighted in Table 19.2.

19.2 Overview of Vaccine Development

19.2.1 History of Vaccine Development

- **Early Vaccines**: Vaccination has traditionally been considered to have originated in the eighteenth century, when Edward Jenner first made use of smallpox vaccine. Ever since then, due to the modernization of science and technologies, the process of development of vaccines greatly improved.
- **Milestones in Vaccine History**: Key events in vaccine history include the development of vaccines against rabies, polio, and measles. Modern methods for producing vaccines were developed in the twentieth century and, with these, mechanisms for regulatory control over their safety and efficacy.

A list of notable vaccine clinical trials with lessons learned and impact on public health is highlighted in Table 19.3.

Table 19.2 List of unique features of vaccine clinical trials

Unique feature(s)	Description
Immunogenicity evaluation	Focused on measuring the immune response triggered by the vaccine
Assessment of serological markers	Monitoring antibody levels and other immune indicators as primary endpoints
Dose and schedule optimization	Investigating various doses and vaccination schedules to determine the most effective regimen
Booster dose investigations	Studies designed to evaluate the need, timing, and efficacy of additional doses to maintain immunity
Cross-protection studies	Evaluating the vaccine's ability to provide protection against different strains or related pathogens
Impact on herd immunity	Analyzing how vaccination affects overall community immunity and disease spread
Cold chain requirements	Ensuring proper storage and transport conditions to maintain vaccine stability and efficacy
Monitoring for adverse events	Detailed tracking of potential vaccine-related side effects, including rare immune reactions
Neutralizing antibody assays	Tests to measure the vaccine's effectiveness in neutralizing the target pathogen
Long-term effectiveness studies	Extended follow-up to assess how long the vaccine remains effective and the need for future boosters

Table 19.3 List of notable vaccine clinical trials with lessons learned and impact on public health

Vaccine	Clinical trial	Key insights	Public health impact
Polio vaccine	Salk Vaccine Trials (1954)	Demonstrated the efficacy of inactivated vaccines in preventing polio	Paved the way for the near-eradication of polio, showcasing vaccination as a vital tool for disease control
Measles vaccine	Measles Vaccine Trials (1963)	Confirmed the vaccine's effectiveness in reducing measles-related complications and mortality	Drastically decreased measles incidence and mortality, contributing to a significant drop in global measles cases
Smallpox vaccine	WHO Smallpox Eradication Campaign (1967–1977)	Proved that mass vaccination could lead to the complete eradication of a disease	Achieved the eradication of smallpox, marking the first successful eradication of a disease through vaccination
Hepatitis B vaccine	HBV Vaccine Trials (1980s)	Showed that vaccination could prevent chronic hepatitis B and associated liver conditions	Led to a significant decline in hepatitis B cases and liver cancer, with global health benefits
HPV vaccine	Gardasil Trials (2000s)	Demonstrated the vaccine's effectiveness in preventing HPV infections and related cancers	Reduced HPV infection rates and cervical cancer incidence, highlighting the role of vaccines in cancer prevention
COVID-19 vaccines	Pfizer-BioNTech and Moderna Trials (2020)	Validated the rapid development and efficacy of mRNA vaccines in addressing a global pandemic	Played a crucial role in managing the COVID-19 pandemic and showcased the potential of mRNA technology for future vaccines
Rotavirus vaccine	RotaTeq and Rotarix Trials (2000s)	Confirmed the effectiveness of vaccines in preventing severe rotavirus gastroenteritis in infants	Reduced hospitalizations and severe cases of rotavirus, significantly benefiting infant health worldwide
Influenza vaccine	Seasonal flu vaccine trials	Highlighted the need for annual updates to match circulating flu strains	Established a model for updating vaccines annually and underscored the importance of ongoing surveillance

19.2.2 The Vaccine Development Pipeline

- **Discovery and Research**: The very basic process of vaccine development involves fundamental research aimed at the identification of antigens and the formulation of a vaccine candidate. This requires substantial basic knowledge regarding the pathogen's biology and the consequent immune response.
- **Preclinical Testing**: Evaluation of a vaccine candidate by laboratory and animal studies, prior to clinical testing, is conducted for its safety and efficiency in provoking an immune response.

- **Manufacturing and Formulation**: Besides the development of a scalable manufacturing process, stability and potency assurance of the vaccine before clinical testing is important. These are crucial steps in the development process.

Differences in 'vaccine development through traditional approach vs during epidemics' are depicted in Table 19.4.

Table 19.4 Differences in 'vaccine development through traditional approach vs during epidemics'

Particulars	Traditional vaccine development	Vaccine development during epidemics/pandemics
Development duration	Usually takes 10–15 years, involving several stages of clinical trials.	Accelerated to a few months to a few years to address urgent health threats.
Research approach	Long-term focus with extensive foundational research and preclinical studies.	Rapid deployment using existing technologies or novel approaches to meet immediate needs.
Clinical trial phases	Detailed and sequential phases (I-IV) with thorough safety and efficacy assessments.	Condensed phases, often merging steps to speed up the evaluation process.
Regulatory procedures	Follow standard regulatory pathways with extensive documentation and review.	Utilizes expedited regulatory processes such as emergency use authorizations to speed up approvals.
Manufacturing scale-up	Incremental scaling up of production facilities over an extended period.	Urgent expansion, sometimes utilizing temporary or existing facilities to quickly increase production capacity.
Funding sources	Typically funded through long-term investments from governments, private sector, or academic institutions.	Often receives emergency funding from governments, international agencies, and public-private partnerships.
Public engagement	Focuses on gradual public education about vaccine benefits and potential side effects.	Requires immediate and ongoing communication to manage public perceptions and misinformation.
Monitoring and surveillance	Long-term surveillance post-marketing to detect rare adverse events.	Enhanced monitoring and rapid assessment to address safety and effectiveness during a crisis.
Vaccine technologies	Includes various established platforms like live attenuated, inactivated, and subunit vaccines.	Frequently employs adaptable technologies such as mRNA and viral vectors due to their rapid development capabilities.
Supply chain management	Established and stable supply chains for routine vaccine distribution.	Needs to rapidly establish and adapt supply chains, often facing challenges related to logistics and material shortages.
Emergency authorization	Typically not used except in specific, exceptional cases.	Frequently used to provide swift access to vaccines during public health emergencies.
Post-marketing research	Continues with long-term studies to evaluate ongoing safety and effectiveness.	Focuses on expedited post-market research due to the urgency of addressing the emergency.

(continued)

Table 19.4 (continued)

Particulars	Traditional vaccine development	Vaccine development during epidemics/pandemics
Community preparedness	Gradual preparedness and planning for vaccine introduction and distribution.	Immediate preparedness efforts, often involving crisis management and coordination with international bodies.
Ethical considerations	Standard ethical guidelines and considerations for participant safety and informed consent.	Heightened ethical considerations due to the urgency and scale of the public health crisis.

Table 19.5 Good manufacturing practices (GMP) in vaccine clinical trials

GMP component(s)	Description
Facility and equipment	Manufacturing sites must adhere to stringent cleanliness and design standards to ensure contamination control and efficient operations
Personnel training and qualification	Personnel must receive specialized training and demonstrate competence to manage production processes and quality control effectively
Material management	Proper handling, labelling, and storage of raw materials, intermediates, and finished products are essential to prevent errors and ensure integrity
Manufacturing processes	Manufacturing protocols must be clearly defined, validated, and consistently followed to ensure uniformity and quality of the vaccine
Documentation and record keeping	Comprehensive records must be maintained for all manufacturing and quality control activities to ensure traceability and compliance
Quality control and testing	Each vaccine batch must be subjected to rigorous testing for attributes such as purity, potency, and sterility to meet predefined standards
Contamination prevention	Implement robust measures to avoid contamination during production, including aseptic techniques and environmental monitoring
Change management	Any modifications to processes, equipment, or materials must be properly evaluated, documented, and approved to ensure they do not compromise quality
Complaint resolution	Establish procedures to handle and investigate product complaints, ensuring corrective actions are implemented when needed
Recall procedures	Develop and maintain effective protocols for recalling products if defects or safety issues arise
Validation and calibration	Regular validation and calibration of equipment and processes are necessary to maintain consistent performance and quality
Supplier and contractor management	Ensure that all external suppliers and contractors meet GMP standards and their performance is continuously monitored and assessed

Good manufacturing practices (GMP) in vaccine clinical trials are highlighted in Table 19.5.

Salient pillars of good manufacturing practices (GMP) in vaccine development are highlighted in Table 19.6.

Important factors to be considered during development of vaccines are highlighted in Table 19.7.

A list of common adjuvant(s) used in development of vaccines is highlighted in Table 19.8.

Table 19.6 Salient pillars of good manufacturing practices (GMP) in vaccine development

GMP	Sterility
	Identity
	Purity
	Potency
	Stability
	Safety

Table 19.7 Important factors to be considered during development of vaccines

Factors	Pathogenic disease structure
	Pathogenic disease diversity
	Pathogenic disease burden
	Life cycle of pathogen
	Life cycle of epidemiology
	Natural immune control
	Natural immune escape
	Pathogenic antigen selection
	Vaccine strategy
	Vaccine formulation
	Vaccine immunogenicity

Table 19.8 List of common adjuvant(s) used in development of vaccines

Adjuvant(s)	Chemical composition	Mechanism	Uses in vaccine(s)
AS01	QS -21 and 3-deacylated monophosphoryl lipid (MPL)	Induces antigen-presenting cells	Malaria
			Zoster
AS03	Emulsion of oil in water with vitamin E	Induces innate immune response including T-cell and B-cell-mediated response	Influenza
AS04	MPL adsorption with aluminum phosphate/ hydroxide	Induces antigen-presenting cells	HPV
			HBV
Alum	Aluminum phosphate/ hydroxide	Induces Th2 immune response	DPT
			Influenza
Virosomes	Phospholipids	Induces Th1 immune response	HAV
			Influenza
MF59	Emulsion of oil in water with squalene	Induces antigen-presenting cells	Influenza

Table 19.9 Quality checkup techniques in vaccine clinical trials

Technique(s)	Description
Preclinical testing	Testing in laboratory settings and on animal models to assess the vaccine's safety and efficacy before human trials.
Good manufacturing practices (GMP)	Standards that ensure products are consistently produced and controlled according to quality standards.
Quality control (QC) testing	Regular testing of raw materials, in-process materials, and finished products to ensure they meet specified quality criteria.
Stability testing	Testing to ensure that the vaccine maintains its effectiveness, safety, and quality throughout its shelf life.
Batch release testing	Testing of each batch of the vaccine before it is released to the market, including potency, sterility, and purity checks.
Clinical trials (phases I-III)	Human trials conducted in phases to assess safety, immunogenicity, and efficacy, with rigorous monitoring and documentation.
Post-marketing surveillance (phase IV)	Ongoing monitoring of the vaccine's performance and adverse events after it has been approved for public use.
Regulatory audits and inspections	Reviews and inspections by regulatory agencies to ensure compliance with regulatory requirements and standards.
Risk management plans	Strategies developed to identify, assess, and mitigate risks associated with the vaccine throughout its lifecycle.
Pharmacovigilance	Continuous monitoring of the vaccine's safety profile and reporting of adverse events to detect potential risks early.

Quality checkup techniques in vaccine clinical trials are highlighted in Table 19.9.

Comparison of 'additives and adjuvants' used in vaccine clinical trials is highlighted in Table 19.10.

19.2.3 Types of Vaccines

- **Live Attenuated Vaccines**: These vaccines take advantage of a weakened form of the pathogen to initiate the immune response. Probably the most well-known example from this category is the measles, mumps, and rubella vaccine.
- **Inactivated Vaccines**: These include the killed form of the pathogen as an antigen to stimulate an immune response. Classic examples are the hepatitis A vaccine and the inactivated poliomyelitis vaccine (IPV).
- **Subunit, Recombinant, and Conjugate Vaccines**: Vaccines use only part of the pathogen, like a protein or carbohydrate, to elicit an immune response. Some very well-known examples include pneumococcal vaccine and HPV vaccine.
- **mRNA Vaccines**: This new technology uses mRNA to instruct cells to make a protein, which then triggers the immune response. The most salient examples of such technology are the vaccines against COVID-19 developed by Pfizer-BioNTech and Moderna.
- **Viral Vector Vaccines**: The pathogen's genetic material is delivered by a harmless virus that serves as the delivery vector. Examples include the Astra Zeneca and Johnson & Johnson COVID-19 vaccines.

Table 19.10 Comparison of 'additives and adjuvants' used in vaccine clinical trials

Particulars	Additive(s)	Adjuvant(s)
Definition	Substances added to vaccines to maintain their stability and potency.	Substances added to vaccines to enhance the body's immune response to the antigen.
Primary purpose	To preserve, stabilize, and ensure the safety and effectiveness of the vaccine.	To boost the immune response, leading to higher and longer-lasting immunity.
Common examples	Preservatives (e.g., thimerosal), stabilizers (e.g., sugars, gelatin), antibiotics (e.g., neomycin).	Aluminum salts (e.g., aluminum hydroxide, aluminum phosphate), oil-in-water emulsions (e.g., MF59, AS03), liposomes.
Mechanism of action	Prevents contamination, stabilizes the vaccine formulation, and prevents degradation.	Enhances the immune response by stimulating the innate immune system, promoting antigen uptake, and increasing antigen presentation.
Usage	Used in both live attenuated and inactivated vaccines to ensure product safety and efficacy.	Mainly used in inactivated and subunit vaccines to enhance immunogenicity.
Regulatory approval	Must meet stringent regulatory requirements for safety and efficacy.	Subject to rigorous testing and approval processes to ensure they are safe and effective.
Safety considerations	Generally recognized as safe when used in recommended amounts, but monitored for potential allergic reactions and side effects.	Monitored for safety, as they can sometimes cause local or systemic reactions, although serious side effects are rare.
Impact on vaccine efficacy	Ensures the vaccine remains effective during storage and administration.	Can significantly enhance the efficacy of vaccines, allowing for lower doses of the antigen and sometimes fewer doses of the vaccine.

Examples of different vaccine platforms are highlighted in Table 19.11.

Pros and cons of technology used in vaccine development are highlighted in Table 19.12.

19.2.4 Stages of Vaccine Development

Vaccine development is a long and cumbersome process that starts from an early discovery phase to post-marketing surveillance. Its phases generally include the following:

(i) **Preclinical Research**: The basis of the process is formed by basic research. Scientists begin the study of pathogen biology and potential antigens which would be able to raise some form of an immune response in the host. A majority of this phase generally involves experiments in vitro and animal studies to study the safety and immune response to potential vaccine candidates.

Table 19.11 Examples of different vaccine platforms

	Type	Example(s)
Vaccine platform(s)	Live attenuated	Yellow fever
		Influenza
		Poliomyelitis
	Whole inactivated	Influenza
		Poliomyelitis
		COVID-19
	DNA	SARS
		COVID-19
		Zika
		MERS
		Lassa fever
	mRNA	COVID-19
		Lassa fever
		Disease X
	Recombinant vectors	COVID-19
		Ebola
		MERS
		Lassa fever
		Nipah
		Zika
		Chikungunya
	Protein based	COVID-19
		Influenza
		MERS
		Nipah

(ii) **Clinical Development**: With promising preclinical data, the vaccine candidate will move into clinical development, consisting of three critical phases of clinical trials.
(iii) **Regulatory Review and Approval**: After clinical trials prove the vaccine's safety and efficacy, the regulatory authorities review the data to conclude whether the use in the general population is allowed or not.
(iv) **Post-marketing Surveillance**: Upon approval, a vaccine also further undergoes monitoring with respect to their continued safety and effectiveness through pharmacovigilance efforts and phase IV studies.

Important differences between vaccine and drug clinical trials are highlighted in Table 19.13.

Differences in vaccine clinical trials with traditional approach and new modern current approaches are highlighted in Table 19.14.

Table 19.12 Pros and cons of technology used in vaccine development

Technology	Pros	Cons
mRNA vaccines	Quick to develop, highly effective, and easy to scale production	Requires specialized cold storage and has limited long-term safety data
Viral vector vaccines	Strong immune response and longer-lasting immunity	Pre-existing immunity to the vector can reduce vaccine effectiveness
Protein subunit vaccines	Offers targeted immune response and is generally safe for people with compromised immunity	Often needs adjuvants and multiple doses for maximum protection
Inactivated vaccines	Established method with a solid safety record	Provides a weaker immune response compared to live vaccines, requiring boosters
Live attenuated vaccines	Delivers strong, long-term immunity with fewer doses	May pose risks for immunocompromised individuals
DNA vaccines	Stable, easy to manufacture, and adaptable for new variants	Limited human data and concerns about potential DNA integration into host cells
Virus-like particle (VLP) vaccines	Mimics the virus to provoke a strong immune response without causing infection	High production costs and complex manufacturing processes
Nanoparticle vaccines	Allows precise delivery of antigens and can enhance immune activation	Expensive and challenging to manufacture on a large scale
Adjuvanted vaccines	Enhances immune response, allowing smaller antigen doses.	May cause local reactions or inflammation due to heightened immune activation
Synthetic peptide vaccines	Cost-efficient with minimal side effects and reduced risk of adverse reactions	Generally produces a weaker immune response, often requiring adjuvants and additional doses

19.3 Phases of Vaccine Clinical Trials

The clinical trial of vaccine comprises of three important phases during its developmental stages before its approval in the market. Each phase of the vaccine clinical trials has distinct aims and objectives.

19.3.1 Phase I Trials: Safety and Immunogenicity

- **Objectives**: The resultant candidate vaccines are primarily tested for safety in Phase I trials among a small group of healthy volunteers, generally 20–100 individuals. Immunogenicity or the extent to which a vaccine can provoke an immune response is also tested.
- **Design**: Most Phase I trials are open-label, where both the researchers and the participants in the trial know what vaccine is being administered. This may also include dose-escalation studies to identify the best dose for the vaccine.

Table 19.13 Important differences between vaccine and drug clinical trials

Aspect	Vaccine clinical trials	Drug clinical trials
Primary aim	Assess immune response and effectiveness in preventing diseases	Evaluate safety, efficacy, and therapeutic benefits for specific conditions
Participant demographics	Typically involve healthy volunteers or targeted populations at risk	Focus on individuals with the specific medical condition being treated
Main outcomes	Immune response indicators (e.g., antibody levels, T-cell activation)	Clinical outcomes (e.g., symptom relief, disease progression)
Study duration	Often shorter for initial evaluations but includes extended follow-up for long-term effects	Generally longer to observe comprehensive therapeutic and safety outcomes
Regulatory processes	May use expedited approval processes (e.g., emergency use authorization) during pandemics	Follow standard approval procedures with detailed data requirements
Safety assessments	Emphasize monitoring for immune-related side effects and long-term safety	Broader safety profile, including potential organ-specific effects
Use of placebo	Commonly used to compare immune responses between vaccinated and unvaccinated groups	Often used to evaluate the drug's effect against no treatment
Blinding methods	Typically involves double-blinding to reduce bias in immune response assessment	Double-blinding is used to minimize bias in evaluating treatment effects
Dosage regimens	Usually involves multiple doses with defined intervals	Can vary widely; may include single or multiple doses depending on the drug
Focus on immunogenicity	Central to the trial, evaluating the ability to provoke an immune response	Not applicable; the focus is on therapeutic efficacy
Challenge studies	May involve exposing participants to pathogens to assess vaccine effectiveness	Not typically used; efficacy is measured through clinical outcomes
Adverse event monitoring	Focuses on vaccine-specific reactions (e.g., injection site reactions)	Includes a range of possible drug-related side effects
Long-term monitoring	Critical for detecting rare or delayed immune-related effects	Important for assessing prolonged safety and therapeutic outcomes
Efficacy evaluation	Determined by the reduction in disease incidence or severity among vaccinated individuals	Assessed through improvements in symptoms or disease progression
Ethical considerations	Balances the risk of adverse reactions with the potential public health benefits of vaccination	Weighs the risk versus benefit for the individual patient

Table 19.14 Differences in vaccine clinical trials with 'traditional approach and new modern current approaches'

Category	Traditional vaccine clinical trials	Modern approaches to vaccine clinical trials
Development duration	Typically spans 10–15 years from initial development to approval	Accelerated timelines, with some vaccines developed within a year (e.g., during health emergencies)
Sequential vs. overlapping phases	Phases (I, II, III) are conducted one after the other	Phases may overlap (e.g., combining phase I/II or II/III) to shorten the process
Vaccine technology	Relies on traditional methods, such as live-attenuated or inactivated vaccines	Employs advanced methods like mRNA, viral vectors, or DNA-based vaccines
Preclinical studies	Extensive animal studies are required before proceeding to human trials	Animal testing is often minimized, with rapid transition to human trials, especially in urgent situations
Production capabilities	Requires large, complex manufacturing setups for mass production	Newer platforms (e.g., mRNA) are easier to scale up and produce quickly
Regulatory pathway	Sequential regulatory reviews, typically at the end of each phase	Rolling reviews allow real-time regulatory evaluations as data becomes available during trials
Participant demographics	Initial trials often focus on limited age groups and health profiles	Broader participant inclusion (varied age, ethnicity, and health conditions) from early trial stages
Flexibility in trial design	Traditional designs follow fixed protocols with limited modifications	Adaptive designs allow protocol changes based on real-time data, enhancing efficiency
Data monitoring	Relies on periodic data collection with limited real-time insights	Continuous data monitoring enabled by digital tools, wearables, and real-time reporting systems
International collaboration	Trials are often localized, with limited cross-border partnerships	Enhanced global cooperation (e.g., COVAX, multinational partnerships) to expedite development
Post-approval surveillance	Primarily focused on long-term safety and efficacy monitoring	Increased reliance on real-world evidence and continuous post-market safety evaluation
Funding mechanisms	Funded mainly by governments or private entities, often over extended periods	Increased public-private partnerships, with rapid emergency funding and collaborative efforts
Approval process	Full approval granted only after all trial phases are completed	Emergency use authorizations (EUA) allow earlier deployment in urgent situations, based on interim data

- **Outcomes**: The main outcomes of Phase I trials are the identification of adverse events, the immune response elicited by the vaccine, and a determination of a safe dosage range.

19.3.2 Phase II Trials: Expanded Safety and Immunogenicity

- **Objective:** Phase II trials extend the safety evaluation to a much larger, more diverse population-group, often amounting to several hundreds. Trials of this nature also provide far more specific information on the immunogenicity of the vaccine and explore the relationship between dosage and response.
- **Design:** Phase II designs are usually randomized and controlled, with the potential to be double-blinded to avoid such biases. Subjects will be assigned to groups, one to receive the candidate vaccine and others to receive placebo controls or another vaccine for comparison.
- **Outcomes:** Phase II trials give a clearer look at the vaccine's safety profile, help to clearly determine the best dosing schedule, and also provide preliminary information regarding its efficacy.

19.3.3 Phase III Trials: Efficacy and Safety

- **Objective:** Phase III trials are the largest, designed to confirm vaccine efficacy-that is, does the vaccine actually prevent the disease in question-in a very large population, with eventual thousands or tens of thousands participating. Safety data will be collected in these trials as well.
- **Design:** In general, Phase III trials are double-blinded, multicentric, randomized, and placebo-controlled studies. They are carried out in a variety of populations with a view to confirming the vaccine's effectiveness among different demographic groups.
- **Outcomes:** The major outcomes of trials in Phase III include but are not limited to the incidence rates of the target disease in those vaccinated as opposed to those who have not been vaccinated, adverse events observed, and a general risk versus benefit assessment seen with the vaccine.

19.3.4 Phase IV Trials: Post-marketing Surveillance

- **Ongoing Safety Monitoring:** Phase IV trials still extend beyond the approval of a vaccine and further assess the safety in general. This phase puts an emphasis on detecting rare adverse events that may not have been observed in trials so far.
- **Effectiveness Studies:** The phase IV trial determines the real-world effectiveness of the vaccine under usual conditions with regard to its impact on actual disease transmission and population health.

- **Long-Term Follow-Up:** It can also evaluate the trials for long-term sustainability of the immune response and thus determine whether booster doses are needed.

Comparison of phases of vaccine clinical trials is highlighted in Table 19.15.

Major goals of different phases of vaccine clinical trials are highlighted in Table 19.16.

19.4 Immunological Considerations in Vaccine Clinical Trials

19.4.1 Understanding the Immune Response to Vaccination

- **Innate vs. Adaptive Immunity:** Vaccination is designed in such a way that it should stimulate both the innate and adaptive immune responses for long-lasting immunity.
- **Humoral and Cell-Mediated Immunity:** Vaccination aims to bring out the humoral response through the production of antibodies, while in most times targeting the vigorous cell-mediated response including the T-cell activation.

Objectives of immunogenicity in vaccine clinical trials are highlighted in Table 19.17.

Table 19.15 Comparison of phases of vaccine clinical trials

Phases			Study participants		Description
Preliminary CTs	I	a	20–100	Healthy	Study in adults
		b			Study in de-escalated population
	II	a	100–300	Varying health status	Human challenge studies
		b			Human non-challenge studies
Pivotal CTs	III	a	1000–3000	Diverse population	Before submission of BLA
		b			After submission of BLA
Post marketing surveillance	IV	In thousand(s)	Pragmatic	Post marketing surveillance (PMS)	

Table 19.16 Major goals of different phases of vaccine clinical trials

Phases of CTs	I	Safety and Immunogenicity
	II	Safety and Immunogenicity
	III	Safety and Efficacy
	IV	Post Marketing Surveillance (PMS)

Table 19.17 Objectives of immunogenicity in vaccine clinical trials

Objectives of immunogenicity CTs
Selection of vaccine formulation(s)
Selection of vaccine posology (primary dose)
Selection of vaccine posology (booster dose)
Comparison with other vaccines
Comparison with ideal setting versus pragmatic
Assessment of lot-to-lot consistency
To support maternal immunization
To support major changes at manufacturing units
Comparison of immune responses at different special population groups

Table 19.18 Immunogenicity in vaccine clinical trials

	Type	Assessment
Immunogenicity	Humoral	ELISA
	Cellular	$CD8^+/CD4^+$
	Functional	In-vitro Neutralization Assays

19.4.2 Biomarkers of Immunogenicity

- **Antibody Titers:** Blood antibody levels are the conventional method of assaying for immunogenicity. Such titers are often accepted as correlates of protection against the disease under consideration.
- **T-Cell Responses:** Assessing T-cell responses gives further details on the vaccine's ability for long-term immunity and protection against infection.

Immunogenicity in vaccine clinical trials is highlighted in Table 19.18.

19.4.3 Durability of Immunity

- **Long-Term Follow-Up Studies:** These post-trial follow-up studies test the persistence of the immune response and, therefore, whether booster doses are required to maintain the protection.
- **Factors Influencing Immunity:** The immune response duration may depend on factors such as age, immunity health status, and previous cases with the pathogen

under investigation. These become very important during follow-up measures in designing trial plans.

19.4.4 Challenges in Measuring Immunogenicity

- **Variability in Immune Responses:** Differences in individual immune responses present challenges with respect to interpreting such immunogenicity data properly. Such variability has to be taken into account during trial design and statistical analysis.
- **Correlates of Protection:** Certain well-defined protection correlates are necessary in order to define the efficacy of any vaccine. With respect to all vaccines, these are sometimes not well described, which may complicate the assessment of vaccine effectiveness.

19.5 Statistical Considerations in Vaccine Clinical Trials

19.5.1 Study Design and Sample Size Calculation

- **Randomization and Blinding:** Double-blind, placebo-controlled, randomized trials are the perfect gold standard for assessing the effectiveness of the vaccine with a minimum scope of bias.
- **Sample Size Determination:** Statistical methods will be applied to arrive at an estimate of the sample size necessary to detect clinically meaningful different incidences between vaccinated and unvaccinated groups.

Design of randomized vaccine clinical trials is highlighted in Table 19.19.

19.5.2 Primary and Secondary Endpoints

- **Choosing Appropriate Endpoints:** The primary endpoint will generally assess the incidence of the target disease, and secondary endpoints could include assessments of immunogenicity, safety, and quality of life.

Table 19.19 Design of randomized vaccine clinical trials

	Comparator	Design
RCT design	When no other vaccines are available	Superiority Clinical Trial
	When other vaccines are available	Non-inferiority Clinical Trial

Table 19.20 Clinical endpoints in vaccine efficacy clinical trials

	Clinical endpoints	Goal/focus
Vaccine efficacy clinical trials	**Primary**	Prevention of clinically apparent infections based on clinical or laboratory criteria
		Clinical symptoms of reactivated latent infections
		Predisposition of chronic asymptomatic infections to later symptomatic infections
		Prediction with sensitive biomarkers for further progression of clinically apparent infections
	Secondary	Number of cases after each dose of vaccine
		Number of cases after booster dose of vaccine
		Number of cases associated with individual strains of organisms
		Number of cases associated with different antigenicity of the organisms
		Number of cases in specific age groups
		Number of cases in specific regions
		Number of cases with different grades of clinical manifestations based on clinical/laboratory criteria

- **Surrogate Endpoints:** Sometimes it is possible, under certain circumstances, to use surrogate endpoints, for example, immune responses, markers in forecasting vaccine efficacy when direct measurement of disease incidence is impracticable.

  Clinical endpoints in vaccine efficacy clinical trials are highlighted in Table 19.20.

19.5.3 Statistical Analysis Methods

- **Intention-to-Treat vs. Per-Protocol Analysis:** While the intention-to-treat analysis includes each participant based on the original treatment assignment regardless of actual treatment adherence, the per-protocol analysis includes only those who completed the study as intended.
- **Handling Missing Data:** Methods for handling missing data include imputation techniques and sensitivity analyses that help ensure the reliability of trial results.

19.5.4 Interim Analyses and Data Monitoring Committees

- **Interim Analysis:** They are performed at regular, predefined intervals throughout the trial to assess safety and efficacy. Such studies may result in the modification of trials or early termination considering success or futility.
- **Role of Data Monitoring Committees (DMCs):** An independent DMC reviews interim analyses and makes recommendations on continuation of the study with

Table 19.21 Trial designs and methodologies in context to vaccine clinical trials

Trial design/methodology	Description
Phased approach	Sequential trials (phase I, II, III) to evaluate safety, efficacy, and optimal dosing progressively
Adaptive design	Flexible trial designs allowing adjustments based on interim data, such as altering sample sizes or modifying protocols
Randomized controlled trials (RCTs)	Participants are randomly assigned to receive either the vaccine or a placebo to eliminate bias and ensure accurate comparisons
Blinding methods	Implementing single or double blinding to keep participants and/or researchers unaware of treatment assignments to prevent bias
Dose-response trials	Studies that test various doses of the vaccine to determine the most effective and safe dose
Booster dose evaluations	Trials assessing the efficacy and timing of additional doses to enhance or prolong immune protection
Cross-sectional analysis	Evaluations conducted at a single point in time to understand vaccine effectiveness and immune response across different groups
Long-term follow-up studies	Extended tracking of participants to assess the durability of the vaccine's protection and identify any long-term effects
Immunogenicity studies	Trials focused on measuring the vaccine's ability to provoke a strong immune response, including antibody production
Real-world effectiveness studies	Observational studies assessing how well the vaccine performs in everyday conditions outside controlled clinical trials
Post-marketing surveillance	Ongoing monitoring after the vaccine is approved to track real-world safety and effectiveness, including rare adverse events

no change, modification of the study, or early termination of the study based on safety and efficacy information.

Trial designs and methodologies in context to vaccine clinical trials are highlighted in Table 19.21.

19.6 Special Populations in Vaccine Clinical Trials

19.6.1 Pediatric Populations

- **Ethical Considerations:** Pediatric trials need to be balanced against the need for vaccine trials in children with the ethical obligation of minimizing the risk of injury. Informed consent by the parents or guardians is the key.
- **Pediatric Immunogenicity:** The Children have a different kind of immune system from adults, and vaccine formulations with schedules should specifically target them. Trials have to rigorously assess the immunogenicity and safety in this demographic.

19.6.2 Pregnant Women

- **Vaccine Safety During Pregnancy:** Pregnant women are not usually allowed to participate in the early-phase trials because of safety issues. However, studying pregnant women should be considered, solely required for comprehensively understanding safety and efficacy in this specific population.
- **Maternal Immunization:** Vaccination during pregnancy can protect both the mother and the fetus; it also has the added advantage of passive immunity to the newborn.

19.6.3 Elderly Populations

- **Age-Related Immune Changes:** Immune function naturally declines with increasing age, as is the increased tendency to develop infections, or may affect vaccine response. Trials should consider such age-related changes.
- **Vaccine Formulation and Dosing:** Higher dosing or the use of adjuvants may be required to induce an adequate immune response in elderly subjects. Trials should test these alternatives to maximally optimize vaccine efficacy in this population.

19.6.4 Immunocompromised Individuals

- **Assessing Vaccine Safety and Efficacy:** Being among the highest risks for severe disease, these immunocompromised individuals have different reaction patterns to vaccines. Trials in this group would be required for keeping a close eye on safety and considering whether modified vaccine regimens may be needed or preferred.
- **Strategies for Inclusion:** Unless specifically targeting those populations, immunocompromised individuals can be included in vaccine studies only through the use of adaptive trial designs and special endpoints that would give due consideration to their safety.

19.7 Vaccine Adverse Events and Safety Monitoring

19.7.1 Types of Vaccine Adverse Events

- **Local Reactions:** These usually consist of redness, pain, and swelling at the site of injection. In general, these are mild in nature and thus resolve spontaneously without the need for any treatment.
- **Systemic Reactions:** Systemic reactions may take the form of fever, tiredness, and general body ache. Most of these are not very serious, though some, like

anaphylaxis, are potentially dangerous and may need immediate medical attention.

19.7.2 Monitoring and Reporting Adverse Events

- **Surveillance Systems:** Surveillance systems are one which collect the data on adverse events occurring after vaccination. These include VAERS (Vaccine Adverse Event Reporting System) in the United States and other similar programs elsewhere in the world.
- **Role of Data Safety Monitoring Boards (DSMBs):** The role of DSMBs is crucial with respect to monitoring safety data during clinical trials. DSMBs have the authority to terminate trials when serious safety issues arise.

19.7.3 Risk Communication and Public Perception

- **Transparent Communication:** There is always the need for effective and correct communication of the risk and benefits associated with the administration of vaccines in order to maintain trust among the public. This is about concern linked to adverse events and the provision of context regarding their frequency and severity.
- **Addressing Misinformation:** Misinformation related to vaccine safety is one of the major factors contributing to the erosion of public confidence. This makes it very crucial that false claims be met with effective risk communication strategies that promote evidence-based information.

19.7.4 Managing Vaccine Hesitancy

- **Understanding the Roots of Hesitancy:** Several reasons—including a lack of trust in institutions, misinformation, and cultural beliefs—may fuel vaccine hesitancy. Unless such factors are identified, targeted interventions will not be possible.
- **Community Engagement:** Community engagement, from design to implementation, in the process of vaccine trials can be used to create an environment of trust and assuage concerns, thus improving vaccine acceptance.

19.8 Ethical Considerations in Vaccine Clinical Trials

Vaccine clinical research involves risks and benefits, and there are various ethical considerations to be taken into consideration. These include:

19.8.1 Informed Consent

- **Importance:** These represent the most important ethical consideration in the informed consent of clinical trials, whereby participants should be informed about the nature of the trial, the possible risks and benefits, and their right to withdraw at any point without any penalties.
- **Challenges:** Informed consent is sometimes a challenge to obtain where access to health care is not good and literacy levels are low. Researchers have to ensure that the type of consent adopted in such cases is indeed free and informed.

19.8.2 Risk-Benefit Analysis

- **Risk Minimization:** This requires the researcher to have critical foresight into the potential risks versus benefits of the candidate vaccine. Although some risks may be inevitable, every precaution should be taken to minimize them, particularly in early-phase trials.
- **Benefit Maximization:** Anticipated benefits of the vaccine at the level of individual participant and public health must outweigh the risks in the trial.

19.8.3 Vulnerable Populations

- **Protection:** Vulnerable populations participating in trials include pregnant women, children, and those with weakened immunity. Other ethical considerations should thus be taken into account since these people could easily be more susceptible to the occurrence of adverse events.
- **Inclusion:** However, this often means such populations are excluded from trials, thus limiting the generalizability of results. Ethics in the design of trials should present a balance between protection and inclusion.

19.8.4 Placebo Use

- **Ethical Dilemma:** Above all, vaccine trials, especially in Phase III, use a placebo. This is one factor that has posed ethical problems in the trials. Whereas placebos play a critical role in establishing efficacy, their use sometimes becomes an issue of contention when an effective vaccine or treatment has already been made available.
- **Alternatives:** The issue of using an active comparator instead of a placebo is ethical in some cases. In the selection of a control group, one needs to provide the rationale considering a specific trial context.

Common ethical challenges in vaccine clinical trials are highlighted in Table 19.22.

Table 19.22 Common ethical challenges in vaccine clinical trials

Ethical challenge(s)	Description
Informed consent for vulnerable groups	Obtaining informed consent from vulnerable populations, such as children, pregnant women, or those with cognitive impairments, is a critical challenge. Protecting these groups while respecting their autonomy is essential
Placebo use in critical situations	Ethical concerns arise when using placebo controls in trials for serious or life-threatening conditions, especially if effective vaccines or treatments already exist, risking harm to participants
Risk vs. benefit evaluation	Striking a balance between the potential risks to trial participants and the broader public health benefits is challenging. This requires ongoing ethical oversight to ensure participant safety is prioritized
Fair access to clinical trials	Ensuring that people from all regions, particularly low-resource settings, have equal access to participate in vaccine trials is crucial. This prevents exploitation and ensures fair distribution of risks and benefits
Post-trial responsibilities	Sponsors and researchers have a duty to provide continued access to effective vaccines for participants after the trial ends, especially in areas where the vaccine may not otherwise be accessible
Building trust with communities	Engaging and involving local communities in the research process is vital to foster trust. Without community buy-in, trials may face resistance, especially in areas with historical mistrust of medical research
Transparency in data sharing	Ethical responsibility demands that trial data, including negative outcomes or adverse effects, be shared transparently with the public and regulatory bodies to support informed decision-making and public trust
Accelerated trials in emergencies	In pandemics or health emergencies, vaccine trials may be fast-tracked, sometimes bypassing standard procedures. This raises ethical concerns about the balance between speed and thorough safety evaluation
Compensation for adverse events	Participants who suffer injury or adverse effects during a trial should be compensated fairly. However, inconsistent policies on compensation across regions raise ethical and legal challenges
Inclusion of marginalized groups	Ensuring participation from underrepresented or marginalized groups in vaccine trials is essential for generalizability, but it must be done ethically, without coercion or exploitation, and with fair access to benefits
Addressing public misinformation	Tackling misinformation and vaccine hesitancy during trials is crucial for public safety. Ethical responsibilities include ensuring that accurate, clear, and timely information reaches the public to prevent harm
Dual-use research concerns	Ethical issues arise when vaccine research, especially using novel technologies, could potentially be repurposed for harmful applications, such as bioweapons. Oversight is needed to manage these dual-use risks responsibly

(continued)

Table 19.22 (continued)

Ethical challenge(s)	Description
Protecting vulnerable communities	Conducting trials in low-resource areas raises concerns of potential exploitation. Ethical guidelines must ensure that participants in these settings are not disproportionately exposed to risks without fair benefits
Reliance on surrogate endpoints	Using surrogate markers to accelerate vaccine approval, while useful, can raise ethical questions if they fail to reliably predict long-term clinical outcomes. Careful justification for their use is essential
Prioritizing access during trials	Ethical dilemmas can arise when deciding who should get priority for receiving vaccines during a trial, particularly during shortages or health crises, requiring careful consideration of fairness and need
Involvement of indigenous groups	Including indigenous populations in trials requires sensitivity to their cultural values and obtaining proper consent. This ensures their participation is respectful and their health needs are ethically addressed
Financial conflicts of interest	Vaccine trials funded by pharmaceutical companies can present conflicts of interest, where profit motives might influence trial outcomes. Ethical oversight is critical to maintaining objectivity and protecting participants
Protecting data privacy	Maintaining the confidentiality of participant data is crucial, especially when dealing with sensitive health information. Compliance with data privacy laws across different jurisdictions is essential to uphold ethical standards
Human challenge studies	Intentionally exposing participants to a pathogen to test a vaccine, as in human challenge trials, accelerates results but raises serious ethical questions about participant safety and potential harm
Equitable sharing of benefits	After a successful trial, ensuring that participants and their communities have access to the benefits, such as the vaccine itself, is a key ethical obligation that prevents exploitation and promotes fairness

19.9 Regulatory Requirements for Vaccine Clinical Trials

Clinical trials of vaccines especially are one of the most widely regulated areas to ensure scientific validity and integrity of the ethics.

Important international guidelines related to vaccine clinical trials are highlighted in Table 19.23.

Table 19.23 Important international guidelines related to vaccine clinical trials

International guideline(s)	Description
ICH E6 (R2) good clinical practice	Provides a unified standard for the European Union, Japan, and the United States to ensure clinical trials are conducted ethically and the data is credible.
WHO guidelines on clinical evaluation of vaccines	Offers comprehensive guidance on the clinical evaluation of vaccines, covering preclinical studies to post-marketing surveillance.
FDA guidance for industry: Development and licensure of vaccines to prevent COVID-19	Specific guidelines for the development, testing, and licensure of COVID-19 vaccines in the United States.
EMA guidelines on clinical trials	European medicines agency's guidelines on conducting clinical trials, focusing on methodological and regulatory aspects.
CIOMS international ethical guidelines	Provides ethical guidelines for biomedical research involving human subjects, ensuring respect for all participants.
GCP (good clinical practice) guidelines	International ethical and scientific quality standards for designing, conducting, recording, and reporting trials involving human participants.
ISO 14155:2020	International standard specifying good clinical practice for the design, conduct, and reporting of clinical investigations of medical devices for human subjects.
WHO good manufacturing practices for pharmaceutical products	Standards to ensure that products are consistently produced and controlled according to quality standards.
UNICEF/WHO guidelines for assessing vaccine quality	Provides a framework for assessing the quality of vaccines, including production and post-production stages.
NIH guidelines for research involving recombinant or synthetic nucleic acid molecules	Ensures safety in research involving recombinant or synthetic nucleic acid molecules.

A list of data to be submitted to regulatory authorities in vaccine clinical trials is highlighted in Table 19.24.

19.9.1 Regulatory Agencies

- **Role of Agencies:** The agencies in-charge like EMA, FDA, and others from the WHO charged with regulatory responsibility play a very responsive role in ensuring that vaccine clinical trials are under strong scrutiny. They set guidelines, review trial protocols, and assess trial data to ensure that vaccines comply with the standards for safety and efficacy.
- **Global Coordination:** Global coordination in the modern, connected world where most of the trials for vaccines take place in a number of countries. In these cases, regulatory agencies have to work together to harmonize requirements and smooth the path for global development and distribution of vaccines.

Table 19.24 List of data to be submitted to regulatory authorities in vaccine clinical trials

Category	Data type	Description
Preclinical data	Laboratory studies	Results demonstrating the vaccine's mechanism of action, safety, and immunogenicity in vitro.
	Animal studies	Data showing safety, immunogenicity, and efficacy in relevant animal models.
Manufacturing information	Production process	Detailed description of the vaccine's manufacturing process, including quality control measures and GMP compliance.
	Batch consistency	Evidence of consistency across multiple production batches, including quality and purity tests.
Clinical trial protocols	Phase I protocols	Study design, objectives, endpoints, inclusion/exclusion criteria, and statistical analysis plans for initial safety trials.
	Phase II protocols	Protocols for dose-finding studies, including safety, immunogenicity, and preliminary efficacy assessments.
	Phase III protocols	Comprehensive study plans for large-scale efficacy and safety trials, including detailed methodology and analysis plans.
Clinical trial data	Phase I data	Safety and immunogenicity results from a small group of healthy volunteers.
	Phase II data	Expanded safety, dose optimization, and preliminary efficacy data from trials in a larger, more diverse population.
	Phase III data	Comprehensive efficacy and safety data from large-scale trials, including subgroup analyses and long-term follow-up.
Safety reports	Adverse event reports	Detailed documentation of all adverse events, including severity, frequency, causality, and management strategies.
	Serious adverse events	Specific reports on serious adverse events, their impact on trial participants, and mitigation measures taken.
Post-marketing surveillance	Pharmacovigilance plan	Strategy for ongoing safety monitoring and reporting of adverse events after the vaccine is approved and marketed.
Statistical analysis	Biostatistical analysis	Statistical evaluation of clinical trial data, including efficacy endpoints, safety data, and subgroup analyses.
Labelling information	Product labeling	Proposed product labels, including indications, dosage, administration, contraindications, and potential side effects.
Regulatory compliance	Compliance documents	Certificates and documentation demonstrating adherence to local and international regulatory standards.

(continued)

Table 19.24 (continued)

Category	Data type	Description
Risk management	Risk management plan	Plans to identify, assess, and mitigate risks throughout the vaccine's lifecycle.
Quality assurance	QA test results	Results of quality assurance tests, including sterility, potency, and stability tests to ensure consistent vaccine quality.
Clinical study reports	Comprehensive study reports	Detailed summaries of methodologies, results, and conclusions from all phases of clinical trials.
Benefit-risk assessment	Benefit-risk analysis	Detailed assessment of the vaccine's benefits versus potential risks, based on all collected data.

19.9.2 Good Clinical Practice (GCP)

- **Definition:** GCP is an international standard by which ethical and scientific quality requirements are defined for designing, conducting, recording, and reporting clinical research studies. Compliance with GCP assures the rights, safety, and well-being of study participants are protected.
- **Implementation:** National regulations adopted by regulatory agencies implement principles and guidelines of GCP. Researchers and trial sponsors are expected to adhere to it throughout the entire research trial process.

Good clinical practices (GCP) in vaccine clinical trials are highlighted in Table 19.25.

19.9.3 Investigational New Drug (IND) Application

- **Purpose:** The IND application to the FDA by the vaccine sponsor should be made prior to the start of clinical trials within the United States. This application will also be required to contain data from preclinical studies, the proposed trial protocol, and information regarding the manufacturing process.
- **Review Process:** FDA reviews the IND for judging the proposed trials to be scientifically sound and ethically acceptable. If the FDA approves the IND, then the sponsor is permitted to conduct clinical trials.

19.9.4 Biologics License Application (BLA)

- **Definition:** A BLA is a formal request for permission to market a biologic product, such as vaccines, in interstate commerce within the United States.

Table 19.25 Good clinical practices (GCP) in vaccine clinical trials

GCP element(s)	Description
Study protocol	Create a comprehensive protocol detailing the trial's objectives, design, methodology, and statistical analysis to guide the study
Informed consent process	Secure informed consent from participants, ensuring they are fully informed about the study's purpose, procedures, risks, and benefits
Ethics committee approval	Obtain approval from an independent ethics committee to ensure the study meets ethical and regulatory standards
Investigator and site selection	Choose qualified investigators and sites with the necessary expertise, resources, and facilities to conduct the trial effectively
Training and competency	Provide thorough training to all trial staff to ensure they understand the GCP guidelines and the specific requirements of the study
Data accuracy and integrity	Maintain high standards of data accuracy and reliability through meticulous data collection, documentation, and validation processes
Participant safety monitoring	Implement robust systems to monitor participant safety, including regular assessments and timely responses to adverse events
Monitoring and quality control	Conduct regular monitoring and quality control checks to ensure compliance with the study protocol and GCP standards
Adverse event reporting	Report all adverse events and serious adverse events promptly to the sponsor, ethics committee, and regulatory bodies as required
Data confidentiality	Ensure participant data is handled with confidentiality and securely stored, accessible only to authorized personnel
Regulatory compliance	Comply with all relevant regulations and guidelines to ensure the trial's legal and ethical conduct

- **Requirements:** The BLA includes usual data from all the clinical trial phases of the vaccine and information on its production, labelling, as well as its intended use. The FDA then assesses the BLA to establish if the vaccine satisfies the required standard in terms of safety, purity, and potency.

19.9.5 Conditional and Emergency Use Authorizations

- **Conditional Approval:** The regulatory agencies grant conditional approval to the vaccine when preliminary results of Phase III trials are available. Here, the vaccine gets permission to be used in targeted populations where further data is to be collected.
- **Emergency Use Authorization (EUA):** EUA allows the use of a vaccine, even though not fully approved as per regulations, during public health emergencies like the COVID-19 pandemic. Although the process of EUA has been accelerated, it requires deep scrutiny on both the safety and efficacy sides concerning the vaccine in question.

Common regulatory challenges in vaccine clinical trials are highlighted in Table 19.26.

Table 19.26 Common regulatory challenges in vaccine clinical trials

Regulatory challenge(s)	Description
Variability in global regulations	Different countries have unique regulatory frameworks for vaccine trials, making it difficult to harmonize protocols and approval processes. This often leads to delays and increased complexity for global trials.
Accelerated approvals in crises	During pandemics or health emergencies, regulators often expedite vaccine approvals. While this addresses urgency, it may compromise the depth of safety and efficacy evaluations, creating potential risks
Post-approval monitoring	Regulatory bodies require continuous post-marketing surveillance to detect long-term adverse effects. Establishing effective systems for this, especially in low-resource settings, is challenging but essential for safety
Safety data collection and reporting	Regulatory agencies must ensure comprehensive reporting of safety data. Inconsistent practices across regions and trial sites complicate data integrity, making safety monitoring a regulatory challenge
Ethical compliance across Borders	Adherence to global ethical standards, such as good clinical practice (GCP), must be ensured while navigating local regulatory requirements. Deviations can delay approvals or halt trials, especially in international studies
Intellectual property and accessibility	Balancing patent protection with the global need for affordable vaccines is a regulatory challenge, especially for developing countries. Negotiating fair licensing agreements can be complex due to varying patent laws
Cold chain and distribution regulations	Regulatory requirements for vaccine storage, transport, and distribution are critical, especially for vaccines that require cold chain management. Non-compliance risks reducing vaccine efficacy and delaying access
Data transparency standards	Ensuring transparency in reporting trial data, including both positive and negative results, is a regulatory priority. Variations in transparency standards across countries can hinder uniform reporting and public trust
Adapting to new vaccine technologies	Regulatory systems must evolve to accommodate novel vaccine platforms (e.g., mRNA, viral vectors), which may not align with traditional approval pathways. Updating guidelines without compromising safety is a regulatory challenge
Coordinated oversight of trial phases	Regulatory agencies must monitor vaccine trials across all phases (I-IV) to ensure safety and efficacy. Coordinating oversight and ensuring consistency across phases, sponsors, and trial sites presents a significant challenge
Emergency use authorizations (EUA)	Issuing EUAs allows for early distribution of vaccines before full regulatory approval. While beneficial in emergencies, it raises concerns about the adequacy of safety and efficacy data under fast-tracked approvals

(continued)

Table 19.26 (continued)

Regulatory challenge(s)	Description
Harmonization of international guidelines	Efforts to standardize regulatory guidelines through international bodies (e.g., WHO, ICH) face challenges due to differences in national regulatory priorities and processes, leading to fragmentation and delays in global vaccine access
Capacity for timely reviews	Regulatory agencies, particularly in low-resource countries, often lack sufficient capacity for timely and thorough review of vaccine applications, contributing to significant delays in vaccine approval and distribution
Compensation and liability mechanisms	Developing clear and consistent frameworks for compensating participants in the event of vaccine-related harm is essential, but varying national policies make it difficult to implement uniform standards for global trials
Regulatory approvals for booster shots	The emergence of new viral variants requires updating vaccines or introducing booster shots. Ensuring that these updates undergo adequate testing while preventing delays in access presents a complex regulatory challenge
Trials in special populations	Regulatory agencies often mandate bridging trials for special populations (e.g., elderly, pregnant women, immunocompromised) to ensure vaccine safety and efficacy, which adds time and complexity to the approval process
Navigating political and public pressure	During public health emergencies, regulators face intense political and societal pressure to expedite vaccine approvals. Balancing scientific rigor with the need for timely solutions is a key regulatory challenge
Complex pharmacovigilance systems	Implementing robust pharmacovigilance systems to track adverse events during and after trials is vital. Inadequate systems or under-reporting can delay the identification of safety issues, complicating regulatory oversight

Comparison of vaccine clinical trials with regulatory approval process in different countries is highlighted in Table 19.27.

Good laboratory practices (GLP) in vaccine clinical trials are highlighted in Table 19.28.

19.10 Special Considerations in Vaccine Clinical Trials

19.10.1 Vaccine Efficacy Vs. Effectiveness

- **Efficacy:** Efficacy is defined as the performance of a vaccine under the controlled environment of a clinical trial. It gives a measure of the reduction in disease incidence among vaccinated participants compared to unvaccinated ones, under ideal conditions.
- **Effectiveness:** Effectiveness regards the performance of the vaccine in the field, where a number of factors, including heterogeneity in the population being vac-

Table 19.27 Comparison of vaccine clinical trials with regulatory approval process in different countries

Description	United States (FDA)	European Union (EMA)	India (CDSCO)	China (NMPA)	Japan (PMDA)
CT phases	Phases 0, I, II, III, IV	Phases 0, I, II, III, IV	Phases I, II, III, IV	Phases I, II, III, IV	Phases I, II, III, IV
Regulatory authority	Food and Drug Administration (FDA)	European medicines agency (EMA)	Central drugs standard control organization (CDSCO)	National Medical Products Administration (NMPA)	Pharmaceuticals and medical devices agency (PMDA)
Pre-clinical testing	Extensive animal studies required	Extensive animal studies required	Extensive animal studies required	Extensive animal studies required	Extensive animal studies required
Application for clinical trials	Investigational new drug (IND) application	Clinical trial application (CTA)	Clinical trial notification (CTN)	Investigational new drug (IND) application	Investigational new drug (IND) application
Review time for initial application	Approximately 6 months	Approximately 1–2 months	Approximately 2–3 months	Approximately 6–12 months	Approximately 6 months
Data safety oversight	Data safety monitoring board (DSMB) required	Data safety monitoring board or equivalent required	Data safety monitoring board or equivalent required	Data safety monitoring board or equivalent required	Data safety monitoring board or equivalent required
Phase III trial requirements	Large, diverse participant groups needed	Large, diverse participant groups needed	Large, diverse participant groups needed	Large, diverse participant groups needed	Large, diverse participant groups needed
Approval pathways	Standard and expedited pathways available	Standard and expedited pathways available	Standard and fast-track pathways available	Standard and fast-track pathways available	Standard and expedited pathways available
Post-marketing surveillance	Extensive monitoring and reporting required	Extensive monitoring and reporting required	Post-marketing studies and adverse event reporting required	Post-marketing studies and adverse event reporting required	Post-marketing studies and adverse event reporting required
Emergency use authorization	Available for public health emergencies	Available for public health emergencies	Available for public health emergencies	Available for public health emergencies	Available for public health emergencies

Table 19.28 Good laboratory practices (GLP) in vaccine clinical trials

GLP element(s)	Description
Laboratory environment	Maintain laboratory facilities to be clean, organized, and designed to prevent contamination, ensuring a controlled environment for testing
Equipment calibration and maintenance	Regularly calibrate and service laboratory equipment to ensure precision and accuracy in test results
Standard operating procedures (SOPs)	Develop and adhere to comprehensive SOPs for all laboratory processes to guarantee consistency and reliability in testing procedures
Staff training and competency	Provide extensive training for laboratory staff on GLP principles, proper equipment use, and safety protocols to ensure competency
Sample handling and storage	Implement robust procedures for the handling, labelling, and storage of samples to maintain their integrity and ensure proper traceability
Data accuracy and integrity	Keep meticulous records of all laboratory work, including test results and observations, to uphold data accuracy and integrity
Quality assurance	Regularly perform quality assurance checks to verify the accuracy and consistency of laboratory results and processes
Safety measures	Follow stringent safety protocols to protect laboratory personnel and prevent contamination or accidents
Equipment servicing	Conduct routine maintenance and inspections of laboratory equipment to ensure optimal functioning
Compliance and audits	Perform regular audits and inspections to ensure adherence to GLP standards and to identify and address any areas needing improvement
Documentation and reporting	Document all laboratory procedures, results, and deviations comprehensively and report them as required by regulatory standards

cinated, differences in storage and administration of the vaccine, adherence to vaccination regimens, affect the outcomes. In general, post-marketing studies or Phase IV trials are designed to measure vaccine effectiveness.

19.10.2 Correlates of Protection

- **Definition:** The correlates of protection involve specific immune responses, such as levels of certain antibodies that must statistically correlate with resistance against infection or disease. Since identification of such a correlate would be important in the manufacture and also in the prediction of long-term efficacy regarding the vaccine, the identification of the correlates of protection is an integral part of vaccine development.
- **Challenges:** Establishment of correlates of protection may broadly be problematic, especially for new pathogens for which the immune response is inadequately recognized. Trials may need to be designed with comprehensive immunological assessments to identify such a correlate.

19.10.3 Herd Immunity and Population-Level Effects

- **Herd Immunity:** A situation wherein the required percentage of the population would have achieved immunity through vaccination or previous infection to a particular disease; hence, reducing the chances of the spread of ailments. The concept of herd immunity should also be considered while researching vaccine trials because of its outcomes.
- **Population-Level Effects:** Apart from providing individual protection, vaccination can have strong effects at the population level, including a reduction in the transmission rate of disease and protection of vulnerable populations. These more general effects are usually considered during post-marketing studies.

19.10.4 Vaccine Adverse Events and Safety Monitoring

- **Adverse Events:** Vaccine trials must monitor adverse events, which have been defined as any undesired health consequence subsequent to vaccination. Thus, anything from injection site soreness to anaphylactic reactions constitutes an adverse event.
- **Safety Monitoring:** The safety monitoring is followed in all the phases of clinical trials, which are even extended to post-marketing surveillance; it will include DSMBs and enhanced reporting systems such as VAERS in the United States.
- **Risk Communication:** Building public trust requires open and transparent communication about the benefits and risks of vaccines, including clear information about potential adverse events and processes put in place to manage them.

Classification of AEFI in vaccine clinical trials has been highlighted in Table 19.29.

Definition of common terms in adverse event following immunization (AEFI) is highlighted in Table 19.30.

Safety surveillance timelines in vaccine clinical trials are highlighted in Table 19.31.

Table 19.29 Classification of AEFI in vaccine clinical trials

Classification	Description
Vaccine product-related reaction	Adverse event caused or precipitated by the inherent properties of the vaccine product.
Vaccine quality defect-related reaction	Adverse event caused by a quality defect of the vaccine product, including its administration device.
Immunization error-related reaction	Adverse event caused by inappropriate vaccine handling, prescribing, or administration.
Immunization anxiety-related reaction	Adverse event arising from anxiety about the immunization itself, rather than the vaccine or its administration.
Coincidental event	Adverse event caused by something other than the vaccine product, immunization error, or anxiety about the immunization.

Table 19.30 Definition of common terms in adverse event following immunization (AEFI)

	Incidence	No. of cases with doses
AEFI	Very common	1:10
	Common	1:10–100
	Uncommon	1:100–1000
	Rare	1:1000–10,000
	Very rare	< 1:10,000

Table 19.31 Safety surveillance timelines in vaccine clinical trials

Adverse event following immunization (AEFI)	Minimum surveillance days after last dose of vaccine
Solicited local and systemic 'adverse events'	7 days
Unsolicited 'adverse events'	21–28 days
Serious 'adverse events'	180 days

Special considerations in vaccine clinical trials are highlighted in Table 19.32.

19.11 Special Considerations in Pandemic Vaccine Trials

19.11.1 Accelerated Development Timelines

- **Challenges of Rapid Development:** The urgency for the response to pandemics means that vaccine development timelines have to be condensed radically-from years to a couple of months. Sometimes, the rapidity of this pace makes proper evaluation of safety and efficacy quite hard.
- **Regulatory Flexibility:** Accelerated approval pathways might, in principle, be allowed by regulatory bodies in the case of pandemics in order to guarantee timely vaccine availability. Examples include emergency use authorizations that can expedite access while maintaining essential safety and efficacy standards.

19.11.2 Global Collaboration and Data Sharing

- **International Partnerships:** Organizations like the Coalition for Epidemic Preparedness Innovations, popularly known as CEPI, and COVAX support cooperative global activities in the development and distribution of vaccines, especially to assist low- and middle-income countries.
- **Data Sharing Initiatives:** Sharing data between researchers, regulators, and public health agencies needs to occur quickly and should be an integral part of accelerating trials of vaccines and dealing with the new challenges emerging effectively during pandemics.

Table 19.32 Special considerations in vaccine clinical trials

Consideration(s)	Description
Trial design	Develop a well-structured trial with control groups, randomization, and blinding to ensure robust, unbiased results
Participant criteria	Select participants carefully based on demographics, health status, and exposure risks to ensure the sample is representative and relevant
Vaccine formulation	Conduct thorough testing of the vaccine formulation for stability, efficacy, and safety before use in clinical trials
Dosage and administration	Determine and standardize the vaccine dose and administration schedule, including any need for booster doses, to optimize effectiveness
Safety monitoring	Establish comprehensive monitoring systems to track, document, and report adverse events for timely intervention and safety assessment
Long-term follow-up	Plan for extended follow-up to assess the long-term safety and effectiveness of the vaccine, including potential late-onset effects
Regulatory adherence	Ensure compliance with all relevant regulatory guidelines and requirements throughout the trial process
Ethical practices	Uphold ethical standards by obtaining informed consent, ensuring a favorable risk-benefit ratio, and protecting participant rights
Manufacturing quality	Follow good manufacturing practices (GMP) to ensure the vaccine is produced consistently and without contamination
Quality assurance	Implement stringent quality assurance measures to verify data accuracy and vaccine performance throughout the trial
Storage and handling	Adhere to specific storage and handling protocols to preserve vaccine potency and prevent degradation
Efficacy assessment	Use appropriate methods to evaluate the vaccine's efficacy, including measuring immune responses and protection against the target disease
Data integrity	Maintain rigorous data management practices to ensure accurate and reliable data collection, analysis, and reporting
Community outreach	Engage with community stakeholders to address concerns, provide information, and encourage participation in the trial
Impact assessment	Assess the potential public health impact of the vaccine, including its role in vaccination programs and overall health policy

19.11.3 Addressing Variant Strains

- **Impact of Variants on Vaccine Efficacy:** The emergence of viral variants, as evidenced during the COVID-19 pandemic, can affect vaccine efficacy. Thus, trials need to be adapted quickly to assess how well the vaccines work against these new strains.
- **Booster Doses and Variant-Specific Vaccines:** Delivery of booster doses or development of vaccines targeting variants could be pursued in studies that aim at improving protection against emerging viral strains.

19.12 Challenges and Innovations in Vaccine Clinical Trials

19.12.1 Rapid Vaccine Development During Pandemics

- **Pandemic Response:** The advent of pandemics, more precisely COVID-19, has ushered in races for vaccine development. The timeline, which often takes 10 to 15 years, is hugely compressed in pandemic cases through accelerated phases of trials and regulation procedures.
- **Innovative Approaches:** Platform technologies such as mRNA vaccines, novel designs of clinical trials, for example, adaptive designs, and international collaboration have greatly facilitated the rapid development, manufacturing, and deployment of vaccines in response to health crises. At the same time, these techniques also introduce new challenges with respect to vaccine safety and public confidence.

19.12.2 Vaccine Hesitancy and Public Perception

- **Vaccine Hesitancy:** The hesitation or refusal to receive the vaccines despite their availability is a real challenge to the initiatives of public health. The clinical trials should help overcome public apprehensions and misinformation in order to encourage vaccinations.
- **Community Engagement:** Trust is apt to build when communities are involved in the trial process-from design to execution-and critically address cultural and social influences for vaccine hesitancy.

19.12.3 Global Vaccine Equity

- **Access to Vaccines:** Equitable access to vaccines remains one of the important challenges to global health. Clinical trials need to be carried out with larger, more diverse populations that represent LMICs to confirm vaccine efficacy and its accessibility in a global sense.
- **Capacity Building:** A substantial infrastructure for clinical trials, along with enhanced research capacity in LMICs, is required to conduct permissible, high-quality studies on vaccines in those regions. Such an initiative would include training of local researchers, establishment or strengthening of ethical review boards, and investment in trial sites.

19.12.4 Adaptive Trial Designs

- **Definition:** Adaptive designs give an advantage of changing the trial protocol based on interim results with adherence to overall integrity of the study. These

designs have especial benefits in vaccine trials at which time new data can arise quite quickly.
- **Advantages:** Adaptive designs can speed up vaccine candidates' testing process by allowing flexibility and efficiency within the trial, which will reduce the tension of time and other resource spendings. What is more important, though, is that for prevention of bias and being in a position to guarantee validity in a trial, proper planning and regulatory monitoring will be required.

19.12.5 Use of Real-World Data and Digital Technologies

- **Real-World Data (RWD):** Real-world data (RWD), through the data gathered from EHRs, for example, adds to these theoretically derived results from clinical trials to include real-world experiences with the safety and performance of vaccines in a very diverse population.
- **Digital Technologies:** Digital technologies, mobile health applications, and wearable devices could be harnessed to extend data collection and monitoring in vaccine trials. These provide possibilities for remote participation, which would further enhance the accessibility and diversity of such trials.

Common challenges encountered in vaccine clinical trials are highlighted in Table 19.33.

A list of innovations in vaccine clinical trials are highlighted in Table 19.34.

Future challenges in vaccine clinical trials are highlighted in Table 19.35.

19.13 Future Directions in Vaccine Clinical Trials

Vaccine clinical trials represent a fast-evolving area, since several technologies and methodologies on the horizon are very likely to radically change the face of current vaccine clinical trials.

Future directions in vaccine clinical trials are highlighted in Table 19.36.

19.13.1 Personalized Vaccinology

- **Definition:** Personalized vaccinology can be defined as a form of vaccinology tailored to fit the characteristics of the person, possibly genetically determined or based on age and condition of the body, among other factors, that could contribute to high efficacy with safety.
- **Potential:** Advances in genomics, immunology, and data analytics are increasingly enabling the creation of personalized vaccines with improved and more specific protection. Clinical trials for these new customized technologies will also need to be reinvented.

Table 19.33 Common challenges encountered in vaccine clinical trials

Challenge(s)	Description
Participant recruitment	Enrolling a diverse and representative participant pool remains difficult, and maintaining their engagement throughout the lengthy trial period poses further challenges
Ethical considerations	Balancing the need for informed consent, especially in placebo-controlled trials, while protecting vulnerable groups such as children, pregnant women, and the elderly is complex
Long-term safety monitoring	Assessing long-term safety and efficacy of vaccines requires extended follow-up, making it hard to detect rare or delayed adverse effects within a limited trial timeframe
Variability in immune response	Individual factors like age, sex, genetic background, and pre-existing conditions can lead to varying immune responses, complicating the evaluation of vaccine performance
Regulatory compliance	Navigating different regulatory requirements across multiple regions can delay trials and increase operational costs due to varying standards and approval timelines
Logistical and operational complexities	Coordinating multi-center trials, ensuring the cold chain for vaccine storage, and maintaining standardized data collection are critical operational challenges
Vaccine hesitancy and mistrust	Public hesitation or mistrust of vaccines can lead to low participation rates in clinical trials, affecting sample sizes and prolonging the study's duration
Placebo control dilemma	Using placebo groups in trials, particularly during pandemics or for serious conditions, raises ethical concerns when effective treatments or vaccines already exist
Financial constraints	Vaccine trials are financially demanding, with high costs for recruitment, monitoring, and long-term follow-up, often dependent on government or industry funding
Viral variants and mutations	The emergence of new viral strains can reduce the efficacy of vaccines developed for earlier variants, complicating ongoing trials and their relevance to future strains
Vaccine storage stability	Maintaining the required temperature and storage conditions for certain vaccines, particularly mRNA-based ones, poses logistical hurdles during trials and distribution
Special population considerations	Trials must account for safety and efficacy in special groups, such as those with compromised immune systems or chronic health conditions, which adds layers of complexity
Data integrity and monitoring	Ensuring high-quality data collection and monitoring for real-time reporting of adverse events is essential for the validity of trial outcomes
Global access and equity	Ensuring that populations in low-resource settings have access to vaccine trials and eventual vaccines presents both logistical and ethical challenges
Adverse event management	Tracking, reporting, and managing adverse events, including rare but serious side effects, requires a comprehensive safety monitoring framework throughout the trial process

Table 19.34 List of innovations in vaccine clinical trials

Innovation(s)	Description	Impact
Adaptive trial designs	Study designs that can be adjusted based on interim results, allowing for real-time modifications	Increases efficiency and allows for flexible response to data
Digital health technologies	Utilization of mobile applications, wearable technology, and electronic health records for participant monitoring	Enhances data collection and enables continuous monitoring
Integration of real-world evidence (RWE)	Incorporating data from everyday clinical settings to complement findings from controlled trials	Provides insights into vaccine performance across various populations
Biomarker-based trials	Trials that utilize biological markers to select participants and predict responses to vaccines	Allows for a more tailored approach and targeted interventions
Machine learning and AI applications	Use of artificial intelligence to analyze trial data, forecast outcomes, and refine trial protocols	Improves data analysis precision and accelerates decision-making
Advanced statistical techniques	Implementation of sophisticated statistical methods for a more reliable interpretation of trial results	Enhances the accuracy and robustness of data analysis
Decentralized clinical trials	Trials conducted remotely using digital tools, reducing the need for physical site visits	Increases participant accessibility and convenience
Human challenge trials	Studies where participants are intentionally exposed to pathogens to evaluate vaccine effectiveness	Speeds up the assessment of vaccine efficacy and safety
Dynamic dose adjustment	Flexible dosing strategies that adjust based on ongoing trial results	Optimizes therapeutic dosing and minimizes adverse reactions
Global multi-regional trials	Trials conducted across various regions to assess vaccine effectiveness and safety on an international scale	Broadens the applicability and safety profile of vaccines

19.13.2 Next-Generation Vaccine Platforms

- **mRNA Vaccines:** mRNA vaccines have proven their potential for rapid vaccine development in the current COVID-19 pandemic. Trials are underway for using mRNA technology against a variety of diseases, including cancer, influenza, and autoimmune disorders.
- **Viral Vectors:** Viral vector vaccines rely on the use of an adapted virus to deliver genetic material from the target pathogen. These are under investigation for new applications. Investigations into clinical trials also study its application in combination with other vaccine platforms to enhance immune responses.
- **Combination Vaccines:** Remarkable research is ongoing to combine vaccines that protect against many diseases in a single formulation to facilitate and improve vaccination schedules and coverage.

Table 19.35 Future challenges in vaccine clinical trials

Challenge(s)	Description	Potential impact
Public vaccine hesitancy	Addressing doubts and misinformation about vaccines to improve public acceptance	Can affect vaccine uptake and public health outcomes
Novel pathogens	Creating vaccines for new or poorly understood pathogens with limited initial data	Demands rapid innovation and flexible development
Equitable access	Ensuring vaccines are available to all populations, especially in under-resourced areas	May lead to inequalities in vaccine distribution and effectiveness
Long-term monitoring	Continuously assessing the safety and effectiveness of vaccines after they are approved	Requires sustained research and surveillance efforts
Regulatory and ethical issues	Navigating complex regulatory standards and ethical dilemmas in vaccine research	Could slow down the approval and deployment of vaccines
Adoption of advanced technologies	Integrating cutting-edge technologies such as gene editing into vaccine development	Requires updating regulatory practices and methodologies
Data protection	Protecting sensitive data collected during trials, especially with increasing digital tools	Ensures compliance with privacy regulations and safeguards participant information
Production scalability	Scaling up production processes to meet global demand while ensuring quality control	Presents challenges in manufacturing and distribution logistics
Handling variants	Adapting vaccines to address new variants and mutations of pathogens	Necessitates ongoing adjustments to vaccine formulations
Cost management	Balancing the high costs of vaccine development and distribution with funding and resource allocation	Affects the affordability and accessibility of vaccines
Inclusive clinical trials	Ensuring that trials include diverse populations to accurately assess vaccine efficacy and safety	Improves the generalizability of trial results across different groups
Supply chain coordination	Managing the complex global supply chain to ensure efficient vaccine distribution and minimize waste	Challenges in logistics and timely delivery
Healthcare system support	Strengthening healthcare infrastructure to support widespread vaccination efforts	Requires additional resources and planning to handle large-scale distribution
Managing side effects	Monitoring and addressing any rare or unexpected side effects that arise from vaccines	Involves robust safety monitoring and response mechanisms
Effective communication	Developing strategies to effectively communicate the benefits and safety of vaccines to the public	Influences public perception and willingness to get vaccinated

Table 19.36 Future directions in vaccine clinical trials

Future direction(s)	Description	Potential benefits
Tailored vaccines	Creating vaccines customized based on individual genetic information or specific health risks	Enhanced effectiveness and minimized side effects
Multi-pathogen vaccines	Developing vaccines that offer protection against several pathogens or their variants simultaneously	Streamlined vaccination processes and broader protection
Nanotechnology applications	Leveraging nanotechnology to improve vaccine delivery systems and enhance immune responses	More precise targeting and potentially increased effectiveness
Genetic vaccine platforms	Advancing the use of mRNA and DNA technologies for faster and more adaptable vaccine development	Quick response to emerging pathogens and flexible vaccine design
Innovative adjuvants	Researching new adjuvants to boost vaccine-induced immune responses and prolong protection	Enhanced vaccine potency and durability
Extended-release vaccines	Designing vaccines with extended release mechanisms to reduce the frequency of booster doses	Simplified vaccination regimens and improved adherence
Broad-Spectrum vaccines	Developing vaccines that provide extensive protection against various strains or related pathogens	Reduced impact of pathogen evolution and greater long-term efficacy
Microbiome-based approaches	Investigating how the microbiome influences vaccine responses and creating vaccines that target microbiome-related factors	Personalized vaccine strategies based on microbiome profiles
Integration of real-world data	Using data from everyday clinical settings to complement and enhance clinical trial findings	Better insight into vaccine effectiveness and safety in diverse populations
Advanced delivery methods	Exploring new methods for vaccine administration, such as oral or patch-based systems	Increased convenience and potential for higher patient compliance
Innovative trial designs	Applying new trial designs, such as adaptive and platform trials, to accelerate vaccine evaluation	More efficient and adaptable vaccine testing processes
Global collaboration	Building stronger international partnerships to share data and resources for vaccine development	Accelerated vaccine research and equitable global access
Updating ethical and regulatory practices	Revising ethical guidelines and regulatory procedures to address modern challenges in vaccine trials.	Streamlined approval processes and adherence to current ethical standards
Predictive analytics	Employing sophisticated modelling and simulation techniques to forecast vaccine performance and guide trial design	More accurate predictions and optimized trial planning
Enhanced public communication	Improving strategies for public education and engagement regarding vaccine benefits and safety	Increased public trust and higher vaccination rates

19.13.3 Universal Vaccines

- **Objective:** The ultimate aim of universal vaccines is to provide variety protection against diverse strains or variants of a pathogen. For instance, the entire group of universal influenza vaccines aims at protection against all strains of flu.
- **Challenges:** Development of universal vaccines is facilitated by deep understanding regarding the process of pathogen evolution and the immune response of an organism. Clinical trials need, therefore, to be conceptualized and constructed in a manner that they can establish the efficacy of vaccines developed against a variety of strains and populations.

19.13.4 Artificial Intelligence (AI) and Machine Learning (ML)

- **AI in Trial Design:** AI and ML are now increasingly being used to optimize the design of clinical trials. Such tools help in predicting the responses of patients and determining suitable geographical areas for the construction of trials. These technologies speed up vaccine tests and also raise their accuracy bar.
- **Data Analysis:** AI and ML are also applied to analyze vast volumes of data from vaccine trials that may remain obscure using traditional methods of analysis.

19.13.5 Regulatory Evolution and Global Standards

- **Adapting to New Technologies**: The regulatory frameworks must change to accommodate more modern technologies, like mRNA and gene-based vaccines, appropriate to the level of safety and efficacy.
- **Global Standards Harmonization:** Indeed, such harmonization on various regulatory standards within various countries would extend greater international cooperation in vaccine trials and facilitate the processes for faster approvals, hence making new vaccines more accessible.

SWOT analysis of vaccine clinical trials is presented in Table 19.37.

19.14 Conclusion

Vaccine clinical trials are absolutely indispensable in ensuring not only that vaccines are safe and effective but also accessible on a global scale. Complexity in these trials requires the highest degree of scientific and ethical standards, by way of comprehensive regulatory oversight to innovative strategy in the meeting of new challenges. As vaccinology continues to evolve, the role of clinical trials will always be central to improvement in public health and protection against infectious diseases. The future of vaccine clinical trials seems brilliant, with the emerging technologies and methodologies just waiting in the wings to transform vaccine

Table 19.37 SWOT analysis of vaccine clinical trials

Particulars	Strengths	Weaknesses	Opportunities	Threats
Scientific advancements	Cutting-edge technologies and innovative methodologies accelerate vaccine development	Complexity of new technologies can extend development timelines	Accelerated responses to emerging diseases through advanced scientific approaches	Rapid advancements may outpace existing regulatory frameworks
Regulatory framework	Established guidelines and frameworks facilitate vaccine approval processes	Regulatory procedures can be lengthy and cumbersome	Potential for streamlined or adaptive regulatory pathways to expedite approvals	Stringent regulations may create delays in vaccine availability
Data collection	Comprehensive methods provide detailed insights into vaccine efficacy and safety	Managing and analyzing extensive data can be resource-intensive	Integration of real-world evidence enhances understanding of vaccine performance across diverse populations	Data privacy issues and cybersecurity threats may arise
Public health impact	Potential to significantly reduce disease burden and prevent outbreaks	Public skepticism and vaccine hesitancy may undermine vaccination efforts	Opportunity to improve global health outcomes and address pressing public health issues	Misinformation and communication challenges can erode public trust
Global collaboration	International partnerships enhance resource sharing and accelerate development	Coordinating across multiple countries can be complex	Enhanced global access to vaccines through collaborative networks and shared resources	Geopolitical tensions may disrupt collaborative efforts
Cost and funding	Availability of funding from various sources supports research and development	High costs associated with vaccine development and clinical trials	Potential for new funding mechanisms and innovative financial strategies	Economic fluctuations could impact funding availability and resources

(continued)

Table 19.37 (continued)

Particulars	Strengths	Weaknesses	Opportunities	Threats
Trial design	Adaptive and flexible trial designs improve efficiency and responsiveness	Complexity in designing trials to meet both regulatory standards and scientific goals	Adoption of innovative trial designs can expedite the evaluation of vaccine candidates	Design challenges or unforeseen issues may affect trial outcomes
Ethical considerations	Strong ethical standards ensure participant safety and integrity of research	Ethical dilemmas may arise in certain trial scenarios	Opportunity to advance ethical practices and enhance transparency in clinical research	Ethical concerns in novel or complex trials may arise
Manufacturing capability	Advanced technologies enable large-scale vaccine production	Scaling production while ensuring quality can be challenging	Potential for improved manufacturing processes to meet global demand efficiently	Production issues or quality control problems may affect vaccine availability
Post-market surveillance	Robust systems for monitoring vaccine safety and effectiveness after approval	Long-term safety and rare adverse reactions may be difficult to detect initially	Opportunity to gather real-world data to refine and improve vaccine use over time	Unanticipated long-term effects could pose risks to public health
Participant recruitment	Broad interest in vaccines enhances recruitment opportunities	Recruitment challenges, including ensuring diverse participation, can impact trial results	Enhanced strategies for recruitment and engagement can improve trial outcomes	Difficulties in recruitment may delay trials and affect data quality
Vaccine development speed	Ability to rapidly develop vaccines for urgent public health needs	Accelerated development may compromise thorough safety assessments	Potential to implement rapid-response frameworks for future outbreaks and health crises	The pressure for quick development might overlook some safety concerns
Innovation in delivery methods	New vaccine delivery methods, such as needle-free options, offer potential benefits	Novel delivery systems may face regulatory approval and validation hurdles	Opportunities for improved administration methods and increased patient compliance	Acceptance and standardization of new delivery methods may face challenges

(continued)

Table 19.37 (continued)

Particulars	Strengths	Weaknesses	Opportunities	Threats
Public engagement	Opportunities to improve public understanding and support for vaccination through education	Public misinformation and misunderstandings can impede engagement efforts	Potential to strengthen public trust and increase vaccine uptake through effective communication	Communication breakdowns may lead to decreased vaccine acceptance and uptake
Global Health impact	Potential to greatly reduce the global disease burden and improve health outcomes worldwide	Variability in healthcare infrastructure and access may limit the overall impact	Opportunity to address global health disparities and promote health equity through vaccination	Inconsistent vaccine access could exacerbate existing health inequalities

development, testing, and distribution processes. Given continuous collaboration, innovation, and adherence to ethical principles, many more highly effective milestones could well be achieved in the field against infectious diseases.

Bibliography and Further Reading

Aqib AI, Anjum AA, Islam MA, Murtaza A, Rehman AU (2023) Recent global trends in vaccinology, advances and challenges. Vaccines (Basel) 11(3):520. https://doi.org/10.3390/vaccines11030520. PMID: 36992104; PMCID: PMC10053289

Centers for Disease Control and Prevention (CDC) (2024) How vaccines are developed and approved for use. [Online]. [cited 2024 March 18]. https://www.cdc.gov/vaccines/basics/test-approve.html

Central Drugs Standard Control Organization (CDSCO) (2024) Draft regulatory guidelines for development of vaccines with special consideration for COVID-19 vaccine. [Online]. [cited 2024 March 18]. https://cdsco.gov.in/opencms/resources/UploadCDSCOWeb/2018/UploadPublic_NoticesFiles/Regulatory_guidelines_for__development_of_Vaccine_20.9.20.pdf

Cunningham AL, Garçon N, Leo O, Friedland LR, Strugnell R, Laupèze B, Doherty M, Stern P (2016) Vaccine development: from concept to early clinical testing. Vaccine 34(52):6655–6664. https://doi.org/10.1016/j.vaccine.2016.10.016. Epub 2016 Oct 18. PMID: 27769596

Deutsche Gesellschaft Für Regulatory Affairs (DGRA) (2024) Overview of the regulatory environment for developing new vaccines including the specific smallpox vaccine and pandemic influenza virus vaccines. [Online]. [cited 2024 March 18]. https://www.dgra.de/media/pdf/studium/masterthesis/master_kaletta_c.pdf

Di Pasquale A, Bonanni P, Garçon N, Stanberry LR, El-Hodhod M, Tavares Da Silva F (2016) Vaccine safety evaluation: practical aspects in assessing benefits and risks. Vaccine 34(52):6672–6680. https://doi.org/10.1016/j.vaccine.2016.10.039. Epub 2016 Nov 8. PMID: 27836435

Doherty M, Buchy P, Standaert B, Giaquinto C, Prado-Cohrs D (2016) Vaccine impact: benefits for human health. Vaccine 34(52):6707–6714. https://doi.org/10.1016/j.vaccine.2016.10.025. Epub 2016 Oct 20. PMID: 27773475

European Medicines Agency (2024) Clinical evaluation of new vaccines -scientific guideline –2023. [Online]. [cited 2023 August 1]. https://www.ema.europa.eu/en/clinical-evaluation-new-vaccines-scientific-guideline#current-version-effective-from-01082023-8042

Excler JL, Saville M, Berkley S, Kim JH (2021) Vaccine development for emerging infectious diseases. Nat Med 27(4):591–600. https://doi.org/10.1038/s41591-021-01301-0. Epub 2021 Apr 12. PMID: 33846611

Goetz KB, Pfleiderer M, Schneider CK (2010) First-in-human clinical trials with vaccines-what regulators want. Nat Biotechnol 28(9):910–916. https://doi.org/10.1038/nbt0910-910. PMID: 20829825; PMCID: PMC7096781

Han S (2015) Clinical vaccine development. Clin Exp Vaccine Res 4(1):46–53. https://doi.org/10.7774/cevr.2015.4.1.46. Epub 2015 Jan 30. PMID: 25648742; PMCID: PMC4313108

Hoos A, Parmiani G, Hege K, Sznol M, Loibner H, Eggermont A, Urba W, Blumenstein B, Sacks N, Keilholz U, Nichol G, Cancer Vaccine Clinical Trial Working Group (2007) A clinical development paradigm for cancer vaccines and related biologics. J Immunother 30(1):1–15. https://doi.org/10.1097/01.cji.0000211341.88835.ae. PMID: 17198079

International Council for Harmonisation of Technical Requirements for Pharmaceuticals for Human Use (ICH) (2024) Efficacy guidelines. [Online]. [cited 2024 March 18]. https://www.ich.org/page/efficacy-guidelines

Iwasaki A, Omer SB (2020) Why and how vaccines work. Cell 183(2):290–295. https://doi.org/10.1016/j.cell.2020.09.040. PMID: 33064982; PMCID: PMC7560117

Kalinke U, Barouch DH, Rizzi R, Lagkadinou E, Türeci Ö, Pather S, Neels P (2022) Clinical development and approval of COVID-19 vaccines. Expert Rev Vaccines 21(5):609–619. https://doi.org/10.1080/14760584.2022.2042257. Epub 2022 Mar 14. PMID: 35157542; PMCID: PMC8935460

Kallon S, Samir S, Goonetilleke N (2021) Vaccines: underlying principles of design and testing. Clin Pharmacol Ther 109(4):987–999. https://doi.org/10.1002/cpt.2207. Epub 2021 Mar 11. PMID: 33705574; PMCID: PMC8048882

Kennedy RB, Ovsyannikova IG, Palese P, Poland GA (2020) Current challenges in vaccinology. Front Immunol 11:1181. https://doi.org/10.3389/fimmu.2020.01181. PMID: 32670279; PMCID: PMC7329983

Koff WC, Burton DR, Johnson PR, Walker BD, King CR, Nabel GJ, Ahmed R, Bhan MK, Plotkin SA (2013) Accelerating next-generation vaccine development for global disease prevention. Science 340(6136):1232910. https://doi.org/10.1126/science.1232910. PMID: 23723240; PMCID: PMC4026248

Liu M, Li Q, Lin J, Lin Y, Hoffman E (2021) Innovative trial designs and analyses for vaccine clinical development. Contemp Clin Trials 100:106225. https://doi.org/10.1016/j.cct.2020.106225. Epub 2020 Nov 21. PMID: 33227451; PMCID: PMC7834363

Lopalco PL, DeStefano F (2015) The complementary roles of phase 3 trials and post-licensure surveillance in the evaluation of new vaccines. Vaccine 33(13):1541–1548. https://doi.org/10.1016/j.vaccine.2014.10.047. Epub 2014 Nov 4. PMID: 25444788; PMCID: PMC4596394

Ministry of Health & Family Welfare, Government of India (MoHFW, GoI) (2020) COVID -19 vaccines: operational guidelines. [Online]. [cited 2024 March 18]. https://www.mohfw.gov.in/pdf/COVID19VaccineOG111Chapter16.pdf

Plotkin SA (2022) Why we need precision vaccinology. Clin Infect Dis 75(Suppl 1):S2–S4. https://doi.org/10.1093/cid/ciac434. PMID: 35738254; PMCID: PMC9376268

Poland GA, Whitaker JA, Poland CM, Ovsyannikova IG, Kennedy RB (2016) Vaccinology in the third millennium: scientific and social challenges. Curr Opin Virol 17:116–125. https://doi.org/10.1016/j.coviro.2016.03.003. Epub 2016 Mar 30. PMID: 27039875; PMCID: PMC4902778

Pollard AJ, Bijker EM (2021) A guide to vaccinology: from basic principles to new developments. Nat Rev Immunol 21(2):83–100. https://doi.org/10.1038/s41577-020-00479-7. Epub 2020 Dec 22. Erratum in: Nat Rev Immunol. 2021 Jan 5;: PMID: 33353987; PMCID: PMC7754704

Preiss S, Garçon N, Cunningham AL, Strugnell R, Friedland LR (2016) Vaccine provision: delivering sustained & widespread use. Vaccine 34(52):6665–6671. https://doi.org/10.1016/j.vaccine.2016.10.079. Epub 2016 Nov 22. PMID: 27884478

Ranga C, Naved T, Thakkar A (2024) Regulatory pathway for the approval of novel candidate vaccine. Int J Pharm Invest 14(2):504–508

Sathyanarayana SD, Fernandes SD, Castelino LJ, Vadakkepushpakath AN, Shriram RG (2020) Vaccines in the United States: a systematic review on history of evolution, regulations, licensing, and future challenges. Clin Exp Vaccine Res 9(2):69–75. https://doi.org/10.7774/cevr.2020.9.2.69. Epub 2020 Jul 31. PMID: 32864362; PMCID: PMC7445324

Serruto D, Rappuoli R (2006) Post-genomic vaccine development. FEBS Lett 580(12):2985–2992. https://doi.org/10.1016/j.febslet.2006.04.084. Epub 2006 May 4. PMID: 16716781

Singh K, Mehta S (2016) The clinical development process for a novel preventive vaccine: an overview. J Postgrad Med 62(1):4–11. https://doi.org/10.4103/0022-3859.173187. PMID: 26732191; PMCID: PMC4944327

Søborg C, Mølbak K, Doherty TM, Ulleryd P, Brooks T, Coenen C, van der Zeijst B (2009) Vaccines in a hurry. Vaccine 27(25–26):3295–3298. https://doi.org/10.1016/j.vaccine.2009.02.030. Epub 2009 Feb 20. PMID: 19460599; PMCID: PMC7172988

Stern PL (2020) Key steps in vaccine development. Ann Allergy Asthma Immunol 125(1):17–27. https://doi.org/10.1016/j.anai.2020.01.025. Epub 2020 Feb 7. PMID: 32044451

Tavares Da Silva F, Di Pasquale A, Yarzabal JP, Garçon N (2015) Safety assessment of adjuvanted vaccines: methodological considerations. Hum Vaccin Immunother 11(7):1814–1824. https://doi.org/10.1080/21645515.2015.1043501. PMID: 26029975; PMCID: PMC4514270

Therapeutic Goods Administration (TGA) (2024) Australian public assessment report for MVC COVID-19 vaccine. [Online]. [cited 2024 March 18]. https://www.tga.gov.au/sites/default/files/2023-09/auspar-mvc-covid-19-vaccine-230907.docx

Thompson A, Komparic A, Smith MJ (2014) Ethical considerations in post-market-approval monitoring and regulation of vaccines. Vaccine 32(52):7171–7174. https://doi.org/10.1016/j.vaccine.2014.10.016. Epub 2014 Oct 23. PMID: 25454882

Wagner R, Meißner J, Grabski E, Sun Y, Vieths S, Hildt E (2022) Regulatory concepts to guide and promote the accelerated but safe clinical development and licensure of COVID-19 vaccines in Europe. Allergy 77(1):72–82. https://doi.org/10.1111/all.14868. Epub 2021 May 21. PMID: 33887070; PMCID: PMC8251031

Wilson-Welder JH, Torres MP, Kipper MJ, Mallapragada SK, Wannemuehler MJ, Narasimhan B (2009) Vaccine adjuvants: current challenges and future approaches. J Pharm Sci 98(4):1278–1316. https://doi.org/10.1002/jps.21523. PMID: 18704954; PMCID: PMC8092333

World Health Organization (WHO) (2024) Clinical evaluation of vaccines. [Online]. [cited 2024 March 18]. https://www.who.int/teams/health-product-policy-and-standards/standards-and-specifications/vaccine-standardization/clinical-evaluation-of-vaccines

Zahid MN, Moosa MS, Perna S, Buti EB (2021) A review on COVID-19 vaccines: stages of clinical trials, mode of actions and efficacy. Arab J Basic Appl Sci 28(1):225–233. https://doi.org/10.1080/25765299.2021.1903144

Zhang C, Maruggi G, Shan H, Li J (2019) Advances in mRNA vaccines for infectious diseases. Front Immunol 10:594. https://doi.org/10.3389/fimmu.2019.00594. PMID: 30972078; PMCID: PMC6446947

Pollard AJ, Bijker EM (2021) A guide to vaccinology: from basic principles to new developments. Nat Rev Immunol 21(2):83–100. https://doi.org/10.1038/s41577-020-00479-7. Epub 2020 Dec 22. Erratum in: Nat Rev Immunol. 2021 Jan 5; PMID: 33353987; PMCID: PMC7754704

[illegible]

Real-World Evidence Studies and Pragmatic Clinical Trials

20

Saibal Das

Abstract

Traditional explanatory clinical trials on well-regulated interventions (drugs, devices) are conducted following strict regulatory requirements that often hinder pre-approval trials to be naturalistic, thereby questioning their generalizability in various settings. Pragmatic (practical or effectivity) trials, on the other hand, aim to approximate the reality of everyday clinical practice and are critical to inform decision-making by patients, clinicians, and policymakers in real-world settings. In this chapter, we have highlighted real-world evidence generation, the drawbacks of explanatory or traditional clinical trials, key differences between explanatory (traditional) and pragmatic trials, dimensions for assessing the level of pragmatism in a clinical trial (pragmatic explanatory continuum indicator summary-2 tool), special designs of pragmatic trials (large simple trial and randomized database studies), and their common pitfalls. Pragmatic trials test interventions and assess patient-centered and hard outcomes in the full spectrum of everyday clinical settings in order to maximize their applicability and generalizability. However, their overt flexibility and heterogeneity, inviting serious risks of biases, sometimes puts their generalizability into question, especially in the era of patient-centered/personalized/precision medicine. Hence, both explanatory and pragmatic trials are essential to maintain the evidence pyramid.

S. Das (✉)
Indian Council of Medical Research – National Institute for Research in Bacterial Infections, Kolkata, India

Department of Global Public Health, Karolinska Institutet, Stockholm, Sweden
e-mail: saibal.das@icmr.gov.in

A. Arivazhahan et al. (eds.), *Introduction to Basics of Pharmacology and Toxicology*,
https://doi.org/10.1007/978-981-95-1920-0_20

Keywords

Real-world evidence · Pragmatic clinical trials · Comparative effectiveness research · Randomized clinical trials

20.1 Introduction

Real-world data in the field of healthcare are the data related to health status and/or healthcare delivery obtained routinely and periodically from various sources. Real-world evidence in medical science is the clinical evidence generated from the use of medical products (drugs, devices, etc.) about their effectiveness and safety derived from the analysis of real-world data. Real-world evidence can also provide substantial information on diverse disease and therapy areas, for example, the natural history of various diseases, effectiveness studies, outcome research, health technology assessment, pharmacoeconomic studies, safety surveillance, etc.

There is a rising global interest in the generation of evidence on the relative benefits and harms of new and existing interventions in the real-world scenario. This piece of evidence can guide patients, clinicians, and policymakers to make informed decisions aiming at improving healthcare at both individual and population levels. Among the various methods available and practiced, real-world evidence can be aptly generated through comparative effectiveness research, which is the generation and synthesis of evidence by comparing the benefits and harms of different interventions to prevent, diagnose, treat, and monitor a clinical condition or to improve the healthcare delivery. Comparative effectiveness research includes, without being limited to, randomized clinical trials (RCTs), observational studies, and systematic reviews. This chapter will be discussing real-world interventional studies.

Clinical trials are performed primarily to evaluate cause-effect relationships. While non-randomized trials have major limitations and biases, RCTs have high internal validity. The results of robustly designed and appropriately conducted RCTs are highly credible and placed at the top of the hierarchy in the evidence pyramid. According to Schwartz and Lellouch, clinical trials can be broadly classified into pragmatic and explanatory types. Pragmatic (naturalistic) trials, in the realm of real-world interventional studies, are intended to evaluate the effectiveness and safety of interventions in everyday routine practice, whereas explanatory trials try to assess whether a particular intervention is effective and safe under optimal conditions (controlled environment). Pragmatic trials generate evidence that is comprehensive and useful to a real-life context. Because the results of explanatory trials cannot often be generalized, of late, pragmatic trials have gained impetus among healthcare workers, researchers, and policymakers.

20.2 Drawbacks of Explanatory or Traditional Clinical Trials

RCTs employ comprehensive designs to control for most of the possible biases (systematic errors) by following specific techniques, such as randomization, blinding, allocation concealment, etc. Clinical equipoise is assumed to exist while designing an RCT. Usually, narrow and strict eligibility criteria are used to recruit a well-defined cohort of participants who could gain maximum benefit from the investigational intervention. Although this experimental design, if appropriately applied, generates statistically reliable and credible results, the applicability of the results to real-life practice may be doubtful. This is because of the very reason that the overall controlled setting ensured throughout the conduct of such trials may not be extrapolated to real-life everyday settings. The same features that lead to the high internal validity of RCTs (controlled environment, well-defined inclusion and exclusion criteria, blinding, etc.) can impede their external validity, i.e., the ability to generalize the findings in different populations and clinical settings.

Trials on well-regulated interventions (drugs, devices) need to be conducted following strict regulatory requirements that often hinder pre-approval trials to be naturalistic or pragmatic. The requirement for clinical trials to be performed following Good Clinical Practice guidelines infers that several trial characteristics, e.g., starting from elaborate informed consent documents to strict monitoring and reporting of solicited and unsolicited adverse events—jeopardize any intention to mimic real-world routine practice. Furthermore, the complexity and intricacy of early- and late-phase trials have increased gradually in recent times, thus drifting away from the real-world scenario (pragmatism). Thus, despite providing the highest level of evidence, RCTs may have questionable applicability and generalizability.

20.3 What Are "Pragmatic Trials"?

Pragmatic (practical) trials aim to approximate the reality of everyday clinical practice and are defined as "trials for which the hypothesis and study design are formulated based on information needed to make a decision". In contrast to explanatory trials that evaluate if and how an intervention works by controlling known biases and confounders to maximize the intervention's effect, pragmatic trials are designed to evaluate interventions in the full range of routine clinical settings to maximize their generalizability and applicability. The research question addressed by such trials is whether an intervention under investigation really works in a real-life context.

Pragmatic trials assess a broad range of outcomes, mostly patient-centered, whereas explanatory trials focus on quantifiable markers (clinical or biological) or symptoms. While explanatory trials try to ensure homogeneity, so that the errors and biases could have a minimum role, pragmatic trials aim towards maximal heterogeneity in all aspects, e.g., settings, participant recruitment, interventions, follow-up plans, outcome assessments, etc. To overcome the inherited heterogeneity leading to a decrease in the effect size, pragmatic trials are large (higher power to detect small effects) and have simple designs.

Pragmatic trials are purposed to replicate routine clinical practice and are crucial to decision-making by patients, clinicians, and policymakers. These trials assess the effectiveness of approved interventions (drugs, devices) and not the investigational (unapproved) ones. The obvious difference between an explanatory trial and a pragmatic trial in real life is often not that distinct, and most trials, by their inherent designs, have both explanatory and pragmatic components. Thrombus Aspiration in ST-Elevation Myocardial Infarction in Scandinavia (TASTE), Post-Myocardial Infarction Free Rx Event and Economic Evaluation (MI FREEE), Antimicrobial catheters for reduction of symptomatic urinary tract infection (UTI) in adults requiring short-term catheterization in hospital, and Corticosteroid Randomization after Significant Head Injury (CRASH) are examples of some landmark pragmatic trials. We have enumerated the key differences of the characteristics between an explanatory (traditional) trial and a pragmatic trial in Table 20.1.

20.4 Key Considerations While Designing a Pragmatic Trial: The PRECIS Tool

There are several key considerations before designing a pragmatic trial. Various important factors in terms of recruitment of investigators and participants, intervention, follow-up, and outcome assessment and analysis need to be considered. The pragmatic explanatory continuum indicator summary (PRECIS) tool was developed to guide investigators in designing trials recognizing the explanatory/pragmatic continuum. The criteria for pragmatism were relaxed in PRECIS-2, and a pragmatic extension to the Consolidated Standards of Reporting Trials (CONSORT) statement was suggested (Table 20.2). Following an objective scoring method, this tool can be used to objectively determine the magnitude of "pragmatism" in any clinical trial.

20.5 Special Designs of Pragmatic Trials

Herein, we will discuss some special designs of pragmatic trials that are sometimes used to generate real-world evidence as a part of comparative effectiveness research.

20.5.1 Large Simple Trials

These are pragmatic trials with less intense data collection. These trials narrowly focus on clearly stated outcomes that are important to patients and clinicians. The trial involving a large sample size, as the name suggests, is powered enough to detect small effect sizes. These trials include a follow-up period and strategy that resemble routine clinical practice. These trials are particularly useful when an expected event rate is low (e.g., a rare adverse effect) or has a delayed latent period

Table 20.1 Key differences between an explanatory (traditional) trial and a pragmatic trial

Characteristics		Explanatory (traditional) trials	Pragmatic trials
Principle	Real-world or naturalistic trend	Not captured	Captured
	Heterogeneity (participants and intervention)	Minimum	Maximum
Environment and setting	Research environment	Controlled and optimal	Real-world
	Settings	Usually academic/ research facilities	Can be in any health facility, including community-based centers
Objectives and endpoints	Objective	Specific	Can be broad
	Endpoints	All	Usually hard and patient-centered
Protocol	Protocol	Complex and elaborate	Simple and brief
Study design	Phase	Early and late phases	Late phase (phase 4)
	Design	Randomized or non-randomized and blinded or open label	Randomized and open label; sometimes, even nonrandomized
	Eligibility criteria	Narrow	Broad
	Intervention(s)	Unapproved and approved	Approved
	Requirements and procedures	Robust and strict	Relaxed
	Adherence	Strict	Flexible
	Monitoring and follow-up	Strict	Flexible
	Sample size	Smaller	Larger
Level of evidence	Internal validity	High	Low
	External validity	Low	High
	Risk of bias	Usually low (if well-designed)	Can be high
Regulatory status	Regulatory guidelines	Robust and exclusive across various disease therapy areas	Evolving

(with a huge attrition rate), when the population is grossly heterogeneous (e.g., diverse demographic characteristics), when several risk factors/predictors need to be assessed, or when several confounding factors need to be adjusted in finding an association. In such circumstances, the complexity, as well as the expense, of a traditional RCT may outweigh its advantages, and large simple trials can help restrict the volume and complexity of data collection to a sizeable limit. It is pertinent to mention here that the term "simple" in the term "large simple trials" refers to the simplicity of the data structure and not to its collection method. It is used in relation to situations where a small number of outcomes are assessed. Hence, the term may not truly reflect the intricacies of performing these studies.

Table 20.2 Dimensions for assessing the level of pragmatism in a clinical trial (PRECIS-2 tool)

Dimensions		Assessment of pragmatism
Recruitment of investigators and participants	Eligibility criteria	Who are the participants?
	Recruitment	How are participants recruited?
	Setting	Where is the trial site?
Intervention and its delivery	Organization	What experience and resources are needed to deliver the intervention?
	Flexibility in delivery	How will the intervention be delivered?
	Flexibility in adherence	What measures are taken to ensure adherence?
Nature of follow-up	Follow-up	How closely the participants will be followed-up?
Nature, determination, and analysis of outcomes	Primary outcome	How relevant is the research question?
	Primary analysis	To what extent are all data included?

Score (in each domain): from 1 to 5 using a 5-point Likert scale
1 very explanatory, *2* rather explanatory, *3* equally pragmatic and explanatory, *4* rather pragmatic, and *5* very pragmatic

20.5.2 Randomized Database Studies

These are a special type of pragmatic trials, where participants are enrolled in a healthcare system with the help of medical records, mostly electronic. Eligible participants are identified by the software, and the comparison between included and excluded participants is facilitated. Database screening or record linkage can be used to identify outcomes of interest that are otherwise evaluated through various routine healthcare processes. Participant recruitment, obtaining informed consent, and collection of participant information are hurdles that need to be addressed, following the regulatory guidelines. Randomized database studies attempt to amalgamate the advantages of randomization and observational database studies. A special type of randomized database study is a registry-based randomized clinical trial, which employs a medical-records registry to identify eligible participants, and form strategies to enroll, randomize, intervene, follow-up, and assess outcomes in these participants.

20.6 Pitfalls of Pragmatic Trials

The principal characteristic feature of a pragmatic trial is its ability to evaluate the effectiveness of an intervention in a real-life setting and guarantee maximum external validity, i.e., the generalizability of results to different settings. But a valid question is often asked—what is the actual definition of "real life" in medical science? Heterogeneities exist across countries, populations, healthcare facilities, and clinical practices. Demonstration of an intervention's effectiveness in a given setting in a pragmatic trial does not ensure that it will also be effective in another one. Is a "one-size-fits-all" approach prudent enough? Furthermore, in the era of patient-centered/personalized/precision medicine, the fact that a single treatment is effective and safe in a routine broad setting may not address the clinical nuances of every specific individual case.

The weak design, particularly the absence of blinding, coupled with the chance of "spin" in interpreting results (due to overt flexible designs) renders pragmatic trials highly susceptible to manifold biases. Their results can be interpreted in multiple ways and the causal link between intervention and any observed outcome becomes considerably weaker as more and more components of an efficacy trial are abandoned. Finally, in very few areas a wholesome and true essence pragmatic trial can really be conducted. Pragmatism is a fundamental attribute or element of the trial that may not be simply dichotomous, i.e., present or absent. Rather, the continuous nature signifies that a majority of the clinical trials have both explanatory and pragmatic aspects. Therefore, many RCTs that are self-labeled as "pragmatic", as available in the literature, may not be strictly pragmatic.

A genuinely "pragmatic trial" should meet two basic criteria. Firstly, it should be extrapolated to routine everyday practice. Secondly, the results should be valid in different settings. In principle, pragmatic trials need to be ideally performed in several sites involving a large sample size of diverse populations. Some trials need not be necessarily pragmatic, while others can naturally have pragmatic features because of the topic of interest and the healthcare context. Trials of truly novel and effective interventions can change treatment practice even without being too pragmatic. Nevertheless, a single trial of any design cannot address all potential questions related to the value of any intervention. A "pragmatic approach" to "pragmatism" is required to accept the characteristics of a pragmatic trial, whenever possible, and when such characteristics do not hinder the quality of the trial and the capacity to address the research question.

20.7 Conclusion

Pragmatic trials reflect routine clinical practice and are critical to inform decision-making by patients, clinicians, and policymakers in real-world settings. While explanatory RCTs assess the efficacy and safety of unapproved and approved interventions, pragmatic trials assess only approved interventions in a broad and flexible real-world setting. There is clearly a hint that the medical science community is inclined to the holistic concept of pragmatism.

Like in any other study concept and design, pragmatic trials do have inherent limitations. However, the whole concept of broadly applicable and generalizable research is very alluring and beneficial to the medical science community. The "pragmatic design" is still an emerging concept, and it will likely be more popular in the coming days. However, this process should not be continued by compromising explanatory (traditional) clinical trials. Both these pillar concepts in evidence-based medicine in medical science are required to provide answers to our research questions.

Take Home Message

- Pragmatic (naturalistic) trials are designed to evaluate the effectiveness and safety of interventions (drugs, devices, etc.) in real-life settings.
- Pragmatic trials are more inclusive (grossly heterogeneous) and have overtly flexible designs.
- These trials test interventions and assess patient-centered and hard outcomes in the full spectrum of everyday clinical settings in order to maximize their applicability and generalizability.
- The flexibility of pragmatic trials, inviting serious risks of biases, sometimes puts their generalizability into question, especially in the era of patient-centered/personalized/precision medicine.

Bibliography

1. Choudhry NK, Avorn J, Glynn RJ et al (2011) Full coverage for preventive medications after myocardial infarction. N Engl J Med 365:2088–2097
2. Collins R, Bowman L, Landray M et al (2020) The magic of randomization versus the myth of real-world evidence. N Engl J Med 382:674–678
3. Dal-Ré R, Janiaud P, Ioannidis JPA (2018) Real-world evidence: how pragmatic are randomized controlled trials labeled as pragmatic? BMC Med 16:49
4. Ford I, Norrie J (2016) Pragmatic trials. N Engl J Med 375:454–463
5. Fröbert O, Lagerqvist B, Olivecrona GK et al (2013) Thrombus aspiration during ST-segment elevation myocardial infarction. N Engl J Med 369:1587–1597
6. Loudon K, Treweek S, Sullivan F et al (2015) The PRECIS-2 tool: designing trials that are fit for purpose. BMJ 350:h2147
7. Patsopoulos NA (2011) A pragmatic view on pragmatic trials. Dialogues Clin Neurosci 13:217–224
8. Pickard R, Lam T, MacLennan G et al (2012) Antimicrobial catheters for reduction of symptomatic urinary tract infection in adults requiring short-term catheterisation in hospital: a multicentre randomized controlled trial. Lancet 380:1927–1935
9. Roberts I, Yates D, Sandercock P et al (2004) Effect of intravenous corticosteroids on death within 14 days in 10008 adults with clinically significant head injury (MRC CRASH trial): randomised placebo-controlled trial. Lancet 364:1321–1328
10. Thorpe KE, Zwarenstein M, Oxman AD et al (2009) A pragmatic-explanatory continuum indicator summary (PRECIS): a tool to help trial designers. J Clin Epidemiol 62:464–475
11. Tunis SR, Stryer DB, Clancy CM (2003) Practical clinical trials. JAMA 290:1624–1632
12. Zuidgeest MGP, Goetz I, Groenwold RHH et al (2017) GetReal Work Package 3. Series: pragmatic trials and real world evidence: paper 1. Introduction. J Clin Epidemiol 88:7–13

Contract Research Organizations: Roles and Responsibilities

21

Anusha Natarajan

Abstract

A contract research organization (CRO) is a specialized service provider that offers critical support to the pharmaceutical sector. Within a CRO, various departments work cohesively to ensure the seamless execution of clinical trials or bioanalytical/bioequivalence (BA/BE) studies. Among these roles, a pharmacologist is responsible for evaluating the medical components of study protocols and ensuring participant safety. Over the last 10 years, India has emerged as a preferred location for global clinical research, attracting numerous international pharmaceutical firms. The contract research industry in India operates under strict scrutiny, with auditors and regulatory inspectors closely monitoring all processes. As per the Clinical Trials Registry-India (CTRI), it is mandatory to register all clinical trials conducted in the country at no cost. This registration must be completed before enrolling the first participant. In a CRO, a pharmacologist often serves as an investigator or principal investigator, overseeing trial conduct. India's prominence as a clinical research hub for multinational pharmaceutical companies stems from multiple advantages. However, despite the growing interest in global clinical research, Indian CROs face certain challenges. Maintaining ethical business practices is crucial, as it fosters trust and strengthens partnerships with sponsors and collaborators.

Keywords

Contract research organization · Indian scenario of CRO · BA/BE study · Clinical research in India

A. Natarajan (✉)
Department of Pharmacology, Jawaharlal Institute of Postgraduate Medical Education & Research (JIPMER), Puducherry, India

A. Arivazhahan et al. (eds.), *Introduction to Basics of Pharmacology and Toxicology*,
https://doi.org/10.1007/978-981-95-1920-0_21

21.1 Introduction

A contract research organization (CRO) is a specialized firm that provides essential support to the pharmaceutical and biotechnology industries. CROs deliver a broad spectrum of outsourced research services, aiding in the drug and medical device development process. Their key services include:

- Product development, formulation, and manufacturing support.
- Clinical trial management, including planning and execution.
- Clinical, medical, and safety monitoring to ensure participant well-being.
- Preclinical and toxicology studies, along with clinical laboratory services for sample analysis.
- Data management, biostatistics, and medical writing for regulatory submissions such as FDA new drug applications (NDA) and abbreviated new drug applications (ANDA).
- Bioavailability and bioequivalence (BA/BE) studies and regulatory affairs assistance.
- Additional support services, including toxicology testing in animal/cell models and protein structure analysis.

The primary objective of a CRO is to assist pharmaceutical and medical device companies in ensuring that clinical trials adhere to federal and state regulations, good clinical practices (GCP), and ethical standards for human subject protection.

21.2 Departments of a CRO

A contract research organization (CRO) operates through specialized departments, each contributing to the efficient execution of clinical trials and BA/BE studies. These departments include:

- Project management—Acts as the primary liaison between sponsors, investigators, and clinical sites. Ensures study sites have the necessary infrastructure, staffing, and resources to conduct trials effectively.
- Quality assurance (QA)—Conducts regular audits to identify and rectify any compliance gaps, ensuring adherence to protocols and implementing corrective/preventive actions.
- Medical writing—Develops study protocols, designs electronic databases for patient data collection, and prepares final reports in compliance with regulatory standards.
- Subject/volunteer management—Handles participant screening, recruitment, and ongoing management to ensure proper trial conduct and retention.
- Clinical pharmacology (including sample processing)—Works closely with investigators to train site teams on study protocols, ensuring alignment with good

clinical practice (GCP). A pharmacologist reviews medical aspects of the protocol and monitors participant safety.
- Bioanalytical laboratory—Processes and analyzes biological samples collected during the study.
- Biostatistics—Applies advanced statistical methods to interpret clinical data and derive meaningful conclusions.
- Regulatory affairs—Ensures trials comply with local and international clinical research regulations.
- Support departments (IT, biomedical engineering, facility management)—Provide technical and operational support for seamless trial execution.

21.3 Prerequisites for CRO

In the past decade, India has attracted itself to be a favorite destination for clinical research by international pharmaceutical companies. In India, for a CRO to be within the business and to satisfy the expectations of global pharmaceutical companies and fulfil the market demand, while also aiding in improving the country's economic standards and market position, well-coordinated efforts are needed from different stakeholders, as shown in Fig. 21.1.

21.3.1 Quality Auditing

The contract research organization (CRO) sector in India operates under rigorous regulatory scrutiny, with constant monitoring by auditors and inspectors. Internal quality audits play a vital role in maintaining operational efficiency and compliance. These audits serve multiple critical purposes:

- To prepare and support both investigators and sponsors with necessary compliance tools.
- To verify strict adherence to established protocols and regulatory guidelines.
- To pinpoint operational areas requiring enhancement or corrective measures.
- To validate compliance with quality management systems and standard operating procedures.
- To confirm implementation of corrective actions from prior audit findings.

The audit process ensures continuous quality improvement while maintaining the highest standards of clinical research practices. This systematic approach helps CROs maintain their credibility and meet the stringent requirements of global regulatory bodies.

21.3.1.1 Types of Audits

Audits can be of two main types, as detailed in Fig. 21.2.

These audits may be of internal or external nature.

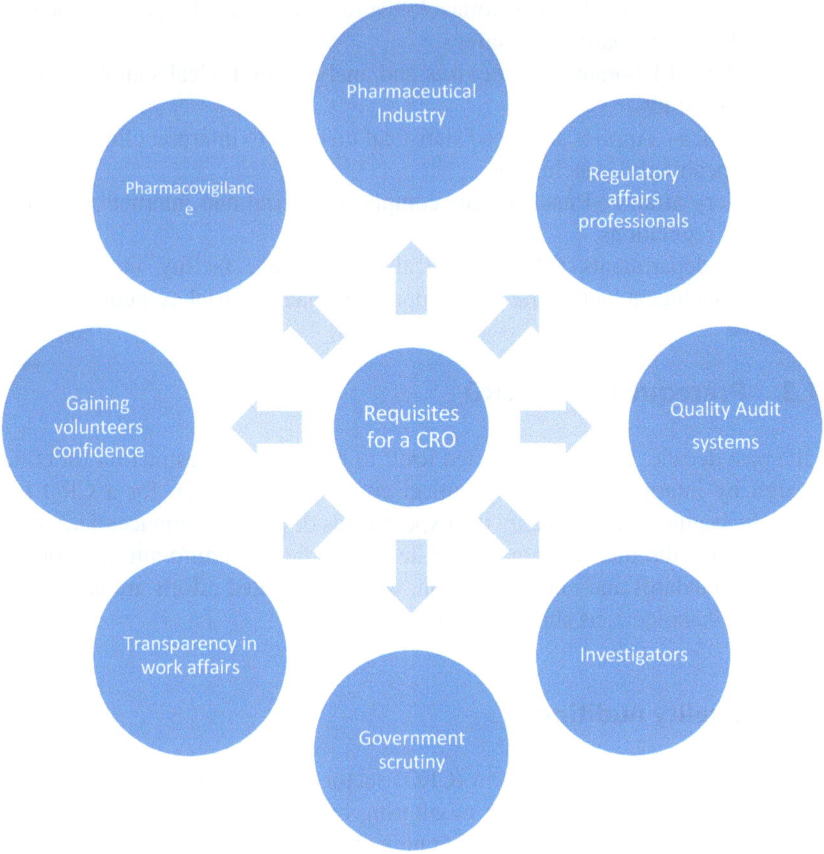

Fig. 21.1 Requisites for a CRO

21.4 Role of a Pharmacologist in CROs

In contract research organizations (CROs), pharmacologists frequently assume the critical role of clinical investigator (CI) or principal investigator (PI). According to ICH-GCP guidelines, an investigator is defined as the individual responsible for conducting clinical trials at a research site. When trials involve a team, the lead investigator assumes the title of principal investigator (PI) and bears ultimate responsibility for all trial-related activities.

Key Responsibilities of a Principal Investigator

1. **Study preparation.**
   - Acquire comprehensive knowledge of the study background (disease pathology, current treatment modalities, and potential treatment side effects).

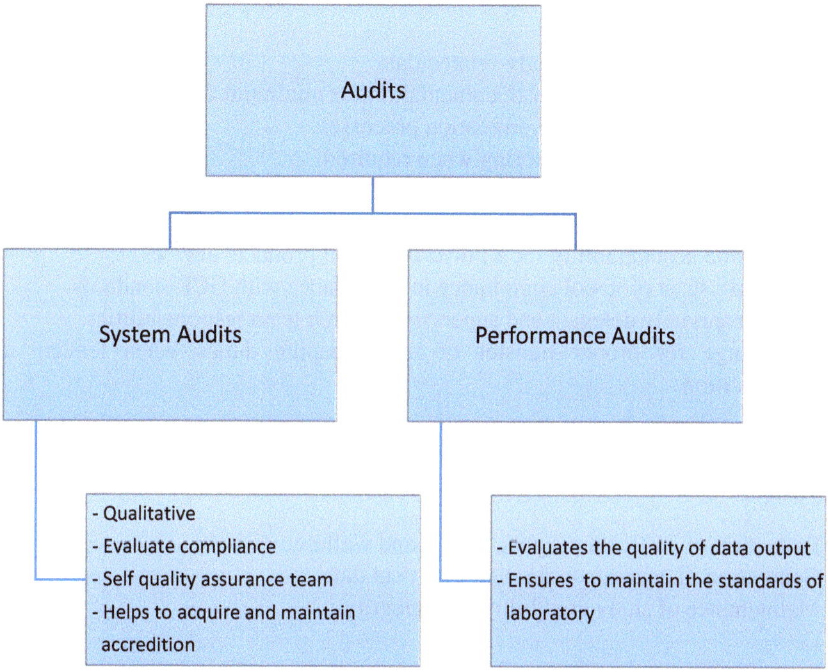

Fig. 21.2 Audits in the CROs

- Thoroughly understand all study protocols and procedures.
- Secure necessary approvals from Institutional Review Board (IRB) or Independent Ethics Committee (IEC).

2. **Participant management.**

- Obtain informed consent from all participants prior to study initiation.
- Ensure strict adherence to eligibility criteria when enrolling patients.
- Monitor and document all treatment effects (therapeutic outcomes and adverse reactions).

3. **Regulatory compliance.**

- Maintain awareness of relevant national regulations affecting study design or participation (drug approval processes, medication importation laws, funding policies).
- Report adverse events and mortality cases to both sponsors and IRB as per protocol requirements.
- Immediately notify relevant parties of any threats to participant safety.
- Submit all protocol amendments for IRB approval.
- Provide regular protocol updates to the IRB.

4. **Data management.**
    - Accurately record all study-related data.
    - Maintain complete study documentation for minimum 2 years post-study.
    - Conduct thorough data verification processes.
    - Facilitate external monitoring when required.
5. **Study oversight.**
    - Assume accountability for all investigational products/devices.
    - Ensure strict protocol compliance in accordance with GCP standards.
    - Appropriately delegate and supervise research team responsibilities.
    - Arrange for proper transfer of recordkeeping duties when leaving an institution.

The principal investigator plays a pivotal role in upholding GCP standards, thereby ensuring:

- Protection of participant rights, safety, and welfare.
- Generation of accurate and reliable clinical data.
- Maintenance of study credibility and integrity.

21.5 CROs: Indian Scenario

India has firmly established itself as a preferred destination for international pharmaceutical companies seeking clinical research services. Several compelling factors contribute to the growing reliance on Indian contract research organizations (CROs):

1. **Skilled workforce**
    - Access to highly qualified professionals across diverse domains including biomedical research, bioinformatics, and biostatistics.
    - Availability of well-trained clinical research personnel with global certifications.
2. **Operational advantages**
    - Cost-effective clinical trial execution without compromising quality standards.
    - Access to treatment-naïve, genetically diverse patient populations.
    - Exceptionally high patient enrolment rates compared to Western countries.
3. **Advanced infrastructure**
    - State-of-the-art healthcare facilities with cutting-edge technology.
    - Well-equipped laboratories meeting international accreditation standards.
    - Modern clinical trial sites with robust data capture systems.

4. **Regulatory framework**
   - Compliance with Trade-Related Aspects of Intellectual Property Rights (TRIPS) agreement since 2005.
   - Strong provisions for data protection and exclusivity.
   - Alignment with international regulatory standards (ICH-GCP, FDA, EMA).
5. **Government support**
   - Attractive fiscal incentives including import duty exemptions.
   - Tax benefits for testing and analysis of new drug entities.
   - Policy initiatives encouraging foreign direct investment in clinical research.

The combination of these factors creates a highly favorable ecosystem for global pharmaceutical companies to conduct efficient, high-quality clinical research while optimizing development costs. India's robust regulatory environment coupled with its vast patient pool positions it as a strategic partner for international drug development programs.

21.6 Ultimatums for CROs in India

While India has emerged as a preferred destination for global clinical research, its CRO sector faces several significant challenges that hinder its full potential:

Key Impediments to Growth

1. Financial limitations
   - Restricted funding opportunities and capital constraints affecting infrastructure development and operational scalability.
2. Regulatory bottlenecks
   - Prolonged drug approval timelines compared to international standards.
   - Understaffing at the Drug Controller General of India (DCGI), leading to delays in regulatory oversight and approvals.
3. Infrastructure and compliance gaps
   - Insufficient number of ICH-GCP-compliant research sites, limiting trial quality and credibility.
   - Rise of nonaccredited CROs, raising concerns about data integrity and ethical standards.
   - Public awareness and participation.
   - Low awareness among potential study participants regarding clinical trial processes and rights.
   - Cultural hesitancy and mistrust toward clinical research in some demographics.

Impact on the Industry

These challenges contribute to:

- Slower trial initiation and completion.
- Reduced competitiveness in the global CRO market.
- Potential compromises in data quality and patient safety.

Addressing these barriers through policy reforms, increased funding, and enhanced training programs could further strengthen India's position as a leading clinical research hub.

21.7 Conclusion

In India's clinical research sector, ethical CROs gain a competitive edge by building trust through compliance with global standards (ICH-GCP, FDA). Their commitment to integrity attracts sponsors and top talent while ensuring sustainable growth. By prioritizing transparency, patient safety, and robust corporate governance, these organizations differentiate themselves in a crowded market. As sponsors increasingly value regulatory adherence and data integrity, ethically driven CROs are positioned to lead India's clinical research evolution. Their focus on quality and compliance not only enhances credibility but also secures long-term partnerships in the global pharmaceutical landscape, making them preferred partners for international trials.

Bibliography

1. Beach J (2001) Clinical trials integrity: a CRO perspective. Account Res 8:245–260
2. Drabu S, Gupta A, Bhadauria A (2010) Emerging trends in contract research industry in India. Contemp Clin Trials 31(5):419–422
3. E6(R2) Good clinical practice: integrated addendum to ICH E6(R1): (2018)
4. Joseph J (2008) Entering the contract research industry in India. Contemp Clin Trials 29:311–313
5. Mukherjee S (2012) Clinical trials and contract research organizations in India. Clin Lab Med 32:315–320
6. Patel R, Patel M (2009) Quality audit: a tool to review quality system. Pharmacol Rev, May, pp 127–129
7. Singh S (2007) Indian pharma enters the global arena. Cell 128:811–814

Bioavailability and Bioequivalence Studies

22

Indumathi Prabath

Abstract

Bioavailability/bioequivalence (BA/BE) studies are the cornerstone for the regulatory approval of generic drugs that significantly reduce medical treatment expenditure, especially in resource-limited settings. Bioavailability studies are conducted to determine the rate and extent of absorption, metabolism, excretion rate, and terminal elimination half-life. Bioequivalence studies justify the interchangeable application of different brands of the same drug. Different regulatory agencies of pharmaceutical companies such as the United States Food and Drug Administration (US-FDA) and the Central Drugs Standard Control Organization of India have laid down the systematic guidelines for the conduct of BA/BE studies in various regions of the world. The main scope of these regulatory guidelines is to ascertain the safety, efficacy, and quality of generic drugs on par with the innovator's small molecules. This chapter briefly discusses the various components of BA/BE studies, namely study subjects and conditions, sample size, study designs, bioanalytical procedures, and bioavailability assessment based on the regulatory recommendations across the world.

Keywords

Bioavailability · Bioequivalence · Generic drugs · Study designs · Bioanalytical · Pharmacokinetics · Regulatory agencies

I. Prabath (✉)
Department of Pharmacology, Chettinad Hospital and Research Institute, Chettinad Academy of Research and Education, Kelambakkam, Tamilnadu, India

A. Arivazhahan et al. (eds.), *Introduction to Basics of Pharmacology and Toxicology*,
https://doi.org/10.1007/978-981-95-1920-0_22

22.1 Introduction and Significance of Bioavailability/ Bioequivalence Studies

Generic drugs play a critical role in minimizing overall health expenditure by the patients and occupy 65% of the global market. Thus, it is essential to ensure generics' quality, safety, and efficacy compared to innovator pharmaceutical products. Drug regulatory authorities like the United States Food and Drug Administration (US-FDA), European Medicines Agency (EMA), and Central Drugs Standard Control Organization of India (CDSCO) emphasize the standards for ensuring the generic drugs' safety, efficacy, and quality by promoting stringent bioavailability and bioequivalence studies. They assure that pharmaceuticals (both generic and innovator products) with the same active drug can be used interchangeably. Based on New Drugs and Clinical Trials Rules 2019, it is mandatory to submit bioavailability and bioequivalence data during the new drug application filing. Bioavailability and bioequivalence (BA/BE) studies evaluate the liberation of the drug from its dosage form and its subsequent absorption into the systemic circulation. These data are obtained by a graph plotting the time versus plasma concentration of the drug. According to Food and Drug Administration Act, a generic drug is bioequivalent to the reference listed drug (RLD) when the "rate and extent of absorption of the drug do not show a significant difference from the rate and extent of absorption of the listed drug when administered at the same molar dose of the therapeutic ingredient under similar experimental conditions in either a single dose or multiple doses" and leads to approval of abbreviated new drug application (ANDA). BA/BE studies compare the two pharmaceutical products containing the same active drug and validate the substitution with therapeutically equivalent drugs in clinical practice. Several guidelines were postulated by different drug regulatory agencies for the proper design, conduct, and analysis of BA/BE studies. It is challenging to demonstrate the bioequivalence of biologics such as animal sera, blood, and plasma derivatives and biotechnologically made drugs.

22.2 Salient Definitions and Pharmacokinetic Terms

- **Bioavailability:** Relative amount of drug from an administered dosage form that enters the systemic circulation and the rate at which the drug appears in the systemic circulation.
- **Bioequivalence:** It is achieved if the extent and absorption rate of a drug product is not significantly different from those of the reference product when administered at the same molar dose under similar conditions in an appropriately designed study.
- **Pharmaceutical equivalents:** Drug products that contain identical amounts of the same active drug molecule in the same dosage form and route of administration, and are available in the same strength or concentration, but need not contain identical inactive substances.

- **Pharmaceutical alternatives:** Drug products that contain the identical therapeutic moiety but not necessarily in the same amount or dosage form or as the same salt or ester.
- **Reference product:** Pharmaceutical product that the Licensing Authority prefers as Designated Reference Product and contains the same active ingredient as the new drug. Mostly, it would be the global innovator product.
- **Therapeutic equivalents:** Pharmaceutical products that contain the same active substance or therapeutic moiety and clinically show the same efficacy and safety.
- **C_{max}:** Maximum drug concentration achieved in systemic circulation following drug administration.
- **C_{min}:** Minimum drug concentration achieved in systemic circulation following multiple dosing at a steady state.
- **T_{max}:** Time required to achieve maximum drug concentration in the systemic circulation.
- **Area under curve (AUC) $_{0\text{-}t}$:** Area under the plasma concentration-time curve, from 0 h to the last quantifiable concentration to be calculated using the trapezoidal rule.
- **$AUC_{0\text{-}\infty}$:** Area under the plasma concentration-time curve, from zero to infinity is calculated as the sum of $AUC_{0\text{-}t}$ plus the ratio of the last measurable concentration to the elimination rate constant.
- **$AUC_{0\text{-}tau}$:** Area under the plasma concentration-time curve over one dosing interval following a single dose for modified release products.
- **Half-life, $T_{1/2}$:** Elimination half-life of a drug is the time necessary to reduce the drug concentration in biological fluids to one-half after equilibrium is reached.

22.3 Specific Dosage Forms Necessitating Mandatory In Vivo Bioequivalence Studies

(i) **Systemic formulations**

- Oral drugs indicated in serious conditions, with a narrow therapeutic range, following pharmacokinetic properties such as incomplete absorption, first-pass metabolism>70%, and nonlinear pharmacokinetics.
- Oral immediate release drugs with high excipient content, low solubility, instability, and poor permeability.
- Transdermal patches, suppositories, and similar products but not administered orally/parenterally.
- Modified release products.
- Fixed-dose combinations for systemic use.

(ii) **Nonsystemic products**

- Oral, nasal, ocular, dermal, rectal, and vaginal pharmaceutical products that are not in solution form.

22.4 Pharmaceutical Products That Do Not Require Bioequivalence Studies

- Parenteral formulations available as an aqueous solution containing the same drug and excipients in the same concentration.
- Oral solutions containing the same active ingredient along with the same excipient.
- Therapeutic gases.
- Reconstituting powders.
- Ophthalmic, otic, and skin pharmaceuticals available as aqueous solutions.
- Inhalational formulations, such as nasal spray with identical active drug and excipient in the same concentration.

22.5 Methods of Bioavailability Assessment

Based on regulatory agencies' recommendations, accurate, sensitive, and reproducible methods are to be used for establishing bioequivalence. This evaluation includes different methods such as comparative pharmacokinetic designs, comparative pharmacodynamic tests, and in vitro studies.

22.5.1 Pharmacokinetic Methods

- Extensively used method of bioequivalence studies and involve estimation of drug level in the biological samples.
- Pharmacokinetic parameters like plasma concentration correlated with the therapeutic effect of the drug.
- These are precise, reliable, and reproducible methods to identify the release of drugs from the pharmaceutical product into the biological circulation.
- Based on regulatory guidelines, systemic exposure is determined in terms of total exposure via $AUC_{0\text{-tau}}$ & $AUC_{0\text{-}\infty}$, peak exposure by C_{max}, and early exposure, which could demonstrate significant clinical differences between test and standard drugs.
- Plasma level-time studies and urinary excretion studies are the two main pharmacokinetic methods.
- Time for peak plasma concentration, peak plasma concentration, and area under the plasma drug concentration-time curve are estimated at the end of plasma level-time studies.
- Cumulative quantity of the excreted drug, rate of drug excretion, and time for maximum urinary excretion are the variables measured in urinary excretion studies. Urinary samples are utilized in BE studies when >40% of the drug is excreted unchanged via the kidney.

22.5.2 Pharmacodynamic Methods

- Drug response is considered to determine the bioequivalence between innovator and generic drugs.
- Pharmacodynamic studies involve the estimation of therapeutic end points related to testing drug's efficacy and safety.
- These study designs are incorporated when the estimation of drugs/metabolites concentration in biological samples is not feasible, there is a deficit of sensitive pharmacokinetic assays and in situations where plasma concentration could not be the optimal surrogate end point for determining the efficacy and safety.
- These methods are really difficult to measure, have high interindividual variability, and are modulated by physiological and environmental factors.
- They should be precise, accurate, specific, and reproducible.
- Time for maximum effect, the area under the pharmacodynamic effect-time curve, and time of onset of effect are the pharmacodynamic parameters measured in this method.
- Double-blinded method should be used and drug responses are to be assessed at repeated time points similar to plasma concentration estimation.
- Crossover or parallel study designs can be utilized for these studies.
- Statistical analysis is performed mostly mimicking the pharmacokinetic method and, in many instances, the acceptable range of bioequivalence criteria is defined based on individual studies.
- Few examples of drugs undergoing pharmacodynamic methods are dry powder inhalers, topical creams, and ointments. In case of bronchodilator, forced expiratory volume in 1 s is fixed as one of the pharmacodynamic end points due to its clinical relevance.

22.5.3 Clinical End Point Studies

- Also termed as comparative clinical trials.
- Well-controlled clinical trials are conducted when no pharmacokinetic or pharmacodynamic methods are available.
- Regulatory agencies have laid down standard guidelines for the conduct of clinical studies to demonstrate bioequivalence.

22.5.4 In Vitro Studies

- Comparative in vitro dissolution studies are sufficient to determine the bioequivalence between different strengths of the drugs that are manufactured by the same pharmaceutical manufacturer, provided the following criteria are met.
- Same chemical composition, the ratio of active ingredients to excipients, manufacturing methods, and equivalence study being performed with at least one strength of the formulation.

- These studies should meet the standards of pharmacopoeia and are usually conducted at 37 ± 0.5 °C and physiological pH. Dosage forms from multiple batches of the same formulation should be tested.
- These studies should be conducted with a minimum of 12 tablets/capsules from each batch, at different time points with uniform intervals, preferably using the same equipment on the same or the next day. A minimum of three aqueous media has to be used for establishing the dissolution profile.
- These studies are conducted to establish the batch-to-batch quality, ensure quality control, and determine the need for BE studies for minor post-approval changes.

22.6 Bioequivalence Study Designs

- Pilot and pivotal studies are the two broad categories of bioequivalence studies.
- Pilot study conventionally precedes pivotal study and used for validation of analytical methods, estimation of sample size, determination of optimal sampling time points, and assessment of pharmacokinetic variability.
- Pivotal study design includes single-dose and multidose pharmacokinetic studies for different formulations such as immediate and modified release dosage forms.
- Single-dose studies are preferred for immediate release and modified release forms, as they precisely assess the liberation and distribution of active ingredients from the drug into the systemic circulation. The maximum strength of the drug is considered for testing in BE studies.
- Multidose study designs or steady-state designs are generally used to evaluate time-dependent pharmacokinetics, and modified release drugs, in conditions where intraindividual variability limits single-dose bioequivalence studies and minimal variability at steady state, enteric-coated tablets with an innovative shell, combination products with special individual drugs and drugs with a long terminal elimination half-life.
- Washout period between the two treatment periods is mandatory and considered to be more than five half-lives of the drugs intended for assessment.
- Crossover study designs, parallel designs, and replicate study designs are the important study designs adapted for bioequivalence studies.
- Two period, two sequence, two-treatment, single-dose crossover study involving healthy subjects is often recommended by FDA for drugs administered for the systemic purpose.

22.6.1 Salient Features of Study Designs

22.6.1.1 Crossover Design

- Exposure of subjects to both the test and reference drugs at two different periods, where each subject acts as his or her control.
- Two treatments are separated by washout period depending on their half-lives.

- Applied for drugs with intra-subject variability significantly lower than intersubject variability and this design is often recommended by most of the regulatory agencies.
- Merits of crossover design: Intersubject variability is reduced leading to minimal interference with error variability. The minimum sample size would be sufficient. Randomization results in the unbiased evaluation of treatment outcomes.
- Demerits: Presence of carryover and period effects because of inadequate washout period. A prolonged study period makes it unsuitable for drugs with a long half-life.

22.6.1.2 Parallel Design

- Test and reference drug formulations are administered to different groups of participants.
- Drugs with a long half-life and high intra-subject variability usually undergo parallel studies. Nevertheless, this study design is mainly limited by significant interindividual variability.
- Advantages: Simple and robust design. Minimal carryover effects and dropouts are observed.
- Disadvantages: Large sample size needed, and mandatory phenotyping required for drugs with polymorphisms.

22.6.1.3 Replicated Design

- Applied for modified release products and highly variable drug products with intrasubject variation coefficient ≥30 and drugs with carryover effects.
- Two sequence and four-period design (TRTR & RTRT), four sequence and four-period design (TTRR, RRTT, TRRT & RTTR), two sequence and three-period design (TRT, RTR), and William's design for three medications are some variations of replicated design. T and R represent test and reference drugs, respectively (Table 22.1).
- Advantages: Facilitates comparison of within-subject variances of test and reference products. The number of participants can be reduced by 50%.
- Disadvantages: Long study duration and more volume of blood collection for bioanalytical purposes. Expensive.

Table 22.1 Four sequence and four-period design

	Period			
Sequence	T	T	R	R
	R	R	T	T
	T	R	R	T
	R	T	T	R

T test, *R* reference

22.7 Study Subjects

- Normal healthy adult volunteers of age ≥18 years and consenting for BABE studies are usually recruited to mitigate the biological variability and detect the difference solely attributed to drugs.
- These studies are allowed to involve both genders, provided the female participants are not pregnant or not likely to conceive during or sometime after the study.
- Elderly subjects (≥60 years) are allowed to participate in case of products meant for geriatric use widely. Male populations are exclusively recruited in the study with teratogenic drugs.
- Drugs with a significant toxicity profile should be evaluated in a stable patient population suffering due to that particular disease and should be preceded by medical examination and laboratory evaluation for the subjects.
- Special laboratory investigations can be performed based on the drug category and safety profile throughout the study. For example, regular ECG monitoring for drugs with potential cardiotoxicity.
- Minimum and maximum number of subjects should be 12 and 24 subjects, based on the guidelines of major regulatory agencies (FDA, EMA, and Canada) whereas, in India, the minimum number of subjects should be 16.
- Level of significance (p value <0.05), error variance (derived from pilot experiments/previous studies/published literature), expected deviation from reference drug and desired power (≥80%) to identify the maximum allowable difference are the various parameters considered for sample size determination. Dropouts can be replaced with new subjects in concordance with the protocol.
- Sequential/add-on studies are also conducted in certain conditions where the statistical significance may not be attained otherwise.
- In general, data of all the subjects should be considered for statistical analysis.
- Phenotyping with/without genotyping should be done for exploratory bioavailability studies, parallel study designs, and crossover studies for safety/pharmacokinetic reasons.

22.8 Study Conditions

Study environment, food and water intake, blood sampling time points, physical activity, and body posture after dosing are the critical study conditions that should be strictly followed in compliance with the study protocol. By minimizing the variability factors, the between-group differences are likely to be attributed exclusively to the difference in drugs exposed between the groups.

22.8.1 Sampling Time Points

- Blood and urine are the frequent samples collected for BA/BE studies. The majority of the studies utilize serum or plasma and whole blood (few studies) for the estimation of drug or metabolites concentration.
- Based on FDA guidelines, 12–18 samples including pre-dose samples should be collected for each subject with each dose.
- For single-dose trials, blood samples should be collected extending up to a minimum of three elimination half-lives.
- Area extrapolated from the last time point to infinity should not exceed 20% of the total AUC. The number of sampling points during the absorption and elimination phases should be three and four, respectively. Three to four samples around the projected T_{max} should also be collected.
- Truncated AUC method is preferred only when it is tedious to calculate terminal elimination rate constant, for example, in the case of drugs undergoing enterohepatic cycling.
- In the case of estimation of urine samples for concentration, it is recommended to collect the samples for seven or more half-lives.

22.8.2 Fasting and fed Conditions

- Fasting for at least 10 h overnight and 4 h post-dose is generally instructed during the single-dose fasting studies.
- For multiple-dose fasting studies, 2 h of fasting pre- and post-dose should be undergone after the intake of the last evening dose.
- Both fasting and fed studies should be conducted for modified release formulation.
- Fed studies are warranted when it is difficult to obtain C_{max} and T_{max} from fasting studies.
- In the fed studies, high-fat breakfasts with 950–1000 Kcal are consumed before dosing based on CDSCO guidelines. The calorie composition of a high-fat breakfast includes at least 50% fat, 15–20% proteins, and the rest from carbohydrates. High-fat breakfast intake should be completed around 15 min before dosing.
- Water intake should be restricted for at least 1 h before and after dosing.
- Drug, either test or reference, should be consumed with an intake of 240 ml water.
- Standardized meals should be provided to all subjects at the scheduled time in every period of the study.
- Alcohol abstinence for 24 h before each study period and until the collection of the last samples of each period should be strictly practiced.

22.8.3 Drugs and Special Conditions Requiring Steady-State Studies

- Drugs with extended elimination half-life and complex to evaluate the plasma concentration.
- In case of the low sensitive assay to determine the terminal elimination phase.
- Highly toxic drugs and drugs requiring multiple-dose therapy. For example, cytotoxic drugs.
- Modified release dosage forms have frequent fluctuation in plasma concentration that needs to be evaluated at a steady state.
- Drugs with high interindividual variability.
- Enteric-coated tablets with innovative coating.
- Nonlinear pharmacokinetics drugs.
- Drugs with significant tissue storage.

22.9 Salient Features of Bioanalytical Procedures

- Predominantly, BA/BE studies involve estimation of the concentration of active drugs in the biological sample. Active and/or inactive metabolites are also measured in some studies where the active drug plasma concentration is very low/negligible, and has limited analytical methods, in the case of unstable drugs, drugs with short half-live and prodrugs.
- Specific enantiomers are estimated when the enantiomers have exclusive pharmacokinetic as well as pharmacodynamic characteristics, nonlinear absorption, and when the primary efficacy or safety is attributed to minor enantiomers.
- Plasma concentration-time curve is widely used to determine the pharmacokinetic parameters, such as C_{max}, T_{max}, $AUC_{0\text{-}t}$, and $AUC_{0\text{-}\infty}$, for assessing the rate and extent of absorption of the study drug.
- In case of steady-state studies, $AUC_{0\text{-}tau}$, C_{max}, C_{min}, and degree of fluctuation are calculated.
- Standardized and validated analytical methods are developed to estimate the drug and/or metabolite concentration in biological fluids such as blood, serum, plasma, or urine.
- Bioanalytical methods are generally validated by two phases such as pre-study and study phases.
- Pre-study phase is conducted before the initiation of the study in which the bioanalytical method is validated using human plasma samples and spiked plasma samples. During this phase, stability of the active drug/metabolite in a biological sample, assay specificity and sensitivity, reproducibility, and accuracy are ensured. Interday variation should lie between 15% and 20% and a minimum of 15% accuracy should be met.
- In the study phase, bioanalytical methods developed are applied to samples collected during BA/BE studies. A standard curve for each analyte was traced to determine its concentration in the unknown samples.

22.10 Key Features of BA/BE Statistical Analysis

- Statistical analysis is performed to confirm the differences between the test and reference groups occurred exclusively due to the difference in the drugs administered and not due to chance.
- Analysis of variance (ANOVA) is the most often employed statistical test for comparing the pharmacokinetic parameters obtained from plasma concentration-time plot and the corresponding variances are derived for subjects, periods, and treatment independently.
- The null hypothesis for this assay is that the pharmaceutical products are bioequivalent and thus, the alternate hypothesis would be that these products are not bioequivalent.
- These BA/BE statistical analyses can be performed using SAS (statistical analysis system) or WinNonlin software, which would test the influence of subject, period, pharmaceutical formulations, and their interactions.
- Geometric mean ratio and log-transformed data are used to detect that the 90% confidence interval of the extent of absorption (AUC_{0-t} and $AUC_{0-\infty}$, and C_{max}) falls within the acceptance limit.
- Exposure matrix C_{max}/AUC and partial area measurements are considered for highly variable drugs, drugs with long elimination $t_{1/2}$, and in cases of special formulations.
- Few most appropriate statistical methods used to determine the interchangeability between test and reference drugs are study power, 75/75 rule, and 90% confidence interval.
- **POWER:** For identifying the proper sample size of the pivotal study, a pilot study with 6–12 subjects can be conducted and this also reveals the variability of the drug and geometric mean ratio between test and reference.
- **75/75 rule:** Two pharmaceutical products are bioequivalent, only if at least 75% of the subjects being evaluated had ratios of pharmacokinetic parameters between 75% and 125% limits and the statistical power could detect a 20% difference between the drugs. This rule was later on superseded by 90% confidence interval approach.
- **90% confidence interval:** In this method, average values of pharmacokinetic parameters of test and reference products were calculated and compared by a 90% confidence interval for the ratio of averages using t-tests. This could probably be the only method that enables the comparison of two products by accounting for the variability inherent within each formulation.

22.11 Criteria for Validating the Bioequivalence

- Ninety percent confidence interval of the area under the curve (AUC) and maximum concentration (C_{max}) of the test drug should lie within 80–125% acceptable bioequivalence range.

- Nonparametric T_{max} 90% confidence interval should fall within a clinically significant range.
- Drugs with a narrow therapeutic index, high toxicity profile, nonlinear pharmacokinetics at therapeutic dose range, and a steep dose-response curve should strictly fall within the acceptable range.

22.12 Summary

The Table 22.2 summarizes the recommendations provided by the different regulatory agencies.

Table 22.2 Recommendations for the conduct of bioavailability/bioequivalence studies by different regulatory agencies

Criteria	CDSCO, India	FDA, USA	EMA, Europe
Participant's gender	Male/female	Both male and female	Either gender
Subject's age	Healthy adult volunteers	≥18 years	≥18 years
Body mass index of subjects (kg/m^2)	Not specified	Not declared	18.5–30
Sample size	Minimum 16	12	Minimum 12
Number of studies	A single-dose, nonreplicated, fasting study Food effect studies at specific conditions	A single-dose, nonreplicated fasting study A food-effect, nonreplicated study	A single-dose, nonreplicated, fasting study Food effect studies are done if SPC[a] of the reference drug denotes food interaction
Fasting timing and duration	Overnight minimum 10 h prior to dosing and 4 h post-dose period	Same as Indian guidelines	Overnight at least 8 h before dosing and 4 h post-dose
Fed study conditions	High-fat breakfast delivering 950–1000 kcal (50% from fat, 15–20% from protein and rest from carbohydrates) should be consumed 15 min prior to dosing	800–1000 calories of high-fat breakfast constituting 150,250 and 500–600 calories from protein, fat, and carbohydrates	Depends on the innovator SPC[a]
Fluid intake, posture, and physical activity	Standard instructions for fluid intake and physical activity should be defined in the protocol	Subjects should take the test drug with 240 mL of water, 1 h water restriction before and after dosing	Standardized volume of at least 150 mL of water should be administered during dosing and water restriction for 1 h pre- and post-dosing should be followed

(continued)

Table 22.2 (continued)

Criteria	CDSCO, India	FDA, USA	EMA, Europe
Sampling of biological matrix	Blood sampling covering minimum 3 elimination half-lives including minimum 3 points during absorption, 3–4 around T_{max}, and 4 points during the elimination phase Urine sample collected for 7 or more half-lives	12–18 blood samples representing absorption, distribution, and elimination phases. Should extend up to 3 or more terminal half-lives of the drug	Sampling around predicted T_{max} $AUC_{0\text{-}t}$ covers at least 80% of $AUC_{0\text{-infinity}}$ Urine samples should be collected for at least three times the terminal elimination half-live
Washout period	Adequate and should be ≥5 half-lives of the drug	Same as CDSCO	Same as CDSCO
Bioequivalence acceptance criteria (90% confidence interval on log-transformed data)	C_{max}, $AUC_{0\text{-}t}$, and $AUC_{0\text{-}\infty}$: 80–125%	Same as CDSCO	C_{max}, $AUC_{0\text{-}t}$: 80–125% $AUC_{0\text{-}\infty}$: not specified

[a]SPC–summary of product characteristics

Bibliography

1. Guidance for industry bioavailability and bioequivalence studies for orally administered drug products—general considerations. US Department of Health and Human Services, Food and Drug Administration, Center for Drug Evaluation and Research (CDER), March 2014
2. Committee for medicinal products for human use. Guideline on the investigation of bioequivalence. European Medicines Agency January 2010
3. Guidelines for bioavailability and bioequivalence studies. Central Drugs Standard Control Organization, Directorate General of Health Services, Ministry of Health and Family Welfare, Government of India, New Delhi, March 2005
4. Mastan S, Latha TB, Ajay S (2011) The basic regulatory considerations and prospects for conducting bioavailability/bioequivalence (BA/BE) studies-an overview. Comp Eff Res 1:1–25
5. Gouthami A, Ramesh M, Nalini M, Nancy MD (2013) A review on general concepts of design and conduct of bioequivalence studies. Int J Phytopharmacol 4(2):74–84
6. Karalis V, Macheras P, Van Peer A, Shah VP (2008) Bioavailability and bioequivalence: focus on physiological factors and variability. Pharm Res 25(8):1956–1962. https://doi.org/10.1007/s11095-008-9645-9. Epub 2008 Jun 13
7. Qayyum A (2012) Bioequivalence studies, vol 39. National University of Sciences and Technology Pakistan, Islamabad, pp 5–9

Part III

Drug Regulations

Indian New Drugs and Clinical Trial Rules 23

Vikneswaran Gunaseelan

Abstract

The New Drugs and Clinical Trials Rules (NDCTR), 2019, introduced by the Central Drugs Standard Control Organization (CDSCO), represent a transformative shift in India's regulatory landscape for clinical research. This chapter provides a comprehensive review of the NDCTR, highlighting its structural framework, key provisions, and implications for stakeholders. The rules, comprising 13 chapters and 9 schedules, aim to streamline clinical trial processes, ensure participant safety, and promote ethical research practices. Key topics include the registration and functioning of ethics committees, regulatory pathways for clinical trials and bioavailability/bioequivalence studies, compensation mechanisms for trial-related injuries, and provisions for accelerated drug approvals in special circumstances. The chapter also discusses the import and manufacture of new drugs, including those not yet approved in India but required for life-threatening conditions. Recent amendments, such as deemed approvals and the registration of clinical research organizations, are also examined. This review serves as a practical guide for researchers, sponsors, and regulatory professionals navigating the evolving clinical trial environment in India.

Keywords

Clinical trial · Regulations · Ethics committee · Guidelines · DCGI · CDSCO

V. Gunaseelan (✉)
Department of Clinical Research, Narayana Health, Bengaluru, India
e-mail: vikneswaran786@gmail.com

A. Arivazhahan et al. (eds.), *Introduction to Basics of Pharmacology and Toxicology*,
https://doi.org/10.1007/978-981-95-1920-0_23

23.1 Introduction

The Central Drugs Standard Control Organization (CDSCO) introduced the New Drugs and Clinical Trials Rules in March 2019, marking a significant update to India's regulatory framework for clinical research. The new rules supersede specific provisions of the 1945 Drug and Cosmetics framework, notably Part Xa and Schedule Y (rule 122DAA). Schedule Y introduced into drugs and cosmetics rules about 30 years ago has seen two major changes, once at the time of publication of ICH GCP guidelines when India entered into Trade-Related Aspects of Intellectual Property Rights (TRIPS) agreement in 2005 and second in 2013 (requiring accreditation of ethics committee and making audio video recording mandatory for consent) finally giving way to the new clinical trial rules of 2019.

The new regulations are drafted with an aim to promote research within the country, provide time-bound review, and create predictability and clarity of the regulatory system. The new clinical trial rules 2019 consists of 13 chapters, which include 107 rules and 8 schedule (schedule 9 added later as amendment). Key features of the updated regulations include provisions for expedited drug approval, expanded terminology, classification of ethics committees into two distinct categories, structured interactions with regulators both before and after submission. In India, the Central Licensing Authority (CLA) is designated by the central government through the appointment of the drugs controller. The CLA holds the authority to delegate responsibilities to the assistant drugs controller as needed (Box 23.1).

Box 23.1: Chapters in NDCT Rules, 2019

Chapter I	Preliminary
Chapter II	Authorities and officers
Chapter III	Ethics committee for clinical trial, bioavailability, and bioequivalence study
Chapter IV	Ethics committee for biomedical and health research
Chapter V	Clinical trial, BA/BE study of new drugs and investigational new drugs
Chapter VI	Compensation
Chapter VII	BA/BE center
Chapter VIII	Manufacture of new drugs or investigational new drugs for CT, BA/BE study or for examination, test, and analysis
Chapter IX	Import of new drugs and investigational new drugs for CT. BA/BE study or for examination, test, and analysis
Chapter X	Import or manufacture of new drug for sales or for distribution
Chapter XI	Import or manufacture of unapproved new drugs for treatment of patients in government hospital and government medical institution
Chapter XII	Amendment of Drug and Cosmetic Rules, 1945
Chapter XIII	Miscellaneous

23.2 Registration and Functioning of Ethics Committee

Under the NDCTR, ethics committees are categorized based on the type of research they oversee. Committees responsible for clinical trials, including bioavailability and bioequivalence studies, must be registered with the Central Licensing Authority (CLA), while those evaluating biomedical and health research are required to register with the Department of Health Research (DHR).

Ethics committee should have minimum of seven members from medical, scientific, and nonscientific areas with at least

- One layperson.
- One woman member.
- One legal expert.
- One independent member from any other field, such as social scientist, philosopher, or ethicist or theologian or representative of nongovernmental voluntary agency.

A minimum of half the committee members must be independent and unaffiliated with the host institution. The chairperson should be a nonaffiliated member, while the member secretary should be affiliated. Medical scientists and clinicians should possess at least postgraduate qualifications.

The members should follow good clinical practice and regulatory guidelines to protect the safety, rights, and well-being of the participants. They should undergo periodic training and development programs. Committee members are required to formally disclose any potential conflicts of interest by signing a declaration.

Functions of the ethics committee are:

- Evaluate and authorize the clinical trial protocol along with all associated documentation.
- To review ongoing trials approved by them at an appropriate interval and monitoring or audit reports submitted by the sponsor.
- To mention the reasons for rejecting or asking for modifications in the protocol and make it available to the CLA.
- To review any serious adverse event and submit its report to CLA complying with the provisions made in Chapter VI.
- To discontinue or suspend trials that are likely to compromise the participants safety or well-being.
- To adhere to regulatory standards and permit inspections by the relevant authorities.

The structure, responsibilities, and operations of ethics committees involved in biomedical and health research must align with the National Ethical Guidelines for Biomedical Research. Any alterations in the structure or membership of a registered ethics committee must be duly reported to the regulatory authority. In case of noncompliance, the designated authority can issue warning to the ethics committee, suspend, or cancel the registration (Box 23.2).

Box 23.2: Forms and Timelines Pertaining to Ethics Committee

Ethics committee registration application	CT form 01
Grant of registration (for CT and BA/BE studies)	CT form 02
Grant of registration (for biomedical and health research)	CT form 03
Validity period for provisional registration	2 years
Validity following main registration	5 years
Appeal in case of rejection of application	Within 60 working days
Renewal of registration	At least 90 days prior

23.3 Regulations for Clinical Trial of New Drug/ Investigational New Drug

Clinical trial of a new drug or an investigational new drug can be undertaken only with the permission of the CLA and approval by the ethics committee. Approval from the Central Licensing Authority (CLA) is contingent upon meeting the following criteria:

- The CLA should be informed about the approval by the ethics committee within 15 working days.
- The study must be listed in the Clinical Trials Registry of India prior to the enrolment of any participants.
- The clinical trial must be carried out strictly according to the approved protocol and in alignment with the principles outlined in the Good Clinical Practice (GCP) guidelines.
- Enrolment status of the study should be updated on a quarterly basis.
- Trial progress reports must be uploaded to the SUGAM portal every 6 months.
- Centers conducting BA/BE studies should be registered with the CLA.
- Notification of trial discontinuation, along with the justification, must be submitted within 30 working days.
- Detailed report of serious adverse events should be submitted within 14 working days of its occurrence to the CLA, ethics committee, and the site.
- The sponsor should provide complete medical care and compensation within 30 working days of communication by the CLA.
- The CLA, if considered necessary, may impose conditions regarding objective, design, study population, assessment, and treatment.
- Allow any person authorized by the CLA to inspect the site with or without prior notice.

- The first patient should be recruited within 1 year of grant of approval of the study, failing which permission should be obtained from the CLA.

When the sponsor fails to comply by the regulations, the CLA can issue warning notice, reject the study results, suspend study temporarily, or even debar the investigator or sponsor from conducting trials in the future depending on the nature of incompliance.

Posttrial Access of an Investigational New Drug

In situations when, after the end of study, there is no alternate treatment available for the patient and the patient is found to benefit from the study drug, the investigator can recommend the sponsor for posttrial access. This should be consented by the patient and approved by the ethics committee.

Clinical Trial of Drugs Discovered in India

The CLA provides faster review for drugs developed and planned to be marketed in India. The application is expected to be assessed and a decision communicated within a 30-day time frame. If the CLA has not replied within this period, then the applicant can consider the permission was granted (automatic approval) and initiate clinical trial. Before initiating the trial, the applicant should notify the CLA about this **via form 4A**.

Approval by Independent Ethics Committee

When a study site does not have its own ethics committee, it can take permission from an ethics committee located at a different site. The ethics committee granting approval must be located either within the same city or within a 50 km radius of the trial site, and it will bear responsibility for monitoring the study's conduct.

Academic Clinical Trial

Under the revised regulations, academic trials—such as those exploring new uses for already approved drugs—are exempt from requiring prior approval from the Central Licensing Authority (CLA). These studies must receive ethics committee approval, and their findings are not permitted to be used for promotional or commercial purposes.

Pre-submission and Post-submission Meeting

The new clinical trial rules have provision for the applicant to request for meeting with the Central Licensing Authority seeking guidance regarding procedure for license, permission for manufacturing, clinical trial, etc. The applicant can do so by making an application in writing along with the documents referred in second schedule. Similarly, the applicant can also seek clarification in person for queries by making an application for post-submission meeting.

Drug Approval in Special Circumstances

The new regulation provides for accelerated drug development in special circumstances like life-threatening conditions, rare diseases, diseases with unmet medical need, disasters, and special defense use. This can be done by two process namely accelerated approval and expedited review.

Under accelerated approval, a drug can be approved for marketing based on surrogate end points instead of the traditional clinical outcomes such as disease progression or mortality. The surrogate markers used should be able to predict disease progression and should be measurable before irreversible morbidity occurs. The approval should be followed by post-marketing clinical trials, which validates the anticipated clinical benefit.

Similarly, when an investigational drug used for a disease (that is life threatening and has unmet medical needs) shows significant clinical efficacy in phase 2 trial, then the drug can be considered for accelerated approval. This approval is conditional upon further clinical trials demonstrating therapeutic benefit in a broader patient population, in accordance with the protocol sanctioned by the regulatory authority.

Furthermore, sponsors may seek an expedited review if specific criteria are met—such as the drug being intended for a life-threatening or rare condition with no existing treatment options, or if it demonstrates clear advantages over current therapies in terms of safety profile or patient adherence According to the New Drugs and Clinical Trials Rules (NDCTR), an orphan drug is defined as one intended to treat a medical condition that affects no more than 500,000 individuals within India (Box 23.3).

Box 23.3: Forms and Timelines Related to Clinical Trial Permission

Application for conducting clinical trial (new drugs)	Form CT-04
Permission to conduct clinical trial (new drugs)	Form CT-06
Notification regarding automatic approval for clinical trial (for drugs developed in India)	Form CT-4A
Application for conducting BA/BE studies	Form CT-05
Permission to conduct BA/BE studies	Form CT-07
Time to review form CT 04	90 working days in general (30 working days for drugs developed in India)
Validity of permission for BA/BE studies	1 year

23.4 Compensation for Trial-Related Injury

It is the responsibility of sponsor to provide compensation in case of serious adverse events related to clinical trials. The sponsor must provide a formal commitment to this requirement when applying for clinical trial authorization. The amount of compensation will be calculated using formula mentioned in seventh schedule. In case of death, the financial compensation should be given to the legal heir. Compensation for research-related injury occurring in academic clinical trials will be reviewed by the ethics committee.

Points that are considered when checking for relatedness of serious adverse events with clinical trial

- Was the adverse effect due to the trial product or any trial-related procedure or due to concomitant medications?
- Was there a deviation of protocol or negligence leading to the event?
- Did the investigational product fail to provide intended effect and was the required standard care not provided?
- Did the child experience any adverse effects in the womb as a result of the parent's involvement in the clinical trial? (Fig. 23.1).

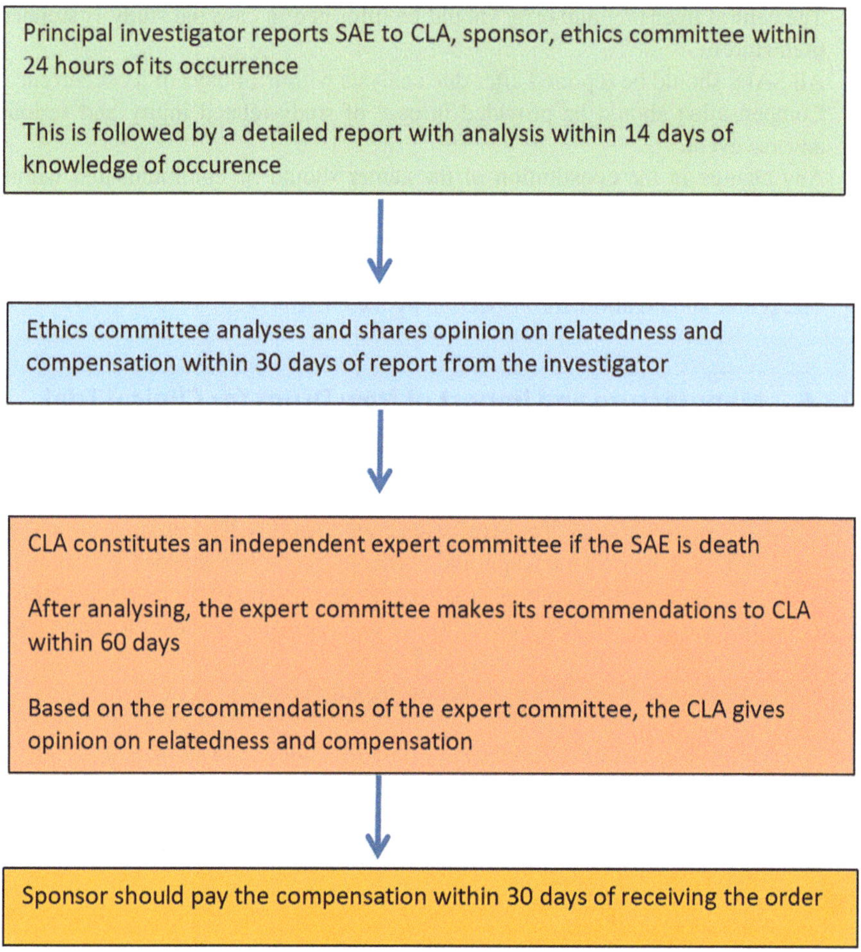

Fig. 23.1 Timeline and procedural flow for addressing compensation in clinical trial-related injuries

23.5 Registration of BA/BE Study Centers

Centers wanting to conduct BA/BE studies should be registered with the CLA using application form CT-08. The registration will remain valid for a duration of 5 years from the date of issuance. Renewal of registration should be made at least **90 days before expiry**. The registration will continue to be in force until further orders, provided the renewal application is made prior to 90 days.

The registration will be granted under the following conditions:

- The facility should have adequately trained and qualified persons.
- The study should be conducted only after the permission of CLA and approval of the ethics committee is obtained.
- The study should be registered with the Clinical Trial Registry of India.
- The study should be conducted as per the approved protocol and Good Clinical Practice guidelines.
- The central licensing authority should be informed in case the study is stopped prematurely.
- All SAEs should be reported after due analysis within 14 days of its occurrence.
- Compensation should be provided in case of study-related injury and serious adverse event.
- Any change in the constitution of the center should be communicated within **30 days**.
- Record should be maintained for up to **5 years or at least 2 years after the expiry date of study drug.**
- The center should allow for inspection by the CLA.

23.6 Manufacture and Import of New Drugs for Clinical Trial or Analysis

A company wanting to manufacture or import new drugs for the purpose of clinical trial or analysis should apply for permission from the CLA. The permission will be valid for 3 years, but under exceptional scenarios it can be extended for an additional 1 year upon written request made by the applicant. After obtaining permission, the permission holder should apply for a license for the same in accordance with the Drugs and Cosmetics Rules, 1945.

The approval is granted under the following stipulations:

1. The drug manufactured should be used only for clinical trial or testing and not to be sold in the market.
2. Manufacturing should follow the good manufacturing process.
3. Record of the number of drugs manufactured and supplied should be maintained.
4. Drugs that are damaged, leftover, expired, or those of substandard quantity should be destroyed and recorded.

5. The permission holder should allow for inspection of the premises by the authorized person.

Drugs manufactured for clinical trial should be kept in containers with label containing the details mentioned in Box 23.4:

Box 23.4. Particulars on the Drug container labels

- Name or code number of the drug.
- Batch or lot number.
- Date of manufacture.
- Use before date.
- Storage condition.
- Name of the center where testing is proposed to be done.
- Manufacturer name and address.

23.7 Manufacture and Import of New Drug for Sale or for Distribution

Authorization from the Central Licensing Authority (CLA) is required to import a new drug intended for commercial sale or distribution. The specific documentation required, along with the necessity for conducting local clinical trials, is determined by the type of drug—such as those containing unapproved new molecules, fixed-dose combinations, or phytopharmaceuticals—as outlined in the Second Schedule.

Scenarios where local clinical trials may not be required are:

1. The medication has received approval and is being distributed in the regions designated by the CLA, with no significant or unforeseen serious adverse effects reported.
2. There is an ongoing global clinical trial in India and the new drug is approved in a country specified by the CLA.
3. There is no evidence suggesting any variation in enzyme or gene involved in Indian population that can alter the pharmacokinetics or pharmacodynamic response of a drug.
4. When there is an undertaking by the applicant to conduct phase IV clinical trial using design approved by the licensing authority.

Relaxations can be made for life-threatening or serious conditions or when there is an unmet need (e.g., drug-resistant tuberculosis) or for rare diseases where there is no available drug or available at high cost.

Authorization will be provided subject to the following terms and conditions:

1. The specifications of the drug should be as approved by the Central Licensing Authority.
2. Labeling should meet the requirements of Drugs and Cosmetics Rules, 1945.
3. Label should contain the warning phrase:
   "To be sold by retail on the prescription of a ... only" in red box
4. Periodic safety update report should be submitted as specified in fifth schedule.
5. No claims other than mentioned should be made.
6. The label and package insert should be approved by the licensing authority.
7. Analysis report should accompany each consignment of import.

Once import approval is secured, the concerned individual must apply for and obtain the corresponding license. Similar process is followed for obtaining permission for manufacturing.

23.8 Importing Unapproved New Drug for Treatment Purpose

Government institutions can obtain permission from the CLA to import a new drug which is not approved in our country but approved in another country for treatment of life-threatening disease or conditions with unmet medical needs. The application should be made in form CT-24 and certified by the Medical Superintendent or Head of the Institution The licensing authority after reviewing the documents if found satisfactory shall grant permission in the form CT-25 with the following conditions:

1. The license (valid for **3 years**) should be displayed where the drug is stocked.
2. The drug should be stored under proper conditions and used exclusively for the treatment of the patient under the supervision of a pharmacist.
3. The pharmacist should maintain records of the drugs and it should be countersigned by the Medical Superintendent.
4. Status of the drug and stock should be updated half yearly to the Central Licensing Authority.
5. All unused, damaged products should be destroyed and recorded.

   Similarly, permission to manufacture a drug in limited quantities can be made for life-threatening disease using form CT-26. Patient consent along with the recommendation of the ethics committee should be included in the application. The permission (1 year validity) will be granted subjected to:

   - The drug should be used only for the purposes specified supervised by a medical officer.
   - The drugs should be kept in accordance with the storage conditions.

- Record should be maintained as specified in the form CT-27 and half yearly report should be submitted.
- Record should contain patient name, address, diagnosis, and dosage details and countersigned by the Medical Superintendent.
- Drugs that are leftover, damaged, or shelf life expired should be destroyed and record should be maintained in this regard.
- The central licensing authority should be informed about any serious adverse events along with the actions taken within 15 days of its occurrence.

23.9 Amendments to New Clinical Trial Rule 2019

Two important amendments have been made since the inception of the new clinical trial rule in 2019 related to deemed approvals and registration of clinical research organization.

Deemed Approvals for Applications
As per this rule, when no communication is made from the CLA within specific time of an application (45 working days for EC registration and 90 days for conducting clinical trial), then the approval for the application can be deemed to be granted. This is applicable for applications related to ethics committee registration, permission for BA/BE studies, permission to manufacture new drug for clinical trial. The applicant, however, must fill and submit automatic approval form (e.g., **CT-02A for ethics committee registration**) before initiating the activity to be kept for official record.

Registration of Clinical Research Organization
Clinical research organizations wanting to conduct clinical trial or bioavailability/bioequivalence study should register with the Central Licensing Authority. Application should be submitted using form CT-07B and approval will be conformed using form CT-07C. The registration will be valid for 5 years. A new schedule (Schedule IX) was added to provide required information.

23.10 Schedules in New Drugs and Clinical Trials Rules, 2019

While the chapters tell what is to be done with respect to conduct of trials, registrations, and permission, the schedules discuss how they must be done. The NDCTR, 2019 contains nine schedules described in Box 23.5:

Box 23.5. The NDCTR, 2019 Schedules and their description

Schedule	Description
First schedule	General principles to be considered for conducting different phases of clinical trial and in special population
Second schedule	Discusses about special situations for accelerated approval, animal studies, fixed-dose combinations, stability testing of new drugs Provides information on data required for applications regarding import/manufacture, clinical trial of new drugs, and phytopharmaceuticals
Third schedule	Discusses regarding conduct of clinical trial, informed consent, responsibilities of the sponsor, investigator, and ethics committee in research **Table 1** Information needed for ethics committee registration **Table 2** Contents of a protocol **Table 3** Checklist for informed consent in a clinical trial **Table 4** Investigator undertaking **Table 5** Information needed for reporting serious adverse event **Table 6** Format of clinical trial report **Table 7** Investigator's brochure **Table 8** Details of prescribing information
Fourth schedule	Discusses about the requirements for bioavailability and bioequivalence study standard operating procedures, clinical pharmacological unit, maintenance of records, and retention of samples
Fifth schedule	Post-market assessment can be conducted in any of the following ways: A. Phase IV (post-marketing) trial—This includes drug interaction studies, safety studies, and studies designed to support approved indications. These are conducted as per the regulatory guidelines with a provision to compensate for trial-related injury. The study drug is usually provided free of cost by the sponsor in this scenario B. Post-marketing surveillance study—These are observational/noninterventional studies conducted for approved indications. The study population are as per recommendations mentioned in the package insert. The regulatory provisions do not apply for these studies C. Through periodic safety update reports
Sixth schedule	Fees for different applications and registration

Seventh schedule	Formulae to determine compensation depends on the nature of serious adverse event as follows: **1. Death** Compensation = (B*F*R)/99.37 B is base amount (8 lakhs) F—depends on the age of trial subject (based on workmen compensation act) R—risk factor depends on disease severity and seriousness When the expected mortality (within 30 days) is 90% or more, then a fixed amount of 2 lakhs is given **2. Injury other than death** **I. Permanent disability** (it is based on the concept that if someone has 100% disability, the compensation should be 90% of the compensation in case of death) Accordingly, compensation = (C*D*90)/(100*100) Where D = percentage of disability C = quantum of compensation due for payment in case of death **II. Congenital anomaly or birth defect:** This includes situation in which any one or both the parent participating in a trial lead to still birth, or deformity. The quantum of compensation in such cases will be 50% of the base amount (i.e., 4 lakhs) along with medical management required. **III. Chronic life-threatening disease and reversible SAE (resolved)** Compensation = 2*W*N Where W = minimum wage per day of the unskilled worker (in Delhi) N = number of days of hospitalization The compensation calculated is based on the number of days of hospitalization. The patient not only loses the wage but will also have other loss such as the wage loss of the attendant, inconvenience, etc.
Eighth schedule	Provides forms for application for permission and grant of registrations
Ninth schedule	Requirements and guidelines for registration of clinical research organization. Specifies the documents required for registration of clinical research organization

Bibliography

1. Annapurna SA, Rao SY (2020) New drug and clinical trial rules, 2019: an overview. Int J Clin Trials 7(4):278–284
2. Jadhav S, Ghool R (2019) New drug and clinical trial rules 2019 – two steps forward and one back. Indian J Pharm Pract 12(3):209–214
3. Central Drugs Standard Control Organization (2019) Drug and clinical trial rules. Central Drugs Standard Control Organization, New Delhi. Available from https://cdsco.gov.in/opencms/export/sites/CDSCO_WEB/Pdf-documents/NewDrugs_CTRules_2019.pdf. Last accessed on 17 Mar 2022
4. Lahiry S, Thakur S, Chakraborty DS (2020) New drugs and clinical trials rules-2019: what academicians need to know. Indian J Dermatol Venereol Leprol 86:445–448
5. Central Drugs Standard Control Organization – Directorate General of Health Services Ministry of Health and Family Welfare Government of India. New Drugs Division. Frequently Asked Questions (FAQs) on New Drugs and Clinical Trials. Available from https://cdsco.gov.in/opencms/resources/UploadCDSCOWeb/2018/UploadPublic_NoticesFiles/faqnd.pdf. Last accessed on 17 Mar 2022

Regulation of Healthcare Products by the United States Food and Drug Administration and Health Canada

24

Neel Shah

Abstract

Evolving medical research and treatment modalities have been channeled into safe and effective therapies for the welfare of the public by means of laws and regulations and their periodic modernizations. A regulated environment also creates a fair place for industry stakeholders to compete. The United States Food and Drug Administration as well as Health Canada, both federal agencies, have been instrumental in bringing new therapies to their respective countries. The granularity of regulations, need for evidence, and associated costs increase as the risks associated with the use of these products increase, with prescription drugs being the most challenging and cosmetics being the least. The International Conference on Harmonization made it possible for countries to develop common guidelines, and for the industry to submit mostly the same dossier to multiple countries. Getting an approval to sell a drug is the start of a journey of continuing compliance and demonstration of adherence to the country's laws and regulations.

Keywords

Food and Drugs Act · Food and Drug Regulations · US-FDA · Health Canada · IND · NDA · NDS · CTA · International conference on harmonization · ICH

N. Shah (✉)
Regulatory Consultant, Concept2Clinic Inc., Richmond Hill, ON, Canada
e-mail: neel.lakshya@gmail.com

A. Arivazhahan et al. (eds.), *Introduction to Basics of Pharmacology and Toxicology*, https://doi.org/10.1007/978-981-95-1920-0_24

24.1 Introduction

The General Inspection Act was passed in Canada in 1874, followed by the Act to Prevent the Adulteration of Food, Drink, and Drugs in 1875 to mitigate adulteration of commodities such as alcohol and grains. The basic version of the "Food and Drugs Act" was passed in 1982, with various updates to it every few years [7].

Across the border, in the United States, the Drug Importation Act was passed in 1848 to control the quality of imported drugs. The first version of the Food and Drugs Act was passed in 1906, which has subsequently undergone multiple modernizations [24].

Over the years, the need to differentiate biologics, prescription drugs, and over-the-counter drugs was identified, as all of them pose different risks in manufacturing as well as safety and efficacy. The need to make quality of drugs more stringent was usually identified after the occurrence of tragedies such as the thalidomide disaster, including the powers given to state agencies to order "stop sale" and recalls. Focus was given on reviewing the safety and efficacy data *before* the sale of medicines. In the last couple of decades, supplements/natural health products, cosmetics, and medical devices have been identified as separate entities requiring a separate set of regulations, usually less stringent than drugs.

Acts are formed by members of the parliament and define the overall outcome that is desired to keep the public safe and healthy, such as the Canadian "Food and Drugs Act" states: "No person shall manufacture, prepare, preserve, package or store for sale any drug under unsanitary conditions" [6]. Further, to give the industry some specifics to prevent "unsanitary" conditions, experts have created the Food and Drug regulations (enabled by the Food and Drugs Act), which elaborate on the need for product licencing (such as submitting a New Drug Submission/ NDS) as well as drug establishment licence requirements (the GMP requirements to manufacture drugs) [5]. Even regulations can be interpreted differently by different stakeholders and hence, for industry to have a uniform, readily available reference, Health Canada (the federal/central regulatory agency for drugs) publishes multiple guidelines under these regulations, such as the labeling requirements for nonprescription drugs guidance document [17] and Labeling of Pharmaceutical Drugs for Human Use [12] (Fig. 24.1).

24.2 Concept of Harmonization: ICH

The huge number of resources (11–14 years and around 10 billion USD) spent through the product lifecycle development cannot be spent for preparing a submission for each country where a company intends to sell their drug. To achieve *harmonization* in meeting standards across countries, and to ensure that safe, effective, and high-quality medicines are developed and registered in the most resource-efficient manner, the **International Conference on Harmonization of Technical Requirements for Registration of Pharmaceuticals for Human Use (ICH)** was established in 1990 by its founding members: the European Commission (EC), the

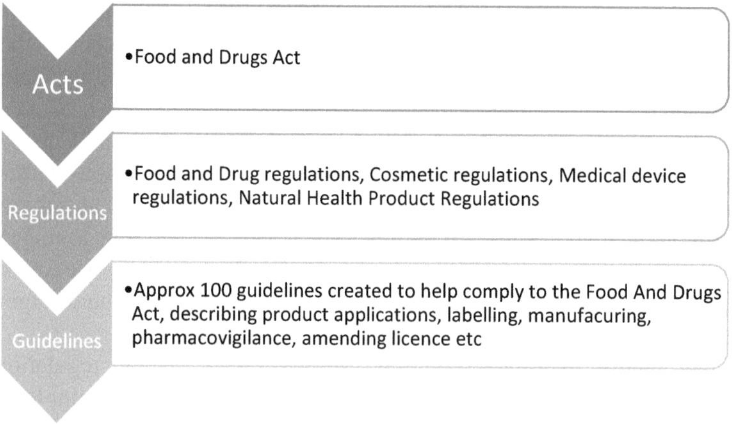

Fig. 24.1 The relationship between Acts, Regulations, and Guidelines in Canada: acts/laws passed by the members of the parliament, regulations made by specific minister under the enabling act, and guidelines made by federal agency to "suggest" ways to comply with the Act and Regulations

US Food and Drug Administration (USFDA), the Pharmaceuticals and Medical Devices Agency (PMDA), Japan, and the respective industry associations of the three countries. Currently, it has got another 12 countries as members and 21 countries as observers [22].

By being members, the regulatory agencies commit to following set standards of pharmaceutical manufacturing, safety and efficacy development, and review process in their country. They also get to create guidelines together for the same and to select topics where harmonization is required, where heterogeneity in the review process exists. All the guidelines that the ICH members create are broadly covered under four headings: Q, S, E, and M (guidelines to demonstrate quality, safety, efficacy of drugs, and multidisciplinary topics). The guideline E14, for example, covers the clinical evaluation of QT interval prolongation of drugs and the guideline Q3A(R2) covers classifying and testing impurities in drug substances [20]. This gives industry a guidance to conduct studies that would be accepted by major regulators around the world.

24.3 Risk-Based Classification of Healthcare Products

Risks related to use of drugs may arise due to lack of efficacy, lack of safety, or due to variability of effect with each dose. **Prescription drugs** are meant to be prescribed after a complete understanding of its indications, conditions of use, and safety information, essentially only by healthcare practitioners. Since they are chemicals or biologics, potentially new to the human body, these need to be backed up by in vitro, animal as well as human studies. The efficacy has also to be proven in phase 2 and 3 studies. The manufacturing data (CMC—chemistry, manufacturing, and controls) must be recorded in detail for both the drug substance (API—active pharmaceutical ingredient) as well as the drug product (finished drug in dosage form) so that same efficacy and safety can be expected throughout the shelf life.

Over-the-counter drugs (as classified in the United States and Canada) need lesser efficacy and safety data since these are meant for not so serious diseases, the general public can be relied upon to understand the instructions and these drugs have been on the market since a long time. The lower cost and time to review these applications help more sellers to enter the market for common diseases such as cough, cold, constipation, allergies, and for use as disinfectants, thus, helping people manage their health in an easier, faster, and affordable way.

Natural health products (identified as NHPs in Canadian regulations) are derived from nature or are synthetic isolates of such substances. Examples include vitamins, minerals, herbal extracts, and probiotics. The counterpart of NHPs in the United States are dietary supplements. Often, the safety and efficacy can be proven by simply attesting to published monographs by Health Canada, or referring to publicly available research or homeopathic textbooks [16]. These can also be authorized for sale based on a long traditional/cultural history of use, such as in Ayurveda [the *Triphala* monograph published by Health Canada [11]] or in Chinese medicine, such as the strengthening Qi energy by use of mushrooms [10]. In most cases, these applications do not undergo detailed review by the USFDA (United States Food and Drug Administration)/Health Canada, with no fees charged and timelines of review ranging from 2 to 7 months by Health Canada and just a notification sufficing for the USFDA.

In the last decade or so, **medical devices** have been receiving greater attention and detailed regulatory pathways have been charted for their review and approval. Medical devices can be classified as per the risk posed: toothbrushes and bandages are examples of class I; an endoscopic stapler or a kit to diagnose pregnancy is class II; a hernia mesh or a hyaluronic acid injection for arthritis is class III; and a stent to treat cardiovascular disease or a kit to diagnose HIV is class IV [14]. Similarly, in United States, the spectrum ranges from Class I to Class III instead of the 4 classes described by Health Canada. While Health Canada requires safety data (clinical studies, biocompatibility data) and efficacy data only for Class III and Class IV devices, the USFDA has even laid a pathway for "generic" devices (510 K pathway), whereby a device can rely upon evidence submitted for devices already approved by the traditional pathway (the "predicate"). The fees and review timelines are much less compared to drugs (e.g., approximately $600 CAD and 15-day review timeline for Class II medical devices by Health Canada).

Lastly, cosmetics are regulated by agencies in a less stringent way by the agencies. The important thing to regulate here is that cosmetics should not make therapeutic claims. For example, a make up to *cover* acne spots would be regulated as cosmetic, but a cream to *treat* acne is a drug. The GMP requirements are not assessed making it possible even for homemade cosmetics to legally enter the market. When it comes to safety, Health Canada maintains a cosmetic "hotlist," where all the restricted ingredients are mentioned [9].

24.4 Regulator's Role in Assessing Safety and Efficacy

Safety and efficacy of drugs (excluding NHPs, supplements, devices, cosmetics) are assessed by the regulatory agency in the following steps (Fig. 24.2):

1. IND: In the Investigational New Drug Application stage (USFDA), the sponsor submits safety data from in vitro and preclinical studies, as well as proof of pharmacological activity, thus, justifying first use in humans. The IND is also a stage for USFDA (along with the research and ethics board) to review protocol of the early clinical trials and for the sponsor to take help from USFDA in developing the same by means of a pre-IND consultation [3]. The IND is "amended" when new protocols are added, moving on from phase I to II and III trials. Unlike one single open IND throughout the drug development, Health Canada requires submission of a separate CTA (Clinical Trial Application) for every clinical trial that is done for all 3 phases of drug development. Both the IND as well as CTA have a review timeline of 30 days.
2. NDS/NDA: New Drug Submission (Health Canada)/New Drug Application (USFDA terminology): In an NDS/NDA application, the regulatory agencies review the clinical trial data coming from the Phase I, II and III studies, whether benefits outweigh risks, whether labeling is adequate for proper use and mitigating risks. Health Canada review timelines are around 340 days for an NDS as of

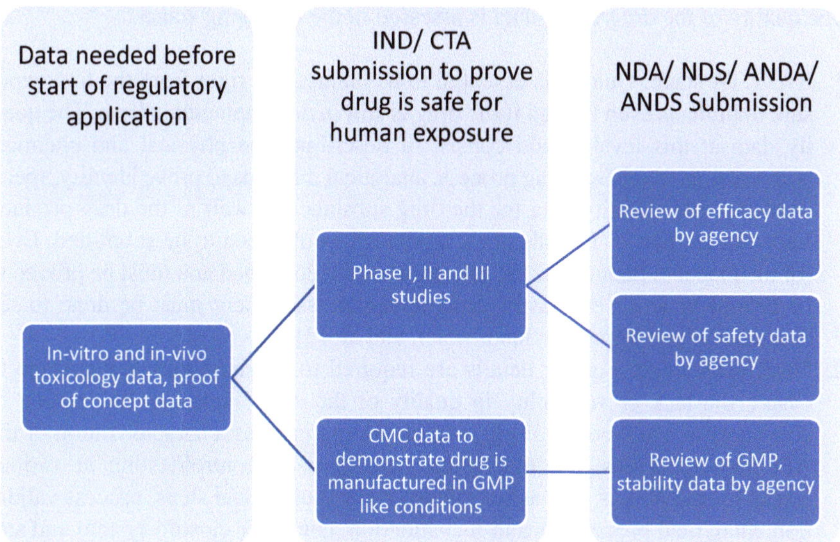

Fig. 24.2 Example of a regulatory pathway for a prescription drug approval by USFDA/Health Canada. The end result may be approval of the drug (issuance of a Drug Identification Number/DIN number by Health Canada and/or National Drug Code/NDC number by USFDA) as well as approval of the facility of manufacturing of the drug. Both review processes (for the drug as well as the facility) can go in parallel. *IND* Investigational New Drug, *CTA* Clinical Trial Application. [8]

2023 (205 days if the drug is approved for priority review), and the fee is $565,000 CAD [13, 18].
3. ANDS/ANDA: Abbreviated NDS/NDA applications are meant for reviews of generic drugs. Biosimilars are, however, not considered generic and need to be reviewed via a full NDS/NDA. Generic applications do not need to have full set of preclinical data and phase I and II studies. Usually, a bioequivalence study comparing the generic to the reference drug is enough. Health Canada review timelines are around 340 days for an ANDS as of 2023 and the fee is $292,000 CAD [13, 18].
4. 505(b)(2) pathway (named after the section in the Food and Drugs Act, USA): Some applications may be for old drugs already approved but may not exactly qualify as generics since they are for a different indication or for a different formulation. For example, Company Y wants to sell extended-release formulation of a drug initially approved for Company X. By means of a 505(b)(2) application, Company Y can rely on data owned by Company X submitted to USFDA in addition to a **clinical** study (not a BA/BE study) done by themselves to prove the efficacy and safety of this extended-release formulation [4]. Such submissions in Canada are submitted under the pathway of "Drug Submissions Relying on Third-Party Data."

24.5 Regulator's Role in Assessing Quality

The quality of the drug/CMC data is assessed in the following stages:

1. IND/CTA stage: Quality is essential to be maintained right from the first exposure to humans even though if the drug is still in developmental phase. The quality data at this level would consist of describing the physical and chemical composition, manufacturing process, analytical methods to prove identity, specifications, and stability data for the drug substance as well as the drug product. Labeling (as part of investigator's brochure) would need to be submitted. Even for the placebo, manufacturing process must be described and must be proven to be devoid of any API. Lastly, environmental assessment must be done to see degradation and impact on land, water, and air [2].
2. NDS/NDA stage: Further details are required to be submitted at this stage to ensure the lack of variability in quality of the drug, including description of characteristics and composition, manufacturing process, characterization of the API and impurities, pharmaceutical development, control/testing at various stages for the API as well as excipients, control of critical steps, process validation, analytical procedures and its validation, container closure system and stability (Fig. 24.3 enlists the names of all the files that have to be submitted) [19].
3. When it comes to "doing it right the first time" for a new molecule/formulation, many countries have adopted the concept of **Quality by Design** (Fig. 24.4) (described in detail in ICH-Q8, Q9, and Q10 guidelines). These guidelines would be applicable to any kind of manufacturing (even for automobiles!) and

TABLE OF CONTENTS FOR QUALITY DOCUMENTS

Module 2: Common Technical Documents Summaries

2.3: Quality Overall Summary (QOS)

- **2.3.S Drug Substance (name, manufacturer)**
  - 2.3.S.1 General Information
  - 2.3.S.2 Manufacture
  - 2.3.S.3 Characterisation
  - 2.3.S.4 Control of Drug Substance
  - 2.3.S.5 Reference Standards or Materials
  - 2.3.S.6 Container Closure System
  - 2.3.S.7 Stability
- **2.3.P Drug Product**
  - 2.3.P.1 Description and Composition of the Drug Product
  - 2.3.P.2 Pharmaceutical Development
  - 2.3.P.3 Manufacture
  - 2.3.P.4 Control of Excipients
  - 2.3.P.5 Control of Drug Product
  - 2.3.P.6 Reference Standards or Materials
  - 2.3.P.7 Container Closure System
  - 2.3.P.8 Stability
- **2.3.A Appendices**
  - 2.3.A.1 Facilities and Equipment
  - 2.3.A.2 Adventitious Agents Safety Evaluation
  - 2.3.A.3 Excipients
- **2.3.R Regional Information**

Module 3: Quality (Body of Data)

3.1: Table of Contents of Module 3

3.2: Body of Data

- **3.2.S Drug Substance (name, manufacturer)**
  - 3.2.S.1 General Information
    - 3.2.S.1.1 Nomenclature
    - 3.2.S.1.2 Structure
    - 3.2.S.1.3 General Properties
  - 3.2.S.2 Manufacture
    - 3.2.S.2.1 Manufacturer(s)
    - 3.2.S.2.2 Description of Manufacturing Process and Process Controls
    - 3.2.S.2.3 Control of Materials
    - 3.2.S.2.4 Controls of Critical Steps and Intermediates
    - 3.2.S.2.5 Process Validation and/or Evaluation
    - 3.2.S.2.6 Manufacturing Process Development
  - 3.2.S.3 Characterisation
    - 3.2.S.3.1 Elucidation of Structure and Other Characteristics
    - 3.2.S.3.2 Impurities
  - 3.2.S.4 Control of Drug Substance
    - 3.2.S.4.1 Specification
    - 3.2.S.4.2 Analytical Procedures
    - 3.2.S.4.3 Validation of Analytical Procedures
    - 3.2.S.4.4 Batch Analyses
    - 3.2.S.4.5 Justification of Specification
  - 3.2.S.5 Reference Standards or Materials
  - 3.2.S.6 Container Closure System
  - 3.2.S.7 Stability
    - 3.2.S.7.1 Stability Summary and Conclusions
    - 3.2.S.7.2 Post-approval Stability Protocol and Stability Commitment
    - 3.2.S.7.3 Stability Data
- **3.2.P Drug Product**
  - 3.2.P.1 Description and Composition of the Drug Product
  - 3.2.P.2 Pharmaceutical Development
    - 3.2.P.2.1 Components of the Drug Product
    - 3.2.P.2.2 Drug Product
    - 3.2.P.2.3 Manufacturing Process Development
    - 3.2.P.2.4 Container Closure System
    - 3.2.P.2.5 Microbiological Attributes
    - 3.2.P.2.6 Compatibility
  - 3.2.P.3 Manufacture
    - 3.2.P.3.1 Manufacturer(s)
    - 3.2.P.3.2 Batch Formula
    - 3.2.P.3.3 Description of Manufacturing Process and Process Controls
    - 3.2.P.3.4 Controls of Critical Steps and Intermediates
    - 3.2.P.3.5 Process Validation and/or Evaluation
  - 3.2.P.4 Control of Excipients
    - 3.2.P.4.1 Specifications
    - 3.2.P.4.2 Analytical Procedures
    - 3.2.P.4.3 Validation of Analytical Procedures
    - 3.2.P.4.4 Justification of Specifications
    - 3.2.P.4.5 Excipients of Human or Animal Origin
    - 3.2.P.4.6 Novel Excipients
  - 3.2.P.5 Control of Drug Product
    - 3.2.P.5.1 Specification(s)
    - 3.2.P.5.2 Analytical Procedures
    - 3.2.P.5.3 Validation of Analytical Procedures
    - 3.2.P.5.4 Batch Analyses
    - 3.2.P.5.5 Characterisation of Impurities
    - 3.2.P.5.6 Justification of Specification(s)
  - 3.2.P.6 Reference Standards or Materials
  - 3.2.P.7 Container Closure System
  - 3.2.P.8 Stability
    - 3.2.P.8.1 Stability Summary and Conclusion
    - 3.2.P.8.2 Post-approval Stability Protocol and Stability Commitment
    - 3.2.P.8.3 Stability Data
- **3.2.A Appendices**
  - 3.2.A.1 Facilities and Equipment
  - 3.2.A.2 Adventitious Agents Safety Evaluation
  - 3.2.A.3 Excipients
- **3.2.R Regional Information**

3.3 Literature References

Fig. 24.3 Contents of Module 3: Quality, taken from "ICH: The Common Technical Document for the registration of pharmaceuticals for human use: Quality—M4Q(R1)". [21]

start by identification of the final "target profile" desired to achieve the set efficacy and safety (such as a transdermal patch which releases a drug, steadily at rate of xx mcg/hour into systemic circulation without dose dumping). Secondly, "critical quality attributes" are identified (such as dissolution rate, microbial limits, identity testing) which must stay within prespecified limits to achieve the "target profile." Lastly, "critical process parameters" and "critical material attributes" are identified which must be monitored to ensure desired quality [23].

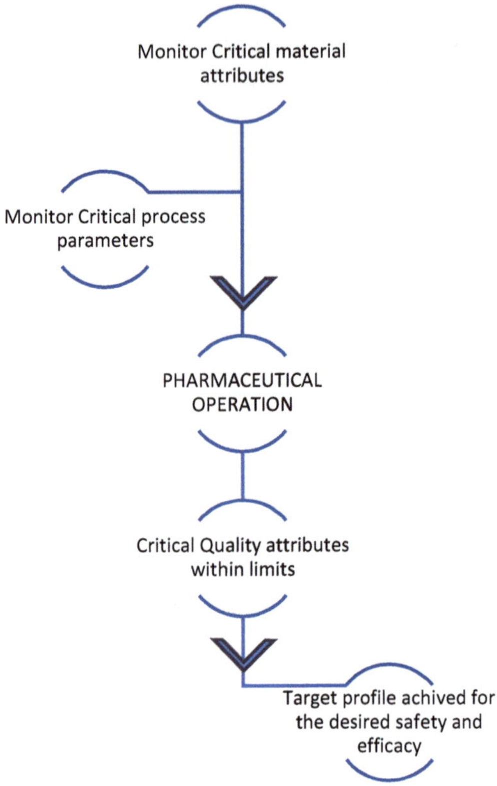

Fig. 24.4 Concept of quality by design. Even though achieving the target profile is the final output, but is also the first step in planning the rest of the design

24.6 Common Technical Document (CTD)

Since, most countries (signatory to the ICH) need the same information about a drug to assess safety, efficacy, and quality, the concept of CTD allows industry to essentially submit this information in the same "format" to each country's regulators (a harmonized electronic submission).

Figure 24.5 shows how data is organized into modules 1, 2, 3, 4, and 5. Module 3 holds all the quality data (Fig. 24.5 shows the file nomenclature), modules 4 and 5 containing the nonclinical and clinical data, respectively. Module 2 contains the summaries of module 3, 4, and 5. The only module which is different for different countries is module 1 (regional module), due to reasons such as labels being in different languages, assessment of the brand name of the drug as per country specific regulations, country specific application forms, product monographs or summary of prescribing information, etc.

All characteristics are specified, such as the naming of the files, creating folders and subfolders to place the documents, creating bookmarks and table of contents within the documents, converting Word files to pdf, setting metadata for the pdf for easily locating information within, and the maximum megabyte size of a single file.

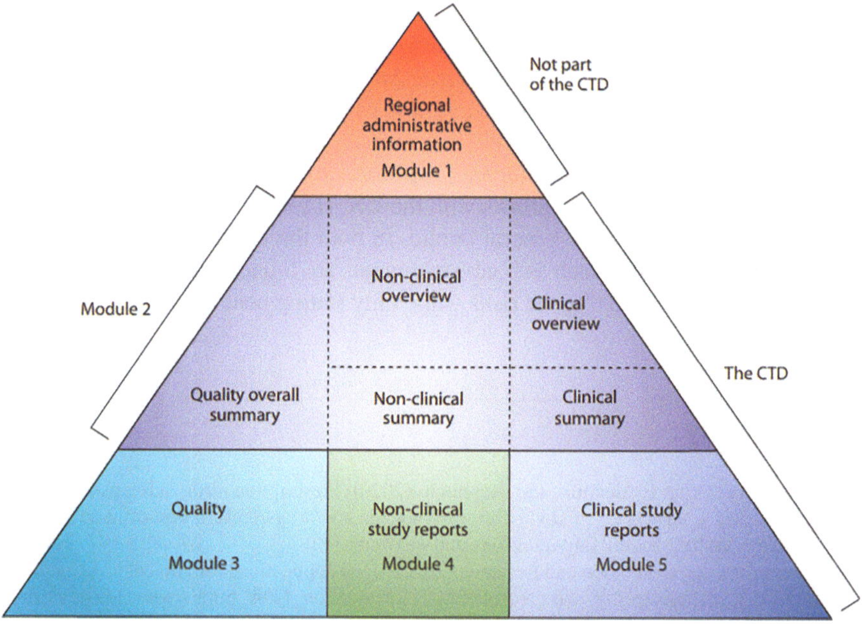

Fig. 24.5 The Common Technical Document triangle, taken from ICH Standards > M4: The Common Technical Document [21]

Around 160 validation rules have been created, and the screening to check adherence to these rules is checked by publishing software [15].

24.7 Post-marketing Regulations

A successful submission results in the issuance of a product licence as well as establishment licence. However, being compliant to the regulations is a continuing process, a drug safe and effective today may not stay the same in the future. Hence, periodic renewals are put in place such as:

- **Annual Drug Notification** (Canada), helping Health Canada maintain a list of drugs that are still marketed or discontinued by the Marketing Authorization Holder (MAH) and the contact details of the MAH.
- **Annual Licence Renewal** (Canada) for each establishment where licensable activities of fabrication, importing, distribution, packaging, labeling, and testing take place, helping Health Canada maintain a list of all licenced establishments around the globe that supply drugs/APIs to Canada and their contact details.
- **NERBY** (New Evidence Required By date) (Canada), where evidence of adhering to GMP has to be submitted every 3–4 years in the form of audit reports for all licenced establishments.

- Periodic Safety Update Reports (PSURs) containing summary of safety data collected worldwide, assessing the benefit-risk profile of the drug.

Advertisement of healthcare products is strictly controlled in Canada, where the Food and Drugs Act prohibits advertising prescription drugs to general public and mandate advertisements to healthcare practitioners to be truthful, consistent, relevant, and transparent. This contrasts with the USFDA, which allows advertisement of prescription drugs to the general public. In both the countries, however, it is a violation of law in cases such as if advertisements are found to be off label, misrepresent data, leave out stating the risks while only stating benefits (lacking "fair balance").[1].

Bibliography

1. Center for Drug Evaluation and Research (2020) Prescription drug advertising | questions and answers. FDA. https://www.fda.gov/drugs/prescription-drug-advertising/prescription-drug-advertising-questions-and-answers
2. Center for Drug Evaluation and Research (2022a) IND applications for clinical investigations: chemistry, manufacturing, and control (CMC) information. FDA. https://www.fda.gov/drugs/investigational-new-drug-ind-application/ind-applications-clinical-investigations-chemistry-manufacturing-and-control-cmc-information
3. Center for Drug Evaluation and Research (2022b) Investigational New Drug (IND) application. FDA, November 29. https://www.fda.gov/drugs/types-applications/investigational-new-drug-ind-application
4. Center for Drug Evaluation and Research (2023) Abbreviated approval pathways for drug product: 505(b)(2) or ANDA? FDA. https://www.fda.gov/drugs/cder-small-business-industry-assistance-sbia/abbreviated-approval-pathways-drug-product-505b2-or-anda
5. Consolidated federal laws of Canada, Food and Drug Regulations (2023) February 15. https://laws-lois.justice.gc.ca/eng/regulations/c.r.c.,_c._870/index.html
6. Consolidated federal laws of Canada, Food and Drugs Act (2023) June 22. https://laws-lois.justice.gc.ca/eng/acts/f-27/
7. Food legislation | The Canadian encyclopedia (n.d.) Retrieved August 12, 2023, from https://www.thecanadianencyclopedia.ca/en/article/food-legislation
8. Health Canada (2001) How drugs are reviewed in Canada [Education and awareness], January 8. https://www.canada.ca/en/health-canada/services/drugs-health-products/drug-products/fact-sheets/drugs-reviewed-canada.html
9. Health Canada (2004a) Cosmetic ingredient hotlist: prohibited and restricted ingredients [Education and awareness], June 18. https://www.canada.ca/en/health-canada/services/consumer-product-safety/cosmetics/cosmetic-ingredient-hotlist-prohibited-restricted-ingredients.html
10. Health Canada (2004b) Product monographs. Mushrooms, July 26 https://webprod.hc-sc.gc.ca/nhpid-bdipsn/atReq.do?atid=mushrooms.champignons&lang=eng
11. Health Canada (2004c). Product monographs. Triphala, July 26. https://webprod.hc-sc.gc.ca/nhpid-bdipsn/atReq.do?atid=triphala&lang=eng
12. Health Canada (2013) Guidance document: labelling of pharmaceutical drugs for human use [guidance], November 1. https://www.canada.ca/en/health-canada/services/drugs-health-products/drug-products/applications-submissions/guidance-documents/labelling-pharmaceutical-drugs-human-use-2014-guidance-document.html
13. Health Canada (2014) Fees for examination of a submission: drugs for human use [guidance], April 1. https://www.canada.ca/en/health-canada/services/drugs-health-products/funding-

fees/fees-respect-human-drugs-medical-devices/pharmaceutical-submission-application-review-funding-fees-drugs-health-products.html
14. Health Canada (2015a) Guidance document—guidance on the risk-based classification system for non-in vitro diagnostic devices (non-IVDDs) [guidance], April 23. https://www.canada.ca/en/health-canada/services/drugs-health-products/medical-devices/application-information/guidance-documents/guidance-document-guidance-risk-based-classification-system-non-vitro-diagnostic.html
15. Health Canada (2015b) Validation rules for regulatory transactions provided to Health Canada in the electronic Common Technical Document (eCTD) format [Notices], August 19. https://www.canada.ca/en/health-canada/services/drugs-health-products/drug-products/applications-submissions/guidance-documents/ectd/notice-validation-rules-regulatory-transactions-submitted-health-canada-electronic-common-technical-document-format-2016-12-1.html
16. Health Canada (2018a) Natural Health Products Management of Applications Policy [policies], June 29. https://www.canada.ca/en/health-canada/services/drugs-health-products/natural-health-products/legislation-guidelines/guidance-documents/management-product-licence-applications-attestations.html
17. Health Canada (2018b) Labelling requirements for non-prescription drugs: guidance document [guidance – legislative], September 28. https://www.canada.ca/en/health-canada/services/drugs-health-products/natural-non-prescription/legislation-guidelines/guidance-documents/labelling-requirements-non-prescription-drugs.html
18. Health Canada (2020) Guidance document: the management of drug submissions and applications [guidance], September 21. https://www.canada.ca/en/health-canada/services/drugs-health-products/drug-products/applications-submissions/guidance-documents/management-drug-submissions/industry/document.html
19. Health Canada (2022) Guidance document: quality (chemistry and manufacturing) guidance: new drug submissions (NDSs) and abbreviated new drug submissions (ANDSs) [consultations; guidance], December 5. https://www.canada.ca/en/health-canada/services/drugs-health-products/drug-products/applications-submissions/guidance-documents/chemical-entity-products-quality/guidance-document-quality-chemistry-manufacturing-guidance-new-drug-submissions-ndss-abbreviated-new-drug-submissions.html
20. ICH Official web site: ICH guidelines (n.d.) Retrieved August 26, 2023, from https://www.ich.org/page/ich-guidelines
21. ICH Official web site: M4: the common technical document (n.d.) Retrieved August 28, 2023, from https://www.ich.org/page/ctd
22. ICH Official web site: Members & observers (n.d.) Retrieved August 26, 2023, from https://www.ich.org/page/members-observers
23. Maguire J, Peng D (n.d.) How to identify critical quality attributes and critical process parameters. US Food and Drug Administration FDA PQRI 2nd conference North Bethesda, MD, USA, 6 Oct 2015
24. Milestones in U.S. Food and Drug Law (2023) FDA. https://www.fda.gov/about-fda/fda-history/milestones-us-food-and-drug-law

Good Clinical Practice

25

Mourouguessine Vimal, Nishanthi Anandabaskar, and M. Shanthi

Abstract

Good clinical practice (GCP) is an "international ethical and scientific quality standard for the design, conduct, performance, monitoring, auditing, recording, analyses and reporting of clinical trials." It is essential in ensuring participant safety and collection of good quality data. Compliance with GCP is a legal mandate in conducting clinical trials. Of the various GCP guidelines, the ICH-GCP guidelines is most commonly followed by the regulators and funders worldwide and will be discussed in detail in this chapter.

Keywords

Good clinical practice · Clinical trials · Ethical standards

M. Vimal
Department of Pathology, Sri Manakula Vinayagar Medical College and Hospital, Puducherry, India

N. Anandabaskar (✉)
Department of Pharmacology, Sri Manakula Vinayagar Medical College and Hospital, Puducherry, Puducherry, India

M. Shanthi
Department of Pharmacology, Sri Manakula Vinayagar Medical College and Hospital, Puducherry, India
e-mail: shanthibabu24@gmail.com

A. Arivazhahan et al. (eds.), *Introduction to Basics of Pharmacology and Toxicology*, https://doi.org/10.1007/978-981-95-1920-0_25

25.1 Introduction to GCP

Good clinical practice (GCP) is an "international ethical and scientific quality standard for the design, conduct, performance, monitoring, auditing, recording, analyses and reporting of clinical trials." It aims at ensuring credible and accurate data generation from research. Also, it aims to protect the research participants' rights, safety, and well-being (refer Fig. 25.1). Adherence to GCP is a legal requirement in conducting clinical trials. Various stakeholders involved in the conduct of clinical trials, like sponsors, investigators and site staff, contract research organizations (CROs), ethics committees, regulatory authorities, and study participants, share the responsibility of ensuring that clinical trials are conducted in accordance with GCP (refer Fig. 25.2).

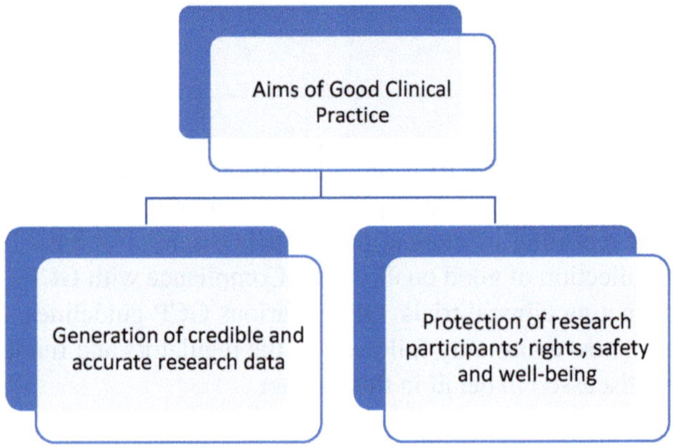

Fig. 25.1 Aims of good clinical practice (GCP)

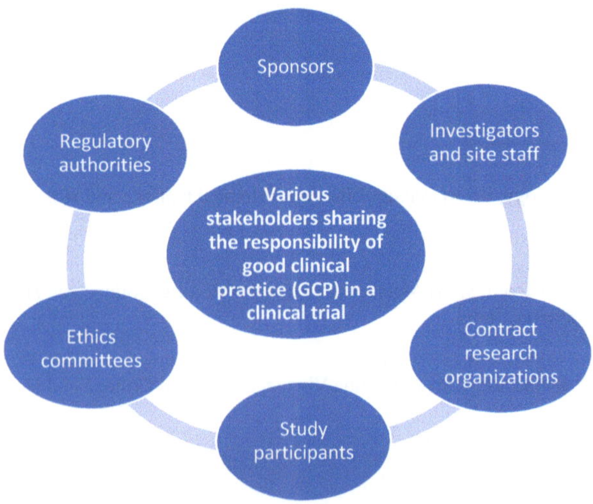

Fig. 25.2 Various stakeholders sharing the responsibility of good clinical practice (GCP) in a clinical trial

25.2 History of GCP

To understand the essence of GCP, it is essential to understand the history behind the development of GCP.

25.2.1 The Pure Food and Drugs Act, 1906

In the United States, Pure Food and Drugs Act of 1906 marks the first milestone in drug regulation. The main aim of this act was to prevent the manufacture, sale, or distribution of adulterated or misbranded food or drugs. However, it could not regulate the false claims made by the pharmaceutical manufacturers.

25.2.2 Sulfanilamide Disaster and Food, Drug, and Cosmetic Act (1937–1938)

Sulfanilamide, an antibacterial drug, showed dramatic cure in the treatment of streptococcal sore throat infections and was used safely for a short while in the form of tablets and powder. In 1937, a new liquid formulation of the drug (elixir) was prepared using diethylene glycol, as a solvent, which unfortunately is a deadly poison. In the absence of mandatory toxicity testing of the new formulation, it was widely sold and led to the death of over 100 people.

This catastrophic event resulted in enactment of the Federal Food, Drug, and Cosmetic Act in 1938. For the first time, manufacturers were legally required to provide evidence for their drugs' safety before marketing.

25.2.3 The Nuremberg Code, 1947

In 1947, the Nuremberg Code was formulated after the unethical experiments conducted by German physicians during World War II at the Nazi war camps. It is a principal document in the ethical conduct of experimentation on humans. It served to uphold basic human rights and prevented the torture of fellow human beings in the name of research. First time in the history of clinical research, it established salient ethical principles like the need for voluntary informed consent from participants, assuring their freedom to withdraw from the study, designing the study based on a sound scientific basis, performing research only by qualified individuals and undertaking measures to minimize the risks to the study participants.

25.2.4 Willowbrook Hepatitis Study (1956–1971)

The children with cognitive impairments institutionalized at the Willowbrook State School in Staten Island, New York, were intentionally exposed to hepatitis virus, in order to investigate the development of the infection and for developing a vaccine against the virus. The study was conducted from 1956 to 1971. The study was justified by the fact that due to the prevalent unsanitary conditions, contracting hepatitis infection was inevitable and also that parental consent was obtained. The study was later criticized for deliberately causing harm to a vulnerable group of people and misusing the prevalent unhygienic conditions in the institution to an experimental advantage. Also, it was found that parents provided consent since it was the only possible way to get their child into the school, which was overpopulated and denied admissions, except for the hepatitis research unit.

25.2.5 Thalidomide Disaster, 1962

Thalidomide, discovered to be an effective antiemetic drug, was used for morning sickness in pregnant women in the late 1950s. However, it was found that babies born to pregnant mothers, who had taken thalidomide, had severe limb deformities called phocomelia. In this medical disaster, more than 10,000 children were born with the birth defect. Later, it was confirmed that thalidomide is a teratogen and it was banned in 1962. This disaster led to the notion that species differences exist in drug response, since mice, the most commonly used experimental animal for screening drug action, were less sensitive to thalidomide, compared to other species like nonhuman primates, rabbits, hamsters, chicken, zebra fish, etc. Since the occurrence of the disaster, there has been a paradigm shift in the drug screening policies to incorporate testing on various animal species and extensive in vitro testing, to avoid such grave mistakes in the future.

25.2.6 Declaration of Helsinki, 1964

In 1964, the World Medical Association developed the Declaration of Helsinki, which served as a foundation for the development of ethical principles outlined in the ICH-GCP guidelines. Its purpose was to guide physicians in ethical conduct of medical research involving human participants. It also stressed that the physicians' prime duty is to promote and protect peoples' health. The general research principles include that the research must be based on sound scientific evidence, should be carried out by well-qualified investigators, with assessment of risks and benefits to participants and undertaking measures to mitigate the risks, and only after obtaining informed consent from the potential participants. Also, it emphasized that participants should have the freedom to withdraw from the research at any time during its conduct. The Declaration of Helsinki was periodically revised to keep pace with the ethical requirements with the advent of new scientific and technological advances, the latest being in the year 2013.

25.2.7 Belmont Report, 1979

The National Commission for the protection of human subjects of biomedical and behavioral research has written the Belmont Report. The national commission was established following the infamous Tuskegee Syphilis Study (1932–1972), in which African black men from Alabama with Syphilis were deliberately left untreated for 40 years, despite the wide availability of an effective treatment (penicillin), leading to several fatalities.

The purpose of the Belmont report is to offer a structured set of principles for resolving ethical issues arising during research on human participants. It outlines the boundaries between clinical research and clinical practice. It describes the three basic ethical principles, namely respect for persons, beneficence, and justice. It also provides insight on the practical application of the ethical principles, such as the requirement for obtaining written informed consent (respect for persons), performing risk-benefit assessment (beneficence) and ensuring fair participant selection (justice).

25.3 GCP Guidelines

The GCP guidelines, in the present form, has evolved through various revisions and amendments from time to time. Initially, the World Health Organization (WHO) GCP guidelines for trials on pharmaceutical products was published in 1995, and subsequently several national and international GCP guidelines were developed by the International Conference on Harmonization (ICH), the International Standards Organization (ISO), the Council for International Organizations of Medical Sciences (CIOMS), the European Agency for the Evaluation of Medicinal Products (EMEA), the United States Food and Drug Administration (USFDA), the Indian Central Drugs Standard Control Organisation (CDSCO), etc. These guidelines underwent multiple revisions to keep pace with the rapid advancements in clinical research.

In India, clinical trials are carried out in compliance with the New Drugs and Clinical Trials Rules, 2019 (refer Chap. 21) and Indian GCP guidelines. The Indian GCP guidelines were formulated based on the WHO, ICH, USFDA, and European GCP guidelines along with the Ethical Guidelines for Biomedical research on Human Subjects issued by the Indian Council of Medical Research (ICMR).

According to the WHO, regulatory authorities of the countries that do not have its own national regulations/guidelines for GCP can adopt the WHO GCP guidelines. In countries where national or adopted international guidelines impose more stringent requirements than the WHO GCP, the more rigorous guidelines should prevail. Currently, the WHO has published a *Handbook for Good Clinical Research Practice (GCP)* in 2005 and it outlines 14 WHO GCP principles (refer Box 25.1).

Box 25.1: The 14 WHO GCP Principles as Mentioned in Its Handbook for Good Clinical Research Practice (GCP)

Principle 1: Ethical Conduct
Principle 2: Research described in a protocol
Principle 3: Risk Identification
Principle 4: Benefit-Risk Assessment
Principle 5: Review by Independent Ethics Committee/ Independent Review Board
Principle 6: Protocol Compliance
Principle 7: Informed Consent
Principle 8: Continuing Review/Ongoing Benefit-Risk Assessment
Principle 9: Investigator Qualifications
Principle 10: Staff Qualifications
Principle 11: Records
Principle 12: Confidentiality/Privacy
Principle 13: Good Manufacturing Practice
Principle 14: Quality Systems.

Of the various GCP guidelines, the ICH-GCP guidelines is most commonly followed by the regulators and funders worldwide and will be discussed in detail in this chapter.

25.3.1 Introduction to ICH-GCP Guidelines

The International Council for Harmonization (ICH) [formerly called the International Conference on Harmonization (ICH)] has formulated the ICH-GCP guidelines to promote regulatory harmonization across key ICH regions, namely Europe, the United States, and Japan, aiming to align the technical requirements for registration of pharmaceuticals for human use. It established a unified standard for mutual acceptance of clinical trial data by the regulatory authorities in Europe, United States, and Japan. It was developed taking into account the prevailing good clinical practice standards of the European Union, Japan, and the United States, along with those of Australia, Canada, the Nordic countries, and the World Health Organization (WHO). The ICH guidelines for regulatory submission requirements of pharmaceutical in human use is categorized into quality, safety, efficacy, and multidisciplinary guidelines, of which the efficacy guideline E6 is on good clinical practice (finalized in May 1996). This harmonized guideline was amended in the year 2016 and its third revision (R3) has been initiated in the year 2019.

Objective of the ICH GCP guidelines: It provides a harmonized set of standards for uniform evaluation and acceptance of clinical trial data by the regulatory authorities of the member countries of ICH.

Scope of the ICH GCP guidelines: It is primarily applicable to interventional clinical trials involving investigational products (drugs, medicines, medicinal products, vaccines, and biologicals) that may or may not be intended to support marketing authorization application.

Structure of the ICH GCP guidelines: It includes principles and annex-1, with the annex-1 elaborating on the principles. It also has appendices on "investigator's brochure, clinical trial protocol and protocol amendment(s), and essential records for the conduct of a clinical trial."

25.3.2 Principles of ICH-GCP Guidelines

ICH-GCP guidelines set forth a general framework governing the conduct of clinical trials, which are applicable across different study types and diverse study settings, and remain relevant even with technological advances. The fundamental principles of ICH GCP include:

1. Clinical trials should be undertaken in accordance with the **ethical principles outlined in the declaration of Helsinki, good clinical practice guidelines, and applicable regulatory requirements**. Upholding the rights, safety, and welfare of the participants is a fundamental ethical obligation. Also, individual participant safety is weighted more than the advancement of science. Performance of risk-benefit analysis of the study, fair participant selection, periodic review of participant safety, ensuring qualified physician is involved in trial-related medical care for participants, and ensuring participants' privacy and confidentiality of their data are highly essential.
2. Participation in clinical trials must be voluntary. Prior to study enrolment, **written informed consent** should be obtained from the participant/legally acceptable representative.
3. Clinical trials must undergo initial and periodic review by an **institutional review board/independent ethics committee (IRB/IEC).** The study must be implemented in strict adherence to the protocol approved by the IRB/IEC.
4. Clinical trials should be **based on scientific grounds** for their intended purpose, in alignment with contemporary scientific evidence and practices.
5. Only **individuals with requisite qualifications** must design and conduct a clinical trial.
6. **Quality** should be an **integral component** of scientific and operational design of a clinical trial, and must be consistently maintained throughout its conduct.
7. Clinical trial approaches and **procedures** should be designed to ensure appropriate balance between **risks to participants and the criticality of the data generated.**
8. The clinical trial **protocol must be clear, concise, and operationally feasible.**
9. Clinical trials should be designed to **produce reliable results.**
10. A clinical trial must have **well-defined and documented roles and responsibilities for each stakeholder** to ensure accountability and compliance.

11. The **investigational products** used in a clinical trial must be **manufactured** as per the **good manufacturing practice (GMP) standards**. Storage, shipping, handling, and disposal of the investigational product should be as per the product specifications and the trial protocol.

25.3.3 Annex-1 of ICH-GCP Guidelines

Annex provides information on how the principles of ICH-GCP could be applied in different types of clinical trials. It includes the following broad topics:

I. Institutional Review Board/Independent Ethics Committee (IRB/IEC).
II. Investigator.
III. Sponsor.
IV. Data governance—investigator and sponsor.

I. **Institutional Review Board/Independent Ethics Committee (IRB/IEC)**

- Every clinical trial must be overseen by an IRB/IEC.
- The IRB/IEC ensures that the rights, safety, and welfare of the clinical trial participants are safeguarded.
- The IRB/IEC should comprise at least five members, including at least one member having nonmedical qualification and one member nonaffiliated to the institution/investigator site.
- The IRB/IEC should function as per its standard operating procedure (SOP) and document all its activities.
- The IRB/IEC reviews the following clinical trial documents:
  - Protocol and its amendments.
  - Informed consent, assent, and related documents.
  - Investigator's brochure.
  - Any additional information relevant to the study that must be disclosed to the trial participant(s).
  - Participant recruitment materials, for example, advertisements, flyers (if used).
  - Details of compensation to be provided to the participants (if any).
  - Periodic updates on safety information.
  - Updated curriculum vitae of investigator(s) and documents to assess his/her qualifications.
  - Any additional documents required by IRB/IEC to perform its designated functions.
- The IRB/IEC reviews the clinical trial documents prior to study initiation and grants approval/recommend modifications/provides disapproval of a trial.

- The IRB/IEC is also entitled to perform continuing review of all ongoing clinical trials at regular intervals as per the risk profile of the trial.
- The IRB/IEC also insists on reporting of
  - Protocol deviations or violations.
  - Protocol amendments.
  - Study progress report/completion report.
  - Serious adverse event reports (as per regulatory requirements).
  - Any newly emerged information that could negatively impact the participants' safety or trial conduct.
- The IRB/IEC should have an archival mechanism for all its records (SOP, member details, submitted and approved protocols and related documents, minutes of the meetings and any correspondences) and make it available for review by the regulatory authority.
- Depending on the regulatory requirements in that region, either the investigator/institution or sponsor must ensure submissions to the IRB/IEC.

II. **Investigator**

- The investigator is responsible for **conducting the clinical trial as per the IRB/IEC approved protocol and in compliance with GCP and regulatory requirements** of that region.
- The investigator must be **well qualified** in terms of education, training, and experience to conduct clinical trials.
- The investigator should **ensure availability of essential resources** (time, qualified staff, infrastructure, and eligible participants) for proper conduct of clinical trial.
- The investigator may **assign trial-related activities** to other persons but he/she is **ultimately responsible** for ensuring participant safety and data credibility.
- Before initiating the study, it is mandatory for the investigator to have obtained **permission from the IRB/IEC** (as per the regulatory requirements of that region, either the investigator or sponsor should document submissions and communications with the IRB/IEC).
- The investigator must ensure that **informed consent is obtained** from the study participants or their legally acceptable representatives, **and properly documented**. Also, he/she is responsible for obtaining assent and parental consent in case the trial involves children.
- The investigator is responsible for **investigational product management** (its storage, inventory management, issuing to participants with explanation of its correct usage and maintenance of related records).
- Only a **qualified healthcare professional**, serving as the investigator or a subinvestigator of the trial, should **take complete responsibility for the participants' medical care and clinical decision-making during the trial.**
- The investigator should ensure **reporting of serious adverse events to the sponsor, IRB/IEC, and central licensing authority** within the stipulated time frame as per the regulatory requirements of that region.

- In case of randomized investigator-blinded trials, the investigator should **comply with protocol-defined randomization procedure** to ensure trial integrity. He/she should also be **trained to perform unblinding** in the event of an emergency to ensure participant safety (investigator should report the occurrence of premature unblinding and the reason for the same to the sponsor).
- The investigator must **uphold the integrity of the trial data** during its generation, recording or reporting.
- The investigator is **accountable for upkeep of trial-related records** and take steps to safeguard them from accidental or premature destruction. It should be archived as per the regulatory requirements of that region and make it available for inspection/audit by monitor, auditor, IRB/IEC, or regulatory authority.
- The investigator must ensure that the **confidentiality of the participants' data** must be **ensured**.
- The investigator shall ascertain that the **data provided to the sponsor are accurate, complete, legible, and reported on time**.
- In case a participant tends to prematurely withdraw from a trial, the investigator should follow appropriate follow-up measures to prevent the loss of essential trial data already gathered, and identify reason for withdrawal while fully respecting the participants' rights.
- On premature suspension/termination of a trial, participants should be duly informed and provided with continued medical oversight and necessary care by the investigator. On investigator terminating the trial, he/she must notify the sponsor, IRB/IEC, and relevant regulatory agencies.
- On study completion, the investigator/institution must **provide a study completion report (summary of trials' outcome) to the IRB/IEC.**

III. **Sponsor**

The sponsor bears the responsibility for upholding participants' safety and maintaining data integrity throughout each stage of the clinical trial.

1. **Trial design**—Sponsor should design the clinical trial with build-in quality measures.
2. **Resources**—Sponsor should ensure availability of sufficient resources for trial conduct.
3. **Allocation of trial-related activities**—Sponsor should assign trial-related tasks by clearly delineating the roles and responsibilities among various persons/agencies.
4. **Qualification and training**—Sponsor should ensure that personnel chosen for various trial related activities are well qualified and trained.
5. **Financing**—The sponsors must document all trial-related financial issues in a written agreement with the investigator/institution.
6. **Agreements**—Before initiating trial-related activities, sponsor should ensure documentation of agreements made with any of the following parties:

- Investigator/institution.
- Service providers.
- Other designated committees (e.g., independent data monitoring committee (IDMC), adjudication committee).

7. **Investigator selection**—It is the sponsor's obligation to select suitable investigator(s)/institution(s) for trial conduct. The sponsor should also provide them with the trial protocol and an up-to-date investigator's brochure and ensure they have adequate time to read and review the documents.
8. **Communication with IRB/IEC and regulatory authority(ies)**—Sponsor should ensure appropriate permissions have been obtained from the IRB/IEC. Sponsor (or sponsor and investigator) is responsible for seeking permission(s) and providing notification(s) to the regulatory authority(ies).
9. **Sponsor oversight**—Sponsor should oversee trial-related activities of investigators and service providers through incorporation of quality assurance and quality control processes. One such measure could be the establishment of an independent data monitoring committee (IDMC) to periodically (or as required) assess the progress of the clinical trial, and safety and efficacy data. The IDMC provides recommendations to the sponsor to continue, modify, or stop the trial.
10. **Quality management**—Sponsor should ensure maintenance of quality throughout all stages of the clinical trial process. Sponsor should adopt a risk-based approach to quality management, which involves identification and management of factors which might adversely affect participant safety and data credibility. The risk management includes various components, which are summarized in Box 25.2.

Box 25.2: Various Components of Risk Management

1. **Risk identification**—the sponsor should identify the factors (risks/hazard) which might adversely affect participant safety and data credibility.
2. **Risk evaluation**—the sponsor should assess the probability of occurrence and extent of the hazard and its impact on participant safety and data credibility.
3. **Risk control**—the sponsor should devise strategies to minimize the risk/hazard (risk mitigation activities). Also, the sponsor should set acceptable ranges within which deviation is acceptable.
4. **Risk Communication**—the sponsor should communicate the recognized risks and planned risk mitigation measures to all relevant stakeholders, including those expected to act and those who might be affected.
5. **Risk Review**—the sponsor must regularly review the implemented risk control strategies to ensure its effectiveness and relevancy in light of the emerging knowledge and experience during the clinical trial conduct.
6. **Risk Reporting**—the sponsor should summarize and report the risks and the remedial measures pertaining to the significant deviations falling outside the acceptable ranges (set during the risk control process). Also, the sponsor should document them in the clinical trial report.

11. **Quality Assurance and Quality Control**

    The sponsor must uphold quality assurance systems and implement quality control procedures to ensure that the trial is conducted in accordance with the approved protocol, GCP guidelines and the relevant regulatory standards.

    - **Quality assurance**—The sponsor should implement strategies to identify protocol deviations/violations, nonadherence to GCP and/or applicable regulatory standards, and facilitate appropriate corrective and preventive measures.
    - **Audit**—The sponsor should conduct audit of the trial (as and when required) by appointing qualified and well-trained auditors, who are independent of the trial.
    - **Quality control**—To ensure credibility of clinical trial data, quality control should be integrated across all stages of data handling. Monitoring and data management processes represent crucial quality control activities in clinical trials.
    - **Monitoring**—Monitoring serves as one of the most crucial quality control activities that aids in ensuring participant safety and data credibility. It should be conducted by individuals independent of the clinical conduct of the trial being monitored. Monitoring may include:
      - Investigator site monitoring—It involves monitoring clinical trial activities at the investigator sites
      - or
      - Centralized monitoring—It involves timely evaluation of ongoing trial data by qualified and trained personnel (e.g., medical monitor, data scientist/data manager, biostatistician) designated by the sponsor.
      - The monitoring report should be submitted promptly to the sponsor to facilitate review and necessary follow-up.

12. **Noncompliance**—The sponsor should take appropriate action(s) if the investigator/institution/service provider are noncompliant with the protocol, SOP, GCP, and/or applicable regulatory requirements. The actions by sponsor include the following:

    - Performing a root cause assessment.
    - Implementing appropriate corrective and preventive actions.
    - Notifying the regulatory authority and/or IRB/IEC (as per local regulations) if the noncompliance significantly impacts participant safety and/or data reliability.
    - Termination of participation by the noncompliant investigator/institution if serious noncompliance persists despite efforts at remediation and this termination should be notified to the regulatory agency and/or IRB/IEC (according to local regulations).

13. **Safety assessment and reporting**—it is the sponsor's obligation to conduct regular assessment of the safety of the investigational product(s). The sponsor should.

    - Periodically review the safety information and update the protocol, Investigator's Brochure, and informed consent documents.
    - Safety reporting—Submit safety updates and periodic reports including changes in Investigator's Brochure, to the regulatory authority. Also, **serious adverse events (SAEs)** and **suspected unexpected serious adverse drug reactions (SUSARs)** should be reported in a timely manner to the IRB/IEC and regulatory authority.
    - Manage an immediate hazard to the participants—Determine the factors contributing to the hazard and implement remedial measures.

14. **Insurance/indemnification/compensation to participants and investigators**—the sponsor should

    - Provide insurance or indemnify (legal and financial coverage) investigator/institution against trial-related liabilities, except in cases of proven malpractice and/or negligence.
    - Make arrangements for provision of compensation and free treatment to the participants in case of any trial-related injury.

15. **Investigational product(s)**

    - **Information on investigational product(s)**—The development and periodic updating of the Investigator's Brochure is the responsibility of the sponsor.
    - **Manufacturing, packaging, labeling, and coding investigational product(s)**—Ensuring good manufacturing practices compliant manufacture of the investigational product (IP) is the obligation of the sponsor. Also, he/she should ensure that the IP is coded and labeled, and appropriately stored.
    - **Supplying and handling investigational product(s)**—The sponsor should supply the IP to the investigator(s)/institution(s) and provide instructions on their handling and storage. He/she must also ensure adequate documentation regarding the supply of the IP and develop mechanisms for retrieval of defective IP and disposal of unused IP.

16. **Data and records**

    - **Data handling**—The sponsor must uphold the integrity and ensure confidentiality of the generated data.
    - **Statistical programming and data analysis**—The sponsor is responsible for verifying the implementation of quality control in statistical programming and data analysis.
    - **Recordkeeping and retention**—The sponsor must maintain all sponsor-specific essential records related to the trial, in compliance with relevant

local regulations. The sponsor must also inform the investigators/institution and service providers to retain the essential records, until the sponsor indicates that further retention is not needed.

- **Record access**—The sponsor must confirm that protocol and contractual agreements mandate the investigators/institutions to provide direct access to the source records for all trial related oversight by auditors, monitors, IEC/IRB members, and regulatory inspectors. In addition, the sponsor must ensure that participants have provided documented informed consent authorizing access to their medical records and trial-related data for the abovementioned purpose.

17. **Reports**

- **Premature termination or suspension of a trial**—In the event of premature termination or suspension of a clinical trial, the sponsor must immediately communicate the decision, along with the justification, to the investigators/institutions, IRB/IEC, and regulatory agency.
- **Clinical trial/study reports**—In case of trial completion, prematurely termination, or undertaking interim analysis, the sponsor should ensure preparation and submission of clinical trial reports to the regulatory authority. Also, the sponsor should give a summary of the trial results to the investigators.

IV. **Data Governance—Investigator and Sponsor**

This section outlines recommendations for the investigators and sponsors to ensure proper management of data integrity, traceability, and security, which facilitate accurate reporting, verification, and interpretation of the clinical trial-related information.

- **Safeguarding blinding in data governance**—In case of blinded clinical trials, safeguarding the blinding during data management and preventing accidental unblinding is highly essential.
- **Data life cycle elements and computerized systems**—Appropriate procedures must be implemented for data governance throughout the entire data life cycle. The data life cycle includes data planning, collecting, analysing, documenting, interpreting, archiving, and publishing.
- When a computerized system is used for data capture,

  - Ensuring system access only to authorized user(s) is essential.
  - Appropriate training needs to be imparted to the personnel involved in handling the computerized system for trial-related activities.
  - Data entry interfaces should support automatic data validation checks to ensure data accuracy.
  - Relevant metadata including audit trails and procedures for its review should be present—the computerized system should record and retain logs of

  - Creation of user account.
  - Modifications to user roles and permissions and user access.
  - Original data entry along with any edits or deletions.
  - Workflow actions in addition to the direct data entry/changes.

- Data integrity should be ensured by performing data verification, validation, reconciliation, and correction of errors and omissions prior to finalizing the data sets for analysis.
- Security of trial data in the computerized system should be ensured—adequate measures should be in place to address user authentication and password control, firewall and antivirus configuration, security patching, system monitoring, and penetration testing should be available.
- Measures must be established for data backup and disaster recovery.
- Technical support for timely management of issues/concerns raised by the user(s) should be available.

25.3.4 Conclusion

Adherence to good clinical practice guidelines is vital to any clinical trial. It upholds the standards of the clinical trial by ensuring participant protection and data integrity. The evolution of GCP guidelines and regulations reveals the unethical practices and human atrocities conducted in the name of research. Thus, to prevent unethical and bogus research, it is a legal mandate to follow GCP guidelines and local regulations in any clinical trial.

Bibliography

1. Vijayananthan A, Nawawi O (2008) The importance of good clinical practice guidelines and its role in clinical trials. Biomed Imaging Interv J 4(1):e5. https://doi.org/10.2349/biij.4.1.e5
2. US Food and Drug Administration. [Internet] Sulfanilamide disaster. Taste of raspberries, taste of death the 1937 elixir sulfanilamide incident. [cited 2023 Oct 6]. Available at: https://www.fda.gov/about-fda/histories-product-regulation/sulfanilamide-disaster
3. Shuster E (1997) Fifty years later: the significance of the Nuremberg code. N Engl J Med 337(20):1436–1440
4. Diamond EF (1973) The Willowbrook experiments. Linacre Q 40(2):9. Available at: https://epublications.marquette.edu/lnq/vol40/iss2/9
5. Vargesson N (2015) Thalidomide-induced teratogenesis: history and mechanisms. Birth Defects Res C Embryo Today 105(2):140–156
6. World Medical Association. [Internet]. Declaration of Helsinki. Ethical principles for medical research involving human subjects. [cited 2023 Oct 6]. Available at: https://www.wma.net/policies-post/wma-declaration-of-helsinki-ethical-principles-for-medical-research-involving-human-subjects/
7. The Belmont Report. [Internet]. Ethical principles and guidelines for the protection of human subjects of research. The National Commission for the Protection of Human Subjects of Biomedical and Behavioral Research. DHEW Publication No. (OS) 78-0012. [cited 2023 Oct 6]. Available at: https://repository.library.georgetown.edu/bitstream/handle/10822/779133/ohrp_belmont_report.pdf?sequence=1&isAllowed=y

8. Adashi EY, Walters LB, Menikoff JA (2018) The Belmont report at 40: reckoning with time. Am J Public Health 108(10):1345–1348
9. Das NK, Sil A (2017) Evolution of ethics in clinical research and ethics committee. Indian J Dermatol 62(4):373–379
10. World Health Organization. [Internet] Handbook for good clinical research practice (GCP): guidance for implementation. [cited 2023 Oct 6]. Available at: https://apps.who.int/iris/bitstream/handle/10665/43392/924159392X_eng.pdf?sequence=1
11. Central Drugs Standard Control Organisation (CDSCO). [Internet] Indian good clinical practice (GCP) guidelines. [cited 2023 Oct 6]. Available at: https://cdsco.gov.in/opencms/opencms/system/modules/CDSCO.WEB/elements/download_file_division.jsp?num_id=MzM5NQ==
12. International Council for Harmonisation of Technical Requirements for Pharmaceuticals for Human Use. ICH harmonised guideline – good clinical practice (GCP)-E6(R3). Internet [cited 2023 Oct 6]. Available at: https://www.ich.org/page/efficacy-guidelines
13. Ravinetto R (2017) The revision of the ICH good clinical practice guidelines: a missed opportunity? Indian J Med Ethics 2(4):255–259

Medical Device and Medical Device Regulations

26

Bikash Ranjan Meher and Vishnoukumaar Sivaji

Abstract

Medical devices play an immensely important role in patient care by enabling effective diagnosis, monitoring, and treatment of many medical conditions. Medical devices are classified into various types on the basis of risk associated with their use. In India, medical devices are classified into four categories, whereas in the United States, it has been classified into three categories. Realizing the significance of safe and effective use of medical devices, regulatory agencies around the world have formulated suitable guidelines for their import as well as their manufacturing. Post-marketing surveillance of medical devices has also been initiated in many countries to avoid any untoward events during the use of medical devices. Union government of India has initiated Materiovigilance Program of India (MvPI) to track the adverse events associated with the use of medical devices, to generate safety data, create awareness among the different stakeholders, and recommend the best practices and interventions to improve the patient's safety.

Keywords

Medical devices · Device regulation · Adverse events · Adverse reactions · Materiovigilance

B. R. Meher (✉)
Department of Pharmacology, All India Institute of Medical Sciences, Bhubaneswar, Odisha, India
e-mail: pharm_bikash@aiimsbhubaneswar.edu.in

V. Sivaji
Teliatry Inc, Richardson, TX, USA

A. Arivazhahan et al. (eds.), *Introduction to Basics of Pharmacology and Toxicology*,
https://doi.org/10.1007/978-981-95-1920-0_26

26.1 Introduction

Medical devices are an indispensable component of healthcare delivery system as they facilitate diagnosis, monitoring, and management of medical ailments. World Health Organization (WHO) has defined medical device as "any instrument, apparatus, implement, machine, appliance, implant, reagent for in vitro use, software, material or other similar or related article used for the diagnosis, prevention, treatment, or alleviation of disease." Examples of medical devices can range from a simple innocuous device like cotton gauze used for wound dressing to highly advanced and sophisticated instruments like cardiac pacemakers, heart-lung machine, magnetic resonance imaging (MRI), and positron emission tomography/computerized tomography (PET-CT). Furthermore, various software applications used in healthcare delivery system are also considered as medical device (software as a medical device, SaMD).

In recent years, the use of medical device in healthcare system has increased exponentially due to evolution in medical technology innovation, and consequently the worldwide medical device market has also grown multifold. Currently, more than 2 million different medical devices are available in the world market, and they are categorized into more than 7000 generic devices groups. The worth of global medical device market has expanded rapidly in the last decade. It was estimated to be valued at approximately 518.46 billion US dollar (USD) in 2023, and is expected to grow 886.80 billion USD by 2032, with a compounded annual growth rate (CAGR) of 6.3% during the said period. The United States is the biggest market for medical device in the world, comprising 40% of the world medtech market. The U.S. medical device market is valued at approximately 450 billion USD in 2022 and is expected to grow further to nearly 1000 billion USD by 2031. With the economic prosperity and advancement in scientific research and innovation, India is also aspiring to become a leading global player in manufacturing and innovation of medical devices by over the next three decades. The size of the Indian medical devices industry was approximately 11 billion USD in 2023 and is expected to become 50 billion USD by 2025. There are nearly 1000 homegrown medical devices manufacturers in India, accounting for 65% of the market.

26.2 Medical Device Regulations in India

26.2.1 Medical Device Classification

Medical devices have been classified in India into four categories following the risk associated with the use of such device, as described in the first schedule of MDR, 2017. Four categories are (1) Class A (low risk), (2) Class B (low to moderate risk), (3) Class C (moderate to high risk), and (4) Class D (high risk).

26.2.2 Medical Device Rules

Like that of conventional drugs, medical devices are used in healthcare delivery system to facilitate the well-being of the patients. Therefore, robust and strict guideline is imperative for the import and manufacturing of medical devices to safeguard the health and ensure safety of patients. India has a robust regulatory guideline for the development of drugs; however, same was not available for medical devices for a long period. To bridge that chasm, Government of India brought Indian Medical Devices Rules (IMDR) 2017. Central Drug Standard Control Organization (CDSCO) developed this all-important regulation, which was further revised in February 2020 as "Medical Devices (Amendment) Rules, 2020" and made operational in 2020, April. The advent of the IMDR has brought clarity in rules and provided much-needed impetus to boost patient safety with respect to the use of medical devices in India. As per the IMDR, rules are applicable to both in vitro diagnostic medical devices and medical devices. The rule has clearly defined about academic clinical study, active diagnostic medical device, active therapeutic medical device, active medical device, investigational medical device, invasive device, academic clinical trial, licensing authority, clinical performance evaluation, recall, etc.

According to the rule laid down in IMDR, the manufacturer of a Class A nonsterile and non-measuring medical device shall upload all the relevant information details about the manufacturer including manufacturing site details as well as details about medical device on the online system for medical devices. Additionally, an undertaking is required to be furnished by the manufacturer that the proposed medical device belongs to Class A nonsterile and non-measuring medical device and it is in accordance with the essential principles checklist of safety and performance of such devices, and the manufacturer shall to adhere with the standards specified in these rules.

Manufacturers interested in the sale or distribution of Class A or Class B in vitro diagnostic medical devices are needed to apply to the respective State Licensing Authority for grant of a license or loan license to manufacture the same. For this, the application can be submitted through an identified online portal of the Ministry of Health and Family Welfare, Government of India, in Form MD-3 and MD-4 for license or loan license, respectively, with the requisite fee amount mentioned in the second schedule of document. Along with the documents, manufacturer is required to furnish an undertaking regarding compliance of quality management system. State Licensing Authority can grant a license to manufacture Class A medical device in Form MD-5 or loan license in Form MD-6 after satisfactory verification of submitted documents. If, due to some reasons, they are not satisfied, then they can reject the application and attribute the reasons for same in writing within 45 days of receiving application.

Audit of the manufacturing site of Class B devices shall be conducted within 90 days' time period from the receipt of application by the Notified Body, and it shall submit the report to the State Licensing Authority within 30 days of the completion of audit. State Licensing Authority can issue license either for sale or for distribution of Class B devices in Form MD-5 or loan license in Form MD-6 if they are satisfied after careful examination of all necessary documents and audit report. Authority can also reject the application if they are not satisfied with the compliance by citing the reasons for such an action, within 20 days from the date of obtaining audit report from the notified body. In case of rejection, concern party or manufacturer can file an appeal before the respective state government within a period of 40 days of receiving rejection. And this issue has to be disposed up within 60 days.

If manufacturer intent to sale or distribute Class C or Class D medical device, then it is required to be applied to the Central Licensing Authority along with a specified fee through an identified online portal of the Central Government for license or loan license for same in Form MD-7 or Form MD-8, respectively. If required, the concern authority can engage an expert from the relevant field for technical verification of the submitted documents. If it was found that the documents are complete and in order, the authority can have an inspection of the manufacturing site by a team of experts if they think necessary or may avail the services of a notified body. After receiving the report, the authority can give a license in Form MD-9 or a loan license in Form MD-10, if satisfied with the compliance of rules. However, authority may reject the application within 45 days from the receipt of inspection report after explaining the reasons for rejection in writing. In case of rejection, the involved party or manufacturer can file an appeal before the central government within a period of 45 days of receiving the rejection. And this issue has to be disposed up within sixty days.

Medical device adverse events (MDAE) are defined as any unexpected or untoward incidence, injury or disease, or an inconvenient clinical sign including abnormal laboratory findings resulting from the use of medical devices. MDAE may occur, if preuse inspection has not been performed diligently, due to user errors, incorrect clinical use, or failure to train. MDAE may be serious or nonserious, expected or unanticipated, frequent or rare.

26.2.3 Materiovigilance

Materiovigilance is defined as surveillance of any unpleasant experiences following the use of medical device by a structured monitoring system. It consists of activities like identification, collection, reporting, and evaluation of all infelicitous incidences and take appropriate corrective actions. Materiovigilance Program of India (MvPI) was initiated by Drugs Controller General of India (DCGI) on July 6, 2015. The main objectives of the program are to develop a pan-India system for reporting suspected MDAE, increase awareness among medical and allied professionals regarding the significance of MDAE reporting, produce robust safety data based on evidences, and share it with the partners, as well as support regulatory agencies in taking appropriate policy decision on the use of medical devices. The Indian Pharmacopeia Commission (IPC), situated at Ghaziabad, Uttar Pradesh, is the National Coordination Center (NCC) of MvPI, whereas CDSCO functions as the regulator of the same. MvPI was initiated to enhance voluntary reporting of

MDAE. For successful implementation of the program, it is essential to know who can report MDAE, what types of MDAE to report, and where to report.

According to the regulation of MvPI, any healthcare professional, such as doctor, nurse, pharmacist, or laboratory technician, can report MDAE. Additionally, manufacturers, importers, and distributors of medical device, biomedical engineer, patients, and common people can also report any suspected MDAE. Any serious or nonserious, expected or unanticipated, frequent or rare adverse events or near-miss incidents associated with the use of any kind of medical equipment's devices and their consumables can be reported. NCC-MvPI has developed few modalities to facilitate reporting of suspected MDAEs. Any suspected MDAEs can be reported by using MDAE reporting form prepared by CDSCO by properly filling all relevant information. This form can be downloaded at free of cost from the website of IPC (www.ipc.gov.in). After filling all required relevant information, duly signed MDAE reporting form can be either deposited in the nearby medical device monitoring center (MDMC) or can be directly dispatched to the National Cordination Centre (NCC). The reporter can also report the suspected adverse event by calling the toll free helpline number provided by the NCC-PvPI (1800-180-3024) or can use ADRMS software for reporting the same.

Like that of pharmacovigilance, casualty assessment is an important aspect of Materiovigilance program. Causality assessment essentially means detecting the strength of association between medical device use and the occurrence of an adverse event. Causality assessment helps in reducing disagreement and building consensus between assessors by establishing a standardized approach. It classifies the likelihood of a relationship between medical devices and adverse events and helps in the improvement of scientific and educational evaluation. However, causality assessment has some limitations as it cannot give a very accurate quantitative measurement of the likelihood of a relationship, it cannot always distinguish valid from invalid cases, and it cannot quantify the contribution of the device to the development or occurrence of an event. Causality assessment has been categorized into Not related, Unlikely, Possible, Probable/Likely, Casual relationship, and Unassessable.

26.3 Medical Device Regulations in the United States

The U.S. Food and Drug Administration (FDA) is responsible for the regulation of drugs and medical devices that are sold in the United States. Center for Devices and Radiological Health (CDRH) is the FDA branch that regulates medical devices.

26.3.1 Device Classification

FDA classifies medical devices into three classes:

- **Class I:** These devices are considered minimal risk and require the least amount of effort to obtain marketing clearance. Most of these devices do not require a

premarket notification. Examples of Class I devices include oxygen mask, bandages, sunglasses, etc.
- **Class II:** These devices are considered moderate risk and most of the time require a premarket notification before they can be marketed. A malfunction of these devices does not cause major bodily harm. Examples of Class II devices include syringes, catheters, powered wheelchair, etc.
- **Class III:** These devices are considered high risk and are usually implanted and/or life sustaining where any malfunction can be life threatening or can lead to severe injury. These devices mostly require a premarket approval, which is the most stringent of all applications for approval. Examples of Class III devices include pacemakers, defibrillators, heart valves, etc.

Medical device manufacturers can use the FDA website to classify their device based on the published product classification database. New devices that have not been classified previously are considered Class III irrespective of the risk. FDA may down-classify such devices once their safety profile has been established and they are found to be lower risk. Alternatively, medical devices manufacturers can choose the de novo process to request the FDA to create a new device classification based on a risk assessment.

26.3.2 Types of Submissions

All medical devices that are not exempt from regulatory approval require either a premarket approval or a premarket notification before they can be legally marketed in the United States. The type of submission depends on the device class. Other types of submissions that apply in specific cases include the investigational device exemption (IDE) and the humanitarian device exemption (HDE).

26.3.2.1 Premarket Notification [510(K)]

Premarket notifications are required for all Class II devices and some Class I devices, and the process is simpler than the more rigorous premarket approval. The application consists of comparing the device to an existing legally marketed device (called the predicate) to establish the claims of substantial equivalence. Two devices are considered to be substantially equivalent if:

- They have the same intended use.
- They have the same technological characteristics.
- Or they have different technological characteristics, but do not raise any questions of safety or efficacy.

FDA makes the determination of whether the device is substantially equivalent to the predicate based on the submitted documentation, which includes bench performance testing, preclinical studies in animal models and in some cases clinical studies. If the FDA finds the device to be substantially equivalent, then the device is cleared for marketing. If the device is found to be not substantially equivalent, then a premarket approval is required.

26.3.2.2 Premarket Approval (PMA)

All Class III devices require premarket approval, which is the most stringent type of submission. In addition to preclinical data that establishes the safety, biocompatibility, and performance in animal models, extensive clinical data is required to demonstrate safety and efficacy in humans. The devices undergo multiple phases of clinical trials after obtaining an IDE. The FDA reviews reports of adverse reactions, device failures, complications, and the outcomes of the study before approving the device for marketing.

26.3.2.3 Investigational Device Exemption (IDE)

An investigational device exemption allows the medical device to be used in clinical studies to obtain safety and efficacy data, which can then be used in support of a PMA. The safety of the device must be established using preclinical studies in order to obtain an IDE. Such devices are labeled stating that they are for investigational use only.

26.3.2.4 Humanitarian Device Exemption (HDE)

Humanitarian device exemption applies to devices that are intended to treat a rare disease or condition that affects less than 4000 people a year in the United States. The regulatory burden is mostly similar to the PMA and includes clinical trials but does not require an evaluation of the efficacy. A device approved under an HDE is called a humanitarian use device.

26.4 Conclusion

Due to the advancement in scientific innovation, the use of medical device has increased substantially in the healthcare system during recent years. Various government around the world including India has realized the importance of it and made specific rules and regulations pertaining to manufacturing, export, and sales of medical devices by manufacturing company which was previously lacking. However, there are still not adequate measures to protect the patients from the untoward occurrences associated with the use of medical devices. Post-marketing surveillance is a good initiative to ensure the safety of medical devices among the device users. The guidance document of MvPI has enacted policy guidelines, and prescribed the role and responsibilities of different stakeholders to enable safety data collection in a systematic manner.

Bibliography

Boosting the Indian medical devices industry (2023). https://pharmaceuticals.gov.in/sites/default/files/Final%20Boosting%20of%20Medical%20Devices%20Industry%20-%20Report%20-%202023.pdf

Guidance Document., Materiovigilance Programme of India (version1. 2)

Gupta SK (2016) Medical device regulations: a current perspective. J Young Pharm 8:6–11. https://ipc.gov.in/images/Guidance_Document_MvPI.pdf

Medical device market. https://www.fortunebusinessinsights.com/industry-reports/medical-devices-market-100085

Medical devices. https://www.who.int/health-topics/medical-devices#tab=tab_1

Medical Devices (Amendment) Rules (2020). https://cdsco.gov.in/opencms/opencms/system/modules/CDSCO.WEB/elements/download_file_division.jsp?num_id=NTU0OQ==

Medical devices market insight. https://www.skyquestt.com/report/medical-devices-market

Medical Devices Rules, Ministry of Health and Family Welfare (2017). https://cdsco.gov.in/opencms/resources/UploadCDSCOWeb/2022/m_device/Medical%20Devices%20Rules,%202017.pdf

Meher BR (2018) Materiovigilance: an Indian perspective. Perspect Clin Res 9(4):175–178

Nomenclature of medical devices. https://www.who.int/teams/health-product-policy-and-standards/assistive-and-medical-technology/medical-devices/nomenclature

Software as a Medical Device (SaMD). https://www.fda.gov/medical-devices/digital-health-center-excellence/software-medical-device-samd

Sun J, Pan J, Jin Y, Zhang Q, Lv Y, Feng J (2022) Establishment of a medical device adverse event management system for hospitals. BMC Health Serv Res 22(1):1406

U.S. Food and Drug Administration (2020). https://www.fda.gov/

Off-Label Use of Drugs

27

Sushil Sharma

Abstract

Off-label uses of drugs are increasingly at the forefront of discussions both in the patients' forum and also in the physician's forum. Off-label drug use refers to the prescription of an approved and marketed medication in a manner that is different from what is approved on the label. The common types of off-label use are the use of a drug for a different indication, different dose, different duration, different route of administration, or different patient population. Off-label drug use is very common and accounts for one-fifth or 20% of all prescriptions and in some cases, it can be very high even up to 80%. When appropriately prescribed, off-label drug use has many advantages and can further the cause of science by discovering new innovative uses for existing drugs. It can also help the physician in providing optimum health care in many diseases/patient groups. However, inappropriate off-label use may expose the patient to a higher risk of adverse effects and potential harm. Off-label drug use demands a heightened standard of care and whenever a physician uses a drug in an off-label manner, the decision must be based on sound scientific evidence and the patient should be made a partner as part of the "shared decision making."

Keywords

Off-label drug use · Drug regulations · Pharmaceutical companies · Evidence-based practice

S. Sharma (✉)
Department of Pharmacology, All India Institute of Medical Sciences (AIIMS), Mangalagiri, Andhra Pradesh, India
e-mail: drsushil.pharma@aiimsmangalagiri.edu.in; drsushilsharma1972@gmail.com

A. Arivazhahan et al. (eds.), *Introduction to Basics of Pharmacology and Toxicology*,
https://doi.org/10.1007/978-981-95-1920-0_27

27.1 Introduction and Background

Before a drug is approved, it has to be proven to be safe and effective for its intended use and hence it is subjected to rigorous scrutiny in the form of in-vitro studies, animal studies, and clinical trials. The regulatory agencies, then analyze the data generated and a decision is then taken regarding its approval for clinical use. Once approved, the company can then market the drug for the uses for which it was investigated and can be used as per the information provided on the approved label. Label normally includes any written material that is disseminated by the manufacturer in the form of a package insert or approved packaging label information. The drug label provides key information, including indications, dosage, frequency of administration, route of administration, age range of patients, duration of treatment, and contraindications for its use. When a drug is used as per the guidelines on the label, it is called on-label use. On-label use assures the physician that the drug has undergone a careful evaluation of its benefits and risks for that use and the decision to use the drug is supported by strong scientific data. Also, there is availability of approved information for healthcare providers on how to use the drug safely and effectively. Issues with insurance, reimbursement, and malpractice are also minimal when the drug is used in an on-label manner.

However, the label has its limitations. This is because it is practically impossible to study or identify all potential uses of a product while it is under the process of approval initially. This makes it impossible for a product to get approved for all indications, dosage forms, and routes of administration, and covering all age groups including children, pregnant women, and lactating mothers. So, there is more to the drug than what is on the label and there could be many more uses of a drug than what are mentioned on the label.

27.2 Off-Label Drug Use: Definition

Considering the limitations of the label, a drug may sometimes be used in a way that is different from that described in the approved label. Off-label drug use refers to the prescription of approved and marketed medication in a manner that is different from what is approved on the label. The common types of off-label use are, the use of a drug for/in:

- Different indication.
- Different dose.
- Different duration.
- Different route of administration.
- Different patient population.

Off-label uses of drugs are increasingly at the forefront of discussions both in the patients' forum and also in the physician's forum. Off-label use is very common and accounts for one-fifth or 20% of all prescriptions and in some cases, it can be very high even up to 80%.

27.3 Reasons for Prescribing Drugs in an Off-Label Manner

As mentioned earlier, it is practically impossible to study or identify all potential uses of a product before approval. Many innovative uses of an approved drug are first identified by observant doctors in an off-label manner based on emerging medical knowledge. Regulatory authorities often take more time and fail to keep pace with ever-evolving clinical practice. The following are a few reasons/situations, which may lead doctors to prescribe drugs in an off-label manner.

(a) **Terminal illness with all approved options exhausted**: Off-label use is often resorted to by a physician if there is no existing standard care or when the existing standard treatment regimen fails, especially if it is a life-threatening or terminal illness. For example, Drugs are often used in an off-label manner in cancers.
(b) **Orphan/rare diseases**: These are diseases that are so rare that companies often lack the financial incentive to invest billions of dollars and the time and effort to develop drugs for these diseases. Only about 5% of rare diseases have approved treatments and for more than 90% of patients suffering from a rare disease, a physician may have no other option but to resort to off-label uses.
(c) **Treatment in special groups**: Certain special populations like pediatric patients or pregnant women are not well represented in many clinical trials, and hence the medication may not have been studied or approved in these patients. Consequently, off-label use may have to be resorted to when these patients are treated with off-label drugs.
(d) **Presumed class effect**: If one drug of a class has been approved for a given indication, then presumed therapeutic equivalence of other drugs of the same class in that indication often propels off-label use of drugs. This is very common in psychiatric conditions.
(e) **Extension to related conditions**: For example, a physician sometimes may feel it appropriate to treat a patient with prediabetes, but due to the paucity of drugs approved for this condition, he/she may use metformin, which is approved for DM.
(f) **Symptom overlap with those of an approved indication**: There could be symptom overlap between conditions, and so if a drug is approved for one of the indications, it may be effective in the other and thus may be used off-label. For example, montelukast, approved for asthma, is used for COPD in an off-label manner.
(g) **Common pathogenesis between the conditions**: Common pathogenesis often forms the basis for selecting a drug for off-label use. IL-1 receptor antagonist-anakinra initially approved for rheumatoid arthritis has been often used off-label in various monogenic inflammatory disorders based on the involvement of

IL-1 in the pathogenesis of these disorders. Similarly, Type II diabetes mellitus (DM) and polycystic ovarian disease (PCOD) are distinct conditions but share a common link in the form of insulin resistance and metabolic syndrome; So, metformin, which is approved for DM is effective and used as off-label for PCOD.

27.3.1 Common Examples of 'Off-Label Drug Use' in Clinical Practice

With so many reasons or grounds for off-label use, it is no surprise that off-label use is indeed very common. The Box 27.1 gives examples of a few drugs and their off-label uses.

Off-label use is not only common and widely used across many patient groups and clinical conditions but in many cases, it may even become a standard of care. Common examples are the use of aspirin for primary prophylaxis of coronary heart

Box 27.1 Drugs with Their Off-Label Use

Drug	Off-label use
Propranolol	Social phobia, performance anxiety, substance disorder and withdrawal symptoms, melanoma
Pethidine	Postanesthetic shivering
Alendronate	Hypercalcemia of malignancy, Crohn's-induced osteoporosis, osteopenia secondary to lung cystic fibrosis, growth hormone deficiency
Sildenafil	Pulmonary hypertension in children
Intranasal desmopressin	Nocturnal enuresis
Selective serotonin receptor inhibitors (SSRIs)	Body dysmorphic disorders, irritable bowel syndrome, menopausal hot flushes, chronic pain
Prazosin	Posttraumatic stress disorders
Anastrozole, letrozole	Height augmentation in boys
Erythromycin	Gastroparesis
Diphenhydramine, trazadone	Insomnia
Pregabalin and gabapentin	Chronic pain disorders
Atypical antipsychotics	Anxiety, insomnia, attention deficit hyperactivity disorder (ADHD), and mood disorders
Antiepileptics	Neuropathic pain, migraine, bipolar disorders, restless leg syndrome
Furosemide	Bronchopulmonary dysplasia
Capecitabine	Radiation sensitizer
Direct oral anticoagulants (DOAC)	Heparin-induced thrombocytopenia, antiphospholipid syndrome
Statins	Hepatocellular carcinoma

disease (CHD) and prevention of preeclampsia, selective serotonin reuptake inhibitors (SSRIs) for premature ejaculation and the use of tricyclic antidepressants for neuropathic pain.

27.3.2 Off-Label Use and Drug Repositioning

Despite widespread and well-accepted off-label use of drugs, the question arises, "Why is approval not obtained by pharmaceutical companies to convert effective off-label uses to on-label uses?" Most of the times, it boils down to money and effort needed. This is because, even when a drug is known to be effective in a clinical condition, there is a regulatory need to provide clinical trial data to justify additional indications. There is a need for at least one phase 3 trial before submitting a supplementary new drug application (sNDA), which might cost between 11 million to over 50 million dollars. Revenues for the new indication may not offset the expense and effort of obtaining approval. Further, limited remaining patent life may discourage innovators and if the patent has already expired the generic medications may not have the requisite funding. Nevertheless, there are examples where additional trials have been undertaken and the label has been expanded by adding new indications (Box 27.2).

Box 27.2 Drugs with Additional Label Indications

Drug	Original indication	New indication
Amantadine	Influenza	*Parkinsonism*
Gabapentin	Epilepsy	*Postherpetic neuralgia*
Propranolol	Hypertension	*Migraine prophylaxis*
Ropinirole	Parkinsonism	*Restless leg syndrome*
Methotrexate	Cancer	*Psoriasis*
Bupropion	Depression	*Smoking cessation*
Indomethacin	Pain, inflammation	*Patent ductus arteriosus*
Minoxidil	Hypertension	*Alopecia*
Duloxetine	Depression	*Fibromyalgia*
Sildenafil	Erectile dysfunction	*Pulmonary arterial hypertension*
Ketoconazole	Anti-fungal	*Cushing's syndrome*

27.4 Strengths and Limitations of Off-Label Use of Drugs

27.4.1 Off-Label Drug Use: Merits and Strengths

(a) **Off-label use acts as a driver of innovation**: The greatest positive attributed to off-label use is that it drives Innovation and furthers the cause of medical science. This is because, as has been discussed earlier, it is not possible to study all potential uses of a drug while it is under initial approval, and many innovative uses of an approved drug are first identified by observant doctors based on emerging medical knowledge. A classic example is propranolol; the FDA initially approved propranolol for the treatment of cardiac arrhythmia in 1968. After its approval, doctors found it to be effective for hypertension and angina pectoris which are its very significant use. Even more unexpectedly, when propranolol was given to patients with arrhythmias or angina who also had migraines, it was discovered to avert migraine attacks. After many years of off-label use for migraine, it was finally approved for this use in 1979. Presently, propranolol is approved and used for a wide range of clinical conditions, which were discovered by the use of this drug in an off-label manner. If off-label use was not allowed, we would probably be using propranolol for only cardiac arrhythmia even now.

(b) **Off-label use provides early access to potentially valuable medications**: For example, paclitaxel was initially approved for treating ovarian cancer, but after reports on breast cancer showed its effectiveness, it was employed for treating breast cancer in an off-label manner for years before this indication was finally approved by regulatory bodies.

(c) **Off-label use is invaluable in the treatment of orphan conditions/rare diseases**: Only a small percentage of orphan diseases have approved medications and more than 90% are treated in an off-label manner, saving hundreds and thousands of lives.

(d) **Off-label use can bring down the cost of therapy**: For example, the rabies vaccine is approved to be given as 1 ml in IM, but studies have shown that when the route is changed from IM to ID the volume of injection can come down to 0.1 ml with almost similar immune response allowing 8–10 pts. to be vaccinated from a single vial; this can be a great help, especially in resource-poor settings and recently even the WHO has approved this change of route.

(e) **Off-label use can greatly expand treatment choices for special groups**: Off-label use expands the treatment choices, in certain special groups like pregnant women and young children, where the availability of approved medications even for many common conditions is minimal. In such cases, off-label use of drugs can allow physicians to treat these special groups with drugs that are not yet approved in them but for which there is evidence of benefit.

27.4.2 Off-Label Drug Use: Limitations and Problems

(a) **Inadequate scientific data for off-label drug use:** Unlike on-label uses, which go through a rigorous process of clinical trials during their approval, off-label uses may not be subject to the same level of scientific testing and review, and hence many off-label uses may lack sound scientific data. Research shows that more than 70% of off-label uses lack strong scientific support.

(b) **Raised risk of adverse drug reactions when drugs are used in an off-label manner:** Off-label use of drugs has a 44% higher risk of adverse effects as compared to approved uses. This could be because, unlike on-label uses where physicians have detailed approved information on how to use the drug safely and effectively, the same detailed info is not available for off-label use. A case in point is "thalidomide," which was widely prescribed off-label by doctors in Europe for treating morning sickness and led to thousands of miscarriages and infants born with severe birth defects.

(c) **Off-label drug use may discourage evidence-based practice:** Off-label use may encourage some health care professionals to try out new treatments based sometimes, on misplaced logic and assumptions and thus may discourage evidence-based medical practice which in turn can cause considerable patient harm. The risk is even more in countries that lack a robust system of checks and balances in this regard.

(d) **Risk of lawsuits against doctors when drugs are prescribed in an off-label manner:** There could be increased risks of lawsuits if the patient perceives that he has been harmed because the physician subjected him to a drug, which is not approved for his condition. The risk for this is even greater if the patient's explicit consent has not been taken regarding the off-label use.

(e) **Reimbursement issues**: Many Insurance firms do not reimburse the costs of the drug if they are used in an off-label manner creating problems for the patients.

27.5 Regulatory Issues in Off-Label Use of Drugs

27.5.1 Global Scenario

Globally, there are different ways, off-label drug use is viewed by regulatory agencies. The USFDA puts the onus of prescribing on to the doctors who "have the responsibility to use the approved drugs safely and effectively for the benefit of the patient." The FDA states clearly "once a drug has been approved for marketing, a physician may prescribe it for uses or in treatment regimens or patient populations that are not included in the approved labelling." However, the USFDA encourages trials for off-label use in children and has provided 6 months of additional exclusivity for such cases. In France, the term "Temporary recommended for use" (RTUs) was introduced by regulators in 2012 under which off-label use of drugs was allowed and controlled. This underwent modification twice and to date, 13 products are allowed to be used as off-label.

In the European Union, Australia, and Japan, off-label use of drugs is legal and allowed to varying degrees. In Italy, off-label use was previously covered under law 648/1996, which was made into a new law in 2014 (79/2014). Under this law, the use of medicines for off-label use is justified even when an alternative treatment is available. In Germany, Federal Joint Committee involving hospitals, insurance companies and doctors has existed since 2004, which looks into the issue of off-label use and updates its list regularly. In the United Kingdom, the General Medical Council regulates the off-label use of medicines. The permission to use a drug off-label is accorded after ensuring no other alternatives available and there is sufficient evidence to use the same. In Japan and Australia, there is no legal hindrance to off-label uses, provided the prescriber can defend with scientific evidence.

27.5.2 Indian Scenario

Indian law does not allow drugs to be prescribed for indications for which they have not been approved. The issue of off-label use was debated in India in 2003 when it was found that letrozole, an anticancer drug was being promoted for infertility. Subsequently, the Drug Controller General of India (DCGI) authorized a probe into media reports that few pharmaceutical companies had endorsed letrozole for treating infertility in women, without valid regulatory permission. Following this controversy, the DCGI asked the Indian Medical Association (IMA) to prepare a report about the various attributes related to the off-label use of medicines. The IMA submitted their report recommending that doctors in India should be allowed to prescribe off-label indications if there is scientific evidence and medical basis for the same. Despite the IMA's positive opinion about off-label prescribing, currently, there are no guidelines from DCGI or CDSCO on off-label prescription in India. Off-label medicines regulation in India remains a grey area and the legal implications are unclear.

27.5.3 Guidelines on Academic Research Involving Off-Label Use of Drugs

In an attempt, to get more objective data on off-label use, the regulations on clinical trials for off-label use of drugs have been relaxed. In India, no express permission from regulatory authorities is needed if the trial is purely intended for academic purposes and not for submitting it for regulatory purposes. For such academic trials, approval from the institution ethics committee (IEC) and registration with the Clinical Trials Registry of India (CTRI) is adequate.

27.5.4 Legal Issues in Off-Label Drug Use: Malpractice and Informed Consent

With the growing trust deficit between doctors and patients, any adverse effect perceived by the patients as being due to drug treatment, has the potential to escalate into a malpractice suit. This is more so if the doctor uses a drug in an off-label manner and the patient develops an adverse effect. To protect against the charge of negligence while using drugs in an off-label manner, the physician must weigh the evidence and ensure that the risk-benefit ratio is favorable. To this effect, off-label use may require a heightened standard of care and a physician needs to obtain reliable, up-to-date information including objective scientific data on the particular off-label use. Even though, informed consent is not a mandatory requirement whenever a drug is being used in an off-label manner, "securing the patients" explicit consent adds an extra level of protection to the physician and reflects a commitment to patient autonomy'.

27.5.5 Regulations on Promotion of Off-Label Use of Drugs

The promotion of off-label use of drugs by pharmaceutical companies is not allowed and is illegal in most countries including India. Even in the United States, the promotion of a drug for off-label use is not permitted as per the Federal Food, Drugs, and Cosmetics Act and companies have been levied heavy penalties for illegally promoting their drugs for off-label use. However, USFDA has provided alternate avenues for pharmaceutical companies like answering the queries of physicians prescribing off-label, distributing reprints of peer-reviewed articles, and sponsoring continuous medical education.

However, globally there is no embargo on the free exchange of information between the scientific community and speakers can discuss off-label during their presentations in conferences and CMEs as long as they are backed by sound data and the deliberations are purely academic.

27.6 Conclusion

Off-label use is very common and when appropriate can help the physician provide optimum health care in many diseases/patient groups. Off-label use of drugs has many advantages and can further the cause of science by discovering new, innovative uses for existing drugs. However, inappropriate off-label drug use may expose the patient to a higher risk of adverse effects. Whenever a physician uses a drug in an off-label manner, the decision should be based on sound scientific evidence and the patient should be made a partner as part of the "shared decision making."

Bibliography

Eguale T, Buckeridge DL, Verma A, Winslade NE, Benedetti A, Hanley JA, Tamblyn R (2016) Association of off-label drug use and adverse drug events in an adult population. JAMA Intern Med 176(1):55–63

Kane B (2009) Off-label drug use: pros and cons. Alb LJ Sci Tech 19:578–586

Meadows WA, Hollowell BD (2008) 'Off-label' drug use: an FDA regulatory term, not a negative implication of its medical use. Int J Impot Res 20(2):135–144

Oberoi SS (2015) Regulating off-label drug use in India: the arena for concern. Perspect Clin Res 6:129–133

Rusz CM, Osz BE, Jitca G, Miklos A, Batrinu MG, Imre S (2021) Off-label medication: from a simple concept to complex practical aspects. Int J Environ Res Public Health 18(19):10447

Wittich CM, Burkle CM, Lanier WL (2012) Ten common questions (and their answers) about off-label drug use. Mayo Clin Proc 87(10):982–990

a drug is being used in an off-label manner. Securing the patient's explicit consent adds an extra level of protection to the physician and reflects a commitment to patient autonomy.

27.5.3 Regulations on Promotion of Off-Label Use of Drugs

[illegible]

27.6 Conclusion

[illegible]

Bibliography

[illegible]

Nonclinical Testing Methods to Assess Safety and Efficacy of New Drugs

28

Snehalata Gajbhiye

Abstract

The nonclinical studies form the important part of drug development. There are number of factors one needs to consider while planning and executing nonclinical studies that include validation of model, fulfilment of good laboratory practice guidelines, and the regulatory requirements. The Institutional Animal Ethics Committee permission is required before carrying out the experimental work. The animal ethical principles of 4Rs must be adhered that include reduction, replacement, refinement, and rehabilitation of animals. Though the regulations have started promoting the use of alternatives to experimental methods to generate data in this regard. The in silico methods, organoids and organ on chip methods, cell culture techniques, etc., still have to undergo validation in order to make use of them routinely in drug development.

Keywords

Experimental studies · Good laboratory practices · Institutional Animal Ethics Committee · CCSEA · In silico models

28.1 Introduction

New drug development encompasses various events including the nonclinical and clinical investigation. The evaluation of nonclinical efficacy and safety includes in vitro, ex vivo, and in vivo assays. With the improvements in scientific technology,

S. Gajbhiye (✉)
Department of Pharmacology, All India Institute of Medical Sciences (AIIMS), Nagpur, Maharashtra, India
e-mail: dr.ssborkar@aiimsnagpur.edu.in

A. Arivazhahan et al. (eds.), *Introduction to Basics of Pharmacology and Toxicology*,
https://doi.org/10.1007/978-981-95-1920-0_28

the methods for assessing the nonclinical activity of compounds have progressed. Also, a lot of emphasis is placed on the reduction of the use of in vivo animals. The animal ethics guidelines mention the usage of animals most rationally and humanely. With the advent of the ARRIVE (Animal Research Reporting of In Vivo Experiments) guidelines, which describe the reporting of research studies, there has been significant progress in the planning and execution of nonclinical studies, as well as in developing sound and scientific experimental design and analysis techniques. Though there are alternative methods to animal experiments coming up, the standardization and validation of these methods are bigger challenges.

28.2 Development of Nonclinical Models

I. **Study design**—During the conduct of the nonclinical studies, the study design needs to be in line with the scientific principles.

1. The animal model chosen for the study must be well-validated and the pathogenetic changes of the disease must be reproduced in animal species.
2. The animal species, strain, age, gender, etc. chosen must be as close to the human clinical condition. For example, the Parkinson's disease model must be produced in the aged animals.
3. The target of the new drug must be present in the animal species and must be modifiable as close to the human target. For example, rabbits are not administered atropine as they produce atropine esterase rendering the drug ineffective.
4. The time at which the drug is administered must be carefully planned. As the administration of the drug before the development of the disease may not represent the human condition and may overamplify the effects of treatment.
5. The recording of behavioral parameters or any other subjective parameter must be done by the study team member who is blinded to treatment allocation in animals. This will remove the researcher's bias.
6. The animal studies that are published do not focus on the safety aspects of the drug; this must be incorporated in the study protocol, and the data must be published.
7. The model must be described in great detail, and the recording of safety parameters must also be specified in methodology. The findings related to efficacy as well as safety must be described in the published paper.

II. **Validation—**There are different criteria to evaluate the validation of the model.

1. Face validity—The model is proposed to have face validity if the symptom/s or sign/s of the disease in humans is developed in the animal model. Also, the model has a higher value if the core symptom can be reproduced in animals.

2. Predictive validity—The model is proposed to have predictive validity if the therapeutically effective drugs for the disease are also effective in the animal model. The predictive validity allows for comparison of standard of care with newer test agents. The graded response (dose-dependent increase in response) of the drug has a higher consideration than the quantal response (all or none effect) of the drug.
3. Construct validity—The model is said to have construct validity if the mechanism used to induce the disease phenotype in animals reflects the currently understood disease pathophysiology.

III. **Statistical consideration.**

1. The number of animals used in animal studies is fixed, and a minimalistic approach is utilized. Also, the sample size is not based on statistical considerations. This may lead to lowered power to detect a difference. Thus, it is recommended that the researchers take into account the sample size estimation as undertaken in clinical studies.
2. If the outcome of interest is "time to event" (e.g., time to develop hypoglycemia), then survival analysis methods are used. However, if the expected number of events is very low and there is censoring of data (i.e., the animals in whom the outcome did not occur till the end of follow-up or they died), then the power of the study is reduced substantially.
3. The sample size determination may be based on the outcome of interest. For example, it could be based on a single continuous outcome for comparing two independent sample (e.g., blood glucose level in untreated versus treated groups), or testing the proportion of animals demonstrating a particular outcome (e.g., % of animals developing convulsion in treated vs untreated group), or to estimate the treatment effect on a particular outcome (e.g., receptor concentration level). Based on the approach, the investigator must choose various ways of estimating sample size.
4. One more problem peculiar in animal studies is about the statistical tests used as the study's sample size is not estimated or may be estimated for a particular outcome. The sample size estimation is based on a defined outcome, thus the statistical assumption states that the test statistic for a particular outcome is less than 0.05 (when $p < 0.05$ is assumed).
5. When the researcher wants to measure two outcomes (e.g., follow-up data of mean blood pressure at different time points), the typical approach is to conduct two separate t-tests, using the same rule of p value <0.05 to determine significance in each test. However, with this approach, type I error will be inflated and, instead of 5%, may double. Few resaerchers carry out multiple t-tests but this may increase the type-I error multiple folds.
6. One of the ways to handle multiple tests is by adjusting the significance level. The significance level can be adjusted by dividing the p value (0.05) by the number of outcomes (n). The outcomes with this new p value (derived by 0.05/n) will be considered to show significant treatment effects. This is called Bonferroni adjustment.

IV. **Decision gates in nonclinical models**—The industry attempts to predict whether the molecule's properties will result in successful development or failure in future clinical trials. The watchful attitude at this stage of drug development can be of financial benefit to the industry, as early failure will save the cost. Some of the examples of the concerned properties and the relevant tests are listed below:

1. Whether sufficient oral bioavailability—Can be tested using PK studies in animals after oral vs IV administration.
2. Whether metabolites are produced and are active or enzymes involved in drug metabolism—In vitro techniques using animal or human hepatocytes, microsomes or enzyme systems, and analysis of metabolites using LC/MS/MS.
3. Where does the drug get distributed, and how long does it stay there—Tissue distribution studies in rats using radiolabeled drug.
4. What route is the drug eliminated—PK studies in animals and radiolabelled drug excretion studies.
5. Whether safety margin is wide—Animal studies for ration of no-effect dose over expected effect dose.
6. Whether the drug has mutagenic or cytogenic potential—Ames bacterial mutagenicity tests.
7. Whether the drug affects cardiovascular function—In vitro studies on isolated rabbit Purkinje fibers and animal studies on cardiac electrophysiology.
8. Whether the drug affects pulmonary function—Rat pulmonary function test or Irwin behavior test.
9. Whether the drug affects gastrointestinal function—Rat gastric motility or irritation studies.
10. Whether the drug affects reproductive function—Segment I, II, and III toxicity studies in animals (explained in detail below).
11. Whether there is potential to develop drug-drug interaction—In vitro studies for inhibition and induction of enzymes with hepatocytes.

V. **Nonclinical studies for drug development in India (NDCT rules 2019)** (Table 28.1).

The data of the following toxicity studies are required before carrying out:

1. *Phase I clinical trials*

   - Single-dose toxicity studies.
   - Dose-ranging studies.
   - Repeat-dose systemic toxicity studies of appropriate duration to support the duration of proposed human exposure.
   - Male fertility study.
   - In vitro genotoxicity tests.
   - Relevant local toxicity studies with proposed route of clinical application (duration depending on proposed length of clinical exposure).

Table 28.1 Characteristics for conduct of nonclinical studies in India

Duration of proposed human administration	Human phase for which study is proposed	Species and duration of study required	Dose level and number of animals	Outcome parameter
Systemic toxicity study for oral and parenteral route				
A single dose or several doses in 1 day, up to 1 week	I, II, III	2 species; 2 weeks	2 g/kg (or 10 times normal dose; whichever is higher) At least 5 animals of either sex At least four graded doses	7 days after parenteral and 14 days after oral administration: Symptoms, signs, and mode of death Macroscopic and microscopic findings Reported outcome—MLD and MTD, LD10, LD 50 with 95% CI, target organ of toxicity, and mortality
>1 week, but up to 2 weeks	I, II, III	2 species; 2 weeks	One rodent (6–10/sex/grp) and one nonrodent (2–3 /sex/group) species Three dose levels should be used with the highest dose having observable toxicity, mid dose between the high and low dose, and the low dose	Behavioral, physiological, biochemical, and microscopic observations. In case of parenteral drug administration, the sites of injection should be subjected to gross and microscopic examination. Initial and final electrocardiogram and fundus examination Reported outcome—Identification of target organ of toxicity and establishment of maximum tolerated dose (MTD)
Up to 2 weeks	Marketing permission	2 species; 4 weeks	Same as above	Same as above
>2 weeks, but up to 4 weeks	I, II, III	2 species; equal to duration of human exposure	One rodent (6–10/sex/group) and one nonrodent (2–3/sex/group) three dose levels should be done with the highest dose having observable toxicity, mid dose between the high and low dose, and the low dose	Cage side observations, body weight changes, food or water intake, blood biochemistry, hematology, and gross and microscopic studies of all viscera and tissues
	Marketing permission	2 species; 12 weeks		

(continued)

Table 28.1 (continued)

Duration of proposed human administration	Human phase for which study is proposed	Species and duration of study required	Dose level and number of animals	Outcome parameter
>4 weeks, but up to 12 weeks	I, II, III	2 species; equal to duration of human exposure	Same as above	Same as above
	Marketing permission	2 species; 24 weeks		
>12 weeks, but up to 24 weeks	I, II, III	2 species; equal to duration of human exposure	One rodent (15–30/sex/group) and one nonrodent (4–6/sex/group) species are needed Daily dosing by proposed clinical route at three graded dose levels should be done. In addition to the control, a "high-dose-reversal" group and its control group	Include signs of intoxication (general appearance, activity, behavior, etc.), body weight, food intake, blood biochemical parameters, hematological values, urine analysis, organ weights, gross and microscopic study of viscera and tissues. Half the animals in "reversal" groups (treated and control) should be sacrificed after 14 days of stopping the treatment. The remaining animals should be sacrificed after 28 days of stopping the treatment or after the recovery of signs or clinical pathological changes
	Marketing permission	2 species; rodent 24 weeks, nonrodent 36 weeks		
>24 weeks	I, II, III	2 species; rodent 24 weeks, nonrodent 36 weeks	One rodent (15–30/sex/grp) and one nonrodent (4–6/sex/group) species are needed At least four groups, including control, should be taken Daily dosing by proposed clinical route at three graded dose levels	Parameters should include signs of intoxication, body weight, food intake, blood biochemistry, hematology, urine analysis, organ weights, gross and microscopic examination of organs and tissues
	Marketing permission	2 species; rodent 24 weeks, nonrodent 36 weeks		

Inhalation (general anesthetics, aerosols) Up to 2 weeks	I, II, III	2 species; 1 month (exposure time 3 h/day, 5 days/week)	Gases and vapors must be exposed whole body level Aerosol must be given by nose only exposure 3 dose groups and vehicle control Exposure and concentration of test substance (limit 5 mg/l) in multiples of human dose	Effects on respiratory rate, findings of bronchial lavage fluid examination, histological examination of respiratory passages and lung tissue
Up to 4 weeks	I, II, III	2 species; 12 weeks (exposure time 6 h/day, 5 days/week)		
>14 weeks	I, II, III	2 species; 24 weeks (exposure time 6 h/day, 5 days/week)		
Dermal Up to 2 weeks	I, II	1 species; 4 weeks	Test substance must be applied with porous gauze dressing shaved skin not less than 10% of body surface area At least 3 dose concentration several fold higher than clinical dosage	The parameters studied are local signs (erythema, edema, and eschar formation) as well as histological examination of sites of application should be used for evaluation of results
	III	2 species; 4 weeks		
>2 weeks	I, II, III	2 species; 12 weeks		
Ocular or optic or nasal Up to 2 weeks	I, II	1 species; 4 weeks	Acute studies—Drug is administered in one eye and the other act as control Repeated dose studies—Separate control group	Changes in cornea, iris, and aqueous humor is done by slit-lamp examination For detecting defects in cornea and conjunctival epithelium, fluorescent dyes (sodium fluorescein, 0.25 to 1.0%) should be used Tonometry must be carried out for detecting changes in intraocular tension Histological examination of eyes should be done after fixation in Davidson's or Zenker's fluid
>2 weeks	III	2 species; 4 weeks		
	I, II, III	2 species; 12 weeks		

(continued)

Table 28.1 (continued)

Duration of proposed human administration	Human phase for which study is proposed	Species and duration of study required	Dose level and number of animals	Outcome parameter
Male fertility test	Phase III in male volunteers	One rodent species (preferably rat) should be used. Dose selection	Three dose groups required including highest dose group showing minimal toxicity in systemic studies and control group Each group should consist of six adult male animals Intended route of clinical use for min 28 days and max 70 days before getting paired with female animals of proven fertility in ratio of 1:2 for mating. Continued therapy of male animals during pairing Pairing should be continued till the detection of vaginal plug or 10 days, whichever is earlier	Female animals getting pregnant should be examined for fertility index after day 13 of gestation All the male animals are sacrificed at the end of the study Weights of each testis and epididymis recorded. Sperms from one epididymis examined for their motility and morphology The other epididymis and both testes should be examined for their histology
Female reproduction and development toxicity studies segment I study	Phase III involving female patients of childbearing age	One species, preferably rats	3 graded doses—Highest (MTD) dose taken in the route intended for therapeutic use 15 males and females per dose level group Both male (for 28 days) and female (for 14 days) receive drug before mating, continue during mating, gestation period, and continued till weaning of pups	Body weight, food intake, clinical signs of intoxication, mating behavior, progress of gestation or parturition period, length of gestation, parturition, postpartum health and gross pathology (and histopathology of affected organs) of dams are recorded Pups from both treated and control groups should be observed for general signs of intoxication, sex-wise distribution in different treatment groups, body weight, growth parameters, survival, gross examination, and autopsy Histopathology of affected organs should be done

Female reproduction and development toxicity studies segment II study	Phase II, III involving female patients of childbearing age	One rodent (preferably rat) and one nonrodent (rabbit) species used	Three dose levels (with control), highest dose should cause minimal toxicity and lowest dose should be in proportion to the intended therapeutic dose and in the route intended for therapeutic use 20 pregnant rats and 12 pregnant rabbits on each dose levels Drug given during organogenesis	Fetus subjected to gross examination, one half of the fetus is examined for skeletal abnormalities and the other half for visceral abnormalities Dams should be observed for signs of intoxication, effect on body weight, effect on food intake, uterus, ovaries examination and uterine contents, number of corpora lutea, implantation sites, resorptions (if any) Fetuses—total number, gender, body length, weight, and gross or visceral or skeletal abnormalities, if any
Female reproduction and development toxicity studies segment III study	Phase III for drugs to be given to pregnant or nursing mothers for long periods or there are indications of possible adverse effects on fetal development	One rodent species (preferably rat)	4 groups along with control with at least 15 animals in each group and in the intended clinical route Drug is given in the last trimester of pregnancy (from day 15 of gestation) and the dose that causes fetal loss should be continued throughout lactation and weaning One male and one female from each litter of F1 gen (15 males and 15 females in each group) is selected at weaning and treated with the dose levels described above throughout their periods of growth to sexual maturity, pairing, gestation, parturition, and lactation	The criteria of evaluation should be the same as described earlier. Animals should be sacrificed and studied for (dams) body weight, food intake, general signs of intoxication, progress of gestation or parturition periods, and gross pathology, if any; and for pups, the clinical signs, sex-wise distribution in dose groups, body weight, growth parameters, gross examination, survival, and autopsy (if needed) and histopathology Mating performance and fertility of F1 generation is evaluated to obtain the F2 generation whose growth parameters should be monitored till weaning

(continued)

Table 28.1 (continued)

Duration of proposed human administration	Human phase for which study is proposed	Species and duration of study required	Dose level and number of animals	Outcome parameter
Allergenicity or hypersensitivity	Phase I, II, III—when there is a cause of concern or for parenteral drugs (including dermal application)	Described under Guinea pig maximization test and local lymph node assay test	Guinea pig maximization test—initially we determine maximum nonirritant and minimum irritant doses The minimum irritant dose should be used for induction A topical minimum irritant dose should be determined for challenge in two males and two females We determine the intradermal induction dose with four dose levels tested by the same route in a batch of four male and female animals (2 of each sex should be given Freund's adjuvant) Later in the main test At least six male and female animals per group should be used in the main study. One test and one control group should be used and one more positive control group. Intradermal induction (day 1) coupled with topical challenge (dayn21) should be done. If there is no response, rechallenge should be done 7 to 30 days after the primary challenge. Local lymph node assay—mice used in this test are either only males or only females. Drug treatment is given on ear skin Three graded doses, the highest being maximum nonirritant dose plus vehicle control is used Minimum of 6 mice per group should be used Test material should be applied on ear skin on three consecutive days and on day 5, the draining auricular lymph nodes should be dissected out	Guinea pig maximization test—erythema and edema (individual animal scores as well as maximization grading) should be used as evaluation criteria (ii) local lymph node assay. On day 5, the draining auricular lymph nodes are dissected out 5 h after i.v. H-thymidine or bromo-deoxy-uridine (BrdU). Increase in H-thymidine or BrdU incorporation is used as the criterion for evaluation of results

Photoallergy or dermal phototoxicity	Phase I, II, III—If the drug or a metabolite is related to an agent causing photosensitivity or the nature of action suggests such a potential	Armstrong or Harber test in Guinea pig	Pretest in eight animals to screen four conc (patch application for 2 h ± 15 min) with and without UV exposure (10 J/cm^2) Main test is performed with 10 test animals and five controls Induction with the dose selected from pretest must use 0.3 ml/patch for 2 h ± 15 min, followed by 10 J/cm^2 of UV exposure This should be repeated on day 0, 2, 4, 7, 9, and 11 of the test Animals should be challenged with the same concentration of test substance between day 20 to 24 of the test with a similar 2 h application, followed by exposure to 10 J/cm^2 of UV light	Pretest observations recorded at 24 and 48 h are used to ascertain highest nonirritant dose. Main test—Examination and grading of erythema and edema formation at the challenge sites should be done 24 and 48 h after the challenge. A positive control like musk ambrette or psoralen should be used
Genotoxicity	Phase III	Invitro test—conducted in bacteria, mammalian cells, mouse lymphomatic assay, Ames Salmonella assay, and chromosomal aberrations (CA) In vivo tests include micronucleus assay (MNA) or CA in rodent bone marrow	In vitro tests—minimum of 3 log doses along with solvent, positive control (cyclophosphamide and mitomycin C) In vivo studies—5 animals/sex/dose groups minimum of 3 log doses along with solvent and positive control (cyclophosphamide with metabolic activation and mitomycin C) should be included	In vitro tests—increased number of aberrations in metaphase chromosomes In vivo tests—bone marrow from both the femora should be taken out, flushed with fetal bovine serum, pelleted and smeared on glass slides Giemsa-may Gruenwald staining should be done and increased number of micronuclei in polychromatic erythrocytes (minimum 1000) is noted

(continued)

Table 28.1 (continued)

Duration of proposed human administration	Human phase for which study is proposed	Species and duration of study required	Dose level and number of animals	Outcome parameter
Carcinogenicity	If expected use >6 months	Rodent species (preferably rat). Drug administered 7 days a week for a fraction of the life span comparable to the fraction of human life span. Period of dosing should be 24 months for rats and 18 months for mice. Each dose group and concurrent control group not intended to be sacrificed early should contain at least 50 animals of each sex. A high dose satellite group for evaluation of pathology other than neoplasia should contain 20 animals of each sex while the satellite control group should contain 10 animals of each sex	The highest dose should be sublethal, and it should not reduce the life span of animals by more than 10% of expected normal. The lowest dose should be comparable to the intended human therapeutic dose or a multiple of it, for example, 2.5x to make allowance for the sensitivity of the species. The intermediate dose to be placed logarithmically between the other two doses	Observations should include macroscopic changes observed at autopsy and detailed histopathology of organs and tissues. Additional tests for carcinogenicity (short-term bioassays, neonatal mouse assay, or tests employing transgenic animals) may also be done. Observation parameters should include signs of intoxication, effect on body weight, food intake, clinical chemistry parameters, hematology parameters, urine analysis, organ weights, gross pathology and detailed histopathology. Comprehensive descriptions of benign and malignant tumor development, time of their detection, site, dimensions, histological typing, etc. should be given

- Allergenicity or hypersensitivity tests (when there is a cause for concern or for parenteral drugs, including dermal application).
- Photoallergy or dermal phototoxicity test (if the drug or a metabolite is related to the drug causing photosensitivity or the nature of action suggests such a potential).

2. *Phase II clinical trials*

   - Repeat-dose systemic toxicity studies of appropriate duration to support the duration of proposed human exposure.
   - In vivo genotoxicity tests.
   - Segment II reproductive or developmental toxicity study (if female patients of childbearing age are going to be involved).

3. *Phase III clinical trials.*

   - Repeat-dose systemic toxicity studies of appropriate duration to support the duration of proposed human exposure.
   - Reproductive or developmental toxicity studies—Segment I (if female patients of childbearing age are going to be involved), and Segment III (for drugs to be given to pregnant or nursing mothers or where there are indications of possible adverse effects on foetal development).
   - Carcinogenicity studies (when there is a cause for concern or when the drug is to be used for more than 6 months).

4. *Phase IV clinical trials.*

   - Provide a summary of all the nonclinical safety data (listed above) already submitted while obtaining the permissions for Phase I, II, and III trials, with appropriate references.
   - In case an application is made for initiating the Phase IV trial, complete details of the nonclinical safety data needed for obtaining the permissions for Phase I, II, and III trials, as per the list provided above must be submitted.

VI. **Nonclinical evaluation of vaccine/biologics**.

- It is important to determine the best species that will be have an immunological response close to humans taking into consideration whether the vaccine is live or the species is susceptible for infection by the wild strain, etc.
- The most commonly used species is rodents and rabbits; however, monkey may be chosen in special circumstances, for example, if the lower species cannot mount an immunological response.
- Mice are used for studying toxicity for the gene transfer-based vaccine.
- For testing of vaccines, the presence of adjuvants, diluents, and the most appropriate species must also be taken into account.
- It may be difficult to find a relevant model, for example, a strain (*S. typhi*) that does not infect animals or if a vaccine binds only human MHC, etc. The solutions for the same could be to develop gene deletion models, which will

cause infection with *S. typhi* or use of mouse-infective *S. enterica* or mice transgenic for a human cell surface receptor might allow immunogenicity testing of vaccine.

- The visual examination of the site and histology is carried out for any local reactogenicity due to the active vaccine or other components of vaccine formulation, for example, diluents, stabilizers, and preservatives.
- Studies must be undertaken to examine the presence of vaccine antigen at injection site or draining lymph node by carrying out immunohistochemistry and its relation to local reactogenicity.
- The most important safety parameters that are considered are cardiovascular system, respiratory system, and central nervous system by carrying out body temperature, locomotion studies, ECG, and respiration measurements. Additional tests are required if the vaccine/adjuvant has specific toxicity, for example, cardiotoxic effect with pertussis vaccine.
- Animals are injected with high dose of unadjuvanted antigen as a representation of the worst-case scenario where high levels of antigen reach systemic circulation. Investigations are carried out immediately to observe the effect of cytokine release, or complement activation.
- Another set of animals are given the usual dose and the immune response is measured along with the safety parameters.

VII. **Good laboratory practice (GLP) guidelines related to nonclinical studies**.

1. GLP is defined as "a quality program related to organizational processes and conditions where non-clinical health and environmental safety are planned, performed, monitored, recorded, reported and archived."
2. GLP is based on the below-mentioned three aspects:

    - Test facility management (TFM): These are the people who have the responsibility for the standard functioning of the operational unit in line with GLP standards. A genuine conviction to meet up the standards will be required from the management.
    - Quality assurance unit (QAU): This is an internal system to ensure that the GLP principles are adhered to in the best possible manner. The members of QAU should not be involved in experimental development, must have access to the different levels of management, and must highlight the deviation from GLP principles in a prompt manner.
    - Study director (SD): The study director takes care of the scientific, administrative, and regulatory aspects of the study. The SD must take care of the scientific standards that are related to every aspect of the study including experimental design.

1. The GLP requirements are mostly related to the implementation of practices that generate quality and maintain data integrity. The primary reason for developing GLP is to fight fraud in data generation and report safety data.

2. The GLP requirements can be broadly summarized in the below-mentioned points:
   - Reproducibility: This can be done by the third party without the active involvement of people involved in the conduct of the study by completely rebuilding the course of the study. This assures that the experiments were conducted in the most scientific manner as required by the regulatory agency.
   - Responsibility: The documentation of responsibility assures that the person responsible for a particular task can be made accountable for the likely error in a particular aspect.
   - Awareness: The raising of awareness toward GLP principles can go a long way in maintaining the desired quality of studies.

VIII. **Animal ethics and CCSEA guidelines.**

1. The Committee for Control and Supervision of Experiments on Animals (CCSEA) is a statutory Committee of the Department of Animal Husbandry and Dairying (DAHD), Ministry of Fisheries, Animal Husbandry and Dairying (MoFAH&D) constituted under the Prevention of Cruelty to Animals (PCA) Act, 1960. It has changed its name from the "Committee for the Purpose of Control and Supervision of Experiments on Animals" (CPCSEA) to the "Committee for Control and Supervision of Experiments on Animals (CCSEA") through its order dated January 06, 2023.
2. CCSEA is duty-bound to take all such measures as may be necessary to ensure that animals are not subjected to unnecessary pain or suffering before, during, or after the performance of experiments on them.
3. According to CCSEA, the Institutional Animals Ethics Committee (IAEC) means a body comprising of a group of persons recognized and registered by the Committee for the purpose of control and supervision of experiments on animals performed in an establishment which is constituted and operated in accordance with procedures specified for the purpose by the Committee.
4. For research involving small animal experimentation the IAEC shall review and accord approval before the start of the study.
5. For approval of experimentation on large animals, it is forwarded to CPCSEA in prescribed manner with the recommendation of IAEC.
6. Animal ethics and welfare is based on the 4R principle which includes—reduction, replacement, refinement, and rehabilitation.
7. The Institutional Animal Ethics Committee (IAEC) has been designed to secure the following objectives:

   (a) The persons carrying out experiments must be duly qualified or the experiments must be performed under the supervision of a duly qualified person, that is, degree holders in Veterinary Science or Medicine or Laboratory Animal Science of a university or an institution recognized by the government for the purpose.

(b) The experiments are performed with due care and humanity, and wherever feasible, the experiments involving operations are performed under anesthesia so that the animals do not feel pain.
(c) If the experiment involves injury to the extent that the recovery process would be painful, the case is considered for euthanasia while still under influence of anaesthesia.
(d) Experiments on animals are avoided if possible and on larger animals avoided if it is possible to achieve the same results with small laboratory animals.
(e) Experiments are not performed merely for developing skills.
(f) Due care is provided to animals before, during, and after experiments.
(g) Suitable records are maintained concerning experiments performed on animals.
(h) The IAEC must monitor all the animal study, obtain periodic reports from study team, visit the animal house facility while the work is being carried out, and ensure compliance with guidelines or law.

8. Composition of IAEC.
9. Institutional Animals Ethics committee shall include eight members as follows:
10. A. IAEC members from the establishment (5 members):

    - One biological scientist.
    - Two scientists from different biological disciplines.
    - One veterinarian involved in the care of animal.
    - One scientist in charge of animal facility of the establishment concerned.

11. Having a veterinarian in IAEC is mandatory for judging level of care and handling of laboratory animals in a given protocol.
12. Nominees from the CPCSEA:

    (i) Main nominee (01).
    (ii) Link nominee (link nominee shall substitute the main nominee in case main nominee).
    (iii) Scientist from outside the institute (01).
    (iv) Socially aware nominee (01).

13. The minimum qualification for the IAEC members is as below:

    (i) B.V.Sc.
    (ii) M.Sc. (Zoology/Animal Sciences/Animal Biotechnology), or
    (iii) M.Sc./M.Tech (Life Sciences, Biological Sciences/Biochemistry/Biotechnology/Biomedical Engineering) with experience in animal handling and animal research, or,

(iv) M. Pharm. with experience in animal handling and animal research, or.
(v) MD/MS with research experience in laboratory animal handling.

14. The IAEC of an establishment is constituted by CPCSEA at the time of registration for a period of 5 years.
15. The committee is required to be reconstituted at the time of renewal of registration, and at least half of the internal IAEC members is required be replaced at the time of renewal.
16. All members should maintain confidentiality of all the deliberations during the meeting and sign a confidentiality form and conflict of interest should be declared by members of the IAEC.
17. IAEC is required to formulate a SOP for its working requirements and follow it in all the meetings.
18. A minimum of six members shall be required to form a quorum of the IAEC meetings. The decisions of IAEC should be undertaken in the meetings and not by the method of circulation of project proposals. The presence of the main nominee of CPCSEA nominee is required to meet a quorum.
19. The chairperson of the IAEC with the help of the member secretary of IAEC shall be responsible for conducting at least two meetings in a calendar year.
20. The decisions of the IAEC will be documented in minutes of meeting and chairperson's approval taken in writing with signature of all the IAEC members present.
21. Decisions of the IAEC will be communicated by the member secretary in writing to CPCSEA within 15 days of conduct of the meeting.

IX. **Alternatives to animal experiments**.

The necessity for beginning alternative methods is there because these methods are time-efficient, cost-effective, and require less manpower.

1. **Computer models (in silico)**—Computers can help to understand the various basic principles of biology. The computer models and specially designed software help to design new drugs based on the receptor-binding sites. The biological action and toxic effect can be predicted using the software programs. Computer Aided Drug Design (CADD) is used to predict the receptor binding site for a new drug molecule. It is also possible to design a new molecule using structure-activity relationship using these software programs.
2. **Organoids and organ on chip**—Organoids are cellular three-dimensional complex structures formed by differentiated stem cells. Organoids of many parts of the human body organs have been successfully established, for example, the brain, liver, lung, breast, and kidney. The normal as well as tumor cells of the organoids can be established. The source of the cells are adult stem cells and pluripotent stem cells. The time, cost,

operability, and success rate of the organoid system in the prediction of the response of the drug is superior.

Organs-on-chips can be defined as a small functional unit that mimics the level of human organs in vitro. Apart from the organs (which are present in the organoids), there is the presence of essential elements necessary for physiological function. Similar to the organoids, the organ-on-chip comprising the normal and tumor cells of many organs have been developed. The main components are irrigation-controlled microchannel, organ-specific stromal cells, and epithelial cells. The organ-on-chip can thus simulate multicellular structure of human organs, tissue interfaces, vascular perfusion systems, chemical ingredients, etc.

3. **Cells and tissue cultures**—The 2D structure of growing cells and tissue along with a suitable growth medium as a monolayer over the surface of the culture plate is a good alternative for animal use. The advantages of these methods are that they are easy, less time consuming, and less expensive. For example, the use of bovine cornea to evaluate the toxicological effect of test chemical irritancy instead of the use of rabbit for Draize test (to check the irritancy of chemicals).
4. **Alternative organisms—**The use of large animals (e.g., dogs and monkey) has higher ethical issues**.** Instead of the use of higher animals, invertebrate organisms must be preferred if it is possible to generate data without compromising the efficacy results. The various alternatives to animal use are:

   (a) Lower vertebrates—These models have genetic relatedness to the higher vertebrates including human. For, example, use of zebra fish, because of its small size, short life cycle, and high fecundity favor its laboratory use.
   (b) Invertebrate—Invertebrate organisms are popularly used in drug development as an alternative for laboratory use of animals. The advantage of the organisms includes short life cycle, small area for housing, simple anatomy, low cost, etc. Numerous models of invertebrate organisms have been developed, which include models of neurodegenerative disorders, muscle dystrophy, and endocrine disorders, muscle dystrophy, endocrine disorder etc. For example, *Drosophila melanogaster* (fruit fly) is one of the most widely studied invertebrates in drug development. Its complete genome has been sequenced and annotated; this encodes >14,000 genes on four chromosomes. Almost 75% of the genes involved in human disorders are believed to have a functional homolog in the fly.
   (c) Microorganisms—Various microbes, including *Saccharomyces cerevisiae*, brewing yeast, etc., are utilized for research. *Saccharomyces cerevisiae* is the most utilized due to its rapid growth, ease of studying endogenous or heterologous proteins, and well-defined genetic system. *S. cerevisiae* helps to understand the fundamental aspects of cellular biology in neurodegenerative diseases like Alzheimer's, Parkinson's, and Huntington's diseases.

Bibliography

Andrade EL, Bento AF, Cavalli J, Oliveira SK, Schwanke RC, Siqueira JM, Freitas CS, Marcon R, Calixto JB (2016) Non-clinical studies in the process of new drug development – part II: good laboratory practice, metabolism, pharmacokinetics, safety and dose translation to clinical studies. Braz J Med Biol Res 49(12):e5646

Brennan FR, Andrews L, Arulanandam AR, Blumel J, Fikes J, Grimaldi C, Lansita J, Loberg LI, MacLachlan T, Milton M, Parker S, Tibbitts J, Wolf J, Allamneni KP (2018) Current strategies in the non-clinical safety assessment of biologics: new targets, new molecules, new challenges. Regul Toxicol Pharmacol. https://doi.org/10.1016/j.yrtph.2018.07.009

Committee for Control and Supervision of Experiments on Animals (CCSEA) (2023) Compendium for CPCSEA. https://ccsea.gov.in/WriteReadData/userfiles/file/Compendium%20of%20CPCSEA.pdf. Accessed 18 Mar 2023

Denayer T, Stohr T, Roy MV (2014) Animal models in translational medicine: validation and prediction. New Horiz Transl Med 2:5–11

New Drugs and Clinical Trials Rules (2019) Ministry of Health and Family Welfare, India. https://cdsco.gov.in/opencms/export/sites/CDSCO_WEB/Pdf-documents/NewDrugs_CTRules_2019.pdf. Accessed 16 Mar 2024

Pugsley MK, Towart R, Authier S, Gallacher DJ, Curtis MJ (2010) Non-clinical models: validation, study design and statistical consideration in safety pharmacology. J Pharmacol Toxicol Methods 62:1–3

Part IV

Novel Drug Therapies

Novel Chemical and Biological Entities in the Past 5 Years

29

Avinash Arivazhahan

Abstract

Each year, regulatory bodies across the world provide marketing approvals for various novel chemical and biological entities. In addition, extended approvals are provided for old entities for new indications based on new trial data that emerge every year (an aspect also called "drug repurposing"). United States Food and Drug Administration (US-FDA) is one of the prime regulatory bodies in the world, and approvals granted by US-FDA are then replicated across other countries' regulatory agencies, with or without additional local data. This chapter lists the significant regulatory approvals granted by the US-FDA in the past 5 years, along with the approved indications and key clinical guidance. This list, however, is not extensive, and does not indicate that these entities are approved across all geographies.

Keywords

New drugs · Drug approvals · US-FDA · FDA · CDSCO · Regulatory

29.1 Introduction

Any drug that finally gets into the market has to undergo several stages of development, as discussed elsewhere in this textbook. Further, the quantum of money that goes into such development is immense. Although the number of new drugs that are approved by regulatory agencies every year is limited, the number of drugs that did not make its way through approval is huge. In addition to new drugs being approved every year, the regulatory agencies also incorporate changes in the labels of existing

A. Arivazhahan (✉)
Medical Affairs & Medical Education, Novo Nordisk India Ltd., Bengaluru, Karnataka, India

A. Arivazhahan et al. (eds.), *Introduction to Basics of Pharmacology and Toxicology*,
https://doi.org/10.1007/978-981-95-1920-0_29

drugs. These label changes can be expansion of clinical indications, black box warnings, milder warnings, ban notices, etc.

Figure 29.1 depicts the total number of new entities approved by US-FDA over the past 5 years.

29.2 US-FDA-Approved Drugs in 2024 (as of Early January)

At the time of writing this chapter, 2024 has just begun, and it has been a promising start with one drug already being approved for molluscum contagiosum (as shown in Table 29.1). Several chemical and biological entities are expected to obtain approval this calendar year.

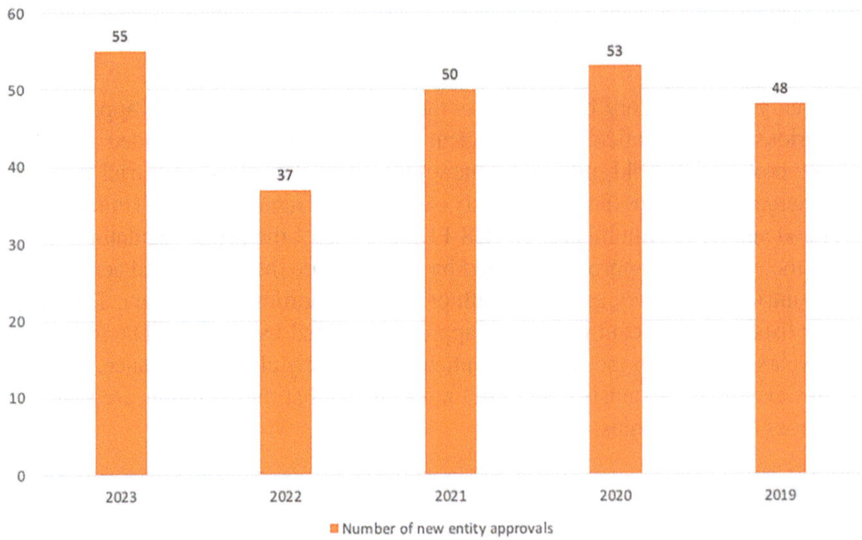

Fig. 29.1 Number of USFDA-approved new entities each year for the past 5 years

Table 29.1 FDA approved entities in 2024 (as of early January)

Drug	Approved indication	Key drug information
Berdazimer	*Molluscum contagiosum*	Berdazimer is a topical formulation (10.3%), which is pharmacologically a nitric oxide-releasing agent. Approval has been granted for use in ages of 1 year and above on the basis of the B-SIMPLE-4 trial

29.3 US-FDA-Approved Drugs in 2023

In the calendar year 2023, there were a total of 55 new approvals granted by the US-FDA, of which the key approvals are detailed in Table 29.2. Looking at the approvals in 2023, the therapy segment of oncology leads the table with 24% of new drugs falling in this bucket, followed by neurology at 16%. Segmentation by the type of new entities shows that 62% of new approval this year fell in the small molecule and small protein class, 31% protein-based therapies, and the remaining being oligonucleotides.

While there were 55 new approvals in 2023 as mentioned earlier, there were also a few key rejections to note: donanemab (for Alzheimer's disease), concizumab (for hemophilia), lebrikizumab (for atopic dermatitis), inbakicept (for bladder carcinoma), among others.

Table 29.2 FDA approved entities in 2023

Drug	Approved indication	Key drug information
Bexagliflozin	Type 2 diabetes mellitus	Bexagliflozin is an oral SGLT-2 inhibitor, which is available as 20 mg dosage. It is approved for use in ages 18 years and above, as an adjunct to diet and exercise
Bimekizumab	Plaque-type psoriasis (moderate to severe grade)	Bimekizumab is a subcutaneous humanized monoclonal antibody (IL-17A and F antagonist), approved for use in adults. It is initially administered every 4 weeks till week 16, and then every 8 weeks
Capivasertib	Breast carcinoma (in combination with fulvestrant)	Capivasertib is an oral kinase inhibitor that is approved in combination with fulvestrant for HR-positive, HER2-negative (following other genetic testing)
Cipaglucosidase alfa-atga	Late onset Pompe's disease	Cipaglucosidase alfa-atga is a lysosomal glycogen-specific enzyme, approved for use in adults (in combination with an enzyme stabilizer). It is an injectable formulation at a dosage of 105 mg
Daprodustat	Anemia secondary to CKD	It is an orally administered hypoxia-inducible factor (HIF) prolyl hydroxlase (PH). It is approved for adults who have been dialyzed for a minimum of 4 months. It is available in multiple doses from 1 mg to 8 mg
Elacestrant	Breast carcinoma	Elacestrant is an orally administered estrogen receptor antagonist approved for ER-positive, HER2-negative, ESR-1-mutated breast cancer, after at least one line of endocrine therapy
Etrasimod	Ulcerative colitis (moderate to severe grade)	Etrasimod is an orally administered sphingosine-1-phosphate receptor modulator, approved for use in adults. It is available at a dosage of 2 mg once a day
Fezolinetant	Postmenopausal hot flushes	Fezolinetant is a neurokinin-3 receptor antagonist, which is orally administered once daily at 45 mg
Fruquintinib	Colorectal cancer	Fruquintinib is an oral kinase inhibitor approved for metastatis colorectal cancer, refractory to multiple earlier therapies

(continued)

Table 29.2 (continued)

Drug	Approved indication	Key drug information
Gepirone	Major depression	Gepirone is a partial 5HT-1A agonist approved for adults with major depressive disorder. It is orally administered once a day
Iptacopan	Paroxysmal nocturnal hemoglobinuria	Iptacopan is an orally administered complement factor B inhibitor, approved for use in adults. It comes with a black box warning of increased risk of serious encapsulated bacterial infections
Lecanemab-irmb	Alzheimer's disease	Lecanemab-irmb is an amyloid beta-directed antibody, conditionally approved with a clause to provide confirmatory trial data. It is dosed intravenously as an infusion
Mirikizumab-mrkz	Ulcerative colitis (moderate to severe grade)	Mirikizumab-mrkz is an IL-23 antagonist, approved for use in adult patients. It is given as intravenous infusions initially, followed by subcutaneous maintenance therapy
Momelotinib	Myelofibrosis in anemia (earlier approved for Child-Pugh C hepatic impairment)	Momelotinib is an oral kinase inhibitor, approved for use in adult patients
Omaveloxolone	Friedrich's ataxia	Omaveloxolone is approved for use in ages 16 years and above. It acts by activating Nrf-2 and inhibiting NF-kB. It is administered orally
Pegunigalsidase alfa-iwxj	Fabry's disease	Pegunigalsidase alfa-iwxj is a lysosomal neutral glycosphingolipid-specific enzyme, approved for use in adults. It is given intravenously as an infusion. It comes with a black box warning for risk of anaphylaxis
Repotrectinib	Lung carcinoma	Repotrectinib is an oral kinase inhibitor approved for ROS1-positive non-small cell lung cancer (NSCLC) therapy in adults
Rezafungin	Candidiasis (invasive) and candidemia	Rezafungin is an intravenously administered echinocandin antifungal, approved for 18 years of age and older. It is however not evaluated in Candida-related endocarditis, meningitis, and osteomyelitis
Ritlecitinib	Alopecia areata	Ritlecitinib is an oral kinase inhibitor, approved for use in patients of 12 years of age and above
Sotagliflozin	Heart failure (earlier approved for type 2 diabetes mellitus)	Sotagliflozin is a dual SGLT inhibitor approved for use in adult patients. It is administered orally
Tofersen	Amyotrophic lateral sclerosis	Tofersen is an antisense oligonucleotide approved for adults with SOD1 mutated amyotrophic lateral sclerosis. It is administered intrathecally. It was conditionally approved, subject to future submission of confirmatory clinical trials

(continued)

Table 29.2 (continued)

Drug	Approved indication	Key drug information
Trofinetide	Rett syndrome	Trofinetide is an analog of IGF-1 that is approved for use in age groups of 2 years and beyond. It can be given orally or via gastrostomy tubes
Vamorolone	Duchenne muscular dystrophy	Vamorolone belongs to the corticosteroid class. It is an oral treatment option that is approved for use in patients of 2 years of age and beyond
Zavegepant	Migraine	Zavegepant is a calcitonin gene-related peptide (CGRP) receptor antagonist for acute treatment of migraine in adult patients. It is administered as a nasal spray
Zilucoplan	Myasthenia gravis	Zilucoplan is a complement inhibitor that is approved for use in adult patients with generalized myasthenia gravis who are AChR-positive. It is given subcutaneously. It carries a black box warning for greater risk of meningococcal infections
Zuranolone	Postpartum depression	Zuranolone is a neuroactive steroid GABA-A-positive modulator approved for use in adults. It is available as oral capsules

29.4 US-FDA-Approved Drugs in 2022

In the calendar year 2022, there were a total of 37 new approvals granted by the US-FDA, of which the key approvals are detailed in Table 29.3. 37 was the least number of new approvals since the year 2016. Looking at the approvals granted in 2022, the therapy segment of oncology leads the table with 31% of new drugs falling in this bucket, followed by neurology at 14%. Segmentation by the type of new entities shows that 53% of new approvals this year fell in the small molecule and small protein class and 25% monoclonal antibody-based therapies.

While there were several new approvals in 2022, there were also a few rejections to note: bardoloxone (for Alport syndrome), zandelisib (for follicular lymphoma), vadadustat (for anemia in CKD), among others.

Table 29.3 FDA approved entities in 2022

Drug	Approved indication	Key drug information
Abrocitinib	Atopic dermatitis (refractory, moderate to severe grade)	Abrocitinib is an oral Janus kinus inhibitor approved for use in patients of 12 years of age and older. It is accompanied with a warning for risk of serious infections, mortality, malignancy, thrombosis, and major adverse cardiac events
Adagrasib	Lung carcinoma	Adagrasib is an oral RAS GTPase inhibitor approved for adults with KRAS G12C mutation-related NSCLC. It holds a conditional approval, subject to future submission of trial data

(continued)

Table 29.3 (continued)

Drug	Approved indication	Key drug information
Daridorexant	Insomnia	Daridorexant is an orexin antagonist approved for use in adult patients. It is an oral agent
Deucravacitinib	Plaque-type psoriasis (moderate to severe grade)	Deucravacitinib is a tyrosine kinase 2 inhibitor that is approved for adult use. It is administered orally
Lenacapavir	HIV-1 infection (MDR)	Lenacapavir is a HIV-1 capsid inhibitor, which is approved for use in adults with multidrug-resistant HIV-1 infection. It is administered as a combination of subcutaneous and oral regimens
Mavacamten	Obstructive hypertrophic cardiomyopathy	Mavacamten is a cardiac myosin inhibitor, which is approved in adults for the treatment of NYHA class II–III obstructive hypertrophic cardiomyopathy. It is administered orally, and is associated with the risk of heart failure
Mirvetuximab soravtansine-gynx	Ovarian carcinoma	Mirvetuximab soravtansine-gynx is a folate receptor-alpha-directed antibody and microtubule inhibitor conjugate. It is approved for use in adult patients with FR-alpha-positive, platinum-resistant epithelial ovarian, fallopian tubal, and primary peritoneal cancers. It is administered intravenously as an infusion. It had received conditional approval, subject to submission of further clinical trial data. It is known to be oculo-toxic, for which it has a label warning
Mosunetuzumab-axgb	Follicular lymphoma	Mosunetuzumab-axgb is a bispecific CD-20-directed CD-3 T cell engager. It is used in adults with relapsed or refractory follicular lymphoma, a type of non-Hodgkin's lymphoma. It holds a warning for cytokine release syndrome development. It is given as intravenous infusion
Oteseconazole	Vulvovaginal candidiasis	Otseconazole is an antifungal from the azole class that is approved for females of nonreproductive potential with recurrent vulvovaginal candidiasis. It is given orally, either alone or with fluconazole
Pacritinib	Myelofibrosis	Pacritinib is an oral kinase inhibitor that has been approved for use in adults with primary or secondary myelofibrosis with a documented low platelet count. It was approved with the condition that further clinical data would be submitted in the future
Spesolimab-sbzo	Pustular-type psoriasis	Spesolimab-sbzo is an IL-36 antagonist, which is indicated in patients of and over 18 years of age for treatment of generalized pustular psoriasis flares. It is given as intravenous infusions
Tapinarof	Plaque-type psoriasis	Tapinarof is an aryl hydrocarbon receptor agonist. It is used topically as a cream for plaque-type psoriasis in adult patients

(continued)

Table 29.3 (continued)

Drug	Approved indication	Key drug information
Teclistamab-cqyv	Multiple myeloma	Teclistamab-cqyv is a bispecific B cell maturation antigen-directed CD3 T cell engager approved for relapsed or refractory multiple myeloma. It is given as subcutaneous injections. It has a warning for cytokine release syndrome and neurological toxicity
Teplizumab-mzwv	Type 1 diabetes mellitus	Teplizumab-mzwv is a first-in-class agent approved for delaying the onset of stage 3 type 1 diabetes mellitus in patients aged 8 years and above. It is administered as a continuous 14-day course intravenously
Tirzepatide	Type 2 diabetes mellitus	Tirzepatide is a GIP-GLP-1 dual receptor agonist, which is approved for use in adults with type 2 diabetes mellitus as an adjunct to diet and exercise. It is given as weekly subcutaneous doses
Tremelimumab	Hepatocellular carcinoma (in combination with durvalumab)	Tremelimumab is a cytotoxic T lymphocyte-associated antigen-4 blocking antibody for unresectable hepatocellular carcinoma, given along with durvalumab. It is given as intravenous infusions
Ublituximab-xiiy	Multiple sclerosis	Ublituximab-xiiy is a CD-20-directed cytolytic antibody. It has been approved for relapsing multiple sclerosis in adult patients. Administration is as intravenous infusions

29.5 US-FDA-Approved Drugs in 2021

In 2021, there were a total of 50 new approvals granted by the US-FDA, of which the key approvals are detailed in Table 29.4. Of all the approvals granted, the therapy segment of rare diseases came out on top with 52% of new drugs falling in this bucket. Further, 52% of the approved drugs were first-in-class with respect to their novel mechanism of action. Also, 58% of the approvals belonged to the small molecule class of drugs.

Table 29.4 FDA approved entities in 2021

Drug	Approved indication	Key drug information
Aducanumab-avwa	Alzheimer's disease	Aducanumab-avwa is an amyloid beta-directed antibody, approved conditionally subject to submission of further clinical data. It is given intervenously as infusions
Amivantamab-vmjw	Lung carcinoma	Amivantamab-vmjw is a bispecific EGF receptor-directed and MET receptor-directed antibody. It is approved for use in adults with NSCLC with EGFR exon 20 mutation. Further trial data submission was mandated for continued approval status

(continued)

Table 29.4 (continued)

Drug	Approved indication	Key drug information
Anifrolumab-fnia	Systemic lupus erythematosus (moderate to severe grade)	Anifrolumab-fnia is a type I interferon receptor antagonist for administration as intravenous infusions in adult patients. It is given once in 4 weeks
Asciminib	Chronic myeloid leukemia	Asciminib is an oral kinase inhibitor that can be used in drug-resistant adult patients with Ph-positive chronic myeloid leukemia. It had received a conditional approval, subject to further submission of clinical trial data
Atogepant	Migraine	Atogepant is a CGRP receptor antagonist, which is indicated for prophylaxis of episodic migraine. It is approved for adults only in oral dosage
Belumosudil	Graft versus host disease	Belumosudil is an oral kinase inhibitor that is approved for ages 12 years and above, for the treatment of chronic graft versus host disease
Belzutifan	von Hippel-Lindau disease, renal cell carcinoma	Belzutifan is a hypoxia-inducible factor inhibitor approved for use in adults as oral tablets. Later in 2023, it also received approval for use in advanced renal cell carcinoma
Casimersen	Duchenne muscular dystrophy	Casimersen is an antisense oligonucleotide approved for intravenous use in patients with DMD gene mutation amenable to exon 45 skipping
Dasiglucagon	Hypoglycemia (severe grade)	Dasiglucagon is an antihypoglycemic agent that is approved for use in patients aged 6 years and above. It is administered subcutaneously
Dostarlimab-gxly	Endometrial carcinoma	Dostarlimab-gxly is a programmed death receptor-1 blocking antibody. It is administered as intravenous infusions in adults
Evinacumab-dgnb	Familial hypercholesterolemia	Evinacumab-dgnb is an angiopoietin-like 3 inhibitor for use in patients aged 5 years and beyond. It is given every 4 weeks as intravenous infusions
Fesinidazole	African trypanosomiasis	Fexinidazole belongs to the nitroimidazole class of antimicrobial agents. It is indicated as an oral agent in patients aged 6 years and beyond
Finerenone	Complicated type 2 diabetes mellitus	Finerenone is a non-steroidal mineralocorticoid receptor antagonist approved for use in adults with type 2 diabetes mellitus and CKD to reduce renal and cardiac adverse endpoints. It is administered orally
Ibrexafungerp	Vulvovaginal candidiasis	Ibrexafungerp is a triterpenoid antifungal agent approved for use in post-menarchal female patients as oral dosing

(continued)

Table 29.4 (continued)

Drug	Approved indication	Key drug information
Inclisiran	Hyperlipidemia	Inclisiran is an siRNA directed toward PCSK9 mRNA that is approved in adults for hyperlipidemia management (initially approved only for familial hypercholesterolemia). It is given subcutaneously every 3 months for first 2 doses, and then every 6 months
Infigratinib	Cholangiocarcinoma	Infigratinib is an oral kinase inhibitor for unresectable cholangiocarcinoma (with a few initiation criteria). It is approved for use in adults, conditionally basis future data that need to be submitted
Melphalan flufenamide	Multiple myeloma (in combination with dexamethasone)	Melphalan flufenamide is an alkylating agent approved for adult patient use. It is administered intravenously. Conditional approval was granted, subject to further clinical trial data submission by the manufacturer
Mobocertinib	Lung carcinoma	Mobocertinib is an oral kinase inhibitor that has received approval for use in adults for NSCLC with EGFR exon 20 mutation. It was approved with the condition that further clinical data would be submitted in the future
Pegcetacoplan	Paroxysmal nocturnal hemoglobinuria	Pegcetacoplan is a complement inhibitor for treatment in adult patients. It is administered subcutaneously twice weekly. It carries a warning for increased susceptibility for encapsulated bacterial infections
Ponesimod	Multiple sclerosis	Ponesimod is a sphingosine 1-phosphate receptor modulator, approved in adult patients as oral dosing
Ropeginterferon alfa-2b-njft	Polycythemia vera	Ropeginterferon alfa-2b-njft is an interferon 2b-based agent, which is approved for use in adults. It is given once in a fortnight subcutaneously
Sotorasib	Lung carcinoma	Sotorasib is an orally administered RAS GTPase family inhibitor approved in adults with KRAS G12C-mutated NSCLC. It was given conditional approval subject to submission of further trial data
Tepotinib	Lung carcinoma	Tepotinib is an oral kinase inhibitor for use in NSCLC with MET exon 14 skipping alterations. It is approved for adult patients
Tezepelumab-ekko	Bronchial asthma	Tezepelumab-ekko is a thymic stromal lymphopoietin blocker for maintenance therapy in severe asthma. It is now approved for patients aged 12 years and beyond. It is administered subcutaneously every 4 weeks
Tivozanib	Renal cell carcinoma	Tivozanib is an oral kinase inhibitor approved for use in adults

(continued)

Table 29.4 (continued)

Drug	Approved indication	Key drug information
Tralokinumab-ldrm	Atopic dermatitis (moderate to severe grade)	Tralokinumab-ldrm is an IL-13 antagonist that is indicated in ages 12 years and above (initially approved for adults only) subcutaneously
Vericiguat	Heart failure	Vericiguat is a soluble guanylate cyclase stimulator approved to reduce cardiac major adverse events in adult patients. It is given orally
Viloxazine	Attention deficit hyperactivity disorder	Viloxazine belongs to the SNRI class, and is approved for oral use in patients aged 6 years and above. It has been given a boxed warning to indicate increased risk of suicidal thoughts and behavior
Voclosporin	Lupus nephritis	Voclosporin is a calcineurin inhibitor that is approved for use in combination with background immunosuppressive regimen in adults as oral dosing. It has received a conditional approval

29.6 US-FDA-Approved Drugs in 2020

In 2020, a total of 53 new approvals were granted by the US-FDA, of which the key approvals are detailed in Table 29.5. Of all the approvals granted, 75% belonged to the small molecule class. The segment of oncology had the maximal number of new approvals, as with many other recent years.

Table 29.5 FDA approved entities in 2020

Drug	Approved indication	Key drug information
Abametapir	Head lice infestation	Abametapir is a topical pediculocide indicated in patients aged 6 months and above
Ansuvimab-zykl	Ebola infection	Ansuviman-zykl is a Zaire ebolavirus glycoprotein (EBOV GP)-directed antibody, approved for use in adult and pediatric patients (including neonates). It is given as an intravenous infusion
Artesunate	Malaria (severe grade)	Artesunate is an injectable antimalarial approved for adult and pediatric use in severe malaria
Avapritinib	Gastrointestinal stromal tumors, systemic mastocytosis	Avapritinib is an oral kinase inhibitor approved initially for gastrointestinal stromal tumors (in adults), and additionally for systemic mastocytosis (in adults). It is administered orally
Belantamab mafodotin-blmf	Multiple myeloma	Belantamab mafodotin-blmf is a B cell maturation antigen-directed antibody and microtubule inhibitor conjugate approved for adult patients' basic conditional approval. It is administered as intravenous infusions

(continued)

Table 29.5 (continued)

Drug	Approved indication	Key drug information
Bempedoic acid	Hyperlipidemia	Bempedoic acid is an adenosine triphosphate-citrate lyase inhibitor, approved for primary hyperlipidemia in adult patients. It is taken orally
Berotralstat	Hereditary angioedema	Berotralstat is a plasma kallikrein inhibitor approved for prophylaxis of hereditary angioedema in patients aged 12 years and above. It is given orally
Capmatinib	Lung carcinoma	Capmatinib is an oral kinase inhibitor for NSCLC in adults
Clascoterone	Acne	Clascoterone is an androgen receptor inhibitor approved for topic therapy for acne vulgaris in patients aged 12 years and beyond
Eptinezumab-jjmr	Migraine	Eptinezumab-jjmr is a CGRP antagonist approved for migraine prophylaxis in adult patients. It is given intravenously as infusions
Fostemsavir	HIV infection	Fostemsavir is a HIV-1 gp120-directed attachment inhibitor, approved for MDR HIV-1 infection. It is indicated orally in adult patients
Isatuximab	Multiple myeloma	Isatuximab is a CD38 cytolytic antibody approved for use in adults with multiple myeloma. It is administered as intravenous infusion
Lactitol	Constipation	Lactitol is an oral osmotic laxative for adult use in chronic idiopathic constipation
Lonafarnib	Premature aging	Lonafarnib is a farnesyltransferase inhibitor approved for use in a few conditions associated with premature aging. Approval is from age of 1 year and above. It is given orally
Lumasiran	Hyperoxaluria	Lumasiran is a HAO-1-directed siRNA for primary hyperoxaluria type 1, approved for adult and pediatric patients as subcutaneous injections
Lurbinectedin	Lung carcinoma	Lurbinectedin is an alkylating agent approved for NSCLC in adult patients as intravenous infusions. It has been granted a conditional approval, subject to submission of further clinical data
Margetuximab-cmkb	Breast carcinoma	Margetuximab-cmkb is a HER2/neu receptor antagonist approved for adult use. It is indicated in HER2-positive breast cancer patients as intravenous infusions
Naxitamab-gqgk	Neuroblastoma (in combination with GM-CSF)	Naxitamab-gqgk is a GD-2 binding antibody approved for ages 1 year and above. It is given as intravenous infusions. It holds a conditional approval, subject to submission of further data
Nifurtimox	Chagas disease	Nifurtimox is a nitrofuran antimicrobial agent approved for use until the age of 18 years from birth. It is given orally.

(continued)

Table 29.5 (continued)

Drug	Approved indication	Key drug information
Oliceridine	Acute pain	Oliceridine is an opioid agonist for acute pain management in adults. It is given intravenously
Opicapone	Parkinson's disease (as adjunct to levodopa/ carbidopa)	Opicapone is a COMT inhibitor approved for Parkinson's disease in patients having "off" episodes. It is administered orally
Osilodrostat	Cushing's disease	Osilodrostat is a cortisol synthesis inhibitor for non-operable Cushing's disease in adult patients. It is administered orally
Ozanimod	Multiple sclerosis, ulcerative colitis	Ozanimod is a sphingosine 1-phosphate receptor modulator initially approved for adults with multiple sclerosis, and later for moderate to severe ulcerative colitis in adults. It is taken orally.
Pemigatinib	Cholangiocarcinoma, myeloid/lymphoid neoplasms	Pemigatinib is an oral kinase inhibitor initially approved for cholangiocarcinoma in adults, and later on for adults with myeloid or lymphoid neoplasms. It holds a conditional approval for the former indication
Pralsetinib	Lung carcinoma, thyroid carcinoma	Pralsetinib is an oral kinase inhibitor initially approved for RET fusion-positive NSCLC in adults (and later on a conditional basis for RET fusion-positive thyroid cancer for patients of 12 years of age and older)
Relugolix	Prostate carcinoma	Relugolix is a GnRH antagonist approved for use in advanced prostate cancer in adults. It is administered orally
Remdesivir	COVID-19	Remdesivir is a SARS-CoV-2 nucleotide analog RNA polymerase inhibitor approved from the age of 28 days and above. It is administered as intravenous infusion
Remimazolam	Procedural sedation	Remimazolam is a benzodiazepine approved for initiation and maintenance of procedural sedation in adults. It is given intravenously for short procedures (30 min or less)
Rimegepant	Migraine	Rimegepant is a CGRP receptor antagonist initially approved for acute migraine treatment, and then also for prophylaxis. It is approved for adult use as oral dosing
Ripretinib	Gastrointestinal stromal tumors	Ripretinib is an oral kinase inhibitor that is approved for adult use for advanced gastrointestinal stromal tumors
Risdiplam	Spinal muscular atrophy	Risdiplam is a survival of motor neuron 2 (SMN2) splicing modifier approved for adult and pediatric use. It is given orally.
Sacituzumab govitecan-hziy	Breast carcinoma, urothelial carcinoma	Sacituzumab govitecan-hziy is a Trop-2-directed antibody, initially approved for triple-negative breast cancer and later also for advanced urothelial cancer in adult patients. It is administered through intravenous route as infusions

(continued)

Table 29.5 (continued)

Drug	Approved indication	Key drug information
Selpercatinib	Lung carcinoma, thyroid carcinoma, solid tumors	Selpercatinib is an oral kinase inhibitor that has been approved initially for NSCLC (adult patients), medullary thyroid cancer (12 years of age and above), and later for RET fusion-positive solid tumors (adult patients).
Selumetinib	Neurofibromatosis	Selumetinib is an oral kinase inhibitor approved for type 1 neurofibromatosis in patients aged 2 years and above.
Somapacitan-beco	Growth failure	Somapacitan-beco is a human growth hormone analog for use in patients of 2.5 years of age and beyond. It is injected subcutaneously.
Tafasitamab-cxix	Large B cell lymphoma	Tafasitamab-cxix is a CD19-directed cytolytic antibody approved conditionally for adult patients. Dosing is as intravenous infusions.
Tazemetostat	Epithelioid sarcoma, follicular lymphoma	Tazemetostat is an orally administered methyltransferase inhibitor with initial approval for epithelioid sarcoma (patients aged 16 years and older), and later for follicular lymphoma (adult patients). It holds conditional approval from FDA.
Tirbanibulin	Actinic keratosis	Tirbanibulin is a microtubule inhibitor for topical use over face and scalp. It is to be applied for 5 consecutive days
Tucatinib	Breast carcinoma	Tucatinib is an oral kinase inhibitor approved for HER2-positive breast cancer. It has received a conditional approval
Vibegron	Overactive bladder	Vibegron is a beta-3 agonist (adrenergic) approved as oral tablets for adult use
Viltolarsen	Duchenne muscular dystrophy	Viltolarsen is an antisense oligonucleotide that has been granted a conditional approval. It is administered through intravenous route as infusions

29.7 US-FDA-Approved Drugs in 2019

A total of 48 new approvals were granted by the US-FDA in 2019, of which the key approvals are detailed in Table 29.6. Of all the approvals granted, 64% belonged to the small molecule class. Majority of the approved molecules belonged to the class of oncology, followed by neurology and hematology.

Table 29.6 FDA approved entities in 2019

Drug	Approved indication	Key drug information
Alpelisib	Breast carcinoma (in combination with fulvestrant)	Alpelisib is an oral kinase inhibitor approved for men and postmenopausal women with HR-positive, HER2-negative breast cancer
Bremelanotide	Hypoactive sexual desire disorder	Bremelanotide is a melanocortin agonist approved for use in premenopausal women. It is given subcutaneously
Brexanolone	Postpartum depression	Brexanolone is a neuroactive GABA-A-positive modulator approved for use in adults as intravenous infusions
Brolucizumab-dbll	Age-related macular degeneration, diabetes-related macular edema	Brolucizumab-dbll is a human VEGF inhibitor approved for use as intravitreal injection -
Caplacizumab-yhdp	Acquired thrombotic thrombocytopenic purpura	Caplacizumab-yhdp is a vWF-directed antibody fragment that has been approved for use in adults. It is given intravenously
Cenobamate	Partial seizures	Cenobamate is a sodium channel blocker that has received approval for use in adults with partial-onset seizures, administered orally
Darolutamide	Prostate carcinoma	Darolutamide is an androgen receptor inhibitor approved as oral tablets in adult patients
Enfortumab vedotin-ejfv	Urothelial carcinoma	Enfortumab vedotin-ejfv is a nectin-4-directed antibody and microtubule inhibitor conjugate approved for use in adult patients in the form of intravenous infusions
Entrectinib	Lung carcinoma, solid tumors	Entrectinib is an oral kinase inhibitor initially approved for NSCLC (adult patients), and then for solid tumors (1 month of age and older) with a few indication criteria. It holds a conditional approval subject to further data submission
Erdafitinib	Urothelial carcinoma	Erdafitinib is an oral kinase inhibitor approved for use in adults with urothelial cancer, subject to submission of further clinical data in the future
Givosiran	Hepatic porphyria	Givosiran is an aminolevulinate synthase 1-directed siRNA approved for acute hepatic porphyria in adult patients, administered subcutaneously
Golodirsen	Duchenne muscular dystrophy	Golodirsen is an antisense oligo nucleotide approved conditionally subject to further data submission by the manufacturer. It is given intravenously as infusions
Istradefylline	Parkinson's disease (as adjunct to levodopa/carbidopa)	Istradefylline is an adenosine receptor antagonist used for adults with Parkinson's disease with "off" episodes. It is to be taken orally

(continued)

Table 29.6 (continued)

Drug	Approved indication	Key drug information
Lasmiditan	Migraine	Lasmiditan is a 5HT-1F agonist for acute management of migraine in adults, given orally
Lefamulin	Community-acquired bacterial pneumonia	Lefamulin is a pleuromutilin antibacterial agent approved for management in adult patients. It is available for administration via oral or intravenous routes
Lemborexant	Insomnia	Lemborexant is an orexin antagonist approved for use in adult patients with insomnia as oral tablets
Lumateperone tosylate	Schizophrenia, bipolar disorder	Lumateperone tosylate is an atypical antipsychotic agent, initially approved for schizophrenia (in adults) and additionally for depressive episodes in bipolar disorders (in adults). It is orally administered
Pitolisant	Narcolepsy	Pitolisant is H3 antagonist/inverse agonist approved in narcolepsy patients with excessive daytime sleepiness. It is approved for use in adults as oral tablets
Risankizumab-rzaa	Plaque-type psoriasis, psoriatic arthritis, Crohn's disease	Risankizumab-rzaa is an IL-23 antagonist approved for use in adults. It is given subcutaneously and as intravenous infusions
Romosozumab-aqqg	Osteoporosis	Romosozumab-aqqg is a sclerostin inhibitor approved for use in postmenopausal women as subcutaneous injections. Upper cap is set at a maximum of 12 monthly doses per patient
Selinexor	Multiple myeloma, B cell lymphoma	Selinexor is an orally administered nuclear export inhibitor, initially approved for multiple myeloma, and later on a conditional basis for B cell lymphoma. Both indications are applicable for adult patients
Siponimod	Multiple sclerosis	Siponimod is a sphingosine 1-phosphate receptor modulator indicated in adult patients as oral dosing
Solriamfetol	Narcolepsy, obstructive sleep apnea	Solriamfetol is a DNRI approved to enhance wakefulness in adults. It is orally administered
Tenapanor	Irritable bowel syndrome	Tenapanor is a sodium-hydrogen exchanger 3 inhibitor approved for adults with constipation predominant type of irritable bowel syndrome. It is given orally
Trifarotene	Acne	Trifarotene is a retinoid approved for topical treatment of acne vulgaris. It has received approval for use in ages 9 years and older

(continued)

Table 29.6 (continued)

Drug	Approved indication	Key drug information
Ubrogepant	Migraine	Ubrogepant is a CGRP receptor antagonist approved for acute treatment of migraine in adult patients. It is administered orally
Upadacitinib	Rheumatoid arthritis, psoriatic arthritis, atopic dermatitis, ulcerative colitis, Crohn's disease, ankylosing spondylitis, axial spondyloarthritis	Upadacitinib is a JAK inhibitor approved for use in patients aged 18 years and above for all indications except atopic dermatitis (12 years and above). It is given orally
Voxelotor	Sickle cell disease	Voxelotor is a HbS polymerization inhibitor approved from ages 4 years and above. It is given as oral formulation. It has received a conditional approval
Zanubrutinib	Mantle cell lymphoma, Waldenstrom's macroglobulinemia, marginal zone lymphoma, chronic lymphocytic leukemia	Zanubrutinib is an oral kinase inhibitor initially approved for mantle cell lymphoma (conditional approval), and later for other indications like Waldenstrom's macroglobulinemia, marginal zone lymphoma (conditional approval), and chronic lymphocytic leukemia. It is only for use in adults

29.8 Conclusion

After a lull period in the previous decade, there has been an influx of several therapeutic, prophylactic, and diagnostic entities that have made their way through the regulatory pathways over the past 5 years. A significant jump in the progress made in the segment of targeted therapies shows promise for the years to come as well. Oncology, immunology, diabetes mellitus, and obesity have been areas of focus for several large-scale pharmaceutical organizations over this period. As evident from the tables in this chapter, kinase inhibitors have stolen the limelight with multiple indications being approved by the FDA. Also, several drugs have been approved through the accelerated approval pathway, with the condition that further data need to be submitted by the manufacturer to the FDA as and when available (in order to maintain the approval status). This is particularly useful for patients who have been waiting for therapies in several disease areas. Also, many of the drugs that belong to the class of targeted therapies have gone beyond the preliminary indication, thereby making these cost-effective and lucrative for the industry also, which ultimately would result in more investments in their research pipelines. Overall, the FDA has also relaxed a few of its strict recommendations and approval pathways, thereby leading to quicker and more efficient approvals.

Disclaimers This chapter is limited to key drug approvals (not exhaustive) that have been granted by the US-FDA over the past 5 years at the time of writing this chapter (2019–2023). Approvals obtained through other regulatory agencies are not included in this chapter, in order to streamline reading convenience. The following key drug approvals are arranged in a reverse chronological manner, and in alphabetical sequencing within each year. Additionally, please note that the information provided in this chapter is for educational purposes only. For detailed information on clinical use, refer to the local prescribing information provided by each individual manufacturer for specific countries and geographies.

Bibliography

Batta A, Kalra BS, Khirasaria R (2020) Trends in FDA drug approvals over last 2 decades: an observational study. J Family Med Prim Care 9(1):105–114

FDA approved drugs at Centerwatch. https://www.centerwatch.com/directories/1067-fda-approved-drugs. Last accessed on 7th January, 2023 at 18:23

New drugs at FDA: CDER's new molecular entities and new therapeutic biological products. https://www.fda.gov/drugs/development-approval-process-drugs/new-drugs-fda-cders-new-molecular-entities-and-new-therapeutic-biological-products. Last accessed on 7th January, 2023 at 18:23

Drug Repurposing

30

Jigar Katwala

Abstract

Drug discovery and traditional drug development are an expensive, time consuming, and risky business. Sometimes, these drugs are a success, while at other times, they are withdrawn, discontinued, or abandoned. Drug repurposing is regarded as a cost-effective and time-efficient method of discovering new therapeutic uses for these drugs. Due to available chemical information and preclinical safety data, the time required to develop these candidates is shorter than for newer molecular entities and costs considerably less. Further, the success rate is higher. This has resulted in many pharmaceutical companies actively directing their efforts toward drug repurposing. The following chapter discusses various strategies, approaches, barriers, challenges, and advantages of drug repurposing.

30.1 Introduction

The traditional drug development research path is usually unpredictable throughout its life cycle. The success rate of developing a new molecular entity is only 2.01% on average. Moreover, new drug development process takes tremendous amount of time and money. The Eastern Research Group (ERG) found that new medicine development takes 11–17 years. An average new drug launch costs $1–2 billion.

J. Katwala (✉)
Medical University of Americas, Nevis, Saint Kitts and Nevis

Department of Pharmacology, Swaminarayan Institute of Medical Sciences & Research, Gujarat, Kalol, Gandhinagar, India
e-mail: drjigarkatwala@gmail.com

A. Arivazhahan et al. (eds.), *Introduction to Basics of Pharmacology and Toxicology*,
https://doi.org/10.1007/978-981-95-1920-0_30

Despite tremendous expenditure and risk in the drug research effort, few new therapeutic medications were licensed since 1995 by FDA. Thus, new drug discovery methodologies are urgently needed.

Drug repurposing has emerged as a promising drug discovery method because of the skyrocketing costs of drug research, and it is frequently used to find therapies for cancer, cardiac disease, neuropathy, infectious diseases, psychosis, rare diseases, and type 2 diabetes mellitus (T2DM). Drug repurposing is also known as drug repositioning, drug profiling, or drug retasking. Drug repurposing was initially introduced in 2004. The National Center for Advancing Translational Sciences (NCATS) defines drug repurposing as "studying the pharmaceuticals that are already approved to treat one disease or condition to see if they are safe and effective for treating other ailments."

Drug repurposing's goal is to give an already approved drug a new label indication. Drugs that have been on the market but whose patents have expired, medications that have been discontinued due to safety issues, and substances that failed to perform as safely and effectively as anticipated in clinical studies are among the active ingredients used in drug repurposing. In essence, drug repurposing refers to the use of licensed or experimental medications for a purpose other than their intended one.

30.2 Drug Repurposing: The Journey

In the past, the majority of drug repurposing was opportunistic and serendipitous. For instance, **sildenafil,** which was first created to treat hypertension and angina pectoris, has now cornered a sizable market for treating erectile dysfunction. Sildenafil's repurposing was based on past clinical experience, but **thalidomide**'s repurposing for multiple myeloma and erythema nodosum leprosum (ENL) was serendipitous. Similarly, checking for off-label uses of an approved drug is another repurposing approach to identify new indications for an approved drug. For example, it has been discovered that the antifungal drug **itraconazole** has an additional antiangiogenesis function. It has currently completed phase 2 studies to examine its efficacy as a second line therapeutic agent in the treatment of lung cancer (NCT02357836) and prostate cancer (NCT00887458). Moreover, drug repurposing also included compounds that were unsuccessful in their experimental studies. For example, failed anticancer drug **saracatinib** significantly reduced symptoms in a mouse model of Alzheimer's disease (AD) and successfully completed phase 1 trials against AD (NCT01864655).

Drug repurposing can be an effective approach to discovery because many existing licensed or experimental drugs already have (a) established formulations and manufacturing processes, (b) extensive pharmacokinetic data, (c) proven therapeutic effectiveness and safety end points in clinical trials phase 1, 2, and 3, and are therefore less likely to fail subsequent trials due to adverse effects as well as phase IV (post-marketing surveillance) safety data. Table 30.1 shows more than 40 approved drugs have already been successfully repurposed for new indications.

Table 30.1 Successfully repurposed drugs

System	Drug name	Original indication	New indication
Cardiovascular	Aspirin	Analgesic	Angina, antiplatelet
	Amphotericin	Antifungal	Antiplatelet
	Colchicin	Gout	Recurrent pericarditis
	Lomitapide	Lipidemia	Familial hypercholesteremia
Neurology	Duloxetine	Depression	Neuropathic pain, anxiety disorders, osteoarthritis, stress incontinence
	Eflornithine	Depression	ADHD
	Bupropion	Depression	Smoking cessation
	Nortriptyline	Depression	Neuropathic pain
	Gabapentine	Epilepsy	Neuropathic pain
	Atomoxetine	PD	ADHD
	Ropinorole	PD	Restless leg syndrome
	Amantadine	Influenza	PD
	Naltrexone	Opioid	Alcohol withdrawal
	Naproxen	Analgesic	AD
	Propranolol	Hypertension	Migraine prophylaxis
	Fingolimod		
Psychiatric	Quetiapine	Schizophrenia	MDD
	Aripiprazole	Schizophrenia	MDD
	Pregabalin, Gabapentin Valporic acid Phenytoin	Epileptic	MDD
	Pramipexole Cabergoline Pergolide	PD	MDD
	Metformin	DM	MDD
	Pioglitazone	DM	MDD
Rare and orphan diseases	Alefacept	Chronic plaque psoriasis	Allogenic solid organ transplant
Infectious diseases	Thalidomide	Morning sickness (withdrawn)	Leprosy
	Zidovudine	Cancer (failed)	AIDS
Dermatology	Minoxidil	Hypertension	Hair loss
	Finasteride	BPH	Hair loss
	Zileuton	Asthma	Acne
	Miltefosine	Cancer	Visceral leishmaniasis
	Methotrexate	Cancer	Psoriasis
	Doxepine	Depression	Antipruritic, insomnia
Obesity	Sibutramine	MDD	Obesity
	Topiramate	Epilepsy	Obesity
Others	Sildenafil	Angina	Erectile dysfunction
	Dapoxetine	Analgesic and depression	Premature ejaculation

(continued)

Table 30.1 (continued)

System	Drug name	Original indication	New indication
Cancer	Arsenic	Syphilis	Leukemia
	Celecoxib	Analgesic	Familial adenomatous polyps
	Disulfiram	Alcoholism	Melanoma
	Thalidomide	Morning sickness	Multiple Myeloma
	Pemetrexed	Mesothelioma	Lung cancer
	Raloxifene	Osteoporosis	Breast cancer
	Retinoic acid	Acne	Acute promyelocytic leukemia
	Everolimus	Immunosuppressant	Pancreatic neuroendocrine tumor
	Imatinib	CML	GIST
	Nelfinavir	HIV	Multiple myeloma
	Sunitinib	GIST, RCC	Pancreatic neuroendocrine tumor
	Trastuzumab	HER-positive breast cancer	HER2-positive metastatic gastric cancer
	Crizotinib	Anaplastic large cell lymphoma	NSCLC
	Aspirin	Analgesic	Colorectal cancer
	Metformin	Type 2 DM	Breast cancer, pancreatic, endocrinal cancer

ADHD Attention deficient hyperactivity disorders, *AD* Alzheimer's disease, *AIDS*acquired immunodeficiency virus, *BPH* benign prostatic hyperplasia, *CML* chronic myeloid leukemia, *MDD* major depressive disorder, *HIV* human immunodeficiency virus, *RCC* renal cell carcinoma, *GIST* gastrointestinal stromal tumor, *NSCLC* non-small cell lung cancer, *PD* Parkinson's disease, *DM* diabetes mellitus

Most of which so far have derived from an understanding of the pharmacology of drugs or retrospective analyses of the clinical effects of a drug when prescribed for its original indications.

The most frequently discussed repurposing drugs in the literature included thalidomide, sildenafil, saracatinib, AZT, aducanumab, sunitinib, ebselen, tamoxifen, raloxifene, and daptomycin.

Thalidomide was discussed as an example of a medication that failed after being introduced on the market in various nations in the middle of the 1950s. It was discontinued due to its teratogenic complications despite being first used for sedation and morning sickness. However, additional research showed that the medication blocked tumor necrosis factor-alpha signaling. As a result, thalidomide was successfully repurposed. It is approved for the treatment of multiple myeloma and erythema nodosum leprosum.

Sildenafil was also reported in the research as a well-known example of a drug that failed to treat angina patients in clinical trials; however, interestingly, research into the drug's peculiar side effects and pretty poor pharmacokinetics for angina led to its eventual use for erectile dysfunction.

After the original drug manufacturers gave up on the antibiotic **daptomycin** when it shut down its infectious illness division, another manufacturer then successfully repurposed it. Daptomycin is now a crucial component of public health care, acting as a helpful last-resort treatment for conditions like methicillin-resistant *Staphylococcus aureus* (MRSA).

Saracatinib was originally developed for multiple oncology indications, but phase II studies showed limited benefit and the drug was deprioritized. The concept of repositioning of this agent came from discoveries of memory impairments in mouse models of AD and data that showed the phosphorylation of the fyn tyrosine kinase was related to Aβ- and tau-associated synaptic dysfunction. The drug is currently being investigated for other indications like bone pain and lymphangioleiomyomatosis through MRC, NIH, and NCATS programs.

The example of **azidothymidine (AZT)** demonstrates how in-depth knowledge of disease and medication mechanisms of action can result in the reapplication of discoveries in completely new applications. In the 1960s, AZT was first considered as a chemotherapy treatment but was later dropped owing to ineffectiveness. However, the NIH teamed up with industry specialists to repurpose the medicine once the antiretroviral action of AZT was discovered during the early stages of the HIV epidemic. This medication thus became the first option of HIV treatment.

An independent monitoring committee's futility study of **aducanumab** revealed that it would not be effective in treating Alzheimer's disease. As a result, the medicine was discontinued. However, a reanalysis of data from two unsuccessful clinical trials revealed encouraging findings, as a subset of individuals treated with the highest dose appeared to demonstrate a statistically significant slowdown of cognitive function and fundamental daily tasks. The drug manufacturer received approval from the FDA to proceed with a regulatory filing, reviving the practically forgotten medication.

On-target repurposing is demonstrated by **sunitinib**. Clinical studies for colorectal, breast, prostate, and non-small cell lung cancer were unsuccessful; however, it was successfully repositioned for the treatment of renal and gastrointestinal stromal tumors. In 2010, it was authorized for the treatment of pancreatic neuroendocrine malignancies following a repurposing initiative.

The National Health Institute Clinical Collection was screened using a pharmacological repurposing technique, and **ebselen** was identified as a possible lithium mimic. Ebselen was not very effective when used as prescribed for stroke. Ebselen, a drug that was never commercialized but may one day be used to treat bipolar illness, was mentioned as being investigated in a 2016 publication.

Despite being a failed orphan medication and contraceptive, **tamoxifen** has shown promise in translational laboratory studies to induce ovulation in infertile women and to treat metastatic breast cancer in postmenopausal women. Tamoxifen, a nonsteroidal antiestrogen, was repurposed and authorized for the treatment of metastatic breast cancer and later for the reduction of breast cancer risk. It is now the accepted practice for long-term adjuvant therapy for estrogen receptor-positive breast cancer (Table 30.2).

It is also important for us to understand a few of the repurposed drugs, which ultimately became unsuccessful for various reasons, as mentioned in Table 30.3.

Table 30.2 Investigational repurposing drugs

System	Drug name	Original indication	New indication
Infectious disease			
	Rosiglitazone	Antidiabetic	Malaria
	Clindamycin	Antibiotic	Malaria in children
	Tinidazole	Antibiotic	Radical cure for malaria
	Dapsone and artesunate combination	Leprosy	Uncomplicated malaria
	Paracetamol	Analgesic	Malaria
	Linezolid	Antibiotic	Multidrug-resistant TB
	Ibuprofen	Analgesic	Extensive drug-resistant TB
	Prednisolone	Corticosteroid	Tuberculous pericarditis
Diabetes	Dextromethorphan	Dry cough	T2DM
	Ranolazine	Antianginal	T2DM
Neurology			
	Bexarotene	T cell lymphoma	AD
	Riluzole	ALS	Mild AD
	Acetritin	Psoriasis	AD
	Carvedilol	Heart failure	AD
	Minocycline	Antibiotic	AD
	Pioglitazone	DM	PD
	Isradipine	Hypertension	PD
	Propranolol	CVS diseases	Vestibular migraine
	Mifepristone	Abortifacient	Bipolar depression
Others	Ofatumumab	CML	Relapsing remitting MS
	Isotretinoin	Acne	Refractory neuroblastoma
	Propranolol	CVS diseases	Osteoporosis
	Lansaprozole	Anti-ulcer	Chronic idiopathic thrombocytopenic purpura
	Eflornithine	Facial hirsutism	African trypanasomiasis

ALS amyotrophic lateral sclerosis, *AD* Alzheimer's disease, *MS* multiple sclerosis, *PD* Parkinson's disease, *DM* Diabetes mellitus, *CVS* cardiovascular disease, *CML* chronic myeloid leukemia, *TB* tuberculosis

30.3 Drug Repurposing is Different from New Drug Development

The four steps of traditional drug development strategies are drug discovery, preclinical research, clinical trials, and post-marketing safety monitoring. An average of 11–17 years is needed to produce a new drug due to regulatory constraints for safety, efficacy, and quality in animal research and clinical trials (Fig. 30.1).

Drug repurposing starts with (1) screening of raw data related to disease-drug targets, followed by (2) compound identification and the establishment of a drug target-disease relationship. Proof of concept is developed using computational diagnostic methods and a wealth of potential evidence. This is followed by (3)

Table 30.3 Unsuccessfully repurposed drugs

Drug	Original indication	Failed indication	Comment
Bevacizumab	Multiple cancer	Gastric cancer	Failed to show efficacy
Bupropion	Depression	Obesity	Due to adverse effects
Naltrexone	Opiods addiction	Obesity	Due to adverse effects
Topiramate	Epilepsy	Inflammatory bowel disease	Successful in rodent study but failed in retrospective cohort
Ceftiaxone	Antibiotic	Amyotrophic lateral sclerosis	Failed phase 3 trial
Latrepirdine	Antihistamine	Huntington's disease	Failed phase 2 trial

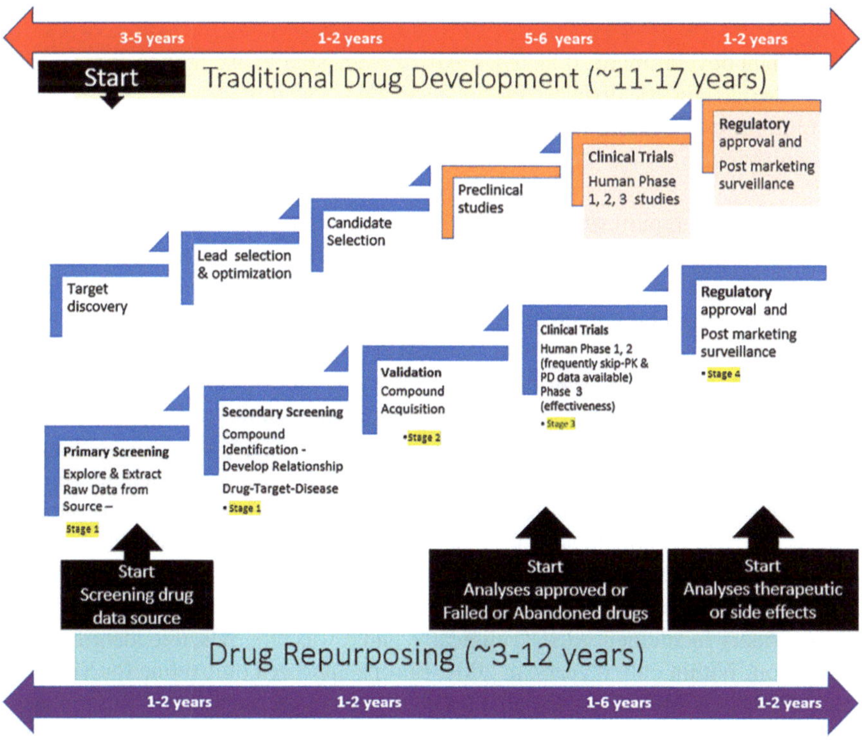

Fig. 30.1 Process of traditional drug development and drug repurposing. (References: Xue et al. (2018), Gns et al. (2019), Jarada et al. (2020), Hua et al. (2022), Repurposing drugs (2017)

experimental validation and compound acquisition. Further, the shortlisted compounds pass through (4) clinical trials for the new indication and (5) enter the market with new labeling. The National Institute of Health (NIH) has proposed two stages of drug repurposing: early and late stages.

Early-Stage Repurposing

- **Screening:** The first step being the screening of approved or marketed drugs against a particular therapeutic target. Searching and extracting large amount of publicly available medical- and health-related data to find evidence or to identify a signal to establish drug-target, drug-drug, drug-disease relationships and build networks by various approaches.
- **Validation:** The shortlisted compounds are further processed for investigation in specific pathophysiological pathways of the disease of interest using in vitro and in vivo methodologies.

Late-Stage Repurposing

- **Clinical development**: It includes experimental studies and human clinical trials for therapeutic effectiveness for the respective indication.
- **Regulatory licensing** for marketing and post-marketing surveillance for safety monitoring.

Overall, drug repurposing takes less time than traditional drug development programs. First, the medications being researched for repurposing are those that have been abandoned or failed because they either did not complete clinical studies or were not successful commercially. These drugs have a known drug profile, which makes for easy regulatory approval from the regulatory authorities, and reduces the time it takes to identify new indications for common or rare diseases. Moreover, these drugs are cost-effective because they are already marketed (Fig. 30.2).

It might shorten the process from 11 to 17 years to roughly 4–11 years by avoiding processes like optimization and preclinical pharmacokinetic, toxicology studies. The earliest stages of clinical trials can be skipped because the drug's effectiveness, safety, and toxicity are already established. These reduce the cost and time required for hectic and expensive initial preclinical and clinical studies. For instance, **duloxetine** was initially approved to treat depression, but in 1998 it was shown to improve stress urinary incontinence (SUI) clinically, and it was repurposed to identify a new indication. Within only 6 years, in 2004, Europe approved duloxetine for SUI.

Similarly, in 2001, a single patient with a gastrointestinal stromal tumor (GIST) was found to respond favorably to **imatinib**, which was created for the treatment of chronic myeloid leukemia (CML). This observation opens a repurposing pathway to identify new indications for imatinib. The US Food and Drug Administration (FDA) later approved imatinib in 2008. It took only 7 years to get a new indication for imatinib.

Another example of the most rapid translation so far is **crizotinib,** a dual MET protooncogene/anaplastic lymphoma kinase (MET/ALK) inhibitor, was initially approved as a MET inhibitor for anaplastic large cell lymphoma, but because of its ALK-inhibiting ability, it was repurposed for NSCLC (non-small cell lung cancer treatment) and authorized in just 4 years.

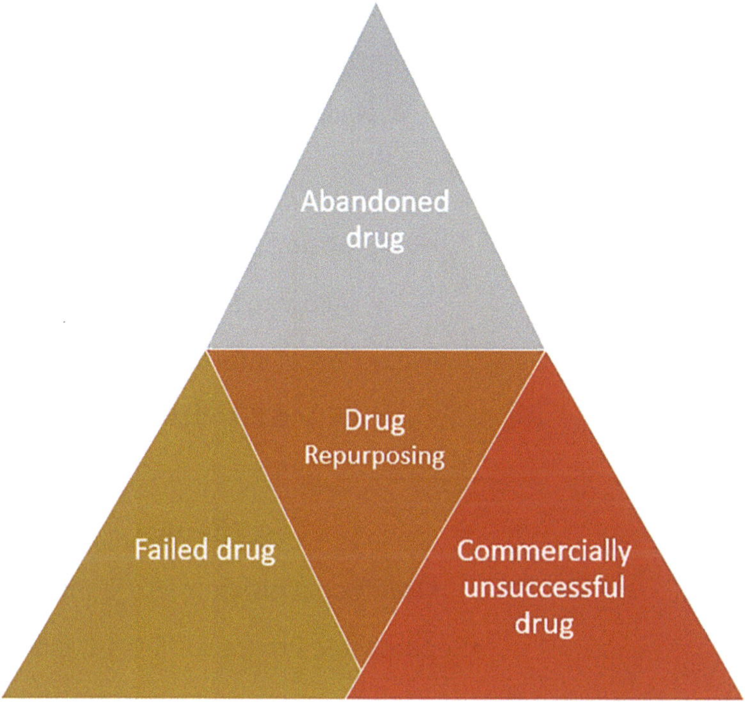

Fig. 30.2 Drug profile for repurposing approach

These turnaround times demonstrate the effectiveness of drug repurposing strategies and are significantly less time consuming than the 13.5-year average currently reported for new medications (Fig. 30.3).

30.4 Drug Repurposing Strategies

Drug repurposing research could be divided into two groups: (i) Drug-based strategies, where discoveries are made using knowledge of drugs, and (ii) Disease-based strategies, where discoveries are made using knowledge of diseases.

30.4.1 Drug-Based Strategies

Drug-related data, such as chemical, molecular, biological, pharmacological, and genetic information, serves as the basis for drug-based techniques that aim to forecast therapeutic potentials and new indications for already available medications. The vast majority of studies under this category share the hypothesis that if two drugs, R1 and R2, have similar profiles and modes of action, and drug R1 is used to cure disease D, then drug R2 can be considered a strong candidate for treating disease D. The profile-based approach and network mapping represent this strategy.

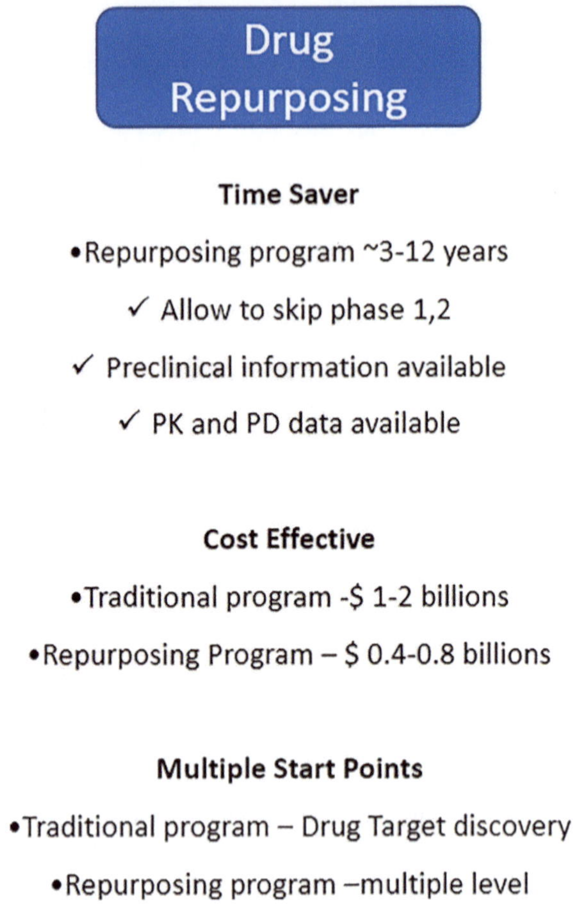

Fig. 30.3 Advantages of drug repurposing

30.4.2 Disease-Based Strategies

Disease-based approaches rely on data about diseases, such as information on phenotypic features, side effects, and indications, as the basis for predicting therapeutic potentials and new indications for already available treatments. The studies under this category share the hypothesis that if two diseases, D1 and D2, have a similar profile and indications, and drug R is used to cure disease D1, then drug R can be considered a strong candidate for curing disease D2. The primary strategy that represents this category is the phenotype strategy (Fig. 30.4). Drug Repurposing Strategies

30.4.3 Data Source

Today's sophisticated technologies have generated a vast amount of data (such as gene expression, drug-disease associations, drug chemical structure profiles, drug-targeted proteins, and phenotypic traits), which has aided in the enormous effort put

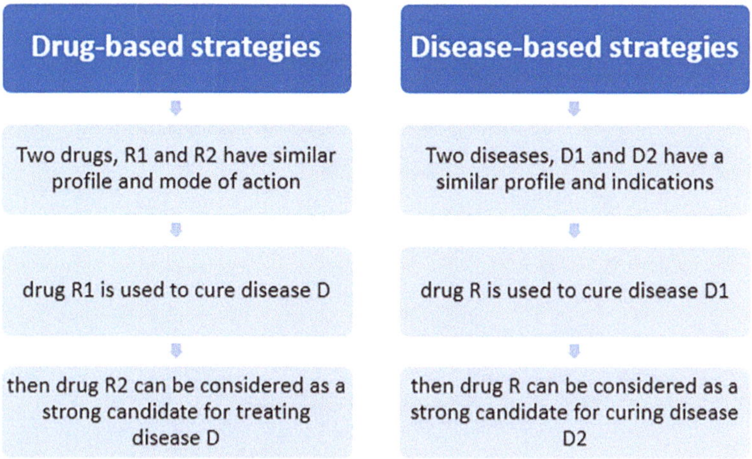

Fig. 30.4 Drug Repurposing Strategies

Table 30.4 Data resource used in drug repurposing research

Drug repurposing strategy	Data source
Chemical structure	PubChem, CheEMBL, DrugBank, DrugCentral, cMAP,STITCH(search tool for interaction of chemical),Therapeutic Target Database(TTD)
Transcriptomic	cMAP, LINCS(Library of Integrated Network-based cellular)
Protein structure	Protein Data Bank(PDB), Protein binding sites(ProBis), Protein-Ligand Interaction(PLIP), UNIPORT(Universal Protein Knowledgebase),
Genomics	GWAS, cMAP, DMAP, Phneome wide association studies, GEO(Gene Expression Omnibus), OMIM(One Mendelian Inheritance in Man)
Network bade	Drug repurposing Hub, Open target, MANTRA(Mode of action by network analysis), KEGG(KyotoEncyclopedia for Genes and Genomes)
Pharmacokinetic data	SwissADME
Clinical trials and adverse effect data	repoDB, repurpose DB, Clinicaltrial.gov, Side effect Resource(SIDER),ADR data base
Toxicity data	Tox cast, FDA label, Drug information panel, Daily Med

forth to create fascinating drug repurposing strategies. Table 30.4 lists the most popular data sources along with a classification of how they categorize drug repurposing strategies.

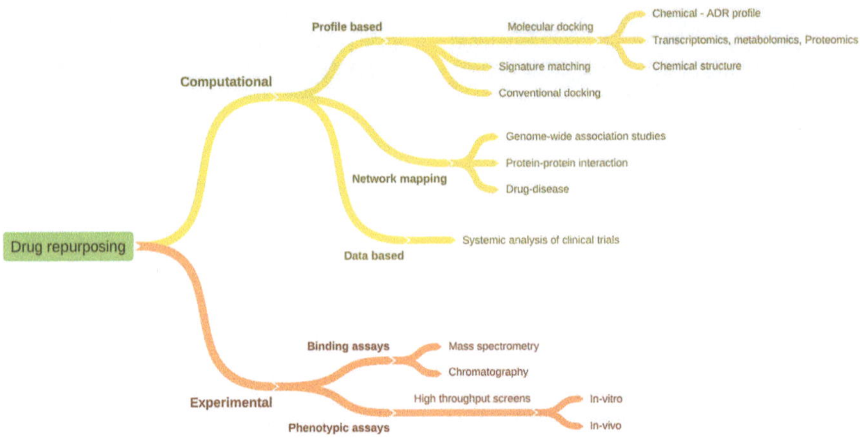

Fig. 30.5 Drug repurposing approaches

30.5 Drug Repurposing Approaches

Finding novel drug-disease relationships is the major challenge in drug repurposing. One of the most important steps in this process is choosing an appropriate strategy. Drug repurposing approaches are divided into two major groups: computational strategies and experimental strategies. Additionally, the hybrid strategy, which combines computational and biological methods, significantly boosts drug repurposing efficiency while cutting costs. Computational methods are far less expensive and more accessible than biological experimental methods (Fig. 30.5).

30.5.1 Computational Drug Repurposing Approach

A computational procedure utilizes various data sources such as genomics, proteomics, transcriptomics, pharmacology, toxicology, and clinical trial data to predict the new use of existing drugs through a systematic drug-target-disease relationship. Computational drug repurposing approaches can be divided into profile-based repurposing, network-based repurposing, and data-based repurposing strategies. Computational methods can also classify based on data mining, machine learning, and network analysis.

30.5.1.1 Profile-Based Drug Repurposing

In a profile-based strategy, the bioactive profile of a drug is combined with other drug or disease profiles. It is divided into three broad categories, such as signature matching, conventional docking, and molecular docking.

Signature Matching

This procedure includes comparison of the "signature" of a drug, such as transcriptomic, proteomic, metabolomic, and chemical structure, and clinical-adverse effect relationship with that of another drug, disease, or clinical phenotype.

Table 30.5 Transcriptomic signature method

Drug	Target-transcriptomic-modifying relevant gene expressions	New proposed disease area
Ketamine	miRNAs like miR-598-5p and miR-451	Mood disorder
Vorinostat	histone deacetylase (HDAC) inhibitors	Depression, anxiety, and schizophrenia
Topiramate	Gene expression signature of inflammatory bowel disease (IBD)	Inflammatory bowel disease

Transcriptomic Signature

This method compares the expression of genes in three different states: healthy, disease, and drug use. A drug is likely to reverse the disease phenotype itself if it can reverse the expression pattern of the genes linked to the condition, which is known as the signature reversion principle (SRP). A strong, negative, correlation between the transcriptomic expression profiles of a drug and a disease would show the potential effect of a drug on the disease (Table 30.5).

Metabolomic Method

The principle of this computational strategy is that a drug can be shared between two different disease treatments with similar pathophysiology. This method recognizes potential druggable targets in different diseases.

Proteomics Generally, drugs produce their therapeutic actions by interacting with protein targets, and it is important to know these interactions to identify new drug-target associations. For example, if a specific protein, which is a causative target of disease A, has a similar local structure to that of protein B, which is a therapeutic target of drug B, we can predict that drug B may be used for disease A. This simple strategy is effective in drug repurposing.

Chemical Structure This procedure creates networks based on shared chemical characteristics since chemical structural similarities may result in the same biological activity. For instance, due to the chemical similarities between chlorcyclizine and the other antipsychotic and antidepressant drugs in this family, they are expected to have similar effects.

Clinical Adverse Event Profile

According to a hypothesis, two drugs with the same side effects might be affecting the same target, protein, or pathway. The phenotype of a drug's side effects may also mirror that of a disease, which would indicate that the drug and the disease may share certain physiology and pathways. Additionally, there could be a shared underlying mechanism that connects adverse events and therapeutic effects. Two drugs for the same disease with distinct mechanisms exhibit the same unusual adverse impact. Cabergoline, an ergot derivative dopamine agonist, caused delusions and was found to have antidepressant-like properties. Another dopamine agonist, pergolide, showed antidepressant effects in Parkinson's disease.

Computational Molecular Docking

This is a strategy to predict binding site complementarity between a ligand (e.g., a drug) and a biological target. In conventional docking, many drugs are tried against a known target that is implicated in the illness (one target and multiple ligands). In inverse docking or molecular docking, a group of targets is examined to see if they are compatible with certain medications to identify novel drug-target interactions (several targets and one ligand). However, the lack of 3D structures of drug targets and structural information on molecules limits the predictability of this strategy (Table 30.6).

30.5.1.2 Network-Based Drug Repurposing

Building networks based on signature matching data, protein interactions, gene expression patterns, disease pathology, or GWAS data is one method used to check for similarities or connections between a drug's side effects and a disease. Some disease-associated genes are not druggable targets. As a result, building and evaluating such networks might be a strategy to identify upstream or downstream genes that can be employed for medication repurposing.

Network-Based Cluster Approach

It aims to find several modules (also known as subnetworks, groups, or cliques) using cluster algorithms according to the topology structures of networks. These modules include various relationships such as drug-disease, drug-drug, or drug-target (PPI network), and drug-protein-disease relationships. The most common network-based cluster approaches include DBSCAN, CLIQUE, STING, and OPTICS.

Network-Based Propagation Approach

It is divided into two types: local approaches and global approaches. These methods for extracting disease-drug relationships and constructing a disease gene network predict novel disease-gene and disease-protein relationships (PPI network). Propagation approaches can be divided into two classes: homogenous and heterogeneous (Table 30.7).

Table 30.6 Molecular docking strategy

Drug	Original action/target	Molecular docking target	New indication
Mecamylamine	Nicotinic receptor antagonist	Glutamatergic receptors	Depression
Dextromethorphan	Antitussive	Glutamatergic receptors	Depression
Mebendazole	Antiparasitic	Inhibit vascular endothelial growth factor receptors	Cancer

Table 30.7 Network-based strategy

Methods	Network	Drug-original indication	Repurpose indication	Pros and cons
Cluster	Drug-protein disease	Lioperidone—schizophrenia	Hypertension	Pros: integrate multiple database Cons: difficult to distinguish between positive and negative network
Cluster	Drug-target-disease	Vismodegib—basal cell ca	Gorlin syndrome	Pros: robust approach Cons: weakly associate
Cluster	Drug-disease	Levodopa—Parkinsonian disease Nimodipine—hypertension Scopolamine —motion sickness	Alzheimer Antidepressant Mood disorder	Pros: reliable Cons: needs more biological information
Propagation	Disease-drug-protein	Methotrexate—antimetabolite Gabapentin—epilepsy	Cancer Neuropathic pain	Pros: robust and efficient Cons: depends on data

Genome-Wide Associated Studies (GWAS)

This strategy is used to identify genetic variations linked to prevalent diseases and to better understand disease biology. It is focused on whether proteins with disease-associated mutations will be the direct targets of drugs treating a disease. Furthermore, this data might lead to the identification of common targets between situations. Pregabalin, gabapentin, nitrendipine, alizapride, mesoridazine, levonorgestrel, diethylstilbestrol, papaverine, scopolamine, ketoconazole, arcaine sulfate, ifenprodil, cycloserine, risperidone, and sulpiride can all be repurposed for MDD, according to the GWAS. When the genes identified in GWAS research are not druggable targets, a network-based technique is useful to identify new targets.

30.5.1.3 Data-Based Drug Repurposing

Systematic Clinical Trial Data Analysis

This approach is based on examining and retrieving important data from many resources, such as EHRs, post-marketing surveillance, and clinical trials. It will result in identifying new indications of a failed or abandoned drug or a new use of an approved drug.

Electronic Health Records

EHRs have a vast amount of structured (diagnosis and pathophysiology data, laboratory test results, and medication prescriptions) and unstructured (patients' symptoms reports and imaging data) data. Systematic analysis of EHRs' data helps identify signals for drug repurposing. EHRs' data has its own limitations and challenges due to ethical issues. Expert assistance is necessary to analyze unstructured

Table 30.8 Electronic health record strategy

Drug	Original indication	Clinical data	New proposed indication
Terbutaline sulfate	Anti-asthmatic	Clinical trials + Lab test result + Genomic signature	Amyotropic lateral sclerosis
Metformin	Antidiabetic	National health insurance of Taiwan research database	Depression and anxiety
Telmisartan	ACEIs	Observational and case control studies	MDD
Pramipexole	Dopamine agonist	Case reports	MDD
Celecoxib	Anti-inflammatory	Retrospective studies	Improve first-line antidepressant action
Valporic acid	Anti-epilepsy	Clinical data	Enhance antidepressant effect
Quetiapine	Antipsychotic	Clinical data	Enhance antidepressant effect, MDD

information. Clinical symptoms can be effectively used for drug repurposing in EHR by combining natural language processing (NLP) and machine learning techniques. EHRs database source: UK clinical practice Research Datalink, Eudra vigilance (a European database of suspected adverse drug reactions), FDA adverse event reporting system (FAERS), and Vigibase (a WHO global data base for adverse drug reactions) (Table 30.8).

Post-marketing Surveillance and Clinical Data

Because they were collected by a pharmaceutical company and for reasons of confidentiality, these data are restricted. Time is changing; recently, in 2016, the European Medical Agency has started to provide this enormous data to private and public users as an analysis signal for drug repurposing.

Novel Sources

There are three novel methods used in this strategy. The first step is to test a variety of chemicals on immortalized human cancer cell lines (CCLs) to see if pharmacological and genomic data match. The second approach identifies the relationship between a patient's genome and their condition by connecting EHR data to DNA biobanks. Patients' online self-reported data about their condition while taking medication is the third novel resource. Novel sources accelerate the drug discovery process, reduce cost, increase patient involvement, and detect the effectiveness of medications.

30.5.2 Experimental Approaches

Binding Assays

Realizing interactions between target and ligand by using different methods such as chromatography and mass spectroscopy. Example of early success is confirmation of cellular target for crizotinib, a tyrosine kinase2 inhibitor.

Phenotypic Screening

This method attempted to identify compounds exhibiting effects of disease consequences in model systems without prior knowledge of the targets they affect. In vitro phenotypic screens using a wide range of high-throughput cell-based assays identified **disulfiram** as a selective antineoplastic agent later validated by genome wide gene expression.

Computational approaches face numerous challenges, including protein flexibility and accuracy of binding affinity prediction, selection of the most relevant protein structure, and receptor druggability. Therefore, it is crucial to develop in silico repurposing methodologies or **Artificial Intelligence (AI)-driven technologies.**

Al-driven technologies can integrate and connect data. AI evolves quickly. It increases drug development's efficiency and cost-effectiveness. The surge in available information from high-throughput screenings (HTS) and omics has advanced AI in drug discovery. Machine learning (ML) is a subset of AI that allows software algorithms to learn from huge datasets, such as those used for drug virtual screening. The FDA, major pharmaceutical corporations, and patient advocacy groups have employed their AI system. **Baricitinib** is an AI based-identified anti-COVID-19 medication. This method merged structured and unstructured biomedical data to target AAK1 inhibition, identifying baricitinib.

Data mining is a more rational approach to the identification of drug candidates for drug repurposing. This technique can be used to generate drug-disease combinations and construct models to forecast future pairs, which will yield new candidates for repurposing through a more rational method.

Text-mining is another data-driven drug repurposing strategy. There are four phases: first, literature search and information retrieval (IR); second, extraction of relevant documents (ERD) to identify biological entities (BE) (proteins, genes, disease, etc.); third, filtration of these concepts to build a knowledge link; and fourth, association of the knowledge graph (KG) to drug-disease and drug-target relationships. This approach is based on Swanson's ABC model, which states that if drug A is related to gene B, and gene B is associated with disease C then drug A may have a connection to disease C. Drug-gene or disease-gene associations are collected from PubMed abstracts based on frequent co-occurrence patterns. Sentence-based networks or drug-disease-gene networks then indicate possible indications of current medications. This technique found that hypertension and arrhythmia medicines such as **diltiazem and quinidine** could treat Alzheimer's. Many different text-mining databases are employed, including static ones like Biovista and DrugQuest and dynamic ones like PubMed, clinicaltrial.gov, and DrugBank. As natural language processing (NLP) techniques have advanced, more and more text-mining tools have been created and are being utilized to find repositionable medications. The text-mining tool faces a challenge due to its limited coverage.

Semantics Approach

Based on the hypothesis that similar targets are linked to similar medications and that similar drugs are linked to similar targets. Semantics-based approaches fully exploit the semantic information contained in huge amounts of literature. As a result, the accuracy of forecasting biological entity relationships has improved.

Massive machine learning algorithms were introduced to improve the performance of drug repositioning in this scenario. Various new methods were used, for instance, Naïve Bayesian, k-nearest neighbors (kNN), random forest, support vector machines (SVM), and deep neural networks for binary classification, multiclass classification, and value prediction.

30.6 Barrier and Challenges to Drug Repurposing

Drug repurposing has received attention recently and accelerates the release of medications for clinical usage. However, it is a complex procedure involving multiple challenges related to regulatory norms, finances, expertise, and data access (Figs. 30.6 and 30.7).

30.6.1 Regulatory Risk

Drug repurposing only decreases, not eliminates, drug development risks. A new compound must still undergo all the regulatory approval processes and prove efficacy and safety standards, which is time consuming, expensive, and complex. Only the preclinical phase is eliminated for repurposed drugs, which can help with early cost savings. However, it can still go through phase 2 and phase 3 clinical trials, which cost a lot of money and eliminate more than half of the compounds.

The problem of intellectual property (IP) is another issue that has to be resolved. IP protection is minimal while repurposing medications. For instance, several

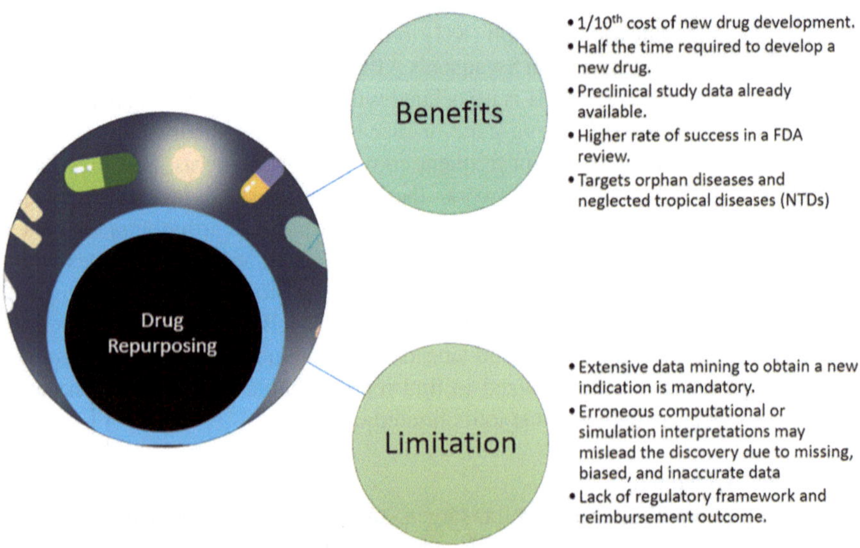

Fig. 30.6 Drug repurposing—benefits and limitation

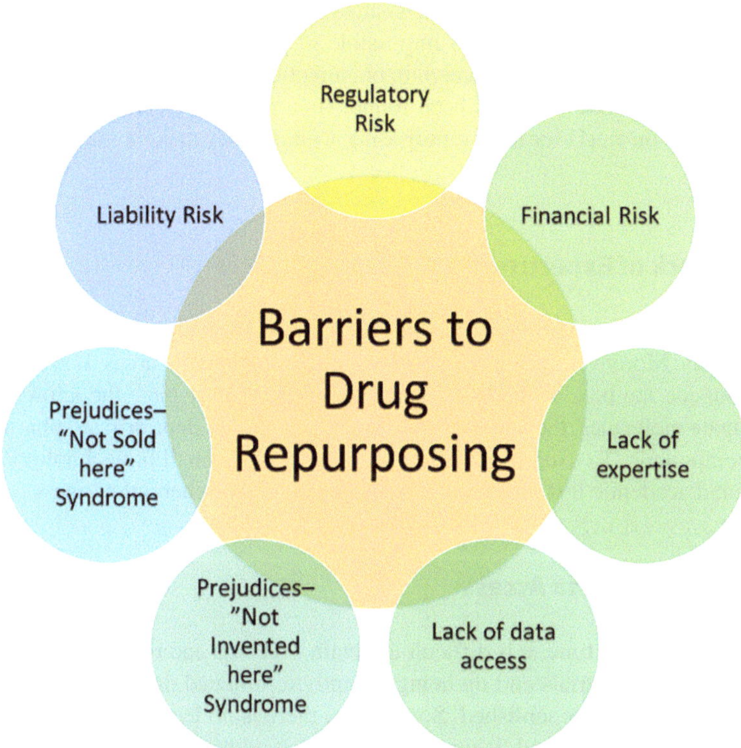

Fig. 30.7 Barriers to drug repurposing

unique drug-targeted disease relationships discovered by repurposing approaches were supported by articles or online databases; yet, due to legal restrictions, it is challenging to apply for IP protection for such relationships. Composition of matter (COM) claims are important IP protections for repurposed drugs. But COM claims can be very difficult to get for a repurposed drug because the patentee must differentiate their patent claims from what is in the public domain and present data. Some repurposed drugs cannot be marketed or sold because of the IP issue. Additionally, material transfer agreements pose a big challenge and are time consuming.

Regulators are not used to different types of applicants than the pharmaceutical industry. There is no appropriate regulatory guideline or timing of interaction for academicians, doctors, and public-private partnerships. The regulatory framework for repurposing, including the processes and data requirements, is still in its infancy.

30.6.2 Financial Risk

The cost of drug repurposing ranges from hundreds of millions to billions of dollars. Moreover, it is challenging for pharmaceutical companies to allocate upfront investment to compounds that were abandoned. For drugs meant to treat rare diseases, or orphan drugs, the population in use is small, hence the company gets a low economic return on investment. It is impossible to predict whether doctors will prescribe, or pharmacists will sell a certain manufacturer's drug in the event that a new purpose for a generic drug has been found. As a result, the company that spent a huge amount on R&D for drug repurposing would either make a minimal profit or lose money.

30.6.3 Lack of Expertise

Pharmaceutical corporations frequently lack experts committed to discontinued compounds. Moreover, they often focus on certain therapeutic areas. It is difficult to think outside the box. Whereas academic researchers may have the knowledge to investigate molecules, they do not have access to a pool of deprioritized pharmaceutical compounds. To overcome a shortage of resources, small biotechnology enterprises and academic institutions may need to acquire commercial partners.

30.6.4 Lack of Data Access

The majority of the time, it is difficult to obtain trial data and results for abandoned medications. Many trials end up being abruptly terminated due to company mergers, with results left unpublished. Sometimes, there is no legal necessity to publish the results. Difficulty in publishing negative trial results or lack of commercial benefit in publishing results on a drug that has been shelved. Companies are reluctant to share abandoned drugs with other companies in case they turn out to be blockbusters. There is a lack of a standard registry for shelved drugs. Additionally, a lot of data is in digital form, which poses a logistical hurdle, and converting it into a user-friendly format is a challenging job. Despite the availability of several medical databases, choosing the best strategy to fully utilize the vast volumes of medical data remains a difficult task.

30.6.5 Prejudices Toward Repurposing

The "not sold here" syndrome refers to companies' reluctance to out-license drugs that have potential for other treatments.

The "not invented here" syndrome refers to the belief that external research and technology are inferior to a company's internal R&D skills and standards and, therefore, unworthy of investigation. External parties may also believe that a supplier keeps the best compounds for themselves and offers lower-value compounds for our license.

30.6.6 Liability Risk

When out-licensing abandoned compounds, drug companies may incur liability risks such as adverse patient events, the requirement to constantly provide the product to the licensee, and lawsuits. To meet the growing demand for liability insurance, the pertussis vaccination cost rose from 17 cents to 11 dollars per dosage, and the number of businesses producing the vaccine reportedly dropped.

Making money from repurposing drugs involves inventing new formulations or dosage forms, creating new compounds with the same therapeutic benefits, or marketing medication in a new geographical area. Another issue is that the medication's effectiveness is dose-dependent. Therefore, during clinical trials, it is essential to determine the proper dose of a repurposed drug for new indications. Investments may be a barrier to repurposing unsuccessful drugs. This problem arises from investors' unwillingness to invest in failing drugs. Additionally, later-stage medication failures have less time to be repurposed before patent expiration. Parallel development approaches can reduce the failure risk. Investments may be a barrier to repurposing unsuccessful drugs. Failure to register an old drug at a reasonable cost result in its commercialization as a high-priced orphan drug. Incentive for clinicians to engage in regulatory activities. Obtaining reimbursement is challenging and time consuming.

30.7 Potential Facilitators of Drug Repurposing

Most of the time, drug repurposing is made easier by collaboration projects, chemical libraries and databases, computational-based methods and tools, regulatory reforms, and tax breaks (Fig. 30.8).

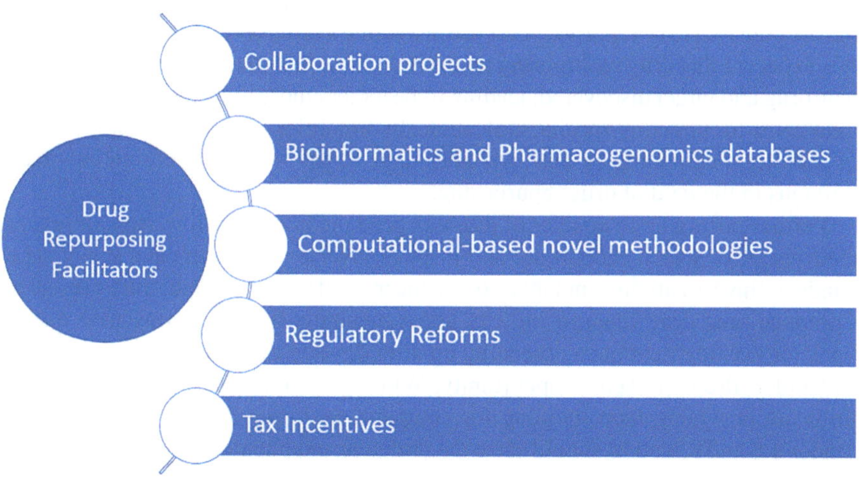

Fig. 30.8 Drug repurposing facilitators

Multi-partner agreements between pharmaceutical companies, academic institutions, nonprofit groups, and biotechnology companies facilitated drug repurposing. Biotechnology companies and academia have knowledge and experience in new fields to study drugs and contribute to innovation. For example, in the United States, the National Institutes of Health's National Center for Advancing Translational Sciences (NIH NCATS) has launched a new drug repurposing model based on three-way collaborations involving public funders, the pharmaceutical sector, and academia researchers. Government funding helps translational research and "de-risks" these drug development programs, which have a small, unprofitable market share. The NIH acts as a trusted intermediary, facilitating deals between researchers and firms. The ECNP Medicines Chest Program provides academic and small industry researchers with promising substances for experimental medicine trials. These collaborative endeavors make drugs, data, human, and financial resources available and handles intellectual property and data sharing, incentives, profit sharing, and registration of successful therapeutic repurposing prospects.

Compound databases and registries provide target and therapeutic profiles, including protein and active site structure and disease biology. Novel computational methods have been developed to predict drug-induced disease responses, validate target and pathway information, and infer novel drug target linkages. A tax incentive for sharing trial data could help develop shelved compounds. Regulatory changes could allow the reuse of safety data. FDA safety discoveries could extend drug availability without affecting risk-benefit analysis.

30.8 The Future of Drug Repurposing

The variety of repurposed drugs listed here demonstrates that every medication, whether withdrawn (such as thalidomide), in clinical trials (such as crizotinib), unsuccessful in clinical trials (such as zidovudine), or approved (such as sunitinib), has the potential to be repurposed for use in treating a different condition (Table 30.1). It is expected that drug repurposing analysis will become standard practice for every new drug and target discovered, leading to faster and more accurate identification of treatments for targeting specific molecular abnormalities. The efficient combination of various methodologies and available data might result in substantial breakthroughs in the field of drug repurposing.

Furthermore, a large number of diseases need medicines to slow, stop, or reverse their progress, which encourages and inspires diverse researchers and scientists to conduct investigations, notably on cancer and orphan and rare diseases. Computational drug repurposing can assist humanity by uncovering new indications for existing treatments, speeding up drug development, and giving withdrawn and failed drugs a second opportunity. While governments and pharmaceutical firms are providing more funding for computational drug repurposing initiatives, academics and scientists should seize the initiative and put more effort into developing innovative, cutting-edge models that will lead to important discoveries and successes.

Bibliography

Gns HS, Gr S, Murahari M, Krishnamurthy M (2019) An update on drug repurposing: re-written saga of the drug's fate. Biomed Pharmacother 110:700–716. https://doi.org/10.1016/j.biopha.2018.11.127

Hua Y, Dai X, Xu Y, Xing G, Liu H, Lu T, Chen Y, Zhang Y (2022) Drug repositioning: Progress and challenges in drug discovery for various diseases. Eur J Med Chem 234:114239. https://doi.org/10.1016/j.ejmech.2022.114239

Jarada TN, Rokne JG, Alhajj R (2020) A review of computational drug repositioning: Strategies, approaches, opportunities, challenges, and directions. J Chem 12(1):46. https://doi.org/10.1186/s13321-020-00450-7

Jourdan J-P, Bureau R, Rochais C, Dallemagne P (2020) Drug repositioning: a brief overview. J Pharm Pharmacol 72(9):1145–1151. https://doi.org/10.1111/jphp.13273

Khataniar A, Pathak U, Rajkhowa S, Jha AN (2022) A comprehensive review of drug repurposing strategies against known drug targets of covid-19. COVID 2(2):148–167. https://doi.org/10.3390/covid2020011

Kim H-S (2022) Drug repositioning: Exploring new indications for existing drug-disease relationships. Endocrinol Metab 37(1):62–64. https://doi.org/10.3803/EnM.2022.1403

Ko Y (2020) Computational drug repositioning: Current progress and challenges. Appl Sci 10(15):5076. https://doi.org/10.3390/app10155076

Krishnamurthy N, Grimshaw AA, Axson SA, Choe SH, Miller JE (2022) Drug repurposing: a systematic review on root causes, barriers and facilitators. BMC Health Serv Res 22(1):970. https://doi.org/10.1186/s12913-022-08272-z

Li YY, Jones SJ (2012) Drug repositioning for personalized medicine. Genome Med 4(3):27. https://doi.org/10.1186/gm326

Mohammad Sadeghi H, Adeli I, Mousavi T, Daniali M, Nikfar S, Abdollahi M (2021) Drug repurposing for the management of depression: where do we stand currently? Life 11(8):774. https://doi.org/10.3390/life11080774

Oprea TI, Bauman JE, Bologa CG, Buranda T, Chigaev A, Edwards BS, Jarvik JW, Gresham HD, Haynes MK, Hjelle B, Hromas R, Hudson L, Mackenzie DA, Muller CY, Reed JC, Simons PC, Smagley Y, Strouse J, Surviladze Z et al (2011) Drug repurposing from an academic perspective. Drug Discov Today Ther Strateg 8(3–4):61–69. https://doi.org/10.1016/j.ddstr.2011.10.002

Pushpakom S, Iorio F, Eyers PA, Escott KJ, Hopper S, Wells A, Doig A, Guilliams T, Latimer J, McNamee C, Norris A, Sanseau P, Cavalla D, Pirmohamed M (2019) Drug repurposing: progress, challenges and recommendations. Nat Rev Drug Discov 18(1):41–58. https://doi.org/10.1038/nrd.2018.168

Repurposing drugs (2017) National Center for Advancing Translational Sciences. https://ncats.nih.gov/preclinical/repurpose

Xue H, Li J, Xie H, Wang Y (2018) Review of drug repositioning approaches and resources. Int J Biol Sci 14(10):1232–1244. https://doi.org/10.7150/ijbs.24612

Zhu S, Bai Q, Li L, Xu T (2022) Drug repositioning in drug discovery of T2DM and repositioning potential of antidiabetic agents. Comput Struct Biotechnol J 20:2839–2847. https://doi.org/10.1016/j.csbj.2022.05.057

Bibliography

[illegible]

Specialized Drug Delivery Systems

31

Kalpana Ramanna Mali

Abstract

Specialized drug delivery systems are of much importance in modern medicine as it targets the specific sites or organs, therefore it enhances the efficacy and reduces adverse effects. Multiple strategies and techniques such as nanoparticles, liposomes, micelles, hydrogels, fast dissolving tablets, prodrugs, and drug-loaded erythrocytes are used in designing and advancing specialized drug delivery systems. These systems offer significant benefit in the field of personalized therapies among various diseases, ranging from inflammatory diseases to cancer, through precise control over pharmacokinetics and targeting techniques. There is need to understand the principles of specialized drug delivery which helps to utilize various pharmaceuticals in improving patient quality of life and outcomes.

Keywords

Specialized drug delivery system · Targeted drug delivery system · Nanoparticles · Hydrogels · Liposomes

31.1 Introduction

Drug delivery (DD) is defined as the formulations, methods, processes, and technologies, needed for transporting a medication to various organs or tissues to attain the expected therapeutic effect. Specialized drug delivery system emphasizes on drug administration with correct dosage, correct time, and correct site with highest safety and efficacy. These novel delivery systems improve the therapeutic efficacy

K. R. Mali (✉)
Department of Pharmacology, All India Institute of Medical Sciences (AIIMS) Bibinagar, Hyderabad, India

A. Arivazhahan et al. (eds.), *Introduction to Basics of Pharmacology and Toxicology*,
https://doi.org/10.1007/978-981-95-1920-0_31

of both new and established medications by providing targeted, controlled, and prolonged release.

31.2 Targeted or specialized Drug Delivery System

Targeting entails the capability to guide the drug-laden system to the desired location of action rather than the whole body or organ. The fundamental concept of drug targeting involves delivering a drug to the intended areas while minimizing its presence in nontargeted areas. The ultimate objective is to enhance the efficacy of treatment while minimizing adverse effects. TDDSs distinguish themselves from conventional or traditional DDSs by achieving targeted release of active ingradient from its dosage form, whereas the latter relies on absorption of drug through cell membranes. The TDDS concept traces back a century ago to Paul Ehrlich's proposition of "magic bullet" concept.

31.2.1 Advantages of Targeted or Specialized Drug Delivery Systems

Enhanced efficacy: By directly delivering drug to targeted organ.

Reduced side effects: By sparing healthy cell or tissue.

Controlled pharmacokinetics: By precisely targeting absorption, distribution, metabolism, and excretion of drug.

Reduction in dose: The desired therapeutic effect can be attained with much lower dose.

Enhanced patient compliance: By decreasing dosage of drug and frequency of drug administration.

Regulated biodistribution: Enhanced penetration and retention, prolonged drug action, increased therapeutic index are the key elements.

31.2.2 Components of Targeted or Specialized Drug Delivery Systems

Drug targeting consists of three interconnected components, namely **drug**, **targeting site**, and **pharmaceutical carrier**.

Drug: It must be effective also chemically and physically compatible with the carrier.

Target: Specific cell, tissue, or organs where drug is going to act.

Pharmaceutical carrier or vehicle: A specially designed system or molecule is crucial for efficiently transporting the drug to selected sites. The ideal drug-targeting complex

- Should exhibit nontoxicity, non-immunogenicity, biochemical inertness, biodegradability, biocompatibility, and physicochemical stability.
- Should have a predictable and controllable release of drug.
- Should be simple, cost-effective, reproducible, and readily eliminated from the body.
- Should have little leakage of drug during transit.

31.2.3 Applications of Targeted or Specialized Drug Delivery Systems

- Cancer treatment: TDDS is revolutionary approach in treatment of cancer to increase the effectiveness and decrease the adverse effects.
- Vaccine adjuvant: TDDS are being explored as vaccine adjuvant to maximize immune response.
- Delivery to ocular and brain tissue: By breaking the challenges of anatomical barriers which are observed in conventional method.
- Delivery to DNA and oligonucleotide: These molecules hold great potential for gene therapy, but their delivery poses significant challenges due to their size, charge, and susceptibility of degradation which can be overcome by TDDS.
- Targeting intracellularly and systemically: These systems are designed to overcome biological barriers.
- Supporting in enzyme immunoassays: TDDS plays pivotal role in increasing the performance of enzyme immunoassay by enhancing sensitivity and specificity.
- Aiding radio imaging: TDDS improves the accuracy of imaging and by delivering radiocontrast directly to specific site thereby increasing the contrast and reducing the background noise.

31.3 Drug Delivery Carriers/Vectors

TDD carriers transport and deliver drugs to target locations, retaining themselves through encapsulation or bonding facilitated by a spacer moiety. These carriers are engineered vectors designed for accurate drug delivery.

Carrier-based drug delivery systems can be divided into four distinct steps:

1. Drug loading (encapsulation/adsorption) on carrier.
2. Transport of drug carrier complex to the target site.
3. Uptake of complex by cell or tissue.
4. Unloading the drug from the carrier.

- Different drug delivery carriers are.

  Liposomes.

Nanoparticles.
Micelles.
Low-density lipoproteins.
Fast dissolving tablets.
Hydrogels.
Prodrugs.
Drug-loaded erythrocytes.
Neutrophils.
Monoclonal antibodies.

31.3.1 Liposomes

Microscopic vesicles composed of lipid bilayers, ranging from 25 nm to 100 μm in diameter. Lipid bilayer encloses an aqueous core and both hydrophilic and lipophilic drugs. Channel proteins within the hydrophobic domain act as size-selective filters. Proteolytic enzymes protect encapsulated drugs within liposomes from premature degradation. Liposomes can be used by oral, topical, and systemic route either in solid, semisolid, or liquid dosage forms. These are widely used in case of infectious diseases, cancer, and for vaccination.

Available liposomal product formulations are amphotericin B, cytarabine, daunorubicin, and doxorubicin.

Further modifications of liposomes are noisome, ufasomes, pharmacosomes, virosomes, cubosomes, ethosomes, transferosomes, and phytosomes.

31.3.2 Miscelles

Drugs are trapped in a core and hydrophilic shell protecting the contents. Moreover, the outer chemical composition of the shell could hinder recognition by the reticuloendothelial system, thus delaying early elimination from circulation.

31.3.3 Hydrogels

These are polymeric hydrophilic networks, which absorbs huge amounts of water or biological fluids. They swell in aqueous environments due to their thermodynamic compatibility with water. Hydrogels regulate drug release in controlled release systems, which can be targeted to specific sites.

31.3.4 Nanoparticles

Nanoparticles (10–200 nm), solid and amorphous or crystalline, increase drug dissolution and solubility by enlarging the surface area. They adsorb and envelope drugs, protecting them from chemical and enzymatic degradation.

The advantages of nanoparticles include the following:

1. Nanoparticles size and their surface characteristics can be manipulated easily to attain drug targeting.
2. They increase efficacy and minimize adverse event through control and sustain release of the drug.
3. It has high capacity of drug loading and preserving the drug activity by incorporating drugs without any chemical reaction.
4. Ligands attachment or magnetic guidance to surface of particles will enhance the site-specific targeting.
5. Nanoparticles can be used for oral, nasal, parenteral, intraocular administration.

The disadvantages of nanoparticles

1. Handling of nanoparticles may become difficult owing to their small size and large surface area, which may lead to particle aggregation.

Nanoparticles are further classified as nanotubes, nano wires, nano shells, nano pores, PEGylated nanoparticles, and dendrimers.

31.3.5 Fast Dissolving Tablet

Oral solid dosage form is designed in such a way that it can be administered in the absence of water. These tablets readily dissolve in saliva within 60 seconds, improving patient compliance.

31.3.6 Drug-Loaded Erythrocytes

Erythrocytes are biocompatible and biodegradable, having a long half-life, therefore can be utilized for loading various drugs. To create carrier erythrocytes, blood samples are taken and erythrocytes are separated from the plasma. The cells are broken through physical and chemical methods to entrap drugs into erythrocytes, which are then resealed, to form "resealed erythrocytes." After administering parenterally, they act like slow-circulating depots, targeting to reticuloendothelial system.

31.3.7 Neutrophils

This system remains an attractive method for transporting diagnostic or therapeutic agents to acute inflammatory areas. These agents can be meticulously purified to include carrier proteins within their granules.

31.3.8 Low-Density Lipoproteins

Malignant cells overexpress LDL receptors, which can be exploited for targeted drug delivery systems. Anticancer molecules with specific physicochemical properties can bind to LDL particles, enabling selective delivery to cancerous cells. Examples include daunamycin and estramustine.

31.3.9 Prodrugs

Targeting prodrugs to specific enzymes or membrane transporters enables site-selective targeting (Table 31.1).

31.3.10 Monoclonal Antibodies

Through advanced hybridoma technology, these are engineered in humanized or chimeric forms. They are coupled with chemotherapeutic drugs, bacterial toxins, radioisotopes, enzymes, and cytokines in the treatment of cancer, increasing their cytotoxic effects (Table 31.2).

Table 31.1 Examples of enzymes and prodrug proposed for cancer therapy

Enzyme	Prodrug	Drug
Xanthine oxidase	Hypoxanthine	Superoxide, hydrogen peroxide
α galactosidase	N-4-galactopyranosyl benzyloxycarbonyl-daunarubicin	Daunarubicine
β glucosidase	Amygdaline	Cyanide
β glucuronidase	Epirubicin-glucuronide	Epirubicin
Cytosine deaminase	5-Flurocytosine	5-Fluorouracil
Alkaline phosphatase	Doxorubicin phosphate	Doxorubicin
Alkaline phosphatase	Etoposide phosphate	Etoposide

Table 31.2 FDA-approved monoclonal antibodies for cancer treatment

Monoclonal antibodies	Indication
Alemtuzumab	Chronic lymphocytic leukemia
Bevacizumab	Brain, breast, colon, kidney, lung cancer
cetuximab	Colon cancer, head and neck cancer
Ibritumomab	Non-Hodgkin's lymphoma
Rituximab	Chronic lymphocytic leukemia, non-Hodgkin's lymphoma
Transtuzumab	Breast, stomach cancer

31.4 Specialized Drug Delivery Systems

31.4.1 Recent Advances in Oral Drug Delivery System

Obstacles to oral administration include stomach acid and enzymatic degradation, osmotic stresses, GI muscle peristalsis, etc. Therefore, there is a need for a specialized delivery system for oral administration.

- Specialized oral delivery devices and methods.
  - Intestinal patches.
  - Nanoparticles.
  - Gastrointestinal microneedles.
  - Micelles.
  - Liposomes.
  - Ion pairing (co-crystals).
  - Absorption enhancers.
  - Efflux pump inhibitors.
  - Pediatric oral drug delivery.

- Intestinal patches

  Mucoadhesive patches adhere to the mucosa GI tract, acting as drug reservoir and protecting the drug against luminal loss. It improves the bioavailability through unidirectional diffusion toward the gastrointestinal mucosa.

  Insulin, calcitonin, and interferon-α investigated for delivery using intestinal patch.
- Gastrointestinal microneedles

  Originally developed for transdermal delivery, microneedles have been adapted for various administration routes such as oral, scalp, perianal, and vaginal routes. Ma et al. (2014) used it for oral vaccine, that is, HIV antigens. Insulin also tried in the form.
- Particulate carriers

  Micelles, microparticles, nanoparticles and liposomes these are the particulate carriers for oral delivery. Micelles are amphiphilic molecules ranging from 5 to

100 nm designed to enhance the solubility of pharmaceuticals and aid its delivery, for example, paclitaxel and doxorubicin micelles.

- Ion pairing
  Also referred as co-crystals are crystalline solids comprising two or more ionic and molecular compounds connected by noncovalent bond, offer a straightforward approach that obviates the necessity for chemical alteration or prodrug development. The bioavailability of drugs can be significantly enhanced by maintaining co-crystals in a supersaturated solution. Research indicated that the solubility of itraconazole co-crystals increased between fourfold and 20fold compared to the crystalline structure of the medication.
- Absorption enhancers
  Various compounds like surfactants, glycerides, cholesterol, salicylates, and bile salts act as absorption enhancers. They enhance bioavailability by increasing permeability. However, strategies that adjust tight junction permeability raise safety issues. Opening tight junctions can facilitate the passage of not only drugs but also other potentially harmful molecules through the intestinal membrane.
- Efflux pump inhibitors
  Coadministering drugs with efflux pump inhibitors can conquer multidrug resistance and enhance bioavailability of medications. Several excipients, including polyethoxylated castor oil, polysorbates, poloxamers, tocopherol polyethylene glycol succinate (TPEGS), and polyethylene glycol (PEG), have been found to modulate efflux transporter function. Cyclosporine A, paclitaxel, and vancomycin, when administered with TPEGS, exhibit improved oral bioavailability.
- Pediatric oral drug delivery
  Children face challenges with swallowing often struggle with large tablets and capsules, as well as formulations with bitter or unpleasant tastes. This issue extends to geriatric and ill adults, including surgical patients or those recovering from comas. Consequently, there is a growing demand for pediatric formulations. While additives deemed safe for adults may not be acceptable for children, due to their unique physiological characteristics and immature tissue functions (Table 31.3).

Table 31.3 Marketed oral pediatric formulations

Oral pediatric formulation	Technology and advantages	Examples
Disintegrating tablets (DTs)	Designed to disintegrate within 1 mi. DTs reduces the need of tablet swallowing	Lansoprazole, ondansetron, desloratadine
Disintegrating films (DFs)	A strip that disintegrates quickly on the tongue	Listerine, phenylephrine, diphenhydramine, ondansetron
Minitablet	It is less than 3 mm diameter	Terbinafine, sodium valproate
Multiparticulates (suspension or sprinkles in apple sauce or yoghurt)	Granules are mixed with food matrices.	Methyl prednisolone, mefloquine, lopinavir, ritonavir)

31.4.2 Transdermal Drug Delivery System (TDDS)

Transdermal system delivers medications through the skin direct into the bloodstream. (Table 31.4 and 31.5)

- Advantages of TDDS.
  1. Bypasses first pass metabolism.
  2. Reduces the adverse effects.
  3. Reduction of variation in plasma concentration of drugs.
  4. Decrease in dosing frequency and thereby improving patient compliance.
  5. Steady infusion of a drug over an extended period of time.
  6. Adverse effects or therapeutic failure commonly linked to intermittent dosing can also be prevented.
- Limitation of TDDS.
- Skin irritation or contact dermatitis

31.4.3 Intranasal Drug Delivery System

Many vaccines and drugs like buserelin, calcitonin, desmopressin, insulin, growth hormone, buprenorphine, steroids (corticosteroids, progesterone, estradiol, testosterone), antihypertensives (nifedipine, hydralazine, nitroglycerine, propranolol), antibiotics, and antivirals are being delivered through the nasal cavity. Studies on various formulations for intranasal drug delivery in the form of nasal spray, nasal pumps, suspensions microemulsion, and mucoadhesive gels have been carried out extensively (Table 31.6 and 31.7).

- Advantages of intranasal drug delivery system:
  Rapid onset of action.
  Enhanced bioavailability.
  Easy and noninvasive administration.
  Bypass first pass metabolism.
  Bypass the blood-brain barrier (BBB).
  Avoiding degradation of drug.
  Less side effects.
  Improved compliance.

- Disadvantages of nasal drug delivery system:
  Restricted delivery of high-molecular-weight drugs.
  Pathological conditions adversely affect the transport.
  Some drugs like budesonide and azelastine causes nasal mucosa irritation

Table 31.4 Techniques enhancing TDDS

Structure-based enhancement techniques	Electric-based enhancement techniques	Velocity-based enhancement techniques	Other enhancement techniques
1.**Transdermal patches**: Subtypes (i) Single layer drug in adhesive (ii) Multilayer drug in adhesive (iii) Vapor patch (iv) Reservoir system (v) Matrix system (vi) Micro reservoir system	**1. Iontophoresis** Passing of current (few milliamperes) to skin using the electrode for example, pilocarpine delivery using iontophoresis to enhance sweating for cystic fibrosis diagnosis and delivery of lidocaine rapid onset of anesthesia.	**1. Needle-free injections** Intraject, Implaject, Jet Syringe, Iject Mini-ject	1. **Transferosomes** Transferosomes contain a component that destabilizes the lipid bilayers
2. **Microfabricated microneedles** (i) Poke with patch approach (ii) Coat and poke approach (iii) Biodegradable microneedles (iv) Hollow microneedles	**2. Ultrasound** Mixing of drug with cream gel or ointment that help to transfer ultrasonic energy to the skin	**2.Powderject** The drug particles are propelled across the skin with the help of high-speed gas flow	**2. Medicated tattoos** Modifying temporary tattoos containing an active drug
3. Macroflux	**3. Photomechanical waves** Penetration of highly permeable drug to the stratum cornea with the help of these waves		**3. Skin abrasion** Removal of the topmost layers of the skin, which enhance permeability of topically applied drug
	4. Electroporation The electrical pulses are considered to form small pores in the stratum cornea, through which transportation of drug occurs		**4. Controlled heat-aided drug delivery (CHADD) system** Applying heat to the skin thereby increasing the temperature and ultimately increase the microcirculation and permeability
	5. Electroosmosis Voltage difference is applied to thus a bulk fluid or volume flow takes place with no concentration gradients		**5. Laser radiation** Exposure of the skin to the laser beam that results in the ablation of the stratum cornea sparing epidermis
			6. Magnetophoretic Magnetic field effect is utilized for diffusion of drug

Table 31.5 Examples of marketed transdermal drug delivery system

Drug	Design
Testosterone	Three-layer patch
Estradiol	Three layer
Estradiol	Three layer
Fentanyl	Four layer
Clonidine	Four layer
Estradiol	Four layer
Nicotine	Multilayer round
Nicotine	Multilayer round
Nicotine	Multilayer rectangular
Nicotine	Multilayer rectangular

Table 31.6 Application of intranasal drug delivery system

Delivery of drugs locally	Delivery of drugs systemically	Delivery of drugs to CNS
To achieve local therapeutic effects such as in case of seasonal rhinitis and nasal congestion due to allergic reactions or infections)	To achieve therapeutic systemic effects, such as migraine, infection prevention, hormone replacement therapy, smoking cessation, and epileptic seizures	The drugs are transported from the nasal mucosa to the CNS through the olfactory and trigeminal nerve fibers via the olfactory epithelium
For example, antihistamines and corticosteroids in rhinitis	For example, propranolol, nifedipine, and nitroglycerin angina pectoris	For example, oxytocin for autism and behavioral therapy, methotrexate and telomerase inhibitors for brain tumors, orexin for narcolepsy, leptin for sleep disorders, and obesity

Table 31.7 Marketed nasal drug for systemic use

Drug	Formulations	Indication
Salmon calcitonin	Spray	Osteoporosis
Desmopressin	Spray	Diabetic insipidus
Buserelin	Spray	Infertility
Nafarelin	Spray	Endometriosis
Oxytocin	Spray	Lactation induction
Protirelin	Spray	Thyroid diagnostics
Zolmitriptan	Spray	Migraine
Sumatriptan	Spray	Migraine
Dihyfroergotamin	Spray	Migraine
Estradiol	Spray	Hormone replacement

31.4.4 Ophthalmic Drug Delivery System

- Challenges in conventional ophthalmic drug delivery (eye drops, ointments, suspensions, and emulsions).

    1. Anterior segment delivery challenges.
       Various factors contribute to the loss of drugs before reaching the cornea, including solution drainage, tear dynamics, lacrimation, evaporation, turnover, dilution, conjunctival absorption, minimal residence time in the cul-de-sac, and the limited permeability of the cornea. To maintain therapeutic levels in the tear film, frequent administration of eye drops is necessary. However, the frequent administration of highly concentrated drugs can lead to toxic effects and cellular damage.
    2. Posterior segment delivery challenges.
       Due to the blood-retinal barrier (BRB), topical ocular medications fail to reach drug targets in the posterior segment.

- Special ophthalmic drug delivery systems.

    1. Liposomes.
       Schaeffer et al. research on indoxole and penicillin G revealed that positively charged liposomes exhibit a higher affinity for the negatively charged corneal surface compared to neutral or negatively charged liposomes.
    2. Niosomes.
       A novel method for delivering cyclopentolate involved the development of a niosomal formulation. This formulation released the drug regardless of pH, leading to a substantial increase in ocular bioavailability.
    3. Nanoparticles/nanospheres.
       Nanocapsules of certain drug (such as betaxolol or carteolol) in an uncharged form within the oily core, enables faster diffusion into the cornea. Moreover, nanoparticles composed of poly-e-caprolactone containing cyclosporin demonstrate enhanced corneal absorption.
    4. Microparticles.
       Efficacy performance is reportedly superior than that conventional dosage forms:
       Methylprednisolone microspheres.
       Pilocarpine-loaded albumin or gelatin microspheres.
       Acyclovir-loaded chitosan microspheres.
    5. Ocular inserts.
       Ocular inserts offer a method for achieving controlled and sustained drug delivery, thereby maintaining optimal drug concentrations in target site. However, they present certain drawbacks including patient non-compliance, challenges with self-insertion, sensations of a foreign body, and potential unintentional loss from the eye. Various techniques have been employed to prepare ocular inserts with different characteristics, such as solubility, erodibility, non-erodibility, and hydrogel composition.

Drug released by ocular insert are pilocarpine, prednisolone, progesterone, chloramphenicol, and tetracyclines

6. Ocular implants.
   Ocular implants are kept intravitreally, specifically at the pars plana through a minor surgical procedure. Nonbiodegradable implants offer more precise control over drug release and longer release durations compared to biodegradable polymers. However, nonbiodegradable systems necessitate surgical removal, which can lead to ocular complications like retinal detachment and intravitreal hemorrhage. Examples of drugs released via this system include ganciclovir (Vitrasert), fluocinolone acetonide (Retisert, Medidur), and dexamethasone (Prosurdex, Surodex).
7. Intravitreal injections.
   Intravitreal injection facilitates targeted drug delivery to specific sites within the eye. However, this method is associated with several side effects, including pain from frequent injections, discomfort, elevated intraocular pressure (IOP), intraocular bleeding, heightened risk of infection, and potential for retinal detachment. The most significant complication associated with intravitreal injections is endophthalmitis, which can lead to loss of vision if not promptly treated. Patient acceptance of this treatment method is often low due to its discomfort and potential complications.
   Common drugs administered via intravitreal injections include penicillins, sulfonamides, dexamethasone, bevacizumab, and ranibizumab.
8. Iontophoresis.
   Ocular iontophoresis delivers drugs anterior as well as posterior segment. Iontophoresis is a noninvasive technique used to transport ionized drugs across membranes using a low electrical current. Several drugs have been successfully administered using this method, including gentamicin, tobramycin, ciprofloxacin, and dexamethasone.
9. Periocular route.
   Administering drugs via the subtenon injection route represents one of the most efficient methods for delivering medications to the posterior segment of the eye. Studies have shown that the subtenon injection route leads to the highest and sustained vitreous concentration of drugs (sodium fluorescein) than that of retrobulbar and subconjunctival routes.

31.4.5 Pulmonary Drug Delivery System

It provides targeted treatment for respiratory diseases. It can be accomplished by incorporating aerosols, metered dose inhalers, dry powder inhalers, and nebulizers, with nanostructures like liposomes, micelles, nanoparticles, and microemulsions.

The success of pulmonary delivery of protein drugs is hindered by lung proteases. Thus, adjuvants like absorption enhancers and protease inhibitors improves the pulmonary absorption of such drugs.

- Miscelles.
- The polymeric micelles have bulky hydrophilic outer shell it evades the mononuclear phagocytic system; therefore, beclomethasone dipropionate-loaded polymeric micelles are very beneficial in delivering hydrophobic corticosteroids for COPD.
- Liposomes.
- Aerosol delivery of liposomal formulations (cyclosporine A) through jet nebulizers have broadened the potential of aerosol-based therapies. Moreover, intratracheal administration of levonorgestrel-encapsulated liposomes have demonstrated enhanced bioavailability in rats.
- Nanoparticles.
- Nanoparticles have been utilized to incorporate drugs such as prednisolone, diazepam, and camptotecin for pulmonary applications.

Bibliography

Homayun B, Lin X, Choi HJ (2019) Challenges and recent progress in oral drug delivery systems for biopharmaceuticals. Pharmaceutics 11(3):129

Keller LA, Merkel O, Popp A (2022) Intranasal drug delivery: opportunities and toxicologic challenges during drug development. Drug Deliv Transl Res:1–23

Mohanraj VJ, Chen YJ (2006) Nanoparticles-a review. Trop J Pharm Res 5(1):561–573

Patel PB, Shastri D, Shelat P, Shukla A (2010) Ophthalmic drug delivery system: challenges and approaches. Syst Rev Pharm 1(2):113

Shingade GM (2012) Review on: recent trend on transdermal drug delivery system. J Drug Deliv Ther 2(1)

Smola M, Vandamme T, Sokolowski A (2008) Nanocarriers as pulmonary drug delivery systems to treat and to diagnose respiratory and non respiratory diseases. Int J Nanomedicine 3(1):1–9

Tewabe A, Abate A, Tamrie M, Seyfu A, Abdela SE (2021) Targeted drug delivery – from magic bullet to nanomedicine: principles, challenges, and future perspectives. J Multidiscip Healthc 2021:1711–1724

Tiwari G, Tiwari R, Sriwastawa B, Bhati L, Pandey S, Pandey P, Bannerjee SK (2012) Drug delivery systems: an updated review. Int J Pharm Investig 2(1):2

Biologicals and Biosimilars

32

Shubham Atal

Abstract

Biologicals or biologics are complex molecules derived from living cells. They include vaccines, therapeutic sera, toxins, antitoxins, blood and blood products, allergenic extracts, monoclonal antibodies, human cells and tissues used for transplantation, gene therapies, and cellular therapies. Since the development of recombinant insulin "humulin" as the first genetically engineered biological medicinal product, they have revolutionized the treatment of many diseases including cancers as targeted therapies. Currently, there are well over 500 biological drugs available worldwide, with many of the top-selling drugs being biologics. However, their manufacture and development are complex, and they are much more expensive than conventional drugs.

"Biosimilars" are generic or alternate versions of biologicals that have come off-patent, having quality, biological activity, safety, and efficacy comparable to an approved biological. They offer the advantages of lower development cost, lesser development period, and increased accessibility. There are well-defined determinants of similarity and interchangeability. In the last two decades, the regulatory agencies across the world have released thorough guidance for rational and scientific development of biologicals and biosimilars. Together, they are fast changing the landscape of modern therapeutics, as "lifesaving" medicines, as well as paving the way for personalized medicine.

S. Atal (✉)
Department of Pharmacology, All India Institute of Medical Sciences (AIIMS), Bhopal, Madhya Pradesh, India
e-mail: shubham.pharm@aiimsbhopal.edu.in

A. Arivazhahan et al. (eds.), *Introduction to Basics of Pharmacology and Toxicology*,
https://doi.org/10.1007/978-981-95-1920-0_32

Keywords

Biologicals · Biosimilars · Regulations · Development

32.1 Introduction

Biologicals or biologics, used interchangeably, are complex molecules derived from natural sources, that is, living cells. Biologicals have revolutionized the treatment of patients with many serious diseases likes hematological (anemia, hemophilia) or autoimmune (rheumatoid arthritis, Crohn's disease) disorders and cancers. The first genetically engineered biological medicinal product in the United States was recombinant insulin "'humulin" in 1982. These products are relatively more difficult to develop, manufacture, and much more expensive than conventional drugs. Currently, over 500 biological drugs have been successfully commercialized in the U.S. (excluding biosimilars), the numbers being higher worldwide. Biologicals are part of a wave of targeted therapies being developed to move toward a personalized medicine approach in treating diseases.

"Biosimilars" are, in simple terms, generic or alternate versions of biologicals that have come off-patent. They have comparable quality characteristics, biological activity, safety, and efficacy to a licensed biological medicine. They offer the advantages of lower development cost, lesser development period, and increased accessibility. Together, biologicals and biosimilars are fast changing the landscape of therapeutics worldwide, and proving to be the modern "lifesaving" medicines in many scenarios.

32.2 Biologicals

32.2.1 Definitions and Facts

- The terms biologicals or biologics or biological medicines or biopharmaceuticals are often used interchangeably.
- A simple practical definition of a biologic is a product whose active ingredient is made in a living system.
- As per the Public Health Service (PHS) Act in the United States, a biological product is defined as a "virus, therapeutic serum, toxin, antitoxin, vaccine, blood, blood component or derivative, allergenic product, or analogous product, applicable to the prevention, treatment, or cure of a disease or condition of human beings."
- As per the Central Drugs Standard Control Organization (CDSCO) in India, biological products, or biologics, are medical products made from a variety of natural sources (human, animal, or microorganism). Biologics are intended to treat diseases and medical conditions, prevent, or diagnose diseases.

- Interchangeable biologics: "Biosimilars" that are approved by the FDA to be substituted by a third party for the reference biologic (detailed later).
- Biologics represent targeted and effective treatment opportunity for patients mainly in areas of oncology, autoimmune diseases, and cardiovascular diseases.
- There are currently approximately 700 marketed biologic products worldwide, with hundreds more under development.
- Commercial aspects.
  - Biological therapies represent a total market value of approximately more than $500 billion.
  - 10 of 20 top-selling drugs are biologics.
  - 8 of 10 best-selling biologics are antibodies.

32.2.2 Types of Biologicals

- As defined, biologicals are structurally complex compounds derived from living material (human, animal, plant, microbe). They are usually comprised of proteins and/or nucleic acids.
- As per CDSCO India, examples of biological products include vaccines; blood and blood products for transfusion and/or manufacturing into other products; allergenic extracts, which are used for both diagnosis and treatment; human cells and tissues used for transplantation (e.g., tendons, ligaments, and bone); gene therapies; cellular therapies; and tests to screen potential blood donors for infectious agents such as HIV.
- A similar description of types of compounds included as biologicals is there in the given definition in the United States, which also mentions "analogous products"; a term not well defined, making the definition broad.
- Common biological medicines or biopharmaceuticals include hormones (insulin, erythropoietin, growth hormones, FSH), enzymes (streptokinase, rasburicase), growth factors (filgrastim, pefilgrastim), and monoclonal antibodies (rituximab, adalimumab, bevacizumab, trastuzumab, etc.)
- Additionally, blood products (coagulation factors), immunological products (vaccines and sera), allergens for testing, and gene and cell therapy products are also categorized as biologicals.
- *Viruses:* Widely used as a platform for the production of therapeutics; key examples are vaccines containing live, dead, and components of viruses; vectors for gene therapy and oncolytic viruses; and, recently, virus-derived proteins as immune modulators.
- *Vaccine:* A suspension containing live, attenuated, modified or killed microorganisms, generally viruses, or tumor antigens, which stimulates the body's immune system to produce specific antibodies, when administered into the body.
- *Therapeutic serum*: Product obtained from blood by removing clot components and blood cells; examples include anti-snake venom, antitoxins like tetanus antitoxin and diphtheria antitoxin, purified immunoglobulins, etc.

- Antitoxin is a product obtained from serum or other body fluid of an immunized animal, which specifically neutralizes the toxin against which the animal is immune.

- *Monoclonal antibodies:* A whole plethora of mABs is completely changing the approach to treatment of cancers, immunological, cardiometabolic, and infectious disorders.
  - mABs are antibodies that have a high degree of specificity (mono-specificity) for an antigen or epitope that are identical because they are produced by a single clone of cells.
  - Produced by hybridoma technology or somatic cell fusion; an antibody producing B cell fused with a myeloma cell to produce a hybrid cell.
  - Different types of antibodies based on their source and composition (Table 32.1). Next-generation antibody formats include bispecifics (e.g., blinatumomab), afucosylated/glyco-engineered mAbs (e.g., obinutuzumab), antibody–drug conjugates (ADCs), and single-domain antibodies.
- *Blood and blood components:* As per WHO, blood products include any therapeutic substances derived from human blood, including whole blood, labile blood components, and plasma-derived medicinal products (e.g., coagulation factors used for hemophilia).
- *Allergenic products*: Used mainly for diagnostic purposes.
  - Allergenic patch tests: Diagnostic test that are applied to the surface of the skin to determine the specific cause of contact dermatitis and to identify the contact allergen.
  - Allergenic extracts: Extracts like natural substances like pollen, animal hair, and food can be used in the diagnosis and treatment of allergic diseases like allergic rhinitis (hay fever), sinusitis, conjunctivitis, and food allergy.

Table 32.1 Types of monoclonal antibodies (mABs)

Type of mAB	Features
Murine (INN infix[a]: –o–)	Entire structure constituted of rodent components Therapeutic response affected by allergic or hypersensitivity response (human antimouse antibody, HAMA)
Chimeric (infix –xi–)	Contains human constant regions with rodent variable regions (~65–70% human content) Less murine antibody response (30%)
Humanized (infix –zu–)	Contains human constant (~90–95%) and variable region except the CDRs (Complimentarity Determining Regions) that are murine Minimal problem of HAMA
Fully human (infix –u–)	Contains human constant and variable regions (no murine sequence); produced via phage display, transgenic mice, or human B-cell cloning Negligible HAMA; lowest immunogenicity among types, anti-drug antibodies (ADA) may still occur

[a]WHO discontinued the antibody "source" infix (–o–/–xi–/–zu–/–u–) in 2017

- *Gene therapy products*: Gene therapy is a technique that seeks to modify or manipulate the expression of a gene or to alter the biological properties of living cells for therapeutic use.
  - Gene therapies can work by several mechanisms such as replacing a disease-causing gene with a healthy copy, inactivating a disease-causing gene or introducing a new or modified gene into the body.
  - Gene therapy products are being studied or used for diseases like cancer, genetic diseases, and infectious diseases.
  - Examples include idecabtagene vicleucel, iltacabtagene autoleucel, tisagenlecleucel, sipuleucel-T, etc.
- *Cellular therapies*: As per FDA, somatic cell therapy is "autologous, allogenic, or xenogenic cells that have been propagated, expanded, selected, pharmacologically treated, or otherwise altered in biological characteristics ex vivo to be administered to human and applicable to the prevention, treatment, cure, diagnosis or mitigation of diseases or injuries."

32.2.3 Mechanism of Action of Biologicals

- Like conventional medicines, biological medicines have mechanisms of action that alter the physiology or pathology of the disease by interacting with the human body system; but usually much more specifically, in a targeted manner.
- *Traditional biologicals:* Biologicals like replacement proteins, cytokines, and hormones are usually developed using recombinant DNA technologies. Examples include growth factors, insulin, erythropoietin (EPO), enzymes, interferon, and granulocyte colony stimulating factor.
- *Advanced targeted biologics:* Monoclonal antibodies are among the most broadly developed targeted biologicals with humira (adalimumab) and rituxan (rituximab) among the first ones to be approved and to become multibillion dollar blockbuster drugs.
- mAbs targeting specific antigens (commonly receptors or cell surface structures) account for 50% of the top 100 drugs currently and are expected to maintain this dominant position in the pharmaceutical market in the coming decades.
- The "recombinant DNA," often used in producing biologics, involves isolating a DNA segment from human cells, modifying it, inserting it into a bacteria or a mammalian cell, and getting that organism or cell to express it.
- There are many steps involved in this process, from locating and cloning the genes that code for proteins, reproducing the proteins associated with the genes, determining the role of the proteins in the disease process, and finally developing a potential therapy.
- A series of cell-based assays are conducted to provide information on how a specific protein changes a biological process. These assays use biological indicators of living organisms or tissues, including cell-based tissue cultures, microarray expression technology, knockout animal models, transgenic animal models, and antisense or antibody technology.

32.2.4 Manufacture and Development of Biologicals

- Genetic engineering and biotechnology are commonly used in the development of biologicals with processes like recombinant DNA technology used for the development of the first biologicals like human insulin.
- Modalities of biologicals are now being developed or explored for therapeutic indications with significant unmet needs, which are beyond the early traditional methods like replacement proteins; these now include highly engineered antibodies, oligonucleotides, fusion proteins, and gene constructs.
- Manufacturing of biologicals is complex with stringent controls and specifications required to ensure safety and efficacy, including addressing their immunogenic potential.
- Specific challenges in development include limitations of study design due to species specificity of therapeutic action, limited delivery options (mostly restricted to subcutaneous or intravenous route).
- The development process for a biological includes genetically engineering a cell to produce the biologic, multiple steps for its purification, and extensive testing to ensure product quality, purity, and stability.
- The heterogeneous nature of the molecules, often composed of hundreds to thousands of amino acids, leads to impurity profile that varies according to the process of manufacturing and testing process utilized.
- While the manufacturing process of chemical drugs is well defined, allowing them to be produced in uniform large quantities, biologics have more complex production processes that often yield small quantities.
- Scaling up the manufacture of biologics from small laboratory quantities used in testing to larger-scale batches is quite difficult and expensive.
- It is also difficult to maintain product purity and batch-to-batch equivalence; these compounds are sensitive to temperature, light, and other physical conditions and enzymatic action.
- They usually require complex bioassays for batch release and stability assessment, as compared to conventional drugs which require chemical tests for identity and purity.
- Well-qualified and experienced personnel should be involved in the production and quality control of biologicals, and they should be trained about safety and hygiene standards.

32.2.4.1 Preclinical and Clinical Development

- Standard preclinical development programs cannot be implemented for these agents as safety studies should be performed in the most pharmacologically relevant species with comparable binding and affinity to humans to identify potential toxicity issues.
- Similarly, the selection of appropriate animal models, including genetically engineered rodents or disease models, or surrogate molecules is important, as is the recognizing and dealing with anti-drug antibodies (ADAs).

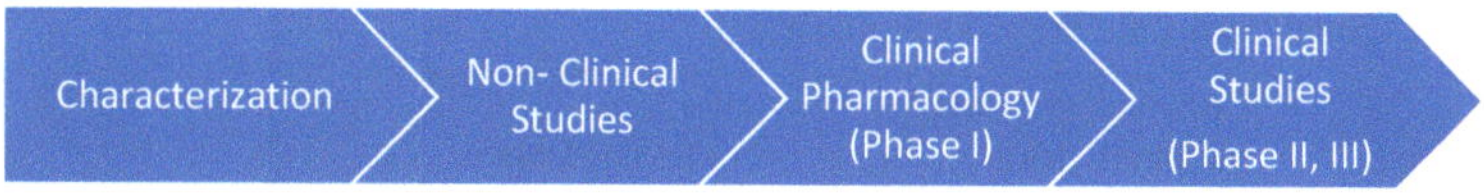
Characterization
Non- Clinical Studies
Clinical Pharmacology (Phase I)
Clinical Studies (Phase II, III)

Fig. 32.1 Development of biologicals

- As live organisms or cultures are used in the production of biologicals, batch to batch variability is introduced, and potency and safety testing is required for each batch.
- Animals used should be regularly monitored, and emphasis is being placed on replacement, reduction, and refinement in the use of animals with development of newer methodologies.
- Like the conventional small molecule therapeutics, the safety and efficacy of biologics should be determined in clinical trials in order to gain approval for each clinical use or indication sought.
- Similar to a conventional investigational drug, an Investigational New Drug Application (IND) is required to be filed in order to administer a biological product to humans.
- Process flow of development of biologicals (Fig. 32.1).
- Analytical characterization is a critical step before the compounds are used for preclinical testing and involves structural and functional characterization (detailed later).
- The FIH (first in human) or phase I studies generally follow the familiar single-ascending dose study followed by a multiple ascending dose study pattern.
- Safety monitoring needs to be hypervigilant due to possibilities of anaphylaxis, immunogenicity, and higher risk of unexpected adverse effects.
- Phase II and III studies follow the same principles and practices as those for the small molecule drugs.

32.2.5 Small Molecule Therapeutics Versus Biologicals

Table 32.2 gives a comparison between conventional small molecule drugs versus the biologicals.

32.2.6 Regulations for Biologicals

- In the last two decades, the regulatory agencies across the world have released thorough guidance for rational and scientific development of biologicals.
- The International Conference on Harmonization (ICH) S6 guidance was the first document in 1997 to provide the best practices for nonclinical approaches to biologic drug development.
- The WHO has published international reference standards for biologicals (referred to as biological therapeutics) to help ensure the consistency of a prod-

Table 32.2 Small molecule drugs vs biological

Characteristic	Conventional small molecule drugs	Biologicals
Origin	Generally obtained through chemical synthetic processes	Derived from living cells or through biological processes
Size	Smaller, usually between 0.1 and 1 kDa	Very large molecules; typically greater than 1 kDa in size
Composition	Tens to hundreds of atoms usually of chemically defined substances (e.g., aspirin contains just 21 atoms)	Thousands of atoms, usually consisting of proteins, carbohydrates, nucleic acids, cells or tissues, or a combination For example, a typical biologic has more than 25,000 atoms
Structure	Simple and well defined	Complex and heterogenous
Production	Synthetically produced through a predictable and consistent chemical process	More complex manufacturing process involving genetically engineering a cell to produce a protein, testing to ensure quality, harvesting, purifying, and stabilizing the protein—Chances of variability high
Stability	Generally, more stable to external influences like heat, light, etc.	Less stable—Generally require specific storage conditions
Administration	Possible by all routes; most drugs can be given orally	Restricted to parenteral routes (SC/IV)
Mechanism	Broad mechanisms of action—May or may not be nontarget specific	Target specific action—Higher efficacy
Response	Generally consistent; linear dose response expected	May be variable; non-linear dose response
Safety	Variable, depending on the type of drug molecule and its action	Relatively better safety profile due to enhanced specificity
Immunogenicity	Rare—Generally not expected	Likely with the action of biologics—Interaction with immune system
Cost	Relatively lower costs	Relatively higher costs
Accessibility	Generally accessible to most populations	Accessibility poorer due to cost and resource constraints, especially in developing world

uct across many batches as well as to allow the comparability of biologicals between manufacturers and/or countries; guidelines have been released for various aspects related to different biotherapeutic products.

- In the United States, the FDA's Center for Biologics Evaluation and Research (CBER) regulates products under a variety of regulatory authorities including the Public Health Service Act (under which biologicals are regulated) and the Food Drug and Cosmetic Act.
- Nondrug biologics are CBER-regulated products; the IND application (as per 21 CFR 312) and NDA (21 CFR 314) are submitted to the CBER.
- Applications for drug biologics including monoclonal antibodies, growth factors, enzymes, immunomodulators, and thrombolytics are reviewed by the FDA's Center for Drug Evaluation and Research (CDER).

- The U.S. CBER and CDER have released addendums concerning the safety evaluation of biologics, and industry guidance as well.
- A complete list of biologicals approved in the United States can be found yearwise on the U.S. FDA portal: https://www.fda.gov/vaccines-blood-biologics/development-approval-process-cber/biological-approvals-year
- In the United States, the Biologics License Application (BLA) is a request for permission to introduce, or deliver for introduction, a biologic product into interstate commerce (21 CFR 601.2).
- In India, the development and approval of biologicals is regulated under the New Drugs and Clinical Trials (NDCT) Rules 2019, and CDSCO is the competent regulatory authority.
- As per the NDCT 2019, "investigational new drug" means a new chemical or **biological entity** or substance that has not been approved for marketing as a drug in any country, and the definition of "new drug" includes a vaccine, recombinant deoxyribonucleic acid (r-DNA)-derived product, living modified organism, monoclonal antibody, stem cell-derived product, gene therapeutic product, or xenografts, intended to be used as drug.

32.3 Biosimilars

32.3.1 Terms and Definitions

- Terms used: Biosimilars, similar biologics (EMA/India), follow-on biologics (FDA).
- The United States. has three options—biologic, biosimilar, interchangeable biologic; most other countries have two options—biologic, biosimilar.
- Considered as "generic equivalent of biologicals."
- Definition: "A Similar Biologic product is that which is similar in terms of quality, safety and efficacy to an approved Reference Biological product based on comparability."
- In Europe: "A biosimilar is a biological medicinal product that contains a version of the active substance of an already authorised reference product in the EEA, and which has shown similarity to the reference product in terms of quality, characteristics, biological activity, safety and efficacy based on a comprehensive comparability exercise."
- In India: "A Similar Biologic product is that which is similar in terms of quality, safety and efficacy to an approved Reference Biological product based on comparability."
- *"Biomimics" or "Biocopies":* Copies of licensed biologic medicines that have not been subjected to rigorous clinical testing or evaluated according to the biosimilar regulatory pathway; nonsimilar biotherapeutic product.
- *"Biobetters"*: Improved versions of the originator biologic.

32.3.2 Biosimilars Versus Generics

- In many ways, biosimilars are to biologics, as generics are to drugs, but there are some key differences between them (Table 32.3):

Table 32.3 Biosimilars vs small molecule generics

Small molecule generics	Biosimilars
Low molecular weight and complexity	High molecular weight and complex 3-D structure
Chemical synthesis	Produced by living organisms
Manufacturing process easy to reverse-engineer	Manufacturing process cannot be replicated
Identical copy of active ingredient	Although required to contain the same primary amino acid sequence, the biosimilar is not identical to the originator, but rather highly similar
Proof of quality and bioequivalence mainly required No substantial clinical data required	After demonstration of quality, some nonclinical and clinical studies are necessary Immunogenic response may be unpredictable and therefore must be tested

- Like biological, biosimilars are also structurally complex compounds where structural variability is acceptable but key functional groups need to be the same.
- Differences in manufacturing processes may also lead to differences in products, provided it does not affect the required "similarity" in quality, safety, or efficacy (Fig. 32.2).

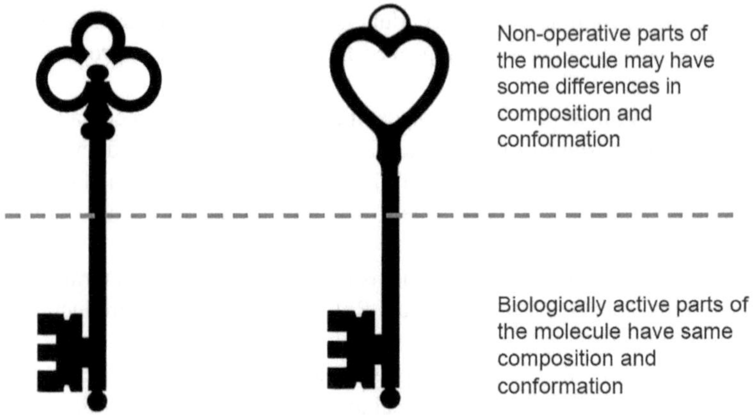

Fig. 32.2 Tertiary structures or "folds" of biosimilars may differ, but the key functional groups remain the same. (Adapted from Webster CJ of BioApprovals. Docket ID: FDA-2018-N-2689. Facilitating Competition and Innovation in the Biological Products Marketplace; Public Hearing; Request for Comments)

32.3.3 Concept and Demonstration of "Similarity"

- Based on different definitions, there are three determinants in the definition of the biosimilar product:
  - It should be a biologic product.
  - The reference product should be an already licensed biologic product.
  - The demonstration of high similarity in safety, quality, and efficacy is necessary.
- Reference product: Reference/innovator biological product licensed inside country or outside used.
- The similarity is to be demonstrated at the levels of "quality, nonclinical, and clinical" using a set of comprehensive comparability exercises.
- Analytical similarity data is the foundation of biosimilar development: extensive structural and functional characterization.
- Preclinical comparability: Pharmacodynamic and toxicological studies.
- Comprehensive clinical comparability: Clinical development program to demonstrate NO clinically meaningful differences between reference and biosimilar.

32.3.4 Biosimilar Development

- Extensive structural and functional characterization is necessary: Data from multiple analytical and biological tests required for complete understanding of the molecule (Fig. 32.3).

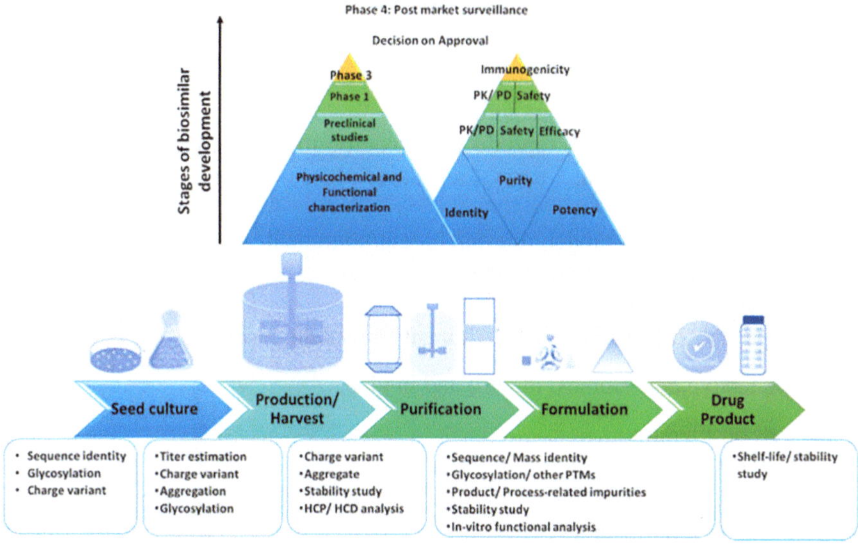

Fig. 32.3 Steps and stages of biosimilar development (From: Nupur et al. 2022)

Part II Drug Discovery and Development

Part III Drug Regulations

Akila Srinivasan Department of Pharmacology, Mahatma Gandhi Medical College and Research Institute (MGMCRI), Sri Balaji Vidyapeeth, Puducherry, India

[illegible]

[illegible]

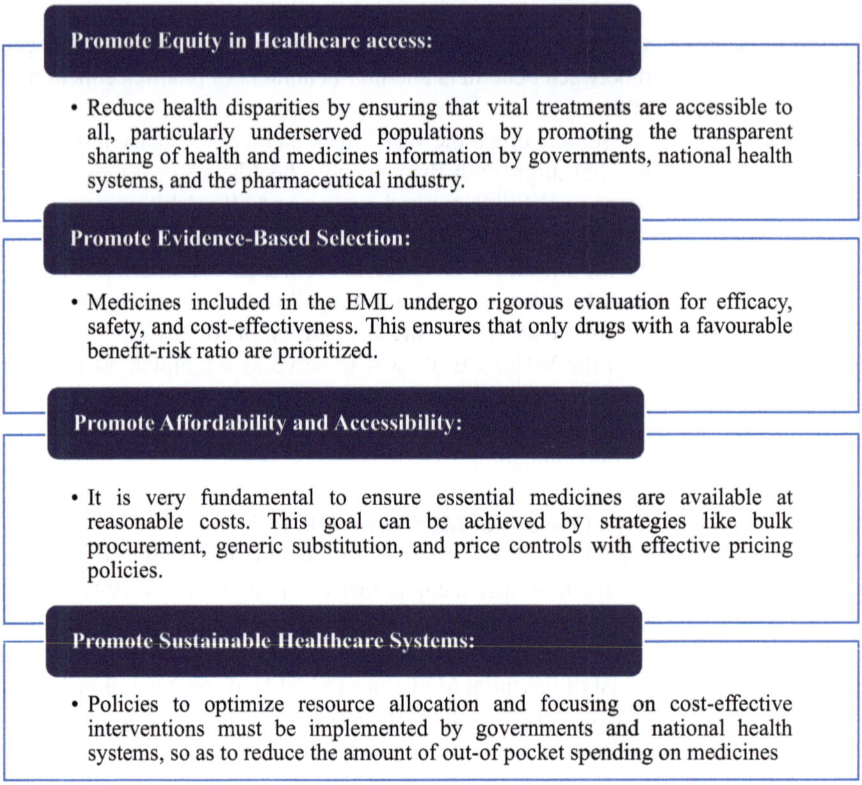

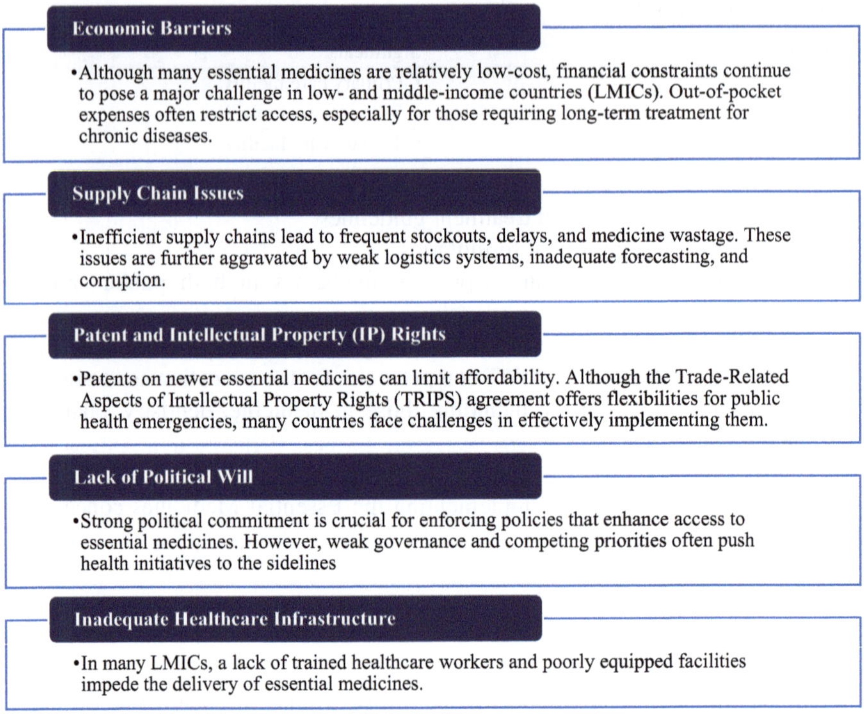

2.2.2.1 Factors Contributing to Irrational Use of Medicines

Factors contributing to Irrational Use of Medicines

Physician related	Patients related	Health care system related	Pharmaceutical and Regulatory related
Inadequate knowledge about evidence-based standard treatment guidelines & rational prescribing practices	Limited understanding on usage of medicines and its work (e.g., stopping antibiotics prematurely)	Lack of availability of Standard Treatment Guidelines	Inadequate Regulatory framework - allows the sale of irrational drug combinations and substandard medicines
Lack of regular upgradation in medical knowledge	Demand for unnecessary antibiotics and pressuring physician to prescribe	Insufficient monitoring of drug prescriptions and dispensing practices	Aggressive marketing & inappropriate drug promotions - influence prescribing practices & compromise rational prescribing
Lack of skills or independent information	Self-medication	Poor Communication Between Providers and Patients	High cost of healthcare drives patients to purchase cheaper but inappropriate/substandard alternatives
Increased work burden	Misconceptions about diseases and treatments	Poor systems for tracking prescribing patterns and patient outcomes	Lack strict regulations on the sale of prescription-only medicines & easy availability of over-the-counter drugs
Failure to explain importance of adhering to prescribed treatments, potential side effects, & proper usage of medicines	Use of traditional remedies or unverified therapies alongside modern medicines	Absence of effective pharmacovigilance systems to detect and prevent adverse drug events or misuse	Availability of Irrational Fixed-Dose Combinations (FDCs) in the market

McCulloch P, Altman DG, Campbell WB et al (2009) No surgical innovation without evaluation: the IDEAL recommendations. Lancet 374(9695):1105–1112. https://doi.org/10.1016/S0140-6736(09)61116-8
[illegible] VM, [illegible] M, [illegible] JP (2017) Shared decision making [illegible]
[illegible]
[illegible]
[illegible]
[illegible]

toxicity. This would also give [illegible] some patients avoid taking drugs due to fear of toxicity.

References

[illegible]

15.6 Conclusion

The frequency of Phase 2 clinical trials is increasing, yet these studies are not small [illegible] controlled Phase 3 trials. Well-designed Phase 2 trials [illegible] [illegible] [illegible] [illegible] [illegible] [illegible] [illegible] [illegible] [illegible] [illegible] Phase 2 designs [illegible] [illegible] development [illegible]

Bibliography

[illegible]

Pollard AJ, Bijker EM (2021) A guide to vaccinology: from basic principles to new developments. Nat Rev Immunol 21(2):83–100. https://doi.org/10.1038/s41577-020-00479-7. Epub 2020 Dec 22. Erratum in: Nat Rev Immunol. 2021 Jan 5; PMID: 33353987; PMCID: PMC7754704

[illegible]

Singh K, Mehta S (2016) The clinical development process for a novel preventive vaccine: an overview. [illegible]

[illegible]

- **Pharmaceutical alternatives:** Drug products that contain the identical therapeutic moiety but not necessarily in the same amount or dosage form or as the same salt or ester.
- **Reference product:** Pharmaceutical product that the Licensing Authority prefers as Designated Reference Product and contains the same active ingredient as the new drug. Mostly, it would be the global innovator product.
- **Therapeutic equivalents:** Pharmaceutical products that contain the same active substance or therapeutic moiety and clinically show the same efficacy and safety.
- $\mathbf{C_{max}}$**:** Maximum drug concentration achieved in systemic circulation following drug administration.
- $\mathbf{C_{min}}$**:** Minimum drug concentration achieved in systemic circulation following multiple dosing at a steady state.
- $\mathbf{T_{max}}$**:** Time required to achieve maximum drug concentration in the systemic circulation.
- **Area under curve (AUC)** $_{\mathbf{0\text{-}t}}$**:** Area under the plasma concentration-time curve, from 0 h to the last quantifiable concentration to be calculated using the trapezoidal rule.
- $\mathbf{AUC_{0\text{-}\infty}}$**:** Area under the plasma concentration-time curve, from zero to infinity is calculated as the sum of $AUC_{0\text{-}t}$ plus the ratio of the last measurable concentration to the elimination rate constant.
- $\mathbf{AUC_{0\text{-}tau}}$**:** Area under the plasma concentration-time curve over one dosing interval following a single dose for modified release products.
- **Half-life,** $\mathbf{T_{1/2}}$: Elimination half-life of a drug is the time necessary to reduce the drug concentration in biological fluids to one-half after equilibrium is reached.

22.3 Specific Dosage Forms Necessitating Mandatory In Vivo Bioequivalence Studies

(i) **Systemic formulations**

- Oral drugs indicated in serious conditions, with a narrow therapeutic range, following pharmacokinetic properties such as incomplete absorption, first-pass metabolism>70%, and nonlinear pharmacokinetics.
- Oral immediate release drugs with high excipient content, low solubility, instability, and poor permeability.
- Transdermal patches, suppositories, and similar products but not administered orally/parenterally.
- Modified release products.
- Fixed-dose combinations for systemic use.

(ii) **Nonsystemic products**

- Oral, nasal, ocular, dermal, rectal, and vaginal pharmaceutical products that are not in solution form.

- *Characterization studies.*
  - Biosimilars must meet the same quality standards as originator products.
  - Physical properties.
  - Protein characterization, amino acid sequence, high order structure and post-translation form.
  - Product-related impurities (amino acid aggregates, oxidized forms, deaminated forms).
  - Process-related impurities and contaminants (host cell protein, residual genomic DNA, reagents, downstream impurities).
  - Receptor binding or cell-based assays.
- Identify critical quality attributes and clinically active components.
- Understanding the relationship between quality attributes and the clinical safety and efficacy profile aids ability to determine residual uncertainty about biosimilarity, and to predict expected "clinical similarity" from the quality data.
- Comprehensive comparability after change in manufacturing process:
  - Companies likely to adapt or improve the manufacturing process several times during the commercial life of a product.
  - A change to manufacturing process must be approved by regulators.
  - Extent of comparability studies following a manufacturing change to a biological medicine will depend on the expected impact on quality, safety, and efficacy of the medicine.
  - Analytical and functional data are usually sufficient, and clinical trials to prove safety and efficacy are not needed; trials are needed only if an impact on safety and efficacy is anticipated.
- *Nonclinical comparability:* Demonstrated through toxicological and pharmacodynamics studies.
- Toxicological studies.
  - Repeated dose toxicity: required.
  - Safety pharmacology, reproductive toxicity, mutagenicity, carcinogenicity: required depending upon repeated dose toxicity and analytical characterization.
  - Choice of animal model: relevant rodent/nonrodent.
  - Route of administration: As intended for use.
  - Duration: 28 days.
  - Dose: 1×, 2×, and 5× of HED (human equivalent dose).
- Pharmacodynamic studies: in vitro and in vivo.
  - Cell proliferation.
  - Cytotoxicity.
  - Neutralizing.
  - Receptor binding assay.
  - In vivo: as required after in vitro studies.
- *Comprehensive clinical comparability:* Clinical studies aim to confirm the characterization work.

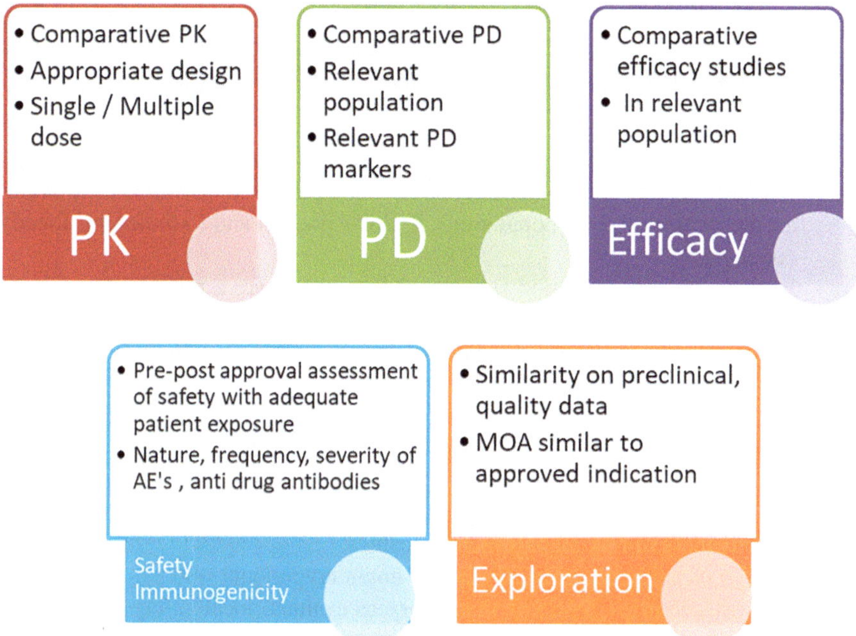

Fig. 32.4 Studies involved in the clinical development program of biosimilars

- Development approach for biosimilars is closer to originators than to generics: require phase 1 PK, phase 3, and 4 studies along with pharmacovigilance.
- Usually take about 7–8 years for development, involving ~500 patients.
- Phase 1 trials: pharmacokinetics, pharmacodynamics, safety, immunogenicity.
- Clinical PK and PD studies should be ideally conducted in healthy subjects if the product can be safely administered to them; considered to be more sensitive in because it is likely to produce less variability compared with a study in patients with potential confounding factors such as underlying and/or concomitant disease and concomitant medications (Fig. 32.4).
- No phase 2 dose finding studies required for biosimilars as it is assumed that similar efficacy will be demonstrated with the same dose regimens for the biosimilar as for the innovator.
- Phase 3 trials: comparative studies against reference biologic showing:
  - Clinical equivalence using sensitive end points.
  - Prespecified and justified equivalence/noninferiority margins.
  - Comparable safety and efficacy in one therapeutic indication.
  - Safety efficacy data may be extrapolated to other indications approved for reference medicine.
- Current FDA and EMA Indian guidance do not mandate performing comparative clinical efficacy trials in every approved indication of the reference product: reduces cost and shortens time for biosimilar development.

- Also called "extrapolation of indications": Biosimilars approved for one indication are granted approval for indications that are held by reference product based on extrapolation of efficacy and safety data.
- *Postauthorization efficacy studies (PAES).*
  - In many other countries, PAES is required in a comparative study design (against innovator) in statistically defined sample size of participants to evaluate the product in local populations, if global phase 1 and 3 studies are already conducted.
  - In India, postauthorization studies for biosimilars are a mix of efficacy and safety, involving at least 200 subjects, with safety as primary end point and efficacy and immunogenicity as secondary end points.
  - Can be randomized or nonrandomized studies.
- *Biosimilar pharmacovigilance:*
  - A postauthorization safety study (PASS) is carried out after a biosimilar has been authorised to obtain further information on its safety, or to measure the effectiveness of risk management measures.
  - PASS's can either be clinical trials or noninterventional studies.
  - In most countries, PASS is mandatory to evaluate local safety on usage of biosimilar.
  - In India: Consists of active post-marketing surveillance (active PMS) involving observational studies of patients prescribed biosimilars for the approved indications.
  - Requirements for the management and reporting of suspected adverse reactions apply equally to biologicals and nonbiological.
  - Specific evaluation of immunogenicity is required during product development and prior to authorization of biotechnological medicines, as it can affect both safety and efficacy of the product.
  - Naming, traceability, specific approaches to case processing, PSURs, RMPs etc. are needed for effective pharmacovigilance.

32.3.5 Concept of "Interchangeability"

- This is a U.S. FDA specific term: Requires specific comparative PK studies and allows automatic substitution between biosimilar and innovator reference in chronic treatments.
- As per FDA definition: "An interchangeable product is a biosimilar product that meets additional requirements outlined by the Biologics Price Competition and Innovation Act." Such a product can be substituted for the reference product without the requiring the prescriber's involvement.
- Interchangeability studies required to produce data sufficient to show that for a biological product that is administered more than once to an individual, the risk in terms of safety or diminished efficacy of alternating or switching between use of the biological product and the reference product is not greater than the risk of using the reference product without such alternation or switch.

- From the FDA's perspectives, interchangeability includes the concept of switching and alternating between an innovative biologic product (R) and its follow-on biologics (T).
- Switching is referred to as not only the switch from "R to T" or "T to R" (narrow sense of switchability), but also "T to T" and "R to R" (broader sense of switchability).
- Alternating is referred to as either the switch from T to R and then switch back to T (i.e., "T to R to or the switch from R to T and switch back to R) (i.e., "R to T to R").
- So, what is the difference between a biosimilar and an interchangeable product?
  - Basically, an interchangeable product, in addition to being biosimilar, meets certain additional requirements—data and information in terms of safety and decreased efficacy, through alternating or switching between products.
  - A prescription from a physician is required to receive a biosimilar, written specifically for that biosimilar whereas for an interchangeable product, the pharmacist is allowed to substitute the interchangeable product for the reference product without consulting the prescriber.

32.3.6 Regulatory Pathways for Biosimilars

- *The United States:* the Affordable Care Act provides an abbreviated licensure pathway for products that are biosimilar or interchangeable with an FDA-licensed biologic reference product.
- FDA guidance for industry: Scientific Considerations in Demonstrating Biosimilarity to a Reference Product (released in April 2015).
- It suggests stepwise approach and consideration of the "totality of the evidence."
- "Stand-alone" and biosimilar development are different: "Abbreviated" development program, 351(k) under the PHS Act.
- A 351(k) application must include information demonstrating that the biological product:
  - Is biosimilar to a reference product.
  - Utilizes the same mechanism(s) of action for the proposed condition(s) of use—but only to the extent the mechanism(s) are known for the reference product.
  - Condition(s) of use proposed in labeling have been previously approved for the reference product.
  - Has the same route of administration, dosage form, and strength as the reference product.
  - Is manufactured, processed, packed, or held in a facility that meets standards designed to assure that the biological product continues to be safe, pure, and potent.
- Scope and magnitude of the clinical studies will depend on the extent of residual uncertainty about biosimilarity.

- *EU biosimilar guideline:* EMA Similar biological medicinal products (CHMP/437/04 Rev. 1), with further guidance available for clinical–nonclinical issues and quality issues (Fig. 32.5).
- Over the next 10 years, biologics in the European Union are expected to lose patent exclusivity predominantly in the domains of oncology (29%), endocrine (11%), and blood and lymphoma (21%) (Fig. 32.6).
- Since the first filgrastim biosimilar approval in 2015, there are currently over 70 biosimilars approved by the U.S. FDA (as of mid 2025); not all of them are available in the market.
- The overall number of approvals by the EMA is higher compared to the FDA's: since somatotropin biosimilar approval in 2006, there have been more than 140 approvals (2025), of whom 14 have been withdrawn post approval.

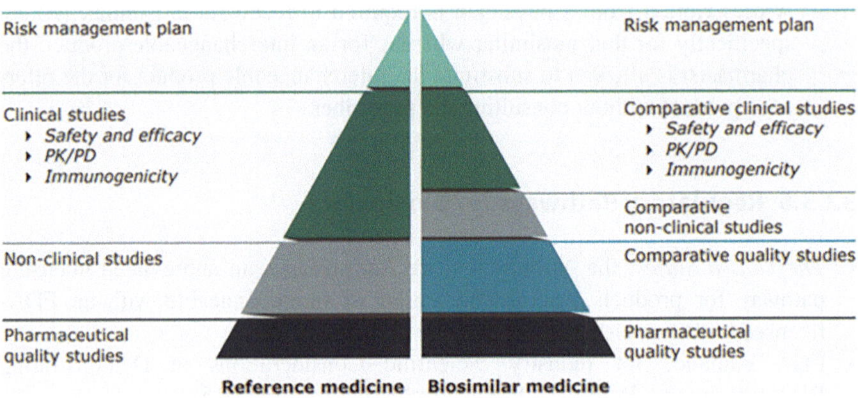

Fig. 32.5 Data requirements for biologics vs biosimilars. (From: EMA: Biosimilars in the EU. Information guide for healthcare professionals)

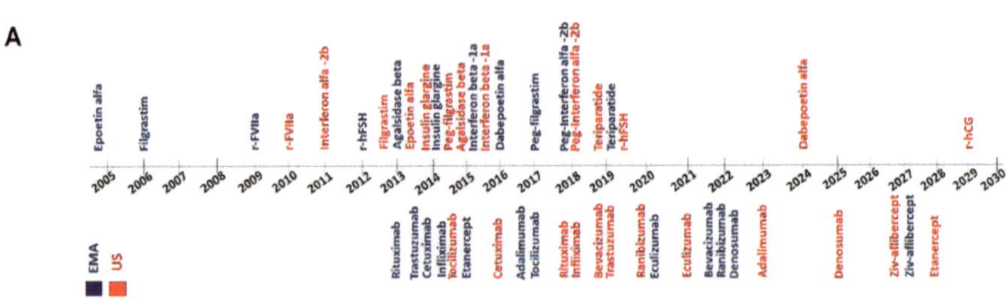

Fig. 32.6 Timeline on patent expirations of reference products in the United States and Europe. (Part reproduction from: Nupur et al. 2022)

32.3.7 Indian Scenario

- There are more than 100 approved biosimilars in India (2023), with at least 50 available in the market, the most of any country globally. Recent trade/industry tallies indicate 130+ biosimilars approved in India, with active marketing varying by product
- The first "similar biologic" was approved and marketed in India for a hepatitis B vaccine in 2000 (before the EU-2006 and US–2015), and the country has demonstrated the greatest acceptance of biosimilars in the world.
- While simple similar biologics, such as insulin and erythropoietin currently hold the majority of market share in the Indian market, the country is soon becoming the fastest growing in the world for mAbs for autoimmune, cardiovascular diseases and oncology.
- The Indian similar biologics market is projected to reach $40 billion by 2030 from being approximately $300 million in 2015.
- Technically, India does not approve biosimilars; the regulatory agency CDSCO approves follow-on brands of biologics as Indian similar biologics, or ISBs.
- Similar biologics approved and marketed in India in the earlier years were not subjected to as rigorous comparative trials as in the EU and United States, but with the development of CDSCO guidelines in 2012, subsequently revised in 2016 in alignment with international agencies, more stringent evaluations have now been implemented.
- As per the revised guidelines, biosimilar applicant in India can use a reference biologic which has been approved in India or any other ICH country if not marketed in India.
- The significant export of similar biologics to highly regulated as well as emerging markets is a testament to improved acceptability.
- Similarly, biosimilar products for trastuzumab, filgrastim and pegfilgrastim were developed in India and are now approved as biosimilars in Europe and beyond.
- There are several reasons for promotion of similar biologics in India—primarily due to low cost of research and development.
- For comparison: Time of development of biosimilar is 8 years in the European Union versus 3 to 5 years in India, and the cost to develop a biosimilar is estimated to be $100–$200 million in the European Union or United States versus $10–$20 million in India; being driven by lower cost of recruiting patients, fewer labour and service fees along with apparently less stringent regulatory requirements.
- Another difference is that there is no requirement for biosimilars to be approved as "interchangeable" to allow switching patients from reference products.
- "National Bio-Pharma Mission"' has been initiated in the country as an industry-academia collaborative mission by the department of biotechnology and the World Bank.

32.4 Conclusion

Biologicals are complex medical products derived from living cells, which have now revolutionized the treatment of many serious diseases across a variety of therapeutic spectrums. Since the approvals of the first biological in the 1980s, their development has been strong with evolution in stringent regulations in parallel. Biosimilars have further paved the way for use of these complex drugs on a broader canvas. These molecules are also known as similar biologics which are similar in terms of quality, safety, and efficacy to an approved reference biological product, and can play an important role in allowing to provide a better healthcare system due to their relative affordability.

However, issues remain on both regulatory and manufacturing sides, particularly in developing countries like India. Overall, stringent guidelines have been able to provide sufficient safeguards when it comes to biosimilars and also streamlined the process for obtaining market authorization. Biosimilars could be considered as interchangeable therapeutic alternatives over original biologics, complex biosimilars, particularly, monoclonal antibodies require more rigorous comparative evaluations.

Future of medicine is expected to revolve around biological and biosimilars in the coming decades.

Bibliography

Andrews L, Ralston S, Blomme E et al (2015) A snapshot of biologic drug development: challenges and opportunities. Hum Exp Toxicol 34(12):1279–1285

Anour R (2014) Biosimilars versus 'biobetters' – a regulator's perspective. GaBIJ 3:166–167

Cornes P (2021) Column: India Struggles to Meet International Biologics Standards. Column: India Struggles to Meet International Biologics Standards (centerforbiosimilars.com). Accessed 28 Aug 2022

Department of Biotechnology (2022) Central Drugs Standard Control Organization. Guidelines on Similar Biologics: Regulatory Requirements for Marketing Authorization in India, 2016. https://www.ibkp.dbtindia.gov.in/DBT_Content_Test/CMS/Guidelines/20181115140059519_Guidelines-on-Similar-Biologics-2016.pdf. Accessed 20 June 2022

Dörner T, Kay J (2015) Biosimilars in rheumatology: current perspectives and lessons learnt. Nat Rev Rheumatol 11(12):713–724

European Medcines Agency (2014) Guideline on similar biological medicinal products. https://www.ema.europa.eu/en/documents/scientific-guideline/guideline-similar-biological-medicinal-products-rev1_en.pdf. Accessed 30 June 2022

European Medcines Agency (2019) Biosimilars in the EU. Information guide for healthcare professionals. https://www.ema.europa.eu/en/documents/leaflet/biosimilars-eu-information-guide-healthcare-professionals_en.pdf. Accessed 30 June 2022

Figg R (2022) How the U.S. Compares to Europe on Biosimilar Approvals and Products In the Pipeline Updated March 14, 2022. https://www.jdsupra.com/legalnews/how-the-u-s-compares-to-europe-on-7635750/ Accessed June 30 2022

Generics and Biosimilars Initiative (2022) 'Similar biologics' approved and marketed in India (2018). https://www.gabionline.net/biosimilars/general/Similar-biologics-approved-and-marketed-in-India. Accessed 25 June 2022

Gherghescu I, Delgado-Charro MB (2020) The biosimilar landscape: an overview of regulatory approvals by the EMA and FDA. Pharmaceutics 13(1):48
Hagen T (2022) Report: Biosimilar Competition in Europe. https://www.centerforbiosimilars.com/view/report-biosimilar-competition-in-europe Accessed 25 June 2022
Jallal B (2017) Realizing the Promise of Biologics. In: Harvard health policy review. http://www.hhpronline.org/articles/2017/4/9/realizing-the-promise-of-biologics. Accessed 22 Apr 2022
Jois R, Mukherjee S, Rajeswari S, Rath PD, Goyal V, Gupta D (2020) Similar biologics in India: a story of access or potential for compromise? Indian J Med Res 152(5):456–467
Kirchhoff CF, Wang XM, Conlon HD et al (2017) Biosimilars: key regulatory considerations and similarity assessment tools. Biotechnol Bioeng 114(12):2696–2705
Makurvet FD (2020) Biologics versus small molecules: drug costs and patient access. Med Drug Discov 9:100075. https://doi.org/10.1016/j.medidd.2020.100075
Markus R, Liu J, Ramchandani M, Landa D et al (2017) Developing the totality of evidence for Biosimilars: regulatory considerations and building confidence for the healthcare community. BioDrugs 31(3):175–187
Meher BR, Balan S, Mohanty RR, Jena M et al (2019) Biosimilars in India; current status and future perspectives. J Pharm Bioallied Sci 11(1):12–15
Morrow T, Felcone LH (2004) Defining the difference: what makes biologics unique. Biotechnol Healthc 1(4):24–29
Mulcahy AW, Hlavka JP, Case SR (2018) Biosimilar cost Savings in the United States: initial experience and future potential. Rand Health Q 7(4):3
Natarajan J, Janani R (2019) A review on regulatory guidelines for biologics in India. J Pharm Sci Res 11(11):3651–3654
Nupur N, Joshi S, Gulliarme D, Rathore AS (2022) Analytical similarity assessment of Biosimilars: global regulatory landscape, recent studies and major advancements in orthogonal platforms. Front Bioeng Biotechnol 10:832059
Pategou J (2021) The opportunities & challenges of India's Biologics Market. The Opportunities Challenges of India's Biologics Market (biosimilardevelopment.com). Accessed 30 Aug 2022
US Food and Drug Administration (2015) Scientific considerations in demonstrating biosimilarity to a reference product. Guidance for Industry. https://www.fda.gov/media/82647/download. Accessed 30 June 2022
US Food and Drug Administration (2022a) Vaccines, blood & biologics. https://www.fda.gov/vaccines-blood-biologics. Accessed 20 Apr 2022
US Food and Drug Administration (2022b) Biosimilar and interchangeable products. https://www.fda.gov/drugs/biosimilars/biosimilar-and-interchangeable-products. Accessed 30 June 2022
Webster CJ of BioApprovals (2022) Docket ID: FDA-2018-N-2689. Facilitating competition and innovation in the biological products marketplace; Public Hearing; Request for Comments. World Health Organization (2022) Health Topics – Biologicals. https://www.who.int/health-topics/biologicals. Accessed 4 May 2022

MIX
Papier aus verantwortungsvollen Quellen
Paper from responsible sources
FSC® C105338

If you have any concerns about our products,
you can contact us on
ProductSafety@springernature.com

In case Publisher is established outside the EU,
the EU authorized representative is:
Springer Nature Customer Service Center GmbH
Europaplatz 3, 69115 Heidelberg, Germany

Printed by Libri Plureos GmbH
in Hamburg, Germany